"Good" carbs, "bad" carbs, simple carbs, complex carbs, net carbs—make carbs work for you!

Carbohydrates are often misunderstood. Most Americans eat about 50 percent of their daily calories as carbs, yet very few people eat enough fiber and almost everyone eats too much sugar. Eating whole grains every day reduces your risk for diabetes, cancer, high blood pressure, high cholesterol, *and* will keep you slimmer. The completely revised and updated *Ultimate Carbohydrate Counter*, 3rd Edition, will help you make simple changes in your diet that will yield big health benefits. Choose the right carbs and choose better health for life.

- Understand carbs—fiber, sugar, and starch—and learn how each affects your health.

- Discover *all* the health benefits of a diet rich in whole grains and fiber, plus try new grains you've never heard of.

- Recognize hidden sources of added sugar in your diet— and how to avoid them.

THE ULTIMATE
CARBOHYDRATE COUNTER
3RD EDITION

THE
ULTIMATE CARBOHYDRATE COUNTER
THIRD EDITION

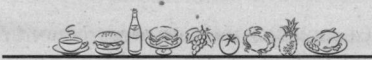

**Karen J. Nolan, Ph.D.
and Jo-Ann Heslin, M.A., R.D.**

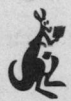

POCKET BOOKS
New York   London   Toronto   Sydney

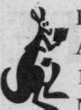
Pocket Books
A Division of Simon & Schuster, Inc.
1230 Avenue of the Americas
New York, NY 10020

Copyright © 1999, 2005 by Annette B. Natow and Jo-Ann Heslin
Revised edition © 2010 by Karen J. Nolan and Jo-Ann Heslin
A previous edition of this work was published as
The Carbohydrate, Fiber, and Sugar Counter.

This Pocket Books paperback edition January 2010

POCKET and colophon are registered trademarks of
Simon & Schuster, Inc.

For information about special discounts for bulk purchases, please contact Simon & Schuster Special Sales at 1-866-506-1949 or business@simonandschuster.com.

The Simon & Schuster Speakers Bureau can bring authors to your live event. For more information or to book an event, contact the Simon & Schuster Speakers Bureau at 1-866-248-3049 or visit our website at www.simonspeakers.com.

Cover photo by Jeffrey Coolidge/Getty

Manufactured in the United States of America

10   9   8   7   6   5   4   3   2   1

ISBN 978-1-4165-7037-0

For Annette.

We continue to build on the foundation
you helped put in place.

ACKNOWLEDGMENTS

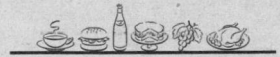

For all her continuous support and help, our agent, Nancy Trichter.

For her suggestions and editing skills, Sara Clemence.

For all her patience, comments and questions—our favorite reviewer, Jean Schwarsin.

Without the tireless cooperation of Stephen Llano and the production department at Pocket Books, *The Ultimate Carbohydrate Counter, 3rd Edition* would never have been completed.

A special thank you to our editor, Micki Nuding.

And, we would like to thank all of our readers for their suggestions and questions. Your input helps us to provide you with the most useful information.

*Since carbohydrates constitute the largest part
of an ordinary diet, their withdrawal changes eating
habits materially, and people find it difficult to be without
the familiar bread, potatoes, cereals, sugars and fruits.*

Mary Swartz Rose, Ph.D.
Feeding the Family
The Macmillan Company, 1919

CONTENTS

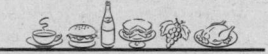

PART ONE

Brand Name, Nonbranded (Generic), and Take-Out Foods
53

PART TWO

Restaurant Chains
453

INTRODUCTION

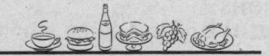

Are you counting carbs?

There are many reasons to watch your carb intake:

Are you trying to lose weight? Some people find a high carb, lowfat, moderate protein intake is the best way to shed pounds. For others, a low carb, moderate fat, high protein intake is more successful. In both cases, changing your carb intake appears to be the key to weight loss.

Are you trying to eat more whole grain foods? Whole grains are rich in important nutrients and fiber that support your immune system, protect you from disease, and help control your weight.

Are you trying to increase your fiber intake? It is estimated that we eat less than half the amount of fiber we need each day. Getting enough fiber helps you lose weight, manage diabetes, relieve constipation, and lowers your risk for heart disease and cancer.

Do you want to eat less sugar? Many experts blame America's continued weight gain, in part, on our very high sugar intake. Many of us, particularly parents, are trying to reduce the amount of sugar our families eat. Knowing which foods are high in sugar can help you achieve this goal.

Is your cholesterol high? Adding whole grains and foods high in fiber can help you bring your cholesterol down.

Do you have a high triglyceride level? Eating more whole grain foods and less sugar can help you lower your triglyceride level.

Have you been diagnosed as prediabetic? This condition is actually a cluster of symptoms that puts you at higher risk for developing diabetes in the future. The best way to prevent this is to lose some weight and monitor the amount of carbohydrates you eat each day, sticking with the good-for-you kind.

Do you have type 2 diabetes? The most effective way to manage type 2 diabetes is to make healthy lifestyle changes. It's important to keep track of the type and amount of carbs you eat each day and to spread out your carb intake throughout the day.

Are you carb loading for an athletic event? High carb meals before a competition can improve performance. High carb foods are easily digested and provide the energy needed to get through a run, swim, or game without becoming fatigued.

The Ultimate Carbohydrate Counter, 3rd Edition can help you count carbs. It gives you the carbohydrate, fiber, and sugar values for over 15,000 foods. It will become your ultimate carb-counting companion.

Make carbs work for you:

- Choose the right whole grain carbs.
- Add more fiber.
- Eat less sugar.

SORTING OUT CARBOHYDRATES

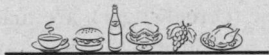

*Carbohydrates, carbs, complex carbs, simple carbs,
"good" carbs, "bad" carbs, net carbs . . .*
Help!

In the last decade, carbs have become a misunderstood nutrient. We went from high carb to low carb to being told to choose specific carbs. Before you can shop and eat wisely, you need to understand carbs.

What Are Carbohydrates?

Carbohydrates are the sugars, starches, and fibers found in food. All plant foods—fruits, vegetables, beans, and grains—are rich in carbohydrates. Fruits have more sugar. Vegetables, beans, and grains have more starch. Both have fiber. Sugars and starches are your body's main sources of fuel (calories).

Sugar

Sugar is an important source of fuel (calories) used by your body. During digestion, sugar molecules enter the bloodstream and travel to your body's cells and to your brain, where they are burned for energy. There are different types of sugar—simple sugars and others that are more complex.

Glucose is a simple sugar found in plants, animals, and in your blood as "blood sugar." It is the only source of energy used by your brain. Fructose (fruit sugar) is another simple sugar.

Other sugars, like sucrose (table sugar), lactose (milk sugar), and maltose (cereal sugar), are made up of two simple sugars that are broken apart in digestion before they can be burned for energy. We'll discuss more about sugar on pages 25 to 34.

Lactose Intolerance

If you experience stomach discomfort, gas, bloating, and diarrhea after eating milk, ice cream, and processed cheese, your body probably lacks the enzyme that breaks down lactose, the naturally occurring sugar in milk. Try yogurt, buttermilk, kefir, and other fermented dairy foods. The friendly bacteria in these foods have already broken down the lactose, which means you won't have discomfort.

Starch

Starch, the main form of carbohydrate found in most plants, is a more complex substance made up of many sugar molecules. During digestion, the larger starch molecule is slowly broken apart to yield smaller sugar fragments, which are sent to the cells in your body and to the brain to be used for energy.

Starch is found in many of the foods we eat, because it can be changed into so many different forms. Corn syrup is made from cornstarch. Modified food starch is used to stabilize gels in yogurt, pudding, whipped toppings, and ice cream. Some starches are used to make light, lower-calorie versions of foods like ice cream, breads, cookies, and cakes by adding more bulk or substance. One type, resistant starch, acts like fiber because it "resists" digestion and is not used by the body for energy. Researchers are currently looking at the health benefits of eating more resistant starch, which is found naturally in potatoes, beans, and cereals.

You Should Know

If you eat more sugar or starch calories than your body needs, the leftover will be stored as fat.

Fiber

Fiber is the carbohydrate that makes up the woody or gummy parts of plants. Our bodies can't digest or absorb fiber, so it is not used as a source of energy in the way that sugars and starches are used. But fiber plays a big role in a healthy diet— it provides protection against a number of diseases and is very important to the health of your digestive tract and immune system. We'll discuss fiber more on pages 18 to 22.

Simple Carbs—Complex Carbs

Simple carbohydrates are foods that contain a lot of sugar— syrups, jelly, honey, soda, and molasses. Complex carbohydrates are foods that contain a lot of starch—whole grains, cereals, beans, and vegetables. Complex carbs are rich in fiber, vitamins, and minerals. Simple carbs are generally poor sources of important nutrients. But there are exceptions. Milk, yogurt, fruits, and some vegetables have a lot of natural sugar yet are rich in important vitamins and minerals. Foods classified as simple carbs—those high in sugar—

can have either natural sugar or added sugar. Simple carbs with natural sugar are the healthier choice.

SORTING OUT CARBOHYDRATE FOODS

Complex Carbs	Simple Carbs
Bagels	*with natural sugar*
Beans	Fruits
Breads	Fruit juice
Cereals	Honey
Corn	Milk
Crackers	Unsweetened yogurt
Grains	
Pasta	*with added sugar*
Peas	Cake
Popcorn	Candy
Potatoes	Cookies
Pretzels	Fruit drinks
Rice	Jellies/jams
Rolls	Gelatin
Squash	Soda
Tortillas	Sweetened yogurt
Vegetables	Sweetened cereal

Good Carbs vs. Bad Carbs

Complex carbs—those foods high in starch—are sometimes called "good carbs." Foods high in sugar or those that are refined, like white flour and pasta, are referred to as "bad carbs." These terms can be misleading and are used more by food marketers than food professionals. There is no question that foods high in sugar like table sugar, candy, cake, cookies, and soda are not the best carb choices. But milk, yogurt, and fruits are also high in natural sugar and they are good choices.

We recommend not worrying about good carbs and bad carbs. Instead, when making choices, pick foods with naturally occurring sugars, like milk and fruit, or those that are less processed, like brown rice and whole wheat bread, more often. Choose foods with added sugars, like soda, candy, cakes, and sweetened cereal, and those that are highly processed, like white rice and white bread, less often.

You Should Know

Most Americans eat about 50% of their daily calories as carbohydrates.
Very few eat enough fiber.
Almost everyone eats too much sugar.
We all need to choose carbs more wisely.

Net Carbs

"Net carbs" or "net impact carbs" are terms that were coined to highlight foods that may help you lose weight. Some food manufacturers use these terms on lower carb brands.

To produce new low carb versions of typically higher carb foods, like bread, cereal, cookies, and energy bars, food companies replace some of the carbohydrates with fiber, glycerin, and sugar alcohols. The reasoning behind these substitutions is that your body does not use these carbs as energy (calories).

This is true for fiber. Your body does not digest fiber, so it provides no calories. Most experts agree that fiber can be subtracted from the total carbohydrate count for a food. Subtracting glycerin and sugar alcohols to arrive at net carb is another story.

Glycerin is a food additive that helps hold moisture in foods and adds some sweetness. It appears on the ingredient list. Sugar alcohols are found on the ingredients listing and may appear on the nutrition facts panel. They often have names that end in "ol"—mannitol, sorbitol, and xylitol. Subtracting glycerin and sugar alcohols to arrive at "net carbs" is more creative math than sound science, because both have calories, though fewer calories than starch or sugar.

Understanding the Glycemic Index

Decades ago, David Jenkins, a researcher at the University of Toronto, coined the term *glycemic index*. This index ranks a food by how quickly it can be converted to glucose and enters your bloodstream. Foods with a high glycemic index— rice, white bread, potatoes—raise blood sugar levels quickly. Foods with a low glycemic index—beans, whole grains, meat, fat—raise blood sugar levels more slowly.

The theory behind the glycemic index is correct. Some foods do raise blood sugar quickly; others do not. But in practice, it's not that simple.

The glycemic index measures the results of eating one food at a time. Straight glucose was given a rating of 100 and individual foods were measured against it. But that's not how people eat.

White bread has a very high glycemic index. But if you add peanut butter, the glycemic index is lowered because peanut butter, a high fat food, has a low glycemic index. The same goes for a baked potato, another high glycemic food. Top it with cheese sauce and broccoli, and the glycemic index drops.

It gets even more complicated. Ripe fruits have a lower glycemic index than unripe fruits. That's right; a hard peach will raise your blood sugar faster than a ripe, juicy one. Cooking pasta al dente is fine. Overcook it, and the glycemic value goes up. Even sugars vary. Glucose is high on the index, but fructose (fruit sugar) is low. There even appears to be an individual reaction. When researchers tested individuals after eating white bread, the glycemic index varied from 44 to 132.

The bottom line: Research into the health effects of the glycemic index is still unfolding. Eating more foods with a low glycemic index may lower the risk for heart disease and help to control diabetes. But if you are trying to lose weight, the best approach is still to reduce calories and increase activity.

GLYCEMIC INDEX OF COMMON FOODS	
High—greater than 70	
White rice	126
Baked potato	121
Cornflakes	119
Rice cakes	117
Jelly beans	114
Carrots	101
White bread	101
Glucose	**100**
Wheat bread	99
Soda	97
Sucrose	92
Cheese pizza	86
Spaghetti	83
Popcorn	79
Corn	78
Banana	76
Orange juice	74

Moderate—between 56 and 69

Peas	68
Orange	62
Bran cereal	60
Apple juice	58
Pumpernickel bread	58

Low—55 and below

Apple	52
Nonfat milk	46
Kidney beans	42
Fructose (fruit sugar)	32
Agave syrup	20

Source: Adapted from *Dietary Reference Intakes for Energy, Carbohydrate, Fiber, Fat, Fatty Acids, Cholesterol, Protein and Amino Acids, Part 1,* Institute of Medicine of the National Academies, The National Academies Press, 2002.

THE WHOLE TRUTH ABOUT WHOLE GRAINS

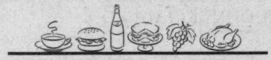

*Only 10% of Americans eat the recommended
3 servings of whole grains every day.*

Eating whole grains every day reduces your risk for diabetes, cancer, high blood pressure, and high cholesterol, *and* will keep you slimmer. Making this one, simple change in your diet can reap some pretty big results. Impressed? You should be, because this is one of the easiest food switches you can make. It's hard to get people to eat more fruits and vegetables. But switching from white bread to whole wheat bread isn't that big a step, and it will yield impressive health benefits.

Those who eat whole grains regularly:

- Weigh less, because whole grains provide a feeling of satisfaction and fullness after eating.

- Have lower total cholesterol and lower bad LDL cholesterol levels because of the fiber and natural plant sterols in whole grains.

- Lower their risk for metabolic syndrome and type 2 diabetes.

- Have healthier bowel function and less trouble with constipation.

- Age well, because whole grains are rich in antioxidants and phytochemicals, which act like bodyguards protecting cells from damaging free radicals that can trigger disease and signs of aging.

- Have lower triglyceride levels, which lowers the risk for heart disease.

- Have a lower occurrence of gum disease.

- May have a lower risk for colon cancer.

- May have lower blood pressure.

When grains are refined, many of these natural health-promoting agents are removed, including fiber, vitamins, minerals, phytosterols, and antioxidants.

One Serving of Whole Grains Equals:

1 slice of 100% whole grain bread
1 cup of whole grain cereal
½ cup cooked whole grain hot cereal or pasta
½ cup cooked brown or wild rice
½ cup any type of cooked whole grain

Whole Grains vs. Fiber

To better understand the difference between fiber and whole grains, let's take a look at the structure of grain. A kernel is the entire grain seed and it's made up of 3 parts: bran, germ, and endosperm. Bran, the outer protective layer, is made up mostly of fiber. The germ can sprout into a new

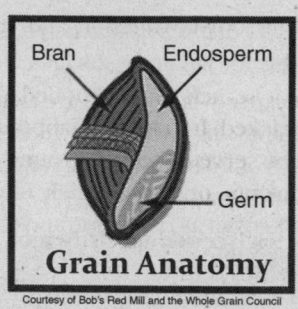

Grain Anatomy

Courtesy of Bob's Red Mill and the Whole Grain Council

plant. The endosperm provides food for the germ to grow if the kernel is planted.

All parts of a whole grain have value. The bran provides fiber and minerals. The endosperm gives you protein and starch. The germ gives you vitamins, minerals, and healthy fats. Eating the entire whole grain gives you the full benefit of all 3. White bread is made from just the endosperm. Whole wheat bread is made from the entire whole wheat kernel.

There are so many ways to eat whole grains. Expand your horizons beyond whole wheat, oatmeal, and brown rice, and try some other whole grain varieties. When you are in a hurry, rely on instant whole grain hot cereals, ready-to-eat whole grain cold cereals, microwave precooked whole grains, instant brown rice, popcorn, or whole grain breads and crackers.

WHOLE GRAINS FROM A TO Z

Amaranth   High in protein and has no gluten.

Barley   A good substitute for rice and more effective at lowering cholesterol than oats.

Brown rice   Easily digested and gluten free, but lower in fiber than most whole grains.

Buckwheat	Unroasted, it's groats; toasted, it's kasha. The base for Japanese soba noodles.
Bulgur	Wheat kernels that are boiled, dried, and cracked. It's used for tabbouleh.
Corn	Can be served popped, ground coarsely into polenta, or ground finely into cornmeal.
Emmer	Also known as farro or grano ferro, an Italian specialty.
Kamut	An heirloom wheat grain with a buttery taste.
Millet	Gluten free, with a mild flavor.
Oats	Regular, instant, or steel cut, oats lower cholesterol.
Quinoa	Cooks quickly into a fluffy grain dish.
Rye	Unique because it has fiber in both the bran and endosperm. Typically made into bread.
Sorghum	Gluten free and can be used popped, as hot cereal, or flour.
Spelt	A high-protein wheat.
Teff	The tiniest whole grain, used to make Ethiopian flatbread; high in iron and calcium.
Triticale	A whole grain hybrid of wheat and rye.
Wheat	High in gluten and very versatile as pasta, flour, seitan, bulgur, cereal, or wheatberries.
Wild rice	The seed of a grass with twice the fiber and protein of brown rice.

Whole Grain Labeling

A recent consumer survey showed 58% of grocery shoppers think whole grains are important.

WHOLE GRAIN STAMPS

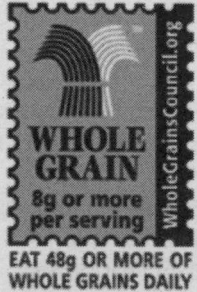 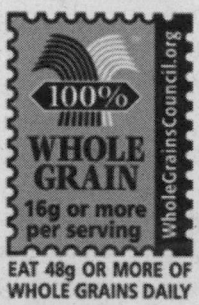

Courtesy Oldways and the Whole Grain Council

More and more foods are displaying the Whole Grain stamp, part of a whole grain awareness program developed by the Whole Grain Council. The Whole Grain stamp can be used on foods providing at least 8 grams of whole grain, which equals a half serving. The 100% Whole Grain stamp is used on products providing at least 16 grams of whole grain, equal to 1 serving. The stamps shown above have the gram value for the minimum amount required to use the stamp on labels. Companies can individualize the value to reflect the exact grams of whole grain in a specific food. These symbols are appearing on more and more foods, and will make it easier to find whole grain foods at a glance when shopping.

This chart will help you sort out whole grain label language.

WHOLE GRAIN LABEL LINGO

Label Terms	What They Really Mean
Brown rice Buckwheat Oats, oatmeal (any type)	All refer to 100% whole grain.

Popcorn
Shredded wheat
Sorghum
Stoneground whole
    (any type of grain)
Teff
Wheatberries
White whole wheat
Whole (any type of grain)
Whole wheat
Whole wheat white flour
Wild rice

Label Terms	What They Really Mean
7-Grain (or any other number-grain) 100% Wheat Cracked wheat Durum wheat Multigrain Organic flour Semolina Wheat flour	May contain some whole grains but are not 100% whole grain foods.

Label Terms	What They Really Mean
Bran (any type) Degermed Enriched flour Honey wheat Refined flour Rice (basmati, converted, white, sticky) Stoneground (without the word whole) Wheat gcrm	Not a whole grain food.

It's White Bread and It's Whole Wheat

*Milder in flavor and less chewy than 100%
whole wheat flour, white whole wheat flour is a
great alternative for diehard white bread fans
and nutritionally equal to whole wheat.*

Let's Talk About Fiber

*A recent consumer survey showed 72% of
grocery shoppers think fiber is important.*

When you eat whole grain foods, you automatically eat
fiber. But, in addition to the naturally occurring fiber found
in whole grains, vegetables, and fruits, many food manufacturers are adding extra fiber to cereals, energy bars, cookies,
and breads. You can even buy fiber-enhanced water.

Ingredients That Signal "Fiber Added"

Inulin
Cellulose
Pectin
FOS (also listed as fructan or fructooligosaccharide)
GOS (also listed as galactooligosaccharide)
Methylcellulose

You already know that fiber comes from the outer layer of
grains, called the bran. Fiber is also found in the woody and
gummy parts of plants.

Fiber isn't digested and has no calories, yet it's important. Why?

Regularly eating more fiber:

- Helps you lose weight.
- Reduces your risk for metabolic syndrome, which increases your risk of heart disease and diabetes.
- Aids in managing diabetes.
- Lowers cholesterol.
- Helps prevent heart disease.
- Helps to lower blood pressure.
- Relieves constipation.
- Stimulates your immune system.
- Reduces the risk for colon, rectal, breast, and endometrial cancer.
- Supports the friendly bacteria that live in your digestive tract.

You Should Know

*Women with the highest fiber intake are 50%
less likely to gain weight in middle age.*

Few Americans eat enough fiber. All the experts agree we need to eat more. We average about 15 grams of fiber a day, only half of what we should be eating.

Kids Need Fiber, Too
Age + 5

*Each day, children 2 and older should eat
the amount of fiber that equals their age + 5.
For a 5-year-old, that would be at
least 10 grams of fiber a day.*

If you normally eat little fiber—and most of us do—add foods rich in fiber to your meals slowly. Fiber-rich foods include beans, berries, bran, fruits, oatmeal, vegetables, and whole grains. Don't go overboard, because it takes your body a little time to adjust to the extra bulk passing through your digestive tract. At first, you may find you are a little gassy, but this passes as you adjust to the higher fiber intake. Drink plenty of fluids. Fiber soaks up fluids like a sponge. This not only helps you feel fuller longer, but helps form soft, easily passed stools.

You Should Know

*High fiber foods have 5 or more grams
of fiber in a serving.
A good source of fiber has 2 or more
grams of fiber in a serving.*

ADD A LITTLE FIBER TO YOUR LIFE

- Eat whole fruits and vegetables instead of drinking juices.
- Eat the fiber-rich skins of cucumbers, apples, pears, potatoes, and zucchini.

- Eat more berries—blueberries, blackberries, raspberries, strawberries.

- Choose whole grains—brown rice, cornmeal, barley, cracked wheat, rye, whole wheat.

- Use whole grain or high fiber cereals—oatmeal, oat flakes, bran, shredded wheat.

- Eat whole wheat bread, bagels, pasta, pretzels, crackers, and rolls.

- Eat beans, lentils, and peas a few times a week.

- Try soybeans in every form—soy nuts, tofu, tempeh, edamame.

- Snack on fig newtons, graham crackers, and popcorn.

- Eat dried fruits and raisins.

- Sprinkle ground flaxseed, bran, or whole wheat granola on cereal or yogurt for a healthy crunch.

- Experiment with higher fiber versions of old favorites, like brown rice, buckwheat noodles, or baked sweet potatoes.

- Have vegetarian meals a few times a week.

- Try some of the new fiber-fortified foods, like high-fiber cereal bars and breads.

You may be wondering, if fiber isn't digested and has no calories, how does it work in your body?

There are trillions of tiny bacteria living in your digestive tract. These helpful little hitchhikers have been with you since birth. Fiber is the food your friendly bacteria live on. A low fiber diet starves your friendly bacteria, and lowers your protection against infection by allowing harmful bacteria to make themselves at home in your body. Eating enough fiber allows your friendly bacteria to thrive and outnumber the harmful invaders. This is your natural resistance against infection and disease, and is especially protective against colon cancer.

Fiber also helps you lose weight. You get the satisfaction of eating and a sense of fullness without calories.

Chew on This

*Eating fiber-rich foods is smarter
than popping a fiber supplement.
Fiber-rich foods are rich in antioxidants,
vitamins, and minerals; supplements are not.*

Gluten Free Foods

Whole wheat foods are a major source of whole grains, but millions of Americans can't eat gluten, a protein found in wheat. About 1% of the population suffers from celiac disease. It is a chronic inflammation of the small intestine that impairs its ability to absorb nutrients, and is triggered by eating gluten. Symptoms of gluten sensitivity can vary widely, from mild discomfort to debilitating fatigue and illness. According to experts in the field, three factors must be present for celiac disease to develop: a genetic predisposition, exposure to gluten, and an initiating event such as pregnancy, a virus, or stress. Once started, celiac disease cannot be cured, but it can be managed by avoiding gluten. Wheat contains the most gluten, but other grains like barley, rye, and triticale contain some, too, and need to be avoided as well.

A larger group of people fit into a category doctors call "gluten sensitive." Their symptoms are milder than those with celiac disease. When people with gluten sensitivity restrict or avoid foods with gluten, they feel better.

It used to be hard to find gluten free foods, but today, more and more products are labeled *gluten free, free of gluten, without gluten,* or *no gluten.* To help you find more gluten free foods, hundreds of brands are listed in the counter section of *The Ultimate Carbohydrate Counter.*

The FDA (Food and Drug Administration) is currently working on a definition for the term *gluten free* to comply with the 2004 Food Allergen Labeling and Consumer Protection Act. Once in place, this definition will help consumers identify gluten free grain foods they can eat, and will help food manufacturers correctly label their products. At the moment, gluten free labeling is voluntary. But stating on the label that a product contains wheat or wheat products is *not* voluntary. This is required as part of the allergy labeling law.

Any food containting wheat also contains gluten. To see if a food you are buying contains wheat, look on the label in the ingredient listing and for the allergy statement that must appear by law. The allergy statement may read *contains wheat, may contain wheat,* or *processed in a facility that also contains wheat (or gluten).*

Foods with Gluten	Gluten FREE Foods
Ale	Amaranth
Barley	Arrowroot
Beer	Beans (all varieties)
Bulgur	Cassava
Communion wafers	Corn (bran, cornmeal)
Cracked wheat	Flax
Farina	Hominy grits
Farro	Millet
Hydrolyzed vegetable protein	Potato, potato starch, and flour
	Quinoa
Kamut	Rice (brown, white, wild, basmati)
Modified food starch	Rice bran

Foods with Gluten	Gluten FREE Foods
Oats*	Rice flours
Pasta	Sorghum
Rye	Soy flour
Seitan	Tapioca and tapioca flour
Semolina	Teff
Spelt	
Triticale	
Vegetarian meat substitutes	
Wheat	

*Oats are gluten free, but some gluten sensitive people may react to them; follow your doctor's advice.

SIMPLE FACTS
ABOUT SUGARS
AND SWEETENERS

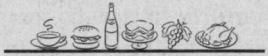

Everyone eats too much sugar.

Most of us enjoy sweets. Babies are born with a preference for sweets. Anthropologists believe that our ability to taste the difference between sweet and bitter plants may have helped early man survive. Sweet tasting foods were usually safe to eat. Bitter tasting foods were often poisonous.

Today, however, our passion for sweets is creating a global epidemic of overweight people. Clearly, we are eating too much sugar. We drink more soda than milk in this country and buy far more sugared drinks than fruit juice. Too many sugary foods can crowd out more nutritious choices.

Studies have shown, over and over, that as sugar intake goes up, vitamin and mineral intake goes down. We should all be eating less sugar, but there is no specific recommendation on how much to eat every day. The U.S. Dietary Reference Intakes suggest 25% of daily calories from added sugar as the maximum. Obviously, people should eat less. The World Health Organization (WHO) has suggested limiting added sugars to no more than 10% of total calories, though some experts feel this amount is unrealistically low.

In both cases, the recommendations are for added sugar, not for sugars found naturally in fruits, milk, grains, and vegetables.

Natural Sugar vs. Added Sugar

Grains, fruits, vegetables, milk, and plain yogurt all contain sugars. These are *natural* sugars and they come along with the vitamins, minerals, and fiber found in the food. In contrast, soda, candy, fruit drinks, cakes, cookies, ice cream, jelly, and syrup offer little more than sweetness and calories. These foods are loaded with *added sugar*.

Americans eat more than 23 teaspoons of added sugars each day. This equals almost 400 sugar calories a day and for some people the amount is even higher. Teenagers eat the most sugar. The way foods are currently labeled for sugar, it can be hard to make the best choices, because the nutrition label lumps together natural sugar and added sugar.

Even though the nutrition label doesn't distinguish between natural and added sugar, the difference is significant. For example, the nutrition label on a quart of milk tells you that one cup has 14 grams of sugar. The label on fruit punch tells you that one cup has 30 grams of sugar. But all of the sugar in milk comes from naturally occurring *lactose,* or milk sugar. Almost all the sugar in fruit punch is added.

So how can you tell natural sugars from added sugars? Check the ingredient listing for the terms below—if they appear, it means sugar has been added to the food. Ingredients are listed in descending order by volume, so the closer an ingredient is to the beginning of the list, the more there is in each serving of food.

SUGAR BY ANY OTHER NAME

Barley malt	Honey
Beet juice	Invert sugar
Brown rice syrup	Maltodextrin
Brown sugar	Malt syrup
Cane syrup	Maple sugar
Corn sweetener	Maple syrup
Corn syrup	Molasses
Crystalline fructose	Muscovado
Dextrose	Raw sugar
Evaporated cane juice	Sorghum
Fructose	Sucrose
Fruit juice concentrate	Sugar in the raw
High fructose corn syrup (HFCS)	Turbinado

Make Good Sugar Choices

*Choose foods with naturally containing
sugars more often.
Choose foods with added sugars less often.*

SOME SURPRISING SUGAR FACTS

- Humans are genetically programmed to like sweets. Both amniotic fluid and breast milk are slightly sweet tasting.

- Sugar does not make kids hyper. Contrary to popular belief, sugar has a calming effect on the brain and acts as a pain reliever in infants.

- Preschoolers average 14 to 17 teaspoons of added sugar every day, mostly from sweetened drinks, desserts, and soda.

- Sugar is not addictive. Sugar cravings are more likely driven by habits.

- A high sugar intake increases triglyceride levels and lowers good HDL cholesterol.

- A high sugar, high refined carb diet increases the risk for cataracts by almost 30% and increases the risk for age-related macular degeneration (AMD).

- A high sugar intake makes it more difficult for people with diabetes to control blood sugar levels.

Healthy Carb to Sugar Ratio

Check the nutrition facts panel and look for a total carbohydrate to sugar ratio of no more than 4 to 1. For example, if a cereal has 24 grams of total carb and 6 or less grams of sugar, there are more complex carbs than simple sugars in the cereal—a good choice.

Liquid Sugar—Sweetened Drinks

Beware of sugar calories in a glass—1 out of every 5 calories Americans consume comes from liquids, and soda is the biggest culprit. The calories in clear drinks—soda, fruit drinks, energy drinks, sports drinks, sweetened coffee and tea—are almost entirely from sugar and they provide very little satisfaction. You don't feel full after drinking sweetened drinks. And, the more you are offered, the more you drink. Up to 20% of our daily calories come from sweet drinks, contributing close to 300 calories a day. Researchers believe that when it comes to weight loss, what you drink may be more important than what you eat.

Portion sizes of sweetened drinks have also increased

dramatically in the last 25 years. We've gone from an 8 ounce bottle of soda to unlimited soda refills served in a quart-sized glass. Sweetened fruit drinks and iced tea often come in 16 ounce bottles, double a traditional serving size. A small coffee has grown from 6 to 10 ounces—and few of us ever order small.

The bottom line

- In small amounts, a sweetened beverage is simply a tasty drink. Drinking larger amounts regularly, especially for children, promotes a high sugar intake and may contribute to weight gain.

- Think of energy drinks as soda with a jolt plus some extra nutrients. They can be very high in sugar calories.

- Soda loads you up with sugar calories, but lets you down when it comes to all other nutrients.

What the Researchers Are Saying

Based on the evidence, experts recommend that children consume no more than one sweetened beverage a week.
There is little room in the diets of children for empty calories from liquid sugar.

High Fructose Corn Syrup (HFCS)

Each day, Americans eat about 50 grams (12 teaspoons) of high fructose corn syrup (HFCS). Many have no idea they're eating so much. HFCS is found in many foods, from ice cream to cereal bars to energy drinks. It's a sugar—nothing more, nothing less. Avoiding it is a simple way to cut down on eating added sugar.

Is HFCS safe? Yes. The FDA listed HFCS as GRAS (Generally Recognized As Safe) in 1983 and reaffirmed the ruling in 1996. High fructose corn syrup has properties that make it useful in food production. It helps cookies, crackers, and cereals stay fresher longer. Ice cream, yogurt, chocolate milk, and cheese spreads with HFCS have a softer texture. It is often combined with no-calorie sweeteners to produce "light" or lower calorie foods. HFCS is added to sports drinks because fructose is efficiently absorbed, providing energy and rehydration needed by athletes.

Over the last 35 years, we've shifted to eating more HFCS and less table sugar. That sounds bad unless you understand that table sugar and high fructose corn syrup are so similar that your body and your taste buds cannot tell the difference. Both have 4 calories in 1 gram. Both are made up of two simple sugars—fructose and glucose. Both are absorbed from your digestive tract at the same rate. If you replace sugar with HFCS in soda, it is simply a swap of one sugar for another. They have the same sweet taste and are equally low in nutrition value.

So why do you often see news stories that link HFCS to our obesity epidemic? High fructose corn syrup started appearing in foods in the 1970s—right around the time our waistlines began to expand. There is no question that overly sweetened foods have contributed to the overweight problem in the U.S. But HFCS, by itself, did not make us fat. Poor food choices and the easy availability of sweet foods are the culprits. In areas of the world where little if any high fructose corn syrup is consumed, obesity is still on the rise. Recent USDA food studies have actually shown the amount of HFCS we eat is going down, but the incidence of obesity still remains high.

> ### What the Researchers Are Saying
> *Overweight adults who drink fructose-sweetened drinks with meals have higher triglyceride levels, increasing their risk for heart disease and diabetes.*

Agave Syrup

The next time you eat a cereal bar or gulp down an energy drink that says "no high fructose corn syrup," take a look at the ingredient list. There's a chance it might contain agave syrup, an increasingly popular sweetener.

Agave comes from the succulent century plant grown in Mexico. Spanish conquistadors fermented its juice into tequila. Agave is processed at low temperatures, making it popular with those eating a raw food diet. It's a plant product, so strict vegetarians use it as a substitute for honey, which is made by bees. And it has a low glycemic value, similar to fructose.

Sweeter than table sugar and thinner than honey, agave syrup comes in two forms, light and dark. The light syrup tastes like simple sugar syrup. The dark variety is similar to honey or very light molasses. A tablespoon has slightly more calories (60) than a tablespoon of sugar (49) but its taste is sweeter, so less can be used. Agave syrup is 90% fructose, which might promote diarrhea if eaten in large amounts.

When a Sugar Isn't a Sugar

Sugar substitutes have been around for decades. Some have calories, others don't, but all have fewer calories than sugar. There are two kinds of sugar substitutes: sugar alcohols like mannitol and sorbitol, and artifical sweeteners like saccharin and aspartame. Sugar alcohols have calories. They are absorbed slowly by the body and have little impact on blood sugar levels. Artificial sweeteners have no calories and don't raise blood sugar.

Each has advantages and drawbacks. A high intake of sugar alcohols can cause diarrhea. Some artificial sweeteners lose their sweetness when heated, so they cannot be used in cooking.

Artificial sweeteners are listed on the food label on the ingredient list. Because they have no calories, they are not required to be listed on the nutrition facts panel. Sugar alcohols do have calories, so they are included both in the ingredient list and as part of the total carbohydrate value on the nutrition label. Some companies list the sugar alcohol content separately on the nutrition label under total carbohydrates. This is done voluntarily.

Sugar Free Shortcomings

194 million Americans regularly eat and drink low calorie and sugar free foods.
Sugar free foods are not always calorie free, so read labels carefully.
Diet soda and sugar substitutes may help satisfy a sweet tooth, but they don't control hunger or cause weight loss.
Sugar free foods have been around for decades, but Americans are still gaining weight.

UNDERSTANDING SUGARS

Common Names	Calories per Gram	Found on the Food Label

When a sugar is a sugar

White sugar	4	Must be listed under
Brown sugar	4	sugar on the nutrition
Honey	4	facts panel and on the
Molasses	4	ingredient list.
Raw sugar	4	
Syrups	4	
High fructose corn syrup (HFCS)	4	
Agave syrup	4	

When a sugar isn't quite a sugar (sugar alcohols)

Trehelose	4	May be listed under total
Sorbitol	3	carbohydrates on the
Mannitol	2	nutrition facts panel and
Xylitol	2	must be listed on the
Isomalt	2	ingredient list.
Lactitol	2	
Maltitol	2	
Erythritol: *Sweet Simplicity, Smart Sweet, Zerose, ZSweet*	<1	

Common Names	Calories per Gram	Found on the Food Label

When a sugar isn't a sugar (artificial and zero calorie natural sweeteners)

Common Names	Calories per Gram	Found on the Food Label
saccharin: *Sweet 'N Low, Sweet Twin, Necta Sweet*	0	Must be listed on the ingredient list.
aspartame: *NutraSweet, Equal, SugarTwin*	4*	
acesulfame-K: *Sunette, Sweet & Safe, Sweet One*	0	
sucralose: *Splenda*	0	
neotame	0	
stevia: *Truvia, PureVia, SweetLeaf, Only Sweet, Stevia In The Raw*	0	

*This sweetener is almost 200 times as sweet as sugar. Even though it does have calories, so little is used in a serving of food that the calorie amount is negligible.

HOW MUCH
SHOULD YOU EAT?

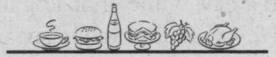

Carbohydrates

How much carb do you need each day?

It's not an easy question to answer. Vegetarians, athletes, and many populations throughout the world base their diets on carbohydrates, getting as much as 80% of their daily calories from carbs. Most food professionals believe that eating 40% or less of your daily calories as carbs would be considered a low carb diet. On average, Americans get approximately 50% of their daily calories from carbs. Over 55% is a high carb diet.

But that still doesn't answer the question. *How much carb do you need each day?*

The FDA says 300 grams of carbs a day is the amount needed by the "typical" consumer. This Daily Value (DV) is used on nutrition labels to compare the amount of carbs in one serving of food. For example, if a cup of cereal has 15 grams of carbohydrate, it would provide 5% of your Daily Value of 300 grams.

The National Academy of Sciences' Recommended Dietary Allowance (RDA) for carbohydrates is no less than 130 grams a day.

It's been estimated that you need at least 50 to 100 grams

of carb a day to prevent ketosis, a condition caused by the incomplete breakdown of fat.

Until long-term studies are done, it's impossible to say what amount of carb is right for you. In the meantime, we'd suggest that you stick with the recommendation of at least 130 grams of carb a day, while choosing more foods high in whole grains and fewer foods high in sugar.

Counting carbs is easy. Decide if you want to eat a low carb, moderate carb, or high carb diet. For a low carb diet, 40% of daily calories or lower is considered a low carb intake. For example, if you eat 1,800 calories a day:

$$40\% \text{ of } 1,800 \text{ calories} = 720 \text{ carb calories}$$

To figure out how many grams of carb to eat a day, you need to know that 1 gram of carb = 4 calories. Using the example above for 1,800 calories:

$$720 \text{ carb calories} \div 4 = 180$$
$$\text{so}$$
$$40\% \text{ of } 1,800 \text{ calories} = 180 \text{ grams carb}$$

For a moderate carb intake, 50% to 55% of daily calories is considered a moderate carb intake. For example if you eat 1,800 calories a day:

$$50\% \text{ of } 1,800 \text{ calories} = 900 \text{ carb calories}$$
$$900 \text{ carb calories} \div 4 = 225$$
$$\text{so}$$
$$50\% \text{ of } 1,800 \text{ calories} = 225 \text{ grams carb}$$

For a high carb intake, over 55% of daily calories or higher is considered a high carb intake. For example if you eat 1,800 calories a day:

$$65\% \text{ of } 1,800 \text{ calories} = 1,170 \text{ carb calories}$$
$$1,170 \text{ carb calories} \div 4 = 292.5$$
so
$$65\% \text{ of } 1,800 \text{ calories} = 293 \text{ grams carb}$$

In every example, you would more than meet the RDA of 130 grams of carb a day and be well above the minimum needed to prevent ketosis.

To set your own target daily carb intake, use the equation below. Your target may change depending on whether you are trying to lose weight, are on a low carb diet, are an athlete who is carb loading, or are eating a high carb, low fat diet.

Your Target Daily Carb Intake Is:

_____ % of _____ calories a day =

_____ carb calories

_____ carb calories ÷ 4 = _____ carb grams

Go to the sections Sorting Out Carbohydrates (pages 4 to 11) and The Whole Truth About Whole Grains (pages 12 to 24) for information on making healthy carb choices.

Fiber

Setting your daily intake of fiber is easy. Simply select your sex and age range on the table below and use that recommendation as your daily target fiber intake.

DAILY FIBER RECOMMENDATIONS

Men

	19–50 years	38 grams of fiber
	50 and older	30 grams of fiber

Women

	19–50 years	25 grams of fiber
	50 and older	21 grams of fiber
	pregnant	28 grams of fiber

Keep in mind that most Americans eat only half of their recommended fiber intake daily. When you start adding fiber to your diet, go slowly and drink plenty of fluids. Go to the section Let's Talk About Fiber (pages 18 to 22) for more information on foods containing fiber and ways to increase the amount of fiber you eat.

Sugar

Without clear-cut recommendations, you need to decide for yourself how much sugar to eat. As we discussed earlier, the World Health Organization (WHO) suggests that 10% of total calories daily should come from added sugar. Some experts feel this may be an unrealistically low amount. The U.S. Dietary Reference Intakes, used to set intake levels for the nutrition label, suggests a maximum of 25% of daily calories from added sugar. We'd recommend eating closer to the WHO recommendation of 10% total calories as sugar, keeping in mind the 25% recommendation as the healthy upper limit.

The guidelines are for "added" sugar. We recommend you use them as a guide to calculate your total daily sugar intake. By counting the foods containing natural sugar and eating fewer foods containing added sugar, you will automatically lower your overall daily sugar intake, which is better for your health.

The following chart gives you both suggested sugar calories and grams of sugar to aim for daily at varying calorie levels. Select the calorie level that is best for you and aim for a daily sugar intake somewhere between the lower and upper limit.

YOUR DAILY TARGET SUGAR INTAKE

Total Calories	Suggested Lower Intake 10% total calories = grams sugar		Upper Limit 25% of total calories = grams sugar	
	Calories	Sugar	Calories	Sugar
2400	240	60	600	150
2200	220	55	550	138
2100	210	53	525	131
2000	200	50	500	125
1900	190	48	475	119
1800	180	45	450	113
1700	170	43	425	106
1600	160	40	400	100
1500	150	38	375	94
1400	140	35	350	88
1300	130	33	325	81
1200	120	30	300	75

Go to the section Simple Facts About Sugars and Sweeteners (pages 25 to 34) to learn more about natural versus added sugar, so you can select foods lower in sugar.

COUNTING CARBS

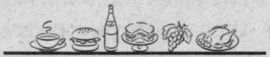

You don't have to be on a diet to count carbs. People with diabetes regularly keep track of how many carbs they eat. Those with high triglycerides may have been told by their doctors to eat moderate amounts of carbohydrates and less sugar. Athletes routinely eat large amounts of carbs to fuel muscles, "carb loading" before a major event. Remember the famous pasta dinners the evening before the New York and Boston Marathons?

The Ultimate Carbohydrate Counter is the best source you can use to count carbs. With over 15,000 foods listed, values for everything you eat are at your fingertips. The easiest way to determine how many carbs you should be eating each day is to go through the following steps.

Setting Your Daily Target Carb Intake

1. Find your target calorie zone.
2. Calculate your daily carb calories.
3. Calculate your daily grams of carb.
4. Select a recommended fiber intake.
5. Select a target sugar range.

1. Find your target calorie zone.

This step is simple. Just write down the amount.

If you are unsure of how many calories you should be eating, think about what weight you'd like to be. If you want to be 130 pounds, then that's your target weight. Next, select the activity factor that best reflects your current activity level. That's your activity factor. Multiply your target weight times your activity factor to find out how many calories you need each day.

Activity factor:

20 = Very active men
15 = Moderately active men or very active women
13 = Inactive men, moderately active women, and people over 55
10 = Inactive women, repeat dieters, seriously overweight people

Calorie equation:

target weight × activity factor =
calories needed each day.

your target weight _____ × your activity factor _____

= _____ calories needed each day

For example, if your target weight is 130 and you are a moderately active woman (factor 13), aged 43, you should be eating between 1,600 and 1,700 calories a day.

130 pounds × 13 (moderately active woman) =
1,690 calories per day

2. Calculate your daily carb calories.

In the section How Much Should You Eat? we discussed how to calculate your daily carb calories (pages 36 to 37). First, you need to decide what percentage of carb you want to eat each day; 40% or lower is considered a low carb eating plan. A moderate carb intake is 50% to 55%. A high carb plan would be more than 55% of your total calories as carb each day.

Let's say you decide to eat 50% of your daily calories as carbs, a moderate carb plan. We have already determined that a 130-pound woman needs about 1,700 calories a day.

Use the following equation to determine your daily carb calories:

_____% of _____ calories a day = _____ carb calories

example: *50% of 1,700 calories a day =*
850 daily carb calories

3. Calculate your daily grams of carb.

In the section How Much Should You Eat? we also discussed how to calculate your daily carb grams (pages 36 to 37). To continue our example, a 130-pound woman eating 1,700 calories a day can eat 850 carb calories, which equals 50% of daily calories as carb.

Use the following equation to determine your daily carb grams:

_____ carb calories ÷ 4 = _____ carb grams

example: *850 carb calories ÷ 4 = 213 daily carb grams*

4. Aim to eat more fiber.

See the table Daily Fiber Recommendations, page 38, to find out how many grams of fiber you should eat each day. For our example, a 43-year-old woman should eat 25 grams, the daily recommendation for women aged 19 to 50.

5. Aim to eat less sugar.

The current recommendation suggests eating between 10% to 25% of your daily calories as sugar. See the chart Your Daily Target Sugar Intake, page 39, to help you select an amount.

Continuing to use the example above, as a 130-pound woman eating 1,700 calories a day, the table on page 39 lists 10% of your daily calories as 170 sugar calories or 43 grams of sugar. The table lists 25% of your daily calories as sugar as 425 sugar calories or 106 grams of sugar.

So for our example, a low sugar intake would be 43 grams of sugar a day. The upper limit for sugar daily would be no more than 106 grams of sugar. Aim toward the lower end.

Your Daily Carb Counting Goals Are:

_____ grams carb

_____ grams fiber

_____ to _____ grams sugar

_____ calories

Now use Your Daily Carb Diary on page 45 to keep track of the carbs and calories you eat. You don't have to track your fiber and sugar intakes daily, but it's a good idea to do it once in a while to see if you're meeting the recommendations.

Your Daily Carb Diary will tell you a lot about how you eat, why you eat, and what you eat. Research has shown that men are more likely to omit items than women, both sexes are more likely to omit snack items, and meat items are more likely to be underestimated. No one else will ever see what you write down, so be honest.

We appreciate that many people eat on a crazy schedule, so the day is broken into 3 periods. This will help you figure out when you do the most eating.

A.M. is from midnight till noon. Many people eat in the middle of the night, so A.M. includes middle-of-the-night noshing, breakfast, coffee break, or morning snack.

Midday is from noon until dinner. It includes lunch and any afternoon or predinner snack, like a drink after work.

P.M. is dinnertime through midnight. It includes your evening meal and afterdinner TV and bedtime snacks.

By subtotaling your carbs and calories 3 times during the day, you can make adjustments for unexpected situations.

YOUR DAILY CARB DIARY

Your Target Calorie Zone _____ Your Daily Carb grams _____

Aim for _____ grams sugar daily Aim for _____ grams fiber daily

Day _____ Date _____

Food	Portion	Calories	Carb	Sugar	Fiber
AM					
AM Totals		_____	_____	_____	_____
MIDDAY					
Midday Totals		_____	_____	_____	_____
PM					
PM Totals		_____	_____	_____	_____
Daily Totals		_____	_____	_____	_____

USING YOUR ULTIMATE CARBOHYDRATE COUNTER

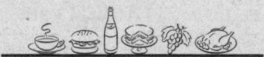

The Ultimate Carbohydrate Counter lists the portion size, calories, carbohydrate, sugar, and fiber values for more than 15,000 foods. Now you can compare the values in your favorite foods and, when necessary, choose substitutes before you go out to shop or eat. This will save you time and help you decide what to buy.

The counter section of the book is divided into two parts: Part One: Brand Name, Nonbranded (Generic), and Take-Out Foods (page 53); and Part Two: Restaurant Chains (page 453). Each part lists foods or restaurant chains alphabetically.

In Part One, for each category, you will find nonbranded (generic) foods listed first, in alphabetical order, followed by an alphabetical listing of brand name foods. The nonbranded listings will help you estimate calorie, carbohydrate, sugar, and fiber values when you don't see your favorite brands. They can also help you to evaluate store brands. Large categories are divided into subcategories, such as canned, fresh, frozen, and ready-to-eat, to make it easier to find what you're looking for. Some categories have "see" and "see also" references to help you find related items.

Because we eat out so often, more than 700 take-out foods are listed in Part One. These are found in the take-out subcategory in many categories throughout this section. Look there for foods you take out or order in, because these foods are not nutrition labeled.

Most foods are listed alphabetically. In some cases, though, foods are grouped by category. For example, a tuna sandwich is found in the SANDWICH category. Other group categories include:

ASIAN FOOD: Page 61
Includes all types of Asian foods except egg rolls and sushi, which are found in the egg rolls and sushi categories.

DELI MEATS/COLD CUTS: Page 195
Includes all sandwich meats except chicken, ham, and turkey, which have their own separate categories.

DINNER: Page 197
Includes all prepared dinners listed by brand name, except pasta dinners, which are found in the pasta dinner category.

LIQUOR/LIQUEUR: Page 267
Includes all alcoholic beverages and mixed drinks except beer, champagne, and wine, which are found in their own separate categories.

NUTRITION SUPPLEMENTS: Page 290
Includes all dieting aids, meal replacements, and drinks, except

energy bars and energy drinks, which
are found in their own separate
categories.

SANDWICHES: **Page 367**
Includes popular sandwich, calzone,
and panini choices.

SNACKS: **Page 385**
Includes a variety of snack items, such
as pork rinds and cheese puffs.

SPANISH FOOD: **Page 404**
Includes all types of Spanish and
Mexican foods except salsa and
tortillas, which are found in their
own separate categories

In Part Two, Restaurant Chains, 87 national and regional restaurant, coffee, doughnut, frozen yogurt, ice cream, pizza,
sandwich, soup, and sushi chains are listed. Brand name
foods are required by federal law to have nutrition information on labels, but in most areas of the country, restaurants
provide this information only voluntarily.

With *The Ultimate Carbohydrate Counter* as your guide,
you will never again wonder how many carbs and calories
are in the foods you eat.

DEFINITIONS

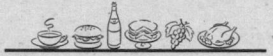

as prep (as prepared): refers to food that has been prepared according to package directions

lean and fat: describes meat with some fat on its edges that is not cut away before cooking, or poultry prepared with skin and fat as purchased

lean only: refers to lean meat that is trimmed of all visible fat, or poultry without skin

not prep (not prepared): refers to food that has not been cooked and may require the addition of other ingredients to prepare

shelf stable: refers to prepared products found on the supermarket shelf that are not canned or frozen, but are packaged and ready-to-eat or are ready to be heated and do not require refrigeration

take-out: describes prepared dishes that you purchase ready-to-eat; those included serve as a guide to the calories, carbohydrates, sugar, and fiber in products you may purchase

ABBREVIATIONS

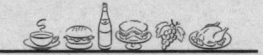

avg	=	average
diam	=	diameter
fl	=	fluid
frzn	=	frozen
g	=	gram
in	=	inch
lb	=	pound
lg	=	large
med	=	medium
mg	=	milligram
oz	=	ounce
pkg	=	package
prep	=	prepared
pt	=	pint
qt	=	quart
reg	=	regular
sec	=	second
serv	=	serving
sm	=	small
sq	=	square
tbsp	=	tablespoon
tr	=	trace
tsp	=	teaspoon
w/	=	with
w/o	=	without
<	=	less than

NOTES

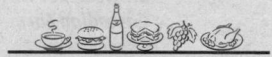

cals = calories

carb = carbohydrates

All carbohydrate, fiber, and sugar values are given in grams.

— (dash) indicates that values are not available

tr (trace) = less than 1 gram of carbohydrate, fiber, or sugar

0 (zero) indicates there are no calories, carbohydrate, fiber, or sugar in that food

Discrepancies in figures are due to rounding of values, product reformulation, and reevaluation. The current labeling law allows rounding. Some of the data listed are analysis data, obtained directly from manufacturers, not from labels; therefore, some values may differ slightly from labels because the values have not been rounded.

PART ONE

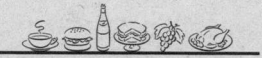

Brand Name, Nonbranded (Generic), and Take-Out Foods

> *Nourishing our bodies needs to be a priority—*
> *healthy meals and snacks deserve a larger*
> *slice of our time-stressed lives.*

FOOD	PORTION	CALS	CARB	SUGAR	FIBER
ABALONE					
breaded & fried	1 serv (3 oz)	162	9	tr	tr
steamed	1 serv (3 oz)	127	6	tr	0
ACAI JUICE					
Arthur's					
Acai Plus	1 bottle (11 oz)	230	45	25	5
Bossa Nova					
Acai Juice Blueberry	8 oz	89	21	18	0
Acai Juice Mango	8 oz	89	23	16	0
Acai Juice Original	8 oz	94	21	18	0
Acai Juice Passion Fruit	8 oz	89	23	18	0
Acai Juice Raspberry	8 oz	89	23	18	0
O.N.E.					
Amazon Acai	1 bottle (11 oz)	157	32	29	3
Zola					
100% Juice	1 box (11 oz)	170	30	29	1
ACEROLA					
fresh	1 (5 g)	2	tr	–	tr
ACEROLA JUICE					
juice	1 cup	56	12	11	1
ADZUKI BEANS					
Arrowhead Mills					
Organic Dried not prep	¼ cup	130	26	1	5
ALCOHOL *(see BEER AND ALE, CHAMPAGNE, LIQUOR/LIQUEUR, MALT, WINE)*					
ALE *(see BEER AND ALE)*					
ALFALFA					
sprouts	½ cup	40	1	tr	tr
ALLIGATOR					
cooked	3 oz	126	0	0	0
ALLSPICE					
ground	1 tsp	5	1	–	tr
ALMONDS					
almond butter w/ salt	2 tbsp	203	7	2	1
almond butter w/o salt	2 tbsp	203	7	–	1

FOOD	PORTION	CALS	CARB	SUGAR	FIBER
almond paste	¼ cup	260	27	21	3
chocolate covered	6 pieces (0.6 oz)	102	6	3	2
dry roasted w/ salt	¼ cup	206	7	2	4
dry roasted w/o salt	¼ cup	206	7	2	4
honey roasted	¼ cup	214	10	–	5
jordan almonds	6 (0.7 oz)	99	14	13	1
oil roasted w/ salt	¼ cup	238	7	2	4
oil roasted w/o salt	¼ cup	238	7	2	4
praline	17 pieces (1.4 oz)	210	21	17	3
yogurt covered	6 pieces (0.8 oz)	122	10	8	1
American Almond					
Marzipan	2 tbsp	130	19	17	1
Arrowhead Mills					
Organic Almond Butter Creamy	2 tbsp	200	6	2	4
Blue Diamond					
Almond Roca Buttercrunch	3 pieces (1.3 oz)	210	19	18	0
Honey Roasted	¼ cup	170	8	4	3
Jalapeno Smokehouse	28 pieces (1 oz)	170	5	1	3
Jordon Pastels	15 pieces (1.4 oz)	180	28	24	2
Lime 'N Chili	28 pieces (1 oz)	170	5	1	3
Maui Onion & Garlic	28 pieces (1 oz)	170	5	1	3
Milk Chocolate Covered	9 pieces (1.4 oz)	230	19	16	3
Salted	¼ cup	170	6	1	3
Smokehouse	28 pieces (1.3 oz)	170	5	1	3
Wasabi & Soy Sauce	28 pieces (1 oz)	170	6	2	3
Whole Natural	¼ cup	180	6	1	3
Yogurt Covered	12 pieces (1.4 oz)	210	21	19	0

FOOD	PORTION	CALS	CARB	SUGAR	FIBER
Eden					
Tamari	3 tbsp (1 oz)	160	8	–	4
Godiva					
Dark Chocolate Almonds	1 pkg (2 oz)	310	23	14	5
Good Sense					
Hickory Smoked	¼ cup	180	4	0	2
Raw Whole	¼ cup	180	6	0	4
Justin's					
Almond Butter Classic	2 tbsp (1.1 oz)	200	6	1	4
Almond Butter Maple	2 tbsp (1.1 oz)	190	8	4	3
Kettle					
Butter Salted	2 tbsp	180	6	0	2
Butter Unsalted	2 tbsp	180	6	0	2
Love'n Bake					
Almond Paste	2 tbsp	140	13	11	2
Almond Schmear	2 tbsp	140	14	11	2
Roasted Butter	2 tbsp	180	6	1	3
Maisie Jane's					
Almond Butter	1 oz	184	6	0	0
Cappuccino	9 pieces (1.4 oz)	220	19	16	2
Chocolate Toffee	9 pieces (1.4 oz)	210	21	19	2
Coffee Glazed	2 tbsp (1 oz)	150	8	3	3
Cowboy BBQ	2 tbsp (1 oz)	140	8	3	3
Mint Chocolate	9 pieces (1.4 oz)	210	20	17	2
Organic Honey Glazed	2 tbsp (1 oz)	160	12	6	4
Tamari	2 tbsp (1 oz)	160	7	1	4
Mrs. May's					
Almond Crunch	1 oz	156	8	3	3
Odense					
Almond Paste	2 tbsp (1.4 oz)	170	24	20	0
Planters					
Chocolate Lovers Dark Chocolate	11 pieces (1.4 oz)	220	18	13	3
Dry Roasted	23 pieces (1 oz)	160	6	2	3
Sunkist					
Accents Italian Parmesan	1 tbsp	40	1	0	0

FOOD	PORTION	CALS	CARB	SUGAR	FIBER
Accents Original Oven Roasted	1 tbsp	40	1	0	0
AMARANTH					
Arrowhead Mills					
Organic Whole Grain not prep	¼ cup	180	31	1	7
ANCHOVY					
boneless	1 oz	60	0	0	0
canned in oil drained	1 can (2 oz)	94	0	0	0
fresh	1 (4 g)	8	0	0	0
Brunswick					
Flat Fillets	1 can (2 oz)	25	0	0	0
Polar					
Rolled Fillets w/Capers In Olive Oil	7 pieces (0.6 oz)	40	0	0	0
ANGLERFISH					
raw	3.5 oz	72	0	0	0
ANISE					
seed	1 tsp	7	1	–	tr
ANTELOPE					
roasted	4 oz	215	0	0	0
APPLE					
CANNED					
sliced sweetened	½ cup	68	17	15	2
Glory					
Fried Apples	½ cup	80	21	11	1
Polar					
Fuji	½ cup	50	12	11	2
DRIED					
chopped	½ cup	104	28	24	4
cooked w/o sugar	½ cup	73	20	17	3
rings	5	78	21	18	3
Bare Fruit					
Chips Cinnamon	1 pkg (0.6 oz)	43	12	10	2
Chukar Cherries					
Cherry Apple Slices	10 (1 oz)	110	28	24	4
Fruit Ripples					
Cinnamon Apple	1 pkg	50	13	10	1
Strawberry Apple	1 pkg	50	13	10	1

FOOD	PORTION	CALS	CARB	SUGAR	FIBER
Mrs. May's					
Fruit Chips	1 pkg	35	8	7	1
Nature's Envy					
Apple Chips Original	1 pkg (0.8 oz)	80	20	17	tr
Sun-Maid					
Apples	¼ cup (1.4 oz)	120	29	22	2
FRESH					
apple	1 sm	55	15	11	3
apple	1 med	72	19	14	3
apple	1 lg	110	29	22	5
candied	1 sm (4.9 oz)	179	40	32	3
candied	1 med (6.5 oz)	234	52	42	4
candied	1 lg (9.8 oz)	357	79	64	6
w/ skin sliced	1 cup	57	15	11	3
w/o skin sliced	1 cup	53	14	11	1
Earthbound Farm					
Organic Slices	1 pkg (2 oz)	30	7	5	1
Eastern Select					
Gala	1 (5.5 oz)	80	22	16	5
Mrs. Prindable's					
Caramel Triple Chocolate	¼ apple (1.7 oz)	120	17	15	1
Caramel Walnut	¼ apple (2 oz)	160	17	15	1
Rainier					
Apple	1 med (5.5 oz)	80	22	16	5
Sullivan					
McIntosh	1 (5.4 oz)	80	22	20	4
FROZEN					
sliced w/o sugar	½ cup	42	11	–	2
Roast Works					
Flame Roasted Fuji	1 serv (5 oz)	90	23	19	2
REFRIGERATED					
Country Crock					
Cinnamon Apples	½ cup (4.4 oz)	130	26	22	1
TAKE-OUT					
baked	1 (6 oz)	128	42	37	4
baked no sugar	1 (5.6 oz)	136	24	18	4
fried apple rings	1 serv (2.7 oz)	91	15	12	2
APPLE JUICE					
cider	1 cup	117	29	27	tr

FOOD	PORTION	CALS	CARB	SUGAR	FIBER
juice + vitamin C & calcium	1 cup	117	29	27	tr
mulled cider	1 serv	265	42	–	6
unsweetened w/o vitamin C	1 cup	117	29	27	tr
Celestial Seasonings					
Cider Apple Caramel Kiss as prep	1 cup	80	21	19	0
Eden					
Organic Juice	8 oz	90	24	12	0
Fizz Ed.					
Green Apple	1 can (8.4 oz)	100	25	21	1
Hansen's					
100% Juice	8 oz	120	28	23	0
Hood					
100% Juice	1 cup	120	31	31	0
Land O Lakes					
Juice	1 cup (8 oz)	120	29	26	0
Nantucket Nectars					
100% Juice Pressed Apple	8 oz	120	30	26	tr
Organic Cloudy Apple	8 oz	120	29	28	0
Phat Phruit					
Green Apple	8 oz	40	11	9	0
Tree Ripe					
Organic 100% Juice	6 oz	80	21	19	0
Tropicana					
Orchard Style	1 bottle (14 oz)	200	50	48	0
Walnut Acres					
Organic Juice	8 oz	110	29	27	0
Zeigler's					
Old Fashioned Cider	8 oz	110	26	21	1
APPLESAUCE					
sweetened	½ cup	97	25	21	2
unsweetened	½ cup	52	14	12	2
Eden					
Organic	½ cup	60	13	10	2
Organic Apple Cherry	½ cup	70	17	12	3
Organic Apple Strawberry	½ cup	60	13	10	2
Organic Cinnamon	1 pkg (4 oz)	70	17	13	2
Langers					
Unsweetened	½ cup	50	13	10	2

FOOD	PORTION	CALS	CARB	SUGAR	FIBER
Mott's					
Healthy Harvest Granny Smith No Sugar Added	1 pkg (3.9 oz)	50	13	11	1
Original	½ cup	110	27	25	1
Single-Serve Cinnamon	1 pkg (4 oz)	100	25	23	1
Single-Serve Natural	1 pkg (4 oz)	50	12	11	1
Musselman's					
Lite	1 pkg (4 oz)	50	12	8	2
Unsweetened	1 pkg (4 oz)	50	12	8	2
Revolution Foods					
Organic Unsweetened	1 pkg (4 oz)	50	13	10	2

APRICOT JUICE

nectar	6 oz	106	27	26	1

APRICOTS

canned heavy syrup	½ cup	91	23	20	3
canned in juice	½ cup	59	15	13	2
canned in water	½ cup	33	8	6	2
canned light syrup	½ cup	80	21	19	2
dried halves	6	51	13	11	2
dried halves cooked w/o sugar	½ cup	106	28	24	3
fresh	1	17	4	3	1
fresh sliced	½ cup	40	9	8	2
frozen sweetened	½ cup	119	30	–	3
Harvest Bay					
Dried	5 (1.4 oz)	60	15	15	3
Mariani					
Ultimate Dried	¼ cup (1.4 oz)	100	24	16	6
Sunsweet					
Dried	6 pieces (1.4 oz)	100	25	17	3

ARROWROOT

raw	1 root (1.2 oz)	21	4	–	tr
raw root sliced	1 cup	78	16	–	2
Bob's Red Mill					
Starch	¼ cup	110	28	0	1

ARTICHOKE
CANNED

hearts in oil	1 serv (3 oz)	100	9	1	4

FOOD	PORTION	CALS	CARB	SUGAR	FIBER
Gertie's Finest					
Tapenade	2 tbsp	29	2	tr	tr
Native Forest					
Organic Hearts Quartered	1 serv (4 oz)	35	6	1	4
Polar					
Hearts	2	18	3	0	2
Hearts Quartered Marinated	1 oz	25	5	0	1
Progresso					
Hearts	2 (4.6 oz)	30	7	2	2
Hearts Marinated	2 (1.1 oz)	60	2	7	0
FRESH					
cooked	1 med	60	13	1	7
hearts cooked	½ cup	42	9	1	5
Ocean Mist					
Lemon	1 (4.2 oz)	60	13	1	6
FROZEN					
cooked	1 cup	42	9	1	5
cooked w/o salt	1 pkg (9 oz)	108	22	2	11
C&W					
Hearts	12 pieces (3 oz)	40	7	1	5
TAKE-OUT					
stuffed	1 (8.8 oz)	397	54	6	10

ASIAN FOOD *(see also* CURRY, DINNER, EGG ROLLS, SAUCE, SOY SAUCE, SUSHI)

FOOD	PORTION	CALS	CARB	SUGAR	FIBER
CANNED					
chow mein chicken w/o noodles	1 cup	194	10	6	2
La Choy					
Chow Mein Beef	1 cup	90	11	2	2
Chow Mein Chicken	1 cup (9.3 oz)	100	10	3	2
Sweet & Sour Noodles	1 cup	150	29	23	5
Teriyaki Chicken	1 cup (8.6 oz)	120	16	7	3
FRESH					
wonton wrapper	1 (0.3 oz)	23	5	–	tr
Frieda's					
Won Ton Wrappers	4 (1 oz)	80	17	1	1
FROZEN					
Contessa					
Chow Mein Chicken w/ Sauce not prep	1¾ cups	320	55	10	3
Curry Chicken w/ Sauce not prep	1¾ cups	240	29	4	2

FOOD	PORTION	CALS	CARB	SUGAR	FIBER
Fried Rice Chicken w/ Sauce not prep	1¾ cups	260	49	5	4
General Tsao Shrimp w/ Sauce not prep	1¾ cups	270	49	17	4
Kung Pao Shrimp w/ Sauce not prep	1¾ cups	200	30	4	3
Low Mein Shrimp w/ Sauce not prep	1¾ cups	250	29	11	2
Stir-Fry Beef w/ Sauce not prep	1¾ cup	190	28	17	4
Stir-Fry Chicken w/ Sauce not prep	1¾ cups	160	18	14	4
Stir-Fry Shrimp w/ Sauce not prep	1¾ cups	120	16	12	2
Sweet & Sour Shrimp w/ Sauce not prep	1½ cups	180	40	12	3
Tandoori Chicken w/ Sauce not prep	1⅓ cups	200	27	2	3
Glutino					
Gluten Free Chicken Pad Thai Peach	1 pkg (7 oz)	370	65	10	3
Healthy Choice					
Five Spice Beef & Vegetables	1 (10 oz)	310	49	17	7
General Tso's Spicy Chicken	1 (10.7 oz)	310	50	10	5
Helen's Kitchen					
Thai Yellow Curry w/ Tofu Steaks & Vegetables & Basmati Rice	1 pkg (9 oz)	280	30	1	2
Joy Of Cooking					
Lo Mein Vegetable	1 cup (7.7 oz)	220	40	6	11
Kahiki					
Beef & Broccoli	1 pkg (10.9 oz)	360	42	4	2
Chicken Fried Rice	1 pkg (10.9 oz)	460	75	2	2
General Tso's Chicken	1 pkg (10 oz)	400	66	23	2
Naturals General Tso's Chicken	1 pkg (10 oz)	330	52	24	3
Naturals Mandarin Orange Chicken	1 pkg (10 oz)	340	58	31	3
Naturals Szechuan Peppercorn Beef	1 pkg (10 oz)	350	35	9	3

FOOD	PORTION	CALS	CARB	SUGAR	FIBER
Naturals Teriyaki Mixed Vegetables	1 pkg (10 oz)	260	51	18	4
Sesame Orange Chicken	1 pkg (10.9 oz)	420	60	15	2
Soothing Lettuce Wraps	4 tbsp (2 oz)	90	9	2	1
Tempura Chicken Nuggets	¾ cup (3.5 oz)	230	10	0	0
Tropical Sweet & Sour Chicken	1 pkg (10.9 oz)	490	82	36	4
Organic Classics					
Thai Chicken Curry	1 pkg (10 oz)	420	50	4	3
Seeds Of Change					
Asian Stir-Fry Noodles	1 pkg (11 oz)	290	55	14	4
Spicy Peanut Noodles	1 pkg (11 oz)	370	53	6	4
Teriyaki Stir Fried Rice	1 pkg (11 oz)	340	56	15	6
Tyson					
Meal Kit Chicken Fried Rice	2½ cups	440	69	15	5
MIX					
Annie Chun's					
Meal Kit Chow Mein Noodles w/ Garlic Black Bean Sauce	⅓ pkg	230	42	8	2
Meal Kit Chow Mein Noodles w/ Peanut Sesame Sauce	⅓ pkg	270	42	8	2
Meal Kit Chow Mein Noodles w/ Scallion Sauce	⅓ pkg	240	39	6	2
Meal Kit Chow Mein Noodles w/ Teriyaki Sauce	⅓ box	210	43	8	2
Meal Kit Soba Noodles w/ Soy Ginger Sauce	⅓ pkg	210	41	8	3
Nissin					
Chow Mein Chicken as prep	½ pkg (2 oz)	240	34	5	2
Chow Mein Thai Peanut as prep	½ pkg (2 oz)	270	35	3	tr
SHELF-STABLE					
Fantastic					
Pad Thai w/ Rice Noodles	1 pkg (7 oz)	400	59	7	5
Thai Lemon Grass w/ Rice Noodles	1 pkg (7.4 oz)	340	48	4	5
Healthy Choice					
Fresh Mixers Sesame Teriyaki Chicken	1 pkg (7.9 oz)	380	69	16	3

FOOD	PORTION	CALS	CARB	SUGAR	FIBER
Fresh Mixers Sweet & Sour Chicken	1 pkg (7.9 oz)	390	78	22	5
Fresh Mixers Szechwan Beef w/ Asian Noodles	1 pkg (6.9 oz)	370	65	18	4
TAKE-OUT					
beef & broccoli	1 cup	221	10	3	3
beef w/ black bean sauce	1 serv (7 oz)	288	6	5	1
buddha's delight w/ cellophane noodles fat choi jai	1 serv (7.6 oz)	211	44	3	2
bun baked red bean	1 (1.1 oz)	102	16	–	1
cha siu bao steamed buns w/ chicken filling	1 (2.3 oz)	160	26	4	tr
chinese garlic chicken	1 cup (5.7 oz)	290	8	3	1
chinese style fried egg noodles w/ seafood & lettuce	1 serv (14 oz)	694	63	1	8
chow mein beef w/o noodles	1 cup	271	12	4	3
chow mein chicken w/ noodles	1 cup (7.7 oz)	273	20	5	2
chow mein noodles	1 cup	237	26	tr	2
chow mein pork w/o noodles	1 cup	284	12	4	3
chow mein shrimp w/o noodles	1 cup	154	11	6	2
chow mein vegetable w/o noodles	1 cup	224	16	8	4
dim sum meat filled	3 pieces (4 oz)	124	11	1	1
egg foo yung beef	1 patty (6 oz)	243	7	3	1
egg foo yung chicken	1 patty (3 oz)	121	4	2	1
egg foo yung pork	1 patty (3 oz)	125	4	2	1
egg foo yung shrimp	1 patty (3 oz)	153	3	2	1
filipino chicken adobo	1 serv (15 oz)	555	45	tr	1
foochow fish ball	1 (1 oz)	36	3	0	1
fried rice	1 cup	333	42	2	1
fried rice beef	1 cup	346	42	1	1
fried rice chicken	1 cup	329	42	1	1
fried rice pork	1 cup	335	42	1	1
fried rice shrimp	1 cup	323	42	2	1
general tsao's chicken	1 cup (5 oz)	296	16	5	1
green beans szechuan style	1 cup	176	16	3	6
indian style fried egg noodles w/ eggs tomato sauce & lime	1 serv (15 oz)	721	80	2	8
korean spicy shredded chicken	1 serv (5 oz)	258	5	5	2

FOOD	PORTION	CALS	CARB	SUGAR	FIBER
kung pao beef	1 cup	410	9	2	2
kung pao chicken	1 cup (5.7 oz)	434	12	4	2
kung pao pork	1 cup	460	12	4	2
kung pao shrimp	1 cup	345	11	3	2
lemon chicken w/o vegetables	1 serv (6.6 oz)	503	26	3	1
lo mein beef	1 cup	286	31	3	3
lo mein chicken	1 cup (7 oz)	280	33	3	3
lo mein meatless	1 cup	234	38	3	3
lo mein pork	1 cup	314	34	3	3
lo mein shrimp	1 cup	236	33	2	4
moo goo gai pan chicken	1 cup (7.6 oz)	272	12	5	3
moo shu pork w/o pancake	1 cup	512	5	2	1
peking duck w/ pancakes & seafood sauce	1 serv (14 oz)	1871	157	39	5
phad thai w/ chicken	1 cup (7 oz)	358	39	5	2
pork w/ chinese cabbage	1 serv (4 oz)	120	1	0	1
sesame seed paste bun	1 (2.5 oz)	220	39	12	2
shrimp chips banh phong tom	6 med	214	20	1	tr
shrimp w/ lobster sauce	1 cup	298	8	2	1
shu mai chicken & vegetable dumplings	6 (3.6 oz)	160	18	6	1
sukiyaki beef	1 cup	165	6	4	1
sukiyaki chicken	1 serv (18 oz)	436	19	7	4
sweet & sour chicken w/o rice	1 cup	670	36	4	2
sweet & sour pork w/ rice	1 cup	268	40	10	2
sweet & sour pork w/o rice	1 cup	231	25	15	2
sweet & sour shrimp	1 cup	480	46	40	1
szechuan chicken	1 cup (5.7 oz)	180	9	2	2
szechuan shrimp & vegetables	1 cup	159	10	3	2
tempura hawaiian fish tofu vegetable	2 cups	285	13	9	2
tempura vegetable	8 pieces	90	8	1	1
teriyaki beef	1 cup	454	13	9	tr
teriyaki chicken w/ rice	1 serv (11 oz)	430	77	10	1
teriyaki shrimp	1 cup	271	14	6	1
thai style pineapple rice w/ ham & pork floss	1 serv (7.7 oz)	408	60	22	6
wonton fried meat filled	1 (0.7 oz)	54	5	tr	tr
wonton meat & shrimp boiled	1 (0.5 oz)	19	2	–	tr

FOOD	PORTION	CALS	CARB	SUGAR	FIBER
ASPARAGUS					
CANNED					
spears	1	3	tr	tr	tr
spears	1 cup	46	6	3	4
Del Monte					
Spears Extra Long	½ cup	20	3	0	1
Gertie's Finest					
White	1 oz	15	3	2	1
Green Giant					
Spears Extra Long	5	20	3	1	1
Native Forest					
White	1 serv (4 oz)	20	3	1	1
Tillen Farms					
Crispy Asparagus Pickled	3 spears	10	1	0	0
FRESH					
cooked	½ cup	20	4	1	2
cooked	4 spears	13	2	1	1
spears raw	4	10	2	1	1
Alpine Fresh					
Fresh Green	5 spears (3.3 oz)	20	5	2	2
Frieda's					
White	⅔ cup	20	4	2	2
Ocean Mist					
Spears	5 (3.3 oz)	25	4	2	2
FROZEN					
cooked	1 pkg (10 oz)	53	6	1	5
cooked	4 spears	11	1	tr	1
C&W					
Spears	7 (3 oz)	20	3	2	tr
Europe's Best					
Spears	7 spears	15	3	2	2
Joy Of Cooking					
Tender	½ cup (3.3 oz)	70	4	1	1
AVOCADO					
california mashed	¼ cup	96	5	tr	4
california peeled & pitted	1	289	15	1	12
florida mashed	¼ cup	69	5	0	1
florida peeled & pitted	1	365	24	7	17

FOOD	PORTION	CALS	CARB	SUGAR	FIBER
Cabilfrut					
Hass fresh	⅕ med (1.1 oz)	55	3	0	3
Earthbound Farm					
Organic Fresh	⅓ med (1 oz)	55	3	0	3
Frieda's					
Fresh Cocktail	1 (1.4 oz)	60	3	0	2
Simply Avo					
Hass Avocado Pulp	2 tbsp	50	3	1	2
Hass Halves	⅙ pkg (1.1 oz)	50	3	0	2
Wholly Guacamole					
Classic	2 tbsp	50	2	0	2
Organic	2 tbsp	50	2	0	2
Pico De Gallo Style	2 tbsp	40	2	0	2
TAKE-OUT					
guacamole	1 serv (2.2 oz)	105	5	1	2
BACON					
bacon grease	1 tbsp	116	0	0	0
beef breakfast strips cooked	3 strips	153	tr	0	0
gammon lean & fat grilled	4.2 oz	274	0	–	0
turkey	2 (0.8 oz)	84	1	0	0
Applegate Farms					
Natural Dry Cured Cooked	2 slices (0.5 oz)	60	0	0	0
Organic Turkey	1 slice (1 oz)	35	0	0	0
Boar's Head					
Fully Cooked Slices	3 (0.5 oz)	70	0	0	0
Butterball					
Turkey Bacon	1 slice (0.5 oz)	25	0	0	0
Hormel					
Real Bits	1 tbsp	25	0	0	0
Jennie-O					
Turkey Bacon	1 slice (0.5 oz)	35	0	0	0
Jimmy Dean					
Lower Sodium	1 slice (0.3 oz)	50	0	0	0
Original	1 slice (0.3 oz)	50	0	0	0
Thick Slice	1 slice (0.5 oz)	80	0	0	0
Oscar Mayer					
Bacon Bits	1 tbsp (7 g)	25	0	0	0
Hardwood Smoked	2 slices (0.5 oz)	70	0	0	0
Lower Sodium	3 slices (0.5 oz)	70	0	0	0
Ready To Serve	3 slices	70	0	0	0

FOOD	PORTION	CALS	CARB	SUGAR	FIBER
Uncured	3 slices (0.5 oz)	60	1	1	0
Tyson					
Hickory Thick Cut	2 pieces (0.8 oz)	140	0	0	0
Wellshire					
Beef Uncured	2 oz	114	0	0	0
Pancetta Sliced	1 slice (0.4 oz)	60	0	0	0
Pork Range Sliced Dry Rubbed	2 slices	30	0	0	0
Uncured Turkey	1 slice (1 oz)	20	0	0	0
BACON SUBSTITUTES					
bacon bits meatless	1 tbsp	33	2	0	1
meatless	1 strip	16	tr	0	tr
Bob's Red Mill					
Bac'Ums	4 tsp	25	2	0	0
Lightlife					
Organic Tempeh Smokey Strips	3 slices (2 oz)	80	6	1	1
Smart Bacon	2 strips (0.8 oz)	45	1	1	1
Worthington					
Stripples	2 strips (0.5 oz)	60	2	0	tr
BAGEL					
cinnamon raisin	1 lg (4 in)	244	49	5	2
cinnamon raisin	1 mini	71	14	2	1
egg	1 lg (4.5 in)	364	69	–	3
low carb	1 (4 oz)	216	42	0	14
mini onion	1 (1.4 oz)	100	20	1	1
oat bran	1 lg (4 in)	227	47	1	3
plain	1 sm (3 in)	190	37	–	2
plain	1 med (3.5 in)	289	56	–	2
plain	1 lg (4.5 in)	360	70	–	3
David's					
Deli Bagels	1 (2.8 oz)	230	46	2	2
Enjoy Life					
Nut Gluten Free Classic Original	1 (3 oz)	270	46	9	3
Natural Ovens					
Blueberry	1 (3 oz)	250	47	13	5
Brainy	1 (3 oz)	230	40	7	8
Whole Wheat	1 (3 oz)	230	40	7	8
New York Style					
Crisps Natural Whole Wheat	6	120	16	1	2

FOOD	PORTION	CALS	CARB	SUGAR	FIBER
Crisps Plain	7	140	17	1	1
Pepperidge Farm					
100% Whole Wheat	1	250	49	9	6
Everything	1	260	53	9	2
Mini 100% Whole Wheat	1	100	20	3	3
Mini Plain	1	110	22	4	1
Sara Lee					
Apple Cinnamon	1 (4 oz)	310	64	16	3
Banana Walnut	1 (4 oz)	350	61	10	4
Blueberry Deluxe	1 (3.3 oz)	260	53	7	2
Blueberry Junior	1 (1 oz)	70	15	2	tr
Blueberry Toaster Size	1 (2.1 oz)	160	34	4	1
Cinnamon Raisin Deluxe	1 (3.3 oz)	260	55	9	4
Heart Healthy 100% Whole Wheat	1 (3.3 oz)	220	47	8	6
Plain	1 (2.1 oz)	160	33	3	1
Sundried Tomato & Basil	1 (4 oz)	300	61	6	2
Whole Grain Plain	1 (3.3 oz)	240	50	6	3
Thomas'					
100% Whole Wheat Mini	1 (1.5 oz)	110	22	3	3
Bagelbread Mini Squares 100% Whole Wheat	1 (2 oz)	150	30	4	4
BAKING POWDER					
baking powder	1 tsp	2	1	0	0
low sodium	1 tsp	5	2	0	tr
Bob's Red Mills					
Baking Powder	1 tsp	5	1	0	0
Calumet					
Double Acting	⅛ tsp	0	0	0	0
Davis					
Baking Powder	1 tsp	0	tr	0	0
BAKING SODA					
baking soda	1 tsp	0	0	0	0
Bob's Red Mill					
Baking Soda	¼ tsp	0	0	0	0
BALSAM PEAR (BITTER GOURD)					
leafy tips cooked w/o salt	1 cup	20	4	1	1
pods raw sliced	1 cup	16	3	—	3
pods sliced cooked w/ salt	1 cup	24	5	2	3

FOOD	PORTION	CALS	CARB	SUGAR	FIBER
BAMBOO SHOOTS					
canned sliced	½ cup	12	2	1	1
fresh sliced cooked w/ salt	½ cup	7	1	–	1
raw sliced	½ cup	20	4	2	2
La Choy					
Bamboo Shoots	½ cup	10	2	0	tr
Polar					
Sliced	½ cup	25	3	1	2
BANANA					
baked	1 (4.5 oz)	163	42	26	4
banana chips	1 oz	147	17	–	2
fresh	1 sm (6 in)	90	23	12	3
fresh	1 med (7 in)	105	27	14	3
fresh	1 lg (8 in)	121	31	17	4
fresh baby	1 extra sm (<6 in)	72	19	10	2
fresh mashed	½ cup	100	26	14	3
fresh sliced	1 cup	134	34	18	4
green fried	1 (3.1 oz)	152	21	11	2
green pickled	½ cup	240	11	6	1
green sliced fried	1 cup	323	45	24	5
powder	1 tbsp	21	5	3	1
red ripe	1 (7 in)	93	24	13	3
red ripe sliced	1 cup	134	34	18	4
whole dried	1 piece (1.2 oz)	130	33	22	2
Bob's Red Mill					
Chips	25 (1.4 oz)	210	26	20	0
Brothers-All-Natural					
Crisps	1 pkg (0.58 oz)	66	16	8	2
Frieda's					
Burro	1 (3 oz)	80	20	13	1
Dried	1 piece (1.2 oz)	130	33	22	2
Goodniks					
Nutty Bananas Crunchy Snack	⅔ cup	230	21	3	3
Kopali					
Organic Dark Chocolate Covered	½ pkg (1 oz)	120	19	17	2

FOOD	PORTION	CALS	CARB	SUGAR	FIBER
Tree Of Life					
Dried Sweetened	½ cup (1.6 oz)	240	27	18	4
TAKE-OUT					
batter dipped fried	1 sm (4 oz)	266	32	9	3
fried dwarf w/ cheese	1 (1.4 oz)	84	10	5	1
fritter	1 (2.3 oz)	197	36	14	2
sliced batter dipped fried	1 cup	335	40	12	3
BARBECUE SAUCE					
barbecue	2 tbsp	52	13	9	tr
low sodium	2 tbsp	52	13	9	tr
Bear-Man					
Black Bear Boogie	2 tbsp	40	8	5	0
Growlin' Grizzly	2 tbsp	60	12	8	tr
Bone Suckin'					
Sauce	2 tbsp	40	10	8	0
Cattlemen's					
Classic	2 tbsp	60	15	10	tr
Honey	2 tbsp	70	17	13	tr
Smokehouse	2 tbsp	60	14	12	tr
David Burke					
Flavor Spray Memphis BBQ	2 sprays	0	0	0	0
Nando's					
Barbecue	1 tbsp	7	2	1	0
Naturally Fresh					
BBQ	2 tbsp	40	10	8	0
Wellshire					
Original	2 tbsp	39	10	4	0
BARLEY					
flour	1 cup	511	110	1	15
pearled cooked	1 cup (5.5 oz)	193	44	tr	6
pearled uncooked	¼ cup	176	39	tr	8
Arrowhead Mills					
Organic Pearled not prep	¼ cup	160	32	1	8
BARRACUDA					
broiled	4 oz	239	tr	tr	0
cooked flaked	1 cup	287	1	tr	0
poached	4 oz	227	0	0	0
TAKE-OUT					
breaded & fried	4 oz	282	5	tr	tr

FOOD	PORTION	CALS	CARB	SUGAR	FIBER
BASIL					
fresh chopped	2 tbsp	1	tr	tr	tr
ground	1 tsp	4	1	tr	1
leaves fresh	5	1	tr	tr	tr
Eden					
Shiso Leaf Powder	1 tsp	0	0	0	0
BASS					
breaded baked	4 oz	205	10	1	1
pickled mero en escabeche	2 oz	156	tr	tr	tr
striped baked	3 oz	105	0	0	0
striped bass farm raised	4 oz	110	0	0	0
BAY LEAF					
crumbled	1 tsp	2	tr	tr	tr
BEAN SPROUTS (see ALFALFA, SPROUTS)					
BEANS (see also individual names)					
CANNED					
baked beans w/ pork & tomato sauce	½ cup	119	24	7	5
Allens					
Original Baked	½ cup	150	29	10	8
Refried Black Beans No Fat Added	½ cup	120	23	1	8
B&M					
Baked Original	½ cup (4.6 oz)	180	31	10	8
Barbeque Baked	½ cup (4.6 oz)	190	39	19	9
Country Style	½ cup (4.6 oz)	170	35	15	7
Vegetarian	½ cup (4.6 oz)	160	31	12	8
Bush's					
Boston Recipe	½ cup	150	31	11	5
Homestyle	½ cup	140	29	12	5
Honey	½ cup	160	32	14	6
Vegetarian Fat Free	½ cup	130	29	12	5
Campbell's					
Pork & Beans	½ cup	140	25	8	7
Eden					
Organic Baked w/ Sorghum	½ cup	150	27	6	7
Gebhardt					
Refried	½ cup	90	16	0	4

FOOD	PORTION	CALS	CARB	SUGAR	FIBER
Refried Fat Free	½ cup	80	17	tr	5
Refried Jalapeno	½ cup	100	17	1	5
Green Giant					
Three Bean Salad	½ cup	80	18	10	3
Las Palmas					
Refried	½ cup	150	23	9	2
Old El Paso					
Refried Fat Free	½ cup	100	18	1	6
Refried Fat Free Spicy	½ cup	100	18	1	6
Pace					
Refried Salsa	½ cup	70	14	4	4
Read					
3 Bean Salad	⅓ cup	60	13	8	2
Rosarita					
Refried	½ cup	120	18	tr	6
Refried Black Beans No Fat	½ cup	110	19	0	8
Refried Fat Free	½ cup	100	19	tr	6
Refried Vegetarian	½ cup	120	19	0	7
Van Camp's					
Baked Beans Homestyle	½ cup	170	33	15	6
Beanee Weenee BBQ	1 can	260	35	12	9
Beanee Weenee Original	1 can	240	29	8	8
Beanee Weenee w/ Chili	1 can	240	26	2	6
Pork And Beans	½ cup	110	23	7	6
Wagon Master					
Pork & Beans	½ cup	130	23	4	9
MIX					
Fantastic					
Instant Black Beans not prep	⅓ cup	160	29	7	7
Instant Refried Beans not prep	¼ cup	130	23	0	8
TAKE-OUT					
frijoles a la charra w/ pork tomatoes & chili peppers	1 cup	341	23	2	5
three bean salad	1 cup	114	15	2	5
BEAR					
simmered	3 oz	220	0	0	0
BEAVER					
roasted	4 oz	240	0	0	0

FOOD	PORTION	CALS	CARB	SUGAR	FIBER
BEE POLLEN					
bee pollen	1 tsp (5 g)	16	2	2	tr
Tree Of Life					
Bee Pollen	1 tsp (7 g)	30	3	0	0
BEEF (see also BEEF DISHES, JERKY, MEATBALLS, VEAL)					
CANNED					
corned beef	1 oz	71	0	0	0
Libby's					
Corned Beef	2 oz	120	0	0	0
Corned Beef Hash	1 cup	420	33	1	3
Potted Meat	¼ cup	120	0	0	0
Roast Beef w/ Gravy	⅔ cup	140	3	0	0
FRESH					
arm pot roast trim 0 fat braised	3.5 oz	297	0	0	0
arm pot roast trim ⅛ in fat braised	3.5 oz	302	0	0	0
beef crumbles 70% lean pan browned	3 oz	230	0	0	0
bottom round roast trim 0 fat braised	4 oz	253	0	0	0
bottom round roast trim 0 fat roasted	3.5 oz	187	0	0	0
bottom round roast trim ½ in fat braised	4 oz	337	0	0	0
bottom round roast trim ⅛ in fat braised	4 oz	280	0	0	0
bottom round roast trim ⅛ in fat roasted	4 oz	247	0	0	0
bottom sirloin butt roast trim 0 fat roasted	3.5 oz	182	0	0	0
brisket flat half trim ⅛ in fat braised	3.5 oz	298	0	0	0
brisket flat trim 0 fat braised	3.5 oz	221	0	0	0
brisket point half trim 0 fat braised	3.5 oz	358	0	0	0
brisket point half trim ¼ in fat braised	3.5 oz	404	0	0	0
brisket point half trim ⅛ in fat braised	3.5 oz	349	0	0	0

FOOD	PORTION	CALS	CARB	SUGAR	FIBER
chuck boston cut roast trim 0 fat roasted	3.5 oz	207	0	0	0
chuck boston cut roast trim ¼ in fat roasted	3.5 oz	242	0	0	0
chuck bottom roast trim 0 fat braised	3.5 oz	334	0	0	0
chuck bottom roast trim ¼ in fat braised	3.5 oz	345	0	0	0
chuck fillet steak trim 0 fat broiled	4 oz	181	0	0	0
chuck top roast trim 0 fat broiled	4 oz	245	0	0	0
club steak trim ½ in fat broiled	4 oz	384	0	0	0
corned beef brisket cooked	3 oz	213	tr	0	0
crosscut shank trim ¼ in fat stewed	1 serv (6.8 oz)	510	0	0	0
delmonico steak trim ¼ in fat broiled	4 oz	409	0	0	0
entrecote steak trim ½ in fat broiled	4 oz	413	0	0	0
eye round roast trim 0 fat roasted	4 oz	190	0	0	0
eye round roast trim ¼ in fat roasted	4 oz	283	0	0	0
eye round roast trim ⅛ in fat roasted	4 oz	236	0	0	0
filet mignon roast trim ¼ in fat roasted	4 oz	376	0	0	0
filet mignon roast trim ⅛ in fat roasted	4 oz	367	0	0	0
filet mignon trim 0 fat broiled	4 oz	247	0	0	0
filet mignon trim ⅛ in fat broiled	4 oz	303	0	0	0
ground 70% lean broiled	3.5 oz	273	0	0	0
ground 75% lean broiled	2.5 oz	195	0	0	0
ground 80% lean broiled	3 oz	234	0	0	0
ground 85% lean pan fried	3 oz	197	0	0	0
ground 90% lean pan fried	3 oz	173	0	0	0
ground 95% lean pan fried	3 oz	139	0	0	0
london broil trim 0 fat broiled	3.5 oz	188	0	0	0

FOOD	PORTION	CALS	CARB	SUGAR	FIBER
london broil trim ¼ in fat broiled	4 oz	260	0	0	0
new york strip steak trim 0 fat broiled	4 oz	219	0	0	0
oxtails cooked	6 pieces (6.3 oz)	472	0	0	0
porterhouse steak trim 0 fat broiled	1 lb	1252	0	0	0
porterhouse steak trim ¼ in fat broiled	1 lb	1492	0	0	0
porterhouse steak trim ⅛ in fat broiled	1 lb	1324	0	0	0
porterhouse steak trim ⅛ in fat broiled	4 oz	337	0	0	0
rib eye roast trim ¼ in fat roasted	3.5 oz	365	0	0	0
rib eye steak trim ⅛ in fat broiled	4 oz	221	0	0	0
rib roast trim ¼ in fat roasted	4 oz	406	0	0	0
rib steak trim ¼ in fat broiled	4 oz	388	0	0	0
round tip roast trim 0 fat roasted	4 oz	213	0	0	0
sandwich steaks thinly sliced	1 serv (2 oz)	173	0	0	0
shell steak trim ¼ in fat broiled	4 oz	366	0	0	0
shortribs lean & fat braised	1 serv (7.8 oz)	1060	0	0	0
skirt steak trim 0 fat broiled	4 oz	289	0	0	0
t-bone steak trim 0 fat broiled	4 oz	280	0	0	0
t-bone steak trim ¼ in fat broiled	1 lb	1388	0	0	0
t-bone steak trim ⅛ in fat broiled	1 lb	804	0	0	0
tip round roast trim ⅛ in fat roasted	4 oz	248	0	0	0
top loin steak boneless trim ⅛ in fat broiled	4 oz	299	0	0	0
top round roast trim 0 fat braised	4 oz	237	0	0	0
top round roast trim ¼ in fat braised	4 oz	281	0	0	0

FOOD	PORTION	CALS	CARB	SUGAR	FIBER
top round roast trim 1/4 in fat roasted	4 oz	265	0	0	0
top round steak trim 1/4 in fat pan fried	4 oz	314	0	0	0
top sirloin steak trim 1/8 in fat broiled	4 oz	275	0	0	0
top sirloin steak trim 1/8 in fat pan fried	4 oz	355	0	0	0
tri-tip roast trim 0 fat roasted	3.5 oz	218	0	0	0
tri-tip steak trim 0 fat broiled	4 oz	300	0	0	0
Laura's Lean					
Eye Of Round	4 oz	135	0	0	0
Ground Beef 92% Lean	4 oz	160	0	0	0
Ground Beef Patties	1 (4 oz)	160	0	0	0
Ground Round 96% Lean	4 oz	140	0	0	0
Sirloin Tip	4 oz	130	0	0	0
Top Round	4 oz	135	0	0	0
Organic Prairie					
90% Lean Ground	4 oz	250	0	0	0
Rumba					
Cheekmeat	4 oz	300	0	0	0
Crosscut Hind Shank	4 oz	190	0	0	0
Marrow Bones	4 oz	290	0	0	0
Oxtail	4 oz	260	0	0	0
Short Ribs	4 oz	400	0	0	0
Shady Brook					
Tri-Tip Roast Rosemary Garlic & Chardonnay	4 oz	180	4	3	0
Tri-Tip Roast Sizzling Ginger	4 oz	210	9	8	0
FROZEN					
patty broiled medium	3 oz	240	0	0	0
Organic Prairie					
Rib Eye Steak	1 (6 oz)	470	0	0	0
READY-TO-EAT					
roast beef spread	1/4 cup	127	2	tr	tr
Applegate Farms					
Organic Roast Beef	2 oz	80	0	0	0
Boar's Head					
Corned Beef Brisket	2 oz	80	0	0	0
Top Round Deluxe	2 oz	80	tr	0	0

FOOD	PORTION	CALS	CARB	SUGAR	FIBER
Top Round Oven Roasted No Salt Added	2 oz	90	0	0	0
Healthy Ones					
Deli Roast Beef	2 oz	70	1	1	0
Oscar Mayer					
Slow Roasted Shaved	¼ pkg (1.8 oz)	60	0	0	0
Sara Lee					
Roast Beef Medium or Rare	2 oz	60	1	0	0
Tyson					
Beef Strips Seasoned	1 serv (3 oz)	130	1	1	0
TAKE-OUT					
roast beef rare	2 oz	70	0	0	0

BEEF DISHES
CANNED
Hormel

FOOD	PORTION	CALS	CARB	SUGAR	FIBER
Corned Beef Hash 50% Reduced Fat	1 cup	290	24	2	2
Libby's					
Hawaiian Corned Beef	2 oz	120	0	0	0
FROZEN					
Quaker Maid					
Sandwich Steaks Pure Beef	1 serv (1.8 oz)	120	0	0	0
Tyson					
Steak Country Fried	1 (3.2 oz)	310	15	1	1
MIX					
Hamburger Helper					
Beef Pasta as prep	1 cup	270	24	1	1
Cheddar Cheese Melt as prep	1 cup	310	30	2	tr
Cheesy Baked Potato as prep	1 cup	310	30	2	2
Chili Cheese as prep	1 cup	340	33	4	1
Double Cheesy Quesadilla as prep	1 cup	350	36	2	tr
Italian Sausage as prep	1 cup	290	29	5	1
Microwave Singles Cheesy Lasagna	1 pkg	210	33	6	1
Philly Cheesesteak as prep	1 cup	320	27	2	1
Salisbury as prep	1 cup	260	27	1	1
Tomato Basil Penne as prep	1 cup	300	31	6	1

FOOD	PORTION	CALS	CARB	SUGAR	FIBER
REFRIGERATED					
Chi Chi's					
For Tacos! Ground Beef	¼ cup	90	5	2	0
Hormel					
Beef Tips & Gravy	½ cup	170	4	3	1
Huxtable's					
Shepherds Pie Beef	1 pkg (10 oz)	270	27	1	3
Tyson					
Chuck Roast w/ Vegetables	1 serv (4 oz)	320	14	0	2
Seasoned Meatloaf	1 serv (5 oz)	320	16	5	0
Steak Tips In Bourbon Sauce	1 serv (5 oz)	180	12	11	0
TAKE-OUT					
beef bourguignonne	1 cup	339	10	3	1
beef satay + peanut sauce	2 skewers	253	6	4	1
bool kogi korean marinated beef ribs	4 oz	190	6	4	0
bracciola	1 roll (4.7 oz)	276	8	1	1
bubble & squeak	5 oz	186	16	–	3
bulgoghi korean grilled beef	1 serv (5.2 oz)	256	5	3	tr
chipped beef on toast	1 slice (5 oz)	226	22	7	1
cornish pasty	1 (8 oz)	847	79	–	3
goulash w/ potatoes	1 cup	298	19	3	2
greek moussaka	1 serv (8.5 oz)	450	12	4	1
kheena	6.7 oz	781	1	–	tr
koftas	5	280	3	–	tr
meatloaf	1 lg slice (5 oz)	294	9	2	1
pepper steak	1 cup	317	5	2	1
pot roast w/ gravy	1 serv (6 oz)	320	4	0	0
samosa	2 (4 oz)	652	20	–	2
shepherds pie	1 serv (7 oz)	282	20	–	2
sloppy joes	1 serv (9 oz)	398	48	5	12
steak & kidney pie w/ top crust	1 slice (5 oz)	400	23	–	1
stew w/ potatoes & vegetables	1 cup	199	22	3	3
stroganoff	1 cup	394	15	2	1
swiss steak w/ sauce	1 serv (8 oz)	234	8	3	1
toad in the hole	1 (4.7 oz)	383	23	–	1
BEEFALO					
roasted	4 oz	213	0	0	0

FOOD	PORTION	CALS	CARB	SUGAR	FIBER
BEER AND ALE					
ale brown	10 oz	77	8	–	0
ale pale	10 oz	88	12	–	0
beer cooler	1 (16 oz)	194	34	–	1
beer light	12 oz can	103	6	tr	0
beer regular	12 oz can	153	13	0	0
black & tan	1 serv (12 oz)	146	13	–	1
black velvet	1 (10 oz)	160	8	–	1
boilermaker	1 serv	216	13	–	1
lager	10 oz	80	4	–	0
mead	1 serv	250	13	–	1
shandy	1 serv	125	12	–	1
stout	10 oz	102	6	–	0
BEETS					
CANNED					
sliced	½ cup	37	9	8	2
Freshlike					
Pickled Sliced	4 slices (1 oz)	20	4	4	0
Greenwood					
Harvard	1 serv (4.4 oz)	100	27	19	1
Pickled	1 oz	25	6	5	0
FRESH					
greens cooked w/o salt	½ cup	19	4	tr	2
sliced cooked	½ cup	37	8	7	2
whole cooked	2 med (3.5 oz)	44	10	8	2
Frieda's					
Beets	½ cup	35	8	5	2

BEVERAGES *(see BEER AND ALE, CHAMPAGNE, COFFEE, DRINK MIXERS, ENERGY DRINKS, FRUIT DRINKS, ICED TEA, LIQUOR/LIQUEUR, MALT, MILKSHAKE, SMOOTHIES, SODA, TEA/HERBAL TEA, WATER, WINE, YOGURT DRINKS)*

FOOD	PORTION	CALS	CARB	SUGAR	FIBER
BISCUIT					
FROZEN					
Jimmy Dean					
Snack Size Sausage On A Biscuit	2	400	24	4	1
MIX					
plain as prep	1 (2 oz)	190	27	–	1
Bisquick					
Heart Smart	⅓ cup	140	27	3	1

FOOD	PORTION	CALS	CARB	SUGAR	FIBER
King Arthur					
Whole Grain Buttermilk not prep	¼ cup	100	19	5	2
REFRIGERATED					
plain baked	1 (1 oz)	93	13	tr	tr
Pillsbury					
Buttermilk	3 (2.2 oz)	150	29	4	1
Flaky Layers	3 (2.2 oz)	160	28	4	1
Grands! Butter Tastin'	1 (2 oz)	190	24	5	tr
Grands! Buttermilk Reduced Fat	1 (2 oz)	170	26	4	tr
Grands! Golden Wheat Reduced Fat	1 (2.1 oz)	180	27	6	2
Grands! Original	1 (2 oz)	190	24	5	tr
Grands! Original Reduced Fat	1 (2 oz)	170	26	5	tr
Perfect Portions Butter Tastin'	1 (1.9 oz)	190	23	4	tr
TAKE-OUT					
buttermilk	1 lg (2.7 oz)	280	37	1	1
oatcakes	2 (4 oz)	115	16	–	1
plain	1 sm (1.2 oz)	127	17	tr	1
tea biscuit	1 (3 oz)	210	30	12	1
w/ egg & bacon	1 (5.3 oz)	458	29	1	1
w/ egg & ham	1 (6.7 oz)	442	30	2	1
w/ egg & sausage	1 (6.3 oz)	581	11	1	1
w/ ham	1 (4 oz)	386	44	1	1
w/ sausage	1 (4.4 oz)	485	40	1	1
BITTERMELON					
Frieda's					
Foo Qua	1 cup	15	3	0	2
BLACK BEANS					
Allens					
Black Beans	½ cup	100	19	1	8
Eden					
Organic Caribbean	½ cup	90	20	1	7
Organic Refried	½ cup	110	18	–	7
Goya					
Black Beans	½ cup (4.3 oz)	90	19	tr	6
Tree Of Life					
Organic	½ cup (4.6 oz)	130	24	1	<6

FOOD	PORTION	CALS	CARB	SUGAR	FIBER
BLACKBERRIES					
canned in heavy syrup	½ cup	118	30	25	4
fresh	½ cup	31	7	4	4
unsweetened frzn	½ cup	48	12	8	4
Cascadian Farm					
Organic frzn	1 cup	80	22	15	7
Oregon					
In Light Syrup	½ cup	120	29	19	6
BLACKBERRY JUICE					
canned	6 oz	65	13	13	tr
BLACKEYE PEAS					
CANNED					
Eden					
Organic	½ cup	90	16	tr	4
TAKE-OUT					
blackeye peas & pork	1 cup	236	25	4	8
BLINTZE					
Golden					
Cheese	1 (2.1 oz)	80	13	5	2
Ratner's					
Cheese	1 (2.2 oz)	100	16	5	0
TAKE-OUT					
cheese	1 (2.7 oz)	160	15	4	tr
BLUEBERRIES					
canned in heavy syrup	½ cup	113	28	26	2
fresh	1 pt	229	58	40	10
fresh	½ cup	41	11	7	2
frzn unsweetened	½ cup	40	9	7	2
C&W					
Ulimate	¾ cup	70	16	3	3
Chukar Cherries					
Puget Sound Dried	¼ cup	160	38	20	5
White Chocolate Covered	3 tbsp (1.4 oz)	223	26	24	tr
De-Lite					
Dried Sweetened	1 oz	86	23	19	4
Eden					
Organic Dried Wild	¼ cup	150	35	21	5

FOOD	PORTION	CALS	CARB	SUGAR	FIBER
Emily's					
Dark Chocolate Covered	¼ cup (1.4 oz)	170	27	22	2
Europe's Best					
Woodland frzn	¾ cup	70	17	13	4
Frieda's					
Dried	¼ cup (1.4 oz)	140	33	17	4
Hodgson Mill					
Dried Wild	¼ cup	120	32	26	6
LiteHouse					
Glaze	3 tbsp	70	17	15	0
Marie's					
Glaze	2 tbsp	40	10	8	0
Oregon					
In Light Syrup	½ cup	110	26	18	2
Sunsweet					
Dried	¼ cup (1.4 oz)	140	33	26	3
Tree Of Life					
Dried	¼ cup (1.5 oz)	150	38	27	4
BLUEBERRY JUICE					
Tart Is Smart					
Wild Blueberry Concentrate	0.5 oz	35	9	7	1
Van Dyk's					
100% Juice	6 oz	74	18	15	0
Walnut Acres					
Organic	8 oz	130	31	28	tr
BLUEFIN					
fillet baked	4.1 oz	186	0	0	0
BLUEFISH					
fresh baked	3 oz	135	0	0	0
BOAR					
wild roasted	3 oz	136	0	0	0
Natural Frontier Foods					
Wild Boar Steaks	1 (4 oz)	170	0	0	0
BOK CHOY (see CABBAGE)					
BONITO					
dried	1 oz	50	0	0	0
fresh	3 oz	117	0	0	0

FOOD	PORTION	CALS	CARB	SUGAR	FIBER

BOTTLED WATER (see WATER)

BOYSENBERRIES
frzn unsweetened	½ cup	33	8	5	4
in heavy syrup	½ cup	113	29	–	3

BRAINS
beef pan-fried	3 oz	167	0	0	0
beef simmered	3 oz	123	0	0	0
lamb braised	3 oz	123	0	0	0
lamb fried	3 oz	232	0	0	0
pork braised	3 oz	117	0	0	0
veal braised	3 oz	116	0	0	0
veal fried	3 oz	181	0	0	0

BRAN
oat	½ cup (1.6 oz)	116	31	–	7
oat cooked	½ cup (3.8 oz)	44	13	–	3
rice	½ cup (2.1 oz)	187	29	–	12
wheat	½ cup (2 oz)	63	19	–	12
Bob's Red Mill					
Rice Bran	2 tbsp	60	8	0	3
Quaker					
Unprocessed	⅓ cup (0.6 oz)	35	11	1	8
Tree Of Life					
Oat Bran	½ cup (1.6 oz)	120	31	1	7
Organic Wheat Bran	¼ cup (1.1 oz)	190	4	1	2

BREAD
CANNED
boston brown	1 slice (1.6 oz)	88	19	5	2
B&M					
Raisin Brown Bread	½ in slice (2 oz)	130	29	16	2

FROZEN
Alexia					
Baguette Garlic	2 pieces (1.6 oz)	130	19	1	tr
Cedarlane					
Organic Mediterranean Stuffed Focaccia	1 piece (4 oz)	295	37	4	1

FOOD	PORTION	CALS	CARB	SUGAR	FIBER
Corbi's					
Chee-Zee Bread Original	½ piece (1.8 oz)	180	21	1	1
Pepperidge Farm					
Garlic	1 slice (2.5 in)	170	24	2	2
Texas Toast Five Cheese	1 slice	150	18	1	1
Whole Grain Texas Toast	1 slice	150	14	1	2
MIX					
cornbread	1 piece (2 oz)	188	29	–	1
READY-TO-EAT					
anadama	1 piece (1.1 oz)	87	16	3	1
baguette whole wheat	2 oz	140	29	tr	1
cassava	1 piece (3.5 oz)	299	71	3	3
challah	1 slice (1.4 oz)	115	19	1	1
cinnamon	1 slice (0.9 oz)	69	13	1	1
cracked wheat	1 slice (1.1 oz)	78	15	–	2
cuban bread	1 slice (1.1 oz)	83	16	1	1
french	1 slice (1.1 oz)	88	17	tr	1
oat bran	1 slice (1.1 oz)	71	12	2	1
oatmeal	1 slice (0.9 oz)	73	13	2	1
pan criõllo	1 piece (0.9 oz)	69	13	tr	tr
pannetone	1 slice (0.9 oz)	86	15	5	1
pita	1 sm (1 oz)	77	16	tr	1
pita	1 lg (2 oz)	165	33	1	1
pita whole wheat	1 sm (1 oz)	74	15	tr	2
pita whole wheat	1 lg (2.2 oz)	170	35	1	5
pumpernickel	1 slice (0.9 oz)	65	12	tr	2
raisin	1 slice (1.1 oz)	88	17	2	1
rye	1 slice (1.1 oz)	83	15	tr	2
seven grain	1 slice (1.1 oz)	80	15	3	2
wheat berry	1 slice (0.9 oz)	65	12	1	1
wheat bran	1 slice (1.3 oz)	89	17	3	1
wheat germ	1 slice (1 oz)	73	14	1	1
white cubed	1 cup	93	18	2	1
whole wheat	1 slice (1 oz)	69	13	6	2
Alvarado Street Bakery					
Sprouted Soy Crunch	1 slice (1.2 oz)	90	15	1	2
Sprouted Whole Wheat	1 slice	90	19	3	3

FOOD	PORTION	CALS	CARB	SUGAR	FIBER
Arnold					
100% Natural Soft Honey Wheat	2 slices (2 oz)	150	28	4	3
Grains & More Double Omega	1 slice	110	19	4	3
Jewish Rye	1 slice	90	17	1	1
Sandwich Thins Multi-Grain	1 (1.5 oz)	100	22	2	5
Sandwich Thins Whole Grain White	1 (1.5 oz)	100	22	2	5
Whole Grains 100% Whole Wheat Double Fiber	1 slice	100	21	3	5
Whole Grains 12 Grain	1 slice	110	21	3	3
Whole Grains 15 Grain	1 slice	110	21	4	3
Whole Grains 7 Grain	1 slice	110	22	4	3
Baker's Inn					
9 Grain	1 slice	100	18	3	2
Cracked Wheat	1 slice	100	18	3	2
Honey White Made w/ Whole Grain	1 slice	110	19	3	1
Honey Whole Wheat	1 slice	100	19	4	2
Potato Made w/ Whole Grain	1 slice	100	18	3	1
Comfort Care					
Cabin Hearth Whole Wheat	1 oz	170	31	7	4
Damascus					
Roll-Up Flax	1 (2 oz)	110	15	1	9
Roll-Up Whole Wheat	1 (2 oz)	110	17	1	7
Earth Grains					
100% Multi Grain Extra Fiber	1 slice	110	19	3	5
Oat & Nut	1 slice	120	20	4	1
Potato	1 slice	110	20	3	tr
Whole Grain Honey	1 slice	110	19	3	2
Whole Wheat Honey	1 slice	110	20	4	5
Ecce Panis					
Classic Ciabatta	⅛ loaf (2 oz)	180	36	tr	tr
Freihofer's					
100% Whole Wheat	1 slice	90	17	3	2
French Meadow Bakery					
Healthy Hemp	1 slice	110	14	1	5
Organic Men's Bread	1 slice	120	10	0	4

FOOD	PORTION	CALS	CARB	SUGAR	FIBER
La Tortilla Factory					
Wraps Smart & Delicious Gluten Free Dark Teff	1 (2.3 oz)	180	31	0	3
Wraps Smart & Delicious Gluten Free Ivory Teff	1 (2.3 oz)	180	30	0	3
Milton's					
100% Whole Wheat	1 slice	110	22	4	5
Buttermilk	1 slice	90	19	3	1
Gourmet White	1 slice	110	23	5	1
Original Multi-Grain	1 slice	120	26	6	3
Potato	1 slice	90	19	3	1
Whole Grain	1 slice	90	16	3	5
Mrs Baird's					
Acti-Fiber Wheat	2 slices (2.2 oz)	160	30	4	4
Whole Grain Wheat Sugar Free	1 slice (1.1 oz)	70	13	0	3
Natural Ovens					
100% Sweet Whole	1 slice	90	16	4	4
Carb Conscious Original	1 slice	80	9	1	4
Healthy Beginnings Better White	1 slice	110	20	3	2
Healthy Beginnings Honey Wheat	1 slice	120	21	3	3
Hunger Filler Whole Grain	1 slice	100	15	2	4
Organic Plus Whole Grain & Flax	1 slice	120	22	3	3
Whole Grain Oat Nut Crunch	1 slice	100	15	2	4
Nature's Own					
100% Whole Wheat	1 slice	50	10	1	2
9 Grain	1 slice	120	24	4	2
Hearty Oatmeal	1 slice	100	18	3	3
Wheat Double Fiber	1 slice	10	10	1	5
Wheat Light	2 slices	80	19	1	5
Wheat N' Fiber	1 slice	60	7	0	2
Whole Wheat w/ Organic Flour	1 slice	100	21	3	3
Nature's Path					
Manna Carrot Raisin	1 slice	130	27	10	5
Manna Millet Rice	1 slice	130	28	9	5
Manna SunSeed	1 slice	160	29	11	7

FOOD	PORTION	CALS	CARB	SUGAR	FIBER
Oroweat					
100% Whole Wheat	1 slice (1.3 oz)	100	19	4	3
Country Potato	1 slice (1.3 oz)	100	20	3	tr
Country Whole Grain White	1 slice (1.3 oz)	90	17	4	1
Double Fiber	1 slice (1.3 oz)	70	16	2	6
Honey Fiber Whole Grain	1 slice (1.3 oz)	80	18	3	4
Russian Rye	1 slice (1 oz)	80	13	tr	tr
Seven Grain	1 slice (1.3 oz)	100	20	4	2
Whole Grain & Flax	1 slice (1.3 oz)	100	17	3	3
Pepperidge Farm					
100% Natural Whole Grain German Dark Wheat	1 slice	100	20	3	3
Breakfast Apple & Grains	1 slice	90	18	5	3
Canadian White	1 slice	100	18	2	1
Carb Style 7 Grain	1 slice	60	8	0	3
Farmhouse Hearty White	1 slice	120	22	4	1
Farmhouse Honey Wheatberry	1 slice	120	22	4	2
Farmhouse Soft 100% Whole Wheat	1 slice	110	19	3	3
Farmhouse Soft Oatmeal	1 slice	120	21	3	1
Honey Flax Whole Grain	1 slice (1.5 oz)	100	19	4	3
Hot & Crusty Italian	1 slice (2 in thick)	150	29	2	1
Jewish Rye Whole Grain Seeded	1 slice	70	14	tr	2
Light Style 7 Grain	1 slice	45	9	1	1
Light Style Oatmeal	3 slices	140	27	2	2
Party Pumpernickel	5 slices	130	23	1	3
Very Thin White	3 slices	120	24	2	1
Whole Grain 100% Soft Whole Wheat Double Fiber	1 slice	100	21	3	6
Whole Grain Honey Oat	1 slice	110	20	4	3
Whole Grain Honey Whole Wheat	1 slice	110	20	4	3
Whole Grain Swirl Cinnamon w/ Raisins	1 slice (1.3 oz)	100	18	5	3
Roman Meal					
Muesli	1 slice (1.5 oz)	110	19	5	2
Original Whole Grain	2 slices (2 oz)	130	25	5	2

FOOD	PORTION	CALS	CARB	SUGAR	FIBER
Rudi's Organic Bakery					
100% Whole Wheat	1 slice	100	19	2	3
14 Grain	1 slice	90	19	2	4
Artisan Country French	1 slice	100	20	1	tr
Artisan Rosemary Olive Oil	1 slice	100	19	0	tr
Low Carb Right Choice	1 slice	45	7	1	2
Spelt Ancient Grain	1 slice	120	20	3	2
Whole Grain Apple N Spice	1 slice	110	24	6	5
S. Rosen's					
Hawaiian	1 slice	110	21	4	0
Rye Black Bavarian	1 slice	100	19	0	1
Sara Lee					
100% Whole Wheat	1 slice	70	13	2	2
Blueberry Crumble	1 slice	180	33	10	4
Cinnamon Raisin	1 slice	190	32	16	3
Classic Wheat	1 slice	70	13	3	2
Delightful Wheat	1 slice	45	9	1	2
Delightful White	1 slice	90	15	1	4
Heart Healthy 100% Whole Wheat Essentials	1 slice	80	14	3	4
Heart Healthy Multigrain	1 slice	100	19	4	2
Honey Wheat	1 slice	70	14	3	1
Honey White	1 slice	100	22	4	tr
Multigrain	1 slice	100	19	4	2
Soft & Smooth 100% Whole Wheat	1 slice	70	12	3	2
Soft & Smooth Whole Grain White	2 slices	150	28	5	3
Sonoma					
Wraps Organic Multi Grain	1 (2.4 oz)	180	27	1	6
Wraps Organic Wheat	1 (2.4 oz)	190	30	2	4
Wraps Orignal White Whole Wheat	1 (2.4 oz)	200	33	1	4
Stroehmann					
100% Whole Wheat	1 slice	90	17	2	3
Dutch Country Twelve Grain	1 slice	100	18	3	2
Potato	1 slice	100	18	3	1
Soft Rye Seeded	1 slice	90	16	tr	1
Sun-Maid					
Raisin Cinnamon Swirl	1 slice (1.2 oz)	100	18	8	1

FOOD	PORTION	CALS	CARB	SUGAR	FIBER
The Baker					
Yoga Bread	1 slice	70	13	2	2
Thomas'					
Breakfast Original	1 slice	90	17	tr	1
Corn	1 slice	110	19	3	1
Sahara Pita Pockets Mini Whole Wheat	1 (1 oz)	70	13	1	2
Swirl Cinnamon Raisin	1 slice	120	21	9	1
Tumaro's					
Wraps Chipotle Chili & Peppers	1 (2.3 oz)	170	34	1	2
Wraps Sun Dried Tomato & Basil	1 (2.3 oz)	170	34	2	2
REFRIGERATED					
Pillsbury					
Italian	⅛ pkg (1.6 oz)	110	21	2	tr
TAKE-OUT					
banana	1 slice (2 oz)	196	33	–	1
chapatis as prep w/ fat	1 (1.6 oz)	95	18	1	3
chapatis as prep w/o fat	1 (2.5 oz)	141	31	–	5
cornbread	1 piece (2.3 oz)	183	27	4	2
cornstick	1 (1.4 oz)	118	18	3	1
focaccia onion	1 piece (4.6 oz)	282	43	2	2
focaccia rosemary	1 piece (3.5 oz)	251	40	1	2
focaccia tomato olive	1 piece (4.7 oz)	270	42	1	2
garlic bread	1 slice (1 oz)	96	13	tr	1
irish soda bread	1 slice (3 oz)	247	48	–	2
italian garlic	1 loaf (11 oz)	990	137	1	8
naan	1 bread (3.5 oz)	286	43	3	2
papadums fried	1 (6 g)	30	2	–	tr
paratha plain	1 (1.6 oz)	136	19	–	2
poori indian puffed bread	1 piece (1.3 oz)	112	16	tr	2
zucchini	1 slice (1.4 oz)	150	19	10	1

FOOD	PORTION	CALS	CARB	SUGAR	FIBER
BREAD COATING					
Don's Chuck Wagon					
Chicken Baking Mix	¼ cup	95	21	0	1
Fish Mix	¼ cup	95	21	0	1
Onion Ring Mix	¼ cup	100	21	0	1
Hodgson Mill					
Vidalia Sweet Onion Mix not prep	¼ cup	100	21	0	1
Zatarain's					
Crispy Seasoned Fish-Fri	2 tbsp	50	11	0	1
BREADCRUMBS					
dry seasoned	¼ cup	115	21	2	2
fresh	¼ cup	30	6	tr	tr
plain	¼ cup	107	19	2	1
4C					
Salt Free Seasoned	⅓ cup	110	23	2	2
Edward & Sons					
Organic Lightly Salted	⅓ cup	110	21	2	1
Organic Panko	⅓ cup	110	21	2	1
Ian's					
Panko Italian	¼ cup	70	15	1	2
Panko Original	¼ cup	71	15	1	1
Panko Whole Wheat	¼ cup	70	14	1	2
Krasdale					
Seasoned	¼ cup	120	21	4	2
Progresso					
Garlic & Herb	¼ cup (1 oz)	110	19	2	1
Plain	¼ cup (1 oz)	110	20	2	1
BREADFRUIT					
fresh	1 sm (13.5 oz)	396	104	42	19
fried	1 cup	379	52	21	9
raw	1 cup	227	60	24	11
BREADSTICKS					
plain	1 lg	41	7	tr	tr
plain	1 sm	21	3	tr	tr
Fattorie & Pandea					
Fornini w/ Sea Salt	5 (1.2 oz)	140	21	1	1
Ferrara					
Slim Thin Torinese Style	6 (0.5 oz)	60	11	1	0

FOOD	PORTION	CALS	CARB	SUGAR	FIBER
Pepperidge Farm					
Garlic frzn	1	160	25	2	1
Pillsbury					
Cornbread Twists	1 (1.4 oz)	140	18	4	0
Original Soft	2 (1.8 oz)	140	25	3	tr
Stella D'Oro					
Mini Cracked Pepper	4 (0.5 oz)	70	11	0	0
Original	1 (0.3 oz)	40	6	0	0
Roasted Garlic	1	45	7	0	0
Sesame	1 (0.4 oz)	50	6	0	0
Sodium Free	1 (0.3 oz)	40	6	0	0

BREAKFAST BARS *(see* CEREAL BARS, ENERGY BARS*)*

BROCCOLI
FRESH

FOOD	PORTION	CALS	CARB	SUGAR	FIBER
chinese broccoli (gai lan) cooked	½ cup	10	2	tr	1
chopped cooked	½ cup (2.7 oz)	27	6	1	3
raab cooked	½ cup	28	3	1	2
raw	1 bunch (1.3 lbs)	207	40	10	16
BroccoSprouts					
Broccoli Sprouts	½ cup	16	2	–	1
Mann's					
Broccoli Wokly	1 serv (3 oz)	25	4	2	2
Broccolini	8 stalks (3 oz)	35	6	2	1
Ocean Mist					
Rapini Broccoli Rabe Chopped Raw	1 cup	9	1	0	1
FROZEN					
chopped cooked	½ cup	26	5	1	3
spears cooked	1 pkg (10 oz)	70	13	4	8
spears cooked	½ cup	26	5	1	3
Birds Eye					
Broccoli & Cheese Sauce	½ cup	90	8	3	1
Steamfresh Cuts	1 cup (3.1 oz)	30	4	2	2
Steamfresh Florets	1 cup (2.3 oz)	30	4	2	2
C&W					
Broccoli & Cheddar Cheese Sauce	1⅓ cups	70	7	3	2

FOOD	PORTION	CALS	CARB	SUGAR	FIBER
Florets	1 cup	30	4	2	2
Cascadian Farm					
Organic Florets	⅔ cup	20	4	2	2
Dr. Praeger's					
Broccoli Bites	2 (2 oz)	110	17	2	2
Green Giant					
Broccoli & Cheese Sauce	⅔ cup	60	7	2	2
Butter Sauce Low Fat	3 spears (4 oz)	40	6	3	2
Cuts as prep	⅔ cup	25	4	2	2
Pasta Broccoli & Alfredo Sauce as prep	1 cup	210	34	6	3
TAKE-OUT					
batter dipped & fried	4 pieces	77	6	1	1
w/ cheese sauce	1 cup	242	16	5	5
BROWNIE					
brownie	1 (2 oz)	227	36	21	1
butterscotch	1 (1.2 oz)	151	19	12	tr
Arrowhead Mills					
Gluten Free as prep	1	160	21	13	tr
Bob's Red Mill					
Gluten Free as prep	1	140	27	17	2
Erin Baker's					
Organic Bite Double Chocolate Chip	1 (1 oz)	90	19	10	2
Organic Bites	1 (1 oz)	100	18	10	2
Foxy's Bake Shop					
Milk Chocolate	½ (1.7 oz)	200	23	18	0
White Chocolate	½ (1.7 oz)	200	23	18	0
French Meadow Bakery					
Gluten Free Fudge	1 (1.3 oz)	150	23	13	1
Glenny's					
100 Calorie 75% Organic	1 (1.45 oz)	100	12	11	7
Joseph's					
Sugar Free	1 (1.5 oz)	150	26	0	1
Laura's Wholesome Junk Food					
Gluten Free Better Brownie	2	120	16	8	2
Nature's Path					
Organic Mix Double Fudge	¹⁄₁₀ pkg	150	31	21	3
Organic Mix HempPlus	¹⁄₁₀ pkg	140	31	20	3

FOOD	PORTION	CALS	CARB	SUGAR	FIBER
Pillsbury					
Traditional Chocolate Fudge	1 (1.4 oz)	150	24	16	tr
Turtle Supreme Bars	1 (1.4 oz)	180	23	15	tr
Sara Lee					
Brownie Bites Chocolate Dipped	1 (0.7 oz)	90	12	8	1
VitaBrownie					
Dark Chocolate Pomegranate	1 (2 oz)	100	21	11	6
Deep Velvety Chocolate	1 (2 oz)	100	23	7	6
BRUSSELS SPROUTS					
FRESH					
cooked	6 pieces	45	9	2	3
Ocean Mist					
Brussels Sprouts	4 (2 oz)	40	6	2	3
Select Gourmet					
Fresh	½ cup	35	8	2	3
FROZEN					
cooked	1 cup	65	13	3	6
Birds Eye					
Steamfresh Baby	10 (2.9 oz)	45	8	2	3
Steamfresh Singles Baby	1 pkg (3.2 oz)	50	9	3	3
C&W					
Petite	10 (3 oz)	45	8	2	3
Green Giant					
Baby & Butter Sauce as prep	½ cup	60	9	3	3
BUCKWHEAT					
groats roasted cooked	½ cup	155	17	1	2
Bob's Red Mill					
Organic Kernels	¼ cup	142	31	0	3
BUFFALO *(see also* JERKY*)*					
burger	3 oz	202	0	0	0
chuck braised	4 oz	205	0	0	0
top round steak broiled	3 oz	313	0	0	0
water buffalo roasted	3 oz	111	0	0	0
Natural Frontier Foods					
Burgers	1 (5 oz)	170	0	0	0
Ground	4 oz	170	0	0	0
Steaks	1 (4 oz)	160	0	0	0

FOOD	PORTION	CALS	CARB	SUGAR	FIBER
BULGUR					
cooked	½ cup	76	17	tr	4
uncooked	½ cup	239	53	tr	13
Bob's Red Mill					
From Soft White Wheat	¼ cup	150	32	0	4
Fantastic					
Tabouli Mix not prep	2 tbsp	70	15	1	4
Near East					
Whole Grain Wheat Pilaf as prep	1 cup	200	40	2	8
Sabra					
Black Bean & Wheat Pilaf	2 oz	45	7	1	2
Cracked Wheat Salad	2 oz	80	12	1	1
Tabouli	2 oz	70	6	1	1
TAKE-OUT					
tabbouleh	1 cup	198	16	2	4
BURBOT (FISH)					
fresh baked	3 oz	98	0	0	0
BURDOCK ROOT					
cooked w/o salt	1 cup	110	26	4	2
cooked w/o salt	1 root (5.8 oz)	146	35	6	3
Frieda's					
Gobo Root	¾ cup	60	15	0	3
BUTTER					
clarified butter	1 tbsp (0.4 oz)	112	0	0	0
clarified butter	¼ cup (1.8 oz)	449	0	0	0
honey butter	1 tbsp (0.6 oz)	85	9	9	0
honey butter	¼ cup (2.5 oz)	338	36	35	tr
light butter whipped salted	1 tbsp (0.3 oz)	48	0	0	0
stick salted	1 stick (4 oz)	810	tr	tr	0
stick salted	1 tbsp (0.5 oz)	102	tr	tr	0
stick salted	¼ cup (2 oz)	407	tr	tr	0
stick unsalted	1 stick (4 oz)	810	tr	tr	0
stick unsalted	1 tbsp (0.5 oz)	102	tr	tr	0
stick unsalted	¼ cup (2 oz)	407	tr	tr	0
whipped salted	1 tbsp (0.3 oz)	67	tr	tr	0
whipped salted	¼ cup (1.3 oz)	271	tr	tr	0
Cabot					
Salted	1 tbsp	100	0	0	0

FOOD	PORTION	CALS	CARB	SUGAR	FIBER
Country Crock					
Spreadable Butter w/ Canola Oil	1 tbsp (0.4 oz)	80	0	0	0
Crystal Farms					
Butter	1 tbsp	100	0	0	0
Whipped	1 tbsp	70	0	0	0
Deerfield					
Creamy	1 tbsp	100	0	0	0
Earth Balance					
Butter Blend Unsalted	1 tbsp	100	0	0	0
Horizon Organic					
European	1 tbsp	100	0	0	0
Land O Lakes					
Light Salted	1 tbsp (0.5 oz)	50	0	0	0
Light Whipped Salted	1 tbsp (0.4 oz)	45	0	0	0
Salted	1 tbsp (0.5 oz)	100	0	0	0
Spreadable w/ Canola Oil	1 tbsp (0.5 oz)	100	0	0	0
Whipped Salted	1 tbsp (0.2 oz)	50	0	0	0
Organic Valley					
European Style	1 tbsp	110	0	0	0
Straus					
Organic European Style Lightly Salted	1 tbsp (0.5 oz)	110	0	0	0
Organic European Style Sweet Butter	1 tbsp (0.5 oz)	110	0	0	0

BUTTERSCOTCH (see also CANDY)
E. Guittard

FOOD	PORTION	CALS	CARB	SUGAR	FIBER
Baking Chips	33 (0.5 oz)	80	10	10	0

CABBAGE (see also COLESLAW)

FOOD	PORTION	CALS	CARB	SUGAR	FIBER
chinese bok choy shredded cooked w/o salt	1 cup	20	3	1	2
chinese pe-tsai shredded cooked w/o salt	1 cup	17	3	–	2
green raw shredded	1 cup	19	4	2	2
green shredded cooked w/o salt	1 cup	34	8	4	3
japanese pickled	½ cup	22	4	1	2
red raw shredded	1 cup	22	5	3	2
red shredded cooked w/o salt	1 cup	44	10	5	4

FOOD	PORTION	CALS	CARB	SUGAR	FIBER
Aunt Nellie's					
Sweet & Sour Red	¼ cup	40	10	8	0
Frieda's					
Baby Bok Choy	⅔ cup	10	2	1	1
Bok Choy	1 cup	10	2	1	1
Gai Choy	1 cup (3 oz)	20	4	1	2
Napa	1 cup (3 oz)	15	3	1	1
Salad Savoy	⅔ cup (3 oz)	25	5	2	3
Tuscan	⅔ cup (3 oz)	20	5	3	2
Glory					
Country Cabbage	½ cup	25	6	3	1
Greenwood					
Red	½ cup	100	24	14	0
TAKE-OUT					
creamed	1 cup	158	13	7	2
kimchee	1 cup	32	6	2	2
stuffed cabbage w/ rice & beef	1 (3.6 oz)	117	9	4	1
sweet & sour red cabbage	4 oz	61	8	–	3
CACAO					
Kopali					
Organic Dark Chocolate Covered Cacao Nibs	½ pkg (1 oz)	140	15	12	2
Navitas Naturals					
Butter	1 tbsp	120	0	0	0
Nibs	1 oz	130	10	0	9
Powder	1 oz	120	18	12	7
Sunfood					
Organic Cacao Beans	1 oz	171	8	0	6
Organic Cacao Nibs	1 oz	171	8	0	6
CACTUS					
fresh cooked w/ fat	1 pad (1 oz)	11	1	tr	1
fresh cooked w/o fat	1 cup (5.2 oz)	22	5	2	3
pricklypear	1 (3.6 oz)	42	10	–	4
Frieda's					
Cactus Pads	¾ cup (3 oz)	20	4	0	1
CAKE *(see also CAKE MIX)*					
battenburg cake	1 slice (2 oz)	204	28	–	1
crumpet	1 (2.3 oz)	131	31	–	2
dutch honey cake	1 slice (0.8 oz)	70	17	8	0

FOOD	PORTION	CALS	CARB	SUGAR	FIBER
eccles cake	1 slice (2 oz)	285	36	–	1
madeira cake	1 slice (1 oz)	98	15	–	1
sponge	1 piece (1.3 oz)	110	23	14	tr
sponge cake dessert shell	1 (0.8 oz)	70	12	7	0
treacle tart	1 slice (2.5 oz)	258	42	–	1
Aunt Trudy's					
Organic Baklava Soy Nut	1 (1.8 oz)	190	29	17	2
Balocco					
Il Panettone	1 serv (3.5 oz)	380	54	27	2
Bellino					
Pandoro	1 (2.8 oz)	330	39	16	1
Chudleigh's					
Apple Blossoms	1 (4 oz)	350	43	19	2
Drake's					
Coffee Cake Low Fat	2 (2.3 oz)	210	44	27	1
El Monterey					
Cheesecake Bites Caramel	1 (2 oz)	180	23	9	0
Cheesecake Bites Raspberry	1 (2 oz)	200	21	6	0
Entenmann's					
All Butter French Crumb	⅛ cake (1.8 oz)	210	29	18	tr
Cheese Cake Deluxe French	⅙ cake (3.8 oz)	390	39	25	tr
Danish Twist Raspberry	⅛ cake	220	28	15	tr
Fudge Iced Golden Cake	⅛ cake	290	41	30	1
Loaf All Butter	⅙ cake (2.4 oz)	220	31	19	0
Marble Loaf	⅛ cake	190	28	16	tr
Marshmallow Iced Devil's Food	⅛ cake	280	40	31	tr
Strawberry Cheese Buns	1 (3 oz)	320	45	26	1
Fillo Factory					
Organic Apple Strudel	1 (4.4 oz)	290	47	15	2
Organic Apple Turnovers	1 (3 oz)	180	30	9	1
Glenny's					
Blondie 100 Calorie 75% Organic	1 (1.45 oz)	100	12	9	7
Gourmet Pastries					
Baklava Walnut	1 piece (1.8 oz)	240	30	18	0

FOOD	PORTION	CALS	CARB	SUGAR	FIBER
Guiltless Gourmet					
Dessert Bowl Bananas Foster Cake	1 pkg (2 oz)	200	42	26	tr
Dessert Bowl Black Velvet Cake	1 pkg (2 oz)	200	42	30	3
Hostess					
100 Calorie Pack Mini Carrot Cake	1 pkg (1.2 oz)	100	20	11	4
100 Calorie Pack Mini Chocolate Cupcakes	1 pkg (1.3 oz)	100	22	10	5
100 Calorie Pack Mini Coffee Cake Cinnamon Streusel	1 pkg (1.2 oz)	100	21	7	5
100 Calorie Pack Mini Golden Cupcakes	1 pkg (1.2 oz)	100	20	11	3
Cup Cakes Chocolate	1 (1.8 oz)	170	30	21	1
Ho Ho's	1	120	18	14	0
Twinkies	1 (1.5 oz)	150	27	19	0
Kellogg's					
Pop-Tarts Apple Cinnamon	1 (1.8 oz)	210	37	17	tr
Pop-Tarts French Toast	1	220	35	15	tr
Pop-Tarts Frosted Cookies & Cream	1	200	35	19	tr
Pop-Tarts Low Fat Frosted Brown Sugar Cinnamon	1 (1.8 oz)	190	38	19	tr
Pop-Tarts Yogurt Blast Strawberry	1 (1.8 oz)	210	37	17	tr
Lance					
Honey Bun	1 (3 oz)	320	47	13	4
Mrs. Freshley's					
Golden Cupcakes Creme Filled	1 pkg (1.3 oz)	100	24	4	5
Mrs. Smith's					
Carrot	1/6 cake (2.9 oz)	300	37	27	2
Cobbler Blackberry	1 serv (4 oz)	260	43	20	2
Singles Heavenly 100 New York Cheesecake	1 (0.9 oz)	100	9	6	0
Nature's Path					
Organic Toaster Pastry Apple Cinnamon	1 (2 oz)	210	40	18	1
Organic Toaster Pastry Blueberry	1 (2 oz)	210	40	18	1

FOOD	PORTION	CALS	CARB	SUGAR	FIBER
Organic Toaster Pastry Frosted Apple Cinnamon	1 (2 oz)	210	39	21	1
Organic Toaster Pastry Frosted Blueberry	1 (2 oz)	200	38	20	1
Organic Toaster Pastry Frosted Strawberry	1 (2 oz)	210	40	19	1
Neuman's					
Date Nut Bread	1 oz	90	17	10	1
Pepperidge Farm					
Chocolate Coconut 3 Layer	⅛ cake	240	33	23	tr
Devil's Food 3 Layer	⅛ cake	220	34	25	tr
Golden 3 Layer	⅛ cake	230	34	25	1
Lemon 3 Layer	⅛ cake	240	34	25	tr
Turnover Apple	1	290	36	13	2
Turnover Peach	1	290	35	16	1
Pillsbury					
Caramel Rolls	1 (1.7 oz)	170	24	10	tr
Cinnamon Rolls w/ Icing	1 (3.5 oz)	310	54	23	1
Cinnamon Rolls w/ Icing Reduced Fat	1 (1.5 oz)	140	24	10	tr
Toaster Strudel	1 (2 oz)	200	28	9	1
Toaster Strudel Blueberry	1 (2 oz)	190	26	9	tr
Toaster Strudel Cream Cheese	1 (2 oz)	200	23	8	tr
Toaster Strudel Raspberry	1 (2 oz)	190	26	9	tr
Toaster Strudel Wildberry	1 (2 oz)	190	25	9	tr
Turnovers Cherry	1 (2 oz)	180	24	12	0
Sara Lee					
Cheesecake Classic French	1 piece (4.7 oz)	410	41	27	1
Cheesecake French Chocolate	1 piece (4.2 oz)	430	52	31	2
Cheesecake French Strawberry	1 piece (4.3 oz)	320	43	26	1
Cheesecake Strawberry Swirl	1 piece (2.9 oz)	290	44	25	1
Cobbler Anytime Apple	1 (4 oz)	350	47	10	1
Coffee Cake Butter Streusel	1 piece (2 oz)	190	25	10	1
Coffee Cake Crumb	1 serv (2 oz)	190	30	18	1
Layer Cake Coconut	1 slice (2.8 oz)	260	33	25	1
Layer Cake Double Chocolate	1 slice (2.8 oz)	260	33	24	2

FOOD	PORTION	CALS	CARB	SUGAR	FIBER
Layer Cake Fudge Golden	1 slice (2.8 oz)	260	34	23	1
Layer Cake Vanilla	1 slice (2.8 oz)	260	32	22	0
Pound Cake All Butter	1 slice (0.6 oz)	240	37	21	1
Pound Cake Free & Light	1 slice (2.5 oz)	200	39	21	1
Weight Watchers					
Lemon w/ Lemon Icing	1 (1 oz)	80	14	10	2
TAKE-OUT					
angelfood	1 slice (2 oz)	143	33	17	tr
apple crisp	1 serv (8.6 oz)	384	76	49	4
apple turnover	1 (6.6 oz)	661	83	30	3
baklava	1 piece (2.7 oz)	334	29	10	2
basbousa namoura	1 piece (1 oz)	60	10	10	2
bean cake	1 cake (1.1 oz)	130	16	7	1
black forest chocolate cherry	1 piece (2.5 oz)	187	27	23	1
boston cream pie	1 slice (3.2 oz)	232	39	33	1
carrot w/ icing	1 slice (4.7 oz)	543	70	52	2
cheesecake	1 slice (4.5 oz)	410	37	28	tr
cheesecake chocolate	1 slice (4.5 oz)	489	49	29	2
chinese moon cake	1 (4.8 oz)	458	92	49	4
coconut mochiko filipino cake	1 piece (2.7 oz)	252	35	11	2
coffeecake iced	1 piece (1.6 oz)	175	24	15	1
cream puff custard filled chocolate frosted	1 (3.9 oz)	293	27	7	1
eclair	1 (3.5 oz)	262	24	7	1
french apple tart	1 (3.5 oz)	302	37	15	2
fruitcake	1 slice (1.5 oz)	139	26	13	2
funnel cake	1 (3.2 oz)	276	29	4	1
gingerbread	1 piece (2.4 oz)	213	35	22	1
jelly roll	1 slice (1.8 oz)	146	28	20	tr
jelly roll lemon filled	1 slice (3 oz)	210	48	29	tr
napoleon	1 (3 oz)	348	25	4	1
napoleon	1 mini (1 oz)	123	9	1	tr
panettone	1/12 cake (2.9 oz)	300	43	21	2
petit fours	2 (0.9 oz)	120	15	12	0

FOOD	PORTION	CALS	CARB	SUGAR	FIBER
pineapple upside down	1 piece (4.2 oz)	387	61	41	1
pound fat free	1 slice (2 oz)	160	35	19	1
sacher torte	1 slice (2.2 oz)	240	30	11	4
strawberry shortcake	1 serv (4.1 oz)	211	40	35	1
strudel apple	1 piece (2.2 oz)	175	26	16	1
strudel cheese	1 piece (2.2 oz)	195	24	14	tr
strudel cherry	1 piece (2.2 oz)	179	29	18	1
sweet potato w/ glaze	1 piece (2.7 oz)	275	39	26	1
tiramisu	1 cake (4.4 lbs)	5732	439	234	3
tiramisu	1 piece (5.1 oz)	409	31	17	tr
torte chocolate ganache (3.5 oz)	1 slice	400	40	24	6
trifle w/ cream	6 oz	291	34	–	1
white w/ coconut icing	1 slice (3.9 oz)	399	71	64	1
zucchini bread	1 slice (1.4 oz)	150	19	10	1
CAKE ICING					
chocolate	¼ cup	269	53	51	1
vanilla	¼ cup	322	64	62	0
Manischewitz					
Dairy Free Chocolate	2 tbsp (1.2 oz)	138	22	19	0
Naturally Nora					
Frosting Mix Chocolate as prep	1/12 pkg	150	24	21	0
Frosting Mix Vanilla as prep	1/12 pkg	170	25	23	0
CAKE MIX					
Bisquick					
Heart Smart	⅓ cup	140	27	3	1
Don's Chuck Wagon					
All Purpose Batter Mix	¼ cup	100	20	0	1
King Arthur					
Cinnamon Buns Kit not prep	½ cup	240	52	23	3
Naturally Nora					
Cheerful Chocolate as prep	1/12 pkg	300	39	21	1

FOOD	PORTION	CALS	CARB	SUGAR	FIBER
Sunny Yellow as prep	1/12 pkg	280	39	23	tr
Surprising Stars as prep	1/12 pkg	300	42	22	tr

CALZONE (see SANDWICHES)

CANADIAN BACON

grilled	2 slices (1.6 oz)	87	1	0	0
Applegate Farms					
Natural	2 slices (2 oz)	90	1	1	0
Boar's Head					
Canadian Bacon	2 oz	70	1	1	0
Celebrity					
98% Fat Free	3 slices (1.8 oz)	60	1	0	0
Organic Prairie					
Hardwood Smoked	1 oz	40	1	1	0
Wellshire					
Sliced	2 oz	20	10	0	0

CANADIAN BACON SUBSTITUTES

Yves					
Meatless Canadian Bacon	2 slices (2 oz)	80	2	tr	0

CANDY

marzipan	1 oz	128	15	–	2
organic dark chocolate w/ raisins & pecans	1.4 oz	220	22	16	3
3 Musketeers					
Bar	1 (2.1 oz)	260	46	40	1
Fun Size	3 bars (1.6 oz)	190	34	30	1
Minis	7 (1.4 oz)	170	32	27	1
Mint	1 bar (1.2 oz)	150	26	22	1
Andes					
Dark Chocolate Covered Cherries	2 (1 oz)	110	19	15	tr
Thins Cherry Jubilee	8 pieces (1.3 oz)	200	22	20	1
Thins Creme De Menthe	8 pieces (1.3 oz)	200	22	20	tr
Annabelle's					
Skinny Hunk Chewy Nougat	1 bar (1 oz)	100	24	25	0
Baby Ruth					
Fun Size	2 bars (1.3 oz)	170	24	20	tr
Snack Bars	2 (1.3 oz)	170	24	20	tr

FOOD	PORTION	CALS	CARB	SUGAR	FIBER
Bartons					
Cashew Toppers	1 (1 oz)	140	14	9	1
Baskin-Robbins					
Soft Candy Mint Chocolate Chip	2 (0.3 oz)	40	7	5	0
Blow Pop					
Regular	1 (0.6 oz)	60	16	12	0
Cadbury					
Milk Chocolate Fruit & Nut	10 blocks (1.4 oz)	200	24	22	1
Milk Chocolate Roast Almond	7 blocks (1.4 oz)	210	21	19	1
Cella's					
Milk Chocolate Covered Cherries	2 (1 oz)	120	20	16	1
Chargers					
Chocolate Covered Espresso Beans	1 pkg (0.5 oz)	60	9	7	tr
Charleston Chews					
Chocolate	1 bar (1.9 oz)	230	43	30	1
Vanilla	1 bar (1.9 oz)	230	44	30	0
Charms					
Fluffy Stuff Cotton Candy	1 pkg (0.6 oz)	70	17	17	0
Sour Balls	1 (5 g)	20	5	3	0
Squares	2 pieces	20	6	4	0
Chew-ets					
Peanut Chews Original Dark	3 pieces	170	22	16	2
Choward's					
Mints All Flavors	3 (5 g)	20	5	5	0
CocoaVia					
Dark Chocolate Blueberry & Almond Bar	1 (0.8 oz)	100	12	9	2
Dark Chocolate Covered Almonds	1 pkg (1 oz)	140	12	8	3
Dark Chocolate Crispy Bar	1 (0.7 oz)	90	11	7	2
Dark Chocolate Original Bar	1 (0.8 oz)	80	12	9	2
Milk Chocolate Almond Bar	1 (0.8 oz)	110	12	10	1
Milk Chocolate Bar	1 (0.8 oz)	110	13	12	0
Milk Chocolate Covered Raisins	1 pkg (1 oz)	150	22	21	1
Crispy Cat					
Roasted Peanut	1 bar (1 oz)	220	29	14	2

FOOD	PORTION	CALS	CARB	SUGAR	FIBER
Dare					
RealFruit Gummies All Flavors	8 pieces (1.4 oz)	120	28	19	0
Dots					
All Flavors	12 (1.5 oz)	140	35	21	0
Dove					
Dark Chocolate Covered Almonds	13 pieces	210	19	16	3
Dark Chocolate Cranberry Almond	⅓ pkg (1.2 oz)	170	20	16	2
Dark Chocolate Miniatures	5 pieces	210	24	19	3
Milk Chocolate	⅓ bar	180	20	18	1
Milk Chocolate Covered Almonds	13 pieces	220	19	16	2
Milk Chocolate Miniatures	5	220	24	22	1
Milk Chocolate Miniatures w/ Caramel	5 pieces	200	24	21	1
Milk Chocolate Roasted Almond	⅓ bar (1.2 oz)	180	18	16	1
E. Guittard					
Bar Quevedo Bittersweet 65% Cocao	1 (2 oz)	290	29	20	5
Bar Sur Del Lago Bittersweet 65% Cacao	1 (2 oz)	290	29	20	5
Emily's					
Espresso Beans Dark Chocolate Covered	26 (1.4 oz)	220	24	21	3
Endangered Species					
Dark Chocolate w/ Espresso Beans	½ bar (1.5 oz)	200	13	11	5
Dark Chocolate w/ Hazelnut Toffee	½ bar (1.5 oz)	220	15	13	4
Milk Chocolate w/ Cherries	½ bar (1.5 oz)	230	22	16	1
Organic Dark Chocolate	½ bar (0.7 oz)	100	12	10	1
Organic Dark Chocolate w/ Tangerine	½ bar (0.7 oz)	100	12	10	1
Organic Milk Chocolate w/ Key Lime	½ bar (0.7 oz)	110	11	10	0
Enjoy Life					
Boom Choco Boom Dark Chocolate Dairy Nut Soy Free	1 bar (1.4 oz)	200	22	17	3

FOOD	PORTION	CALS	CARB	SUGAR	FIBER
Equal Exchange					
Organic Chocolate Espresso Bean	1 bar (1.4 oz)	216	22	17	3
Organic Milk Chocolate	1 bar (1.4 oz)	230	19	12	1
Organic Very Dark Chocolate	1 bar (1.4 oz)	220	18	11	5
Ethel's					
Truffles Assorted	4	200	17	9	1
Fauchon					
Assortment Truffles	3 pieces (1.3 oz)	160	19	16	2
Ferrero					
Rocher	3 pieces (1.3 oz)	220	16	15	1
Rondnoir	3 pieces (1.4 oz)	220	21	16	2
Figamajigs					
Fig Candy Drops Dark Chocolate Covered	1 pkg (1.4 oz)	150	29	21	3
Fig Candy Drops Orange & Yellow Chocolate Covered	1 pkg (1.4 oz)	150	32	26	2
Frooties					
Chewy Candy Fruit Flavored	12 pieces (1.3 oz)	104	29	21	0
Fruitzels					
Assorted	7 pieces	120	29	19	0
Ghirardelli					
Squares Milk Chocolate w/ Caramel Filling	3 (1.6 oz)	220	27	24	tr
Squares Mint Indulgence	3 (1.6 oz)	210	30	26	2
Squares 60% Cacao Dark Chocolate	4 (1.5 oz)	220	23	23	3
Squares 60% Cacao Dark Chocolate w/ Caramel	3 (1.6 oz)	220	25	18	3
Godiva					
Truffles Assorted	2 pieces (1.4 oz)	210	20	17	2
Green & Black's					
Organic Chocolate Fairtrade Maya Gold	1 bar (3.5 oz)	526	48	43	8
Organic Dark Chocolate	1 bar (3.5 oz)	551	36	29	12

FOOD	PORTION	CALS	CARB	SUGAR	FIBER
Organic Dark Chocolate Mint	1 bar (3.5 oz)	478	51	44	9
Organic Dark Chocolate w/ Hazelnuts & Currants	1 bar (3.5 oz)	513	45	40	9
Organic Milk Chocolate	1 bar (3.5 oz)	523	54	48	4
Organic Milk Chocolate Caramel	1 bar (3.5 oz)	495	56	53	3
Organic Milk Chocolate Raisins & Hazelnuts	1 bar (3.5 oz)	556	47	42	3
Organic Milk Chocolate Whole Almonds	1 bar (3.5 oz)	578	38	35	5
Organic White Chocolate	1 bar (3.5 oz)	573	54	51	tr
Guylian					
Twists Milk Chocolate Truffle	5 pieces (1.2 oz)	230	15	14	1
Twists Original Praline	4 pieces (1.2 oz)	200	19	17	1
Hammond's					
Root Beer Drops	3 (0.6 oz)	60	14	12	0
Hershey's					
Bliss Dark Chocolate	3 (0.8 oz)	100	12	10	2
Bliss Milk Chocolate	6 (1.5 oz)	210	24	22	1
Cacao Reserve 65% Cacao Dark	3 blocks (1.3 oz)	180	18	12	4
Cacao Reserve 35% Cacao Milk Chocolate w/ Hazelnuts	3 sq (1.3 oz)	220	18	16	1
Miniature Assorted	5 (1.5 oz)	210	25	22	2
Nuggets Milk Chocolate	4	230	24	21	1
Sticks Special Dark	1 (0.4 oz)	60	7	6	tr
Joyva					
Halvah Chocolate Covered	1 serv (2 oz)	380	20	19	3
Junior					
Caramels	1 box (1.4 oz)	170	35	32	tr
Mints	1 box (1.4 oz)	170	35	32	tr
Kellogg's					
Fruit Flavored Snacks Hello Kitty	10 pieces	100	26	17	0
Fruit Flavored Snacks Winnie The Pooh	1 pkg	80	21	14	0
Fruit Streamers Watermelon Madness	1 pkg (0.8 oz)	80	17	10	0

FOOD	PORTION	CALS	CARB	SUGAR	FIBER
Fruit Twistables Triple Cherry Explosion	1 pkg (0.8 oz)	70	17	10	0
Gamester Rolls All Varieties	1 pkg (0.7 oz)	80	16	10	0
Yogos Crazy Berries	1 pkg (0.8 oz)	90	18	15	0
KitKat					
Bar	1 (0.5 oz)	73	9	7	tr
Kopali					
Organic Dark Chocolate Covered Espresso Beans	½ pkg (1 oz)	120	17	15	2
Lance					
Peanut Bar	1 (2.3 oz)	340	29	19	3
Legacy Chocolates					
Truffles Assorted	1 piece (0.5 oz)	90	6	4	1
Let's Do Organic					
Black Licorice Bars	1 (0.9 oz)	80	20	11	tr
Black Licorice Chews	8 (1.4 oz)	130	30	18	tr
Gummi Bears	1 pkg (0.9 oz)	80	22	18	0
Lindt					
Lindor Truffles Swiss Dark Chocolate	3 (1.4 oz)	240	17	16	2
Petits Desserts Assorted	4 (1.3 oz)	210	20	17	tr
Love Candy					
Dark Chocolate	1 bar (1.5 oz)	190	21	15	1
Milk Chocolate	1 bar (1.5 oz)	200	22	15	tr
Yogurt Supreme	1 bar (1.5 oz)	190	23	7	tr
M&M's					
Almond	1 pkg (1.3 oz)	200	21	18	2
Dark Chocolate	1 pkg (1.7 oz)	240	33	27	2
Milk Chocolate	1 pkg (1.7 oz)	240	34	31	1
Minis	1 pkg (1.1 oz)	150	21	19	1
Peanut	1 pkg (1.7 oz)	250	30	25	2
Peanut Butter	1 pkg (1.6 oz)	240	26	22	2
Mamba					
Fruit Flavor	6 (0.9 oz)	170	36	19	0
Sour	6 (0.9 oz)	100	22	11	0
Milkfuls					
Candy	6 (1.4 oz)	170	35	23	0
Milky Way					
Bar	1 (2 oz)	260	41	35	1
Fun Size	2 bars (1.2 oz)	150	24	20	0

FOOD	PORTION	CALS	CARB	SUGAR	FIBER
Midnight	1 bar (1.8 oz)	220	36	29	1
Midnight Minis	5 (1.4 oz)	180	29	24	1
Milk Chocolate Covered Caramels	5 (1.5 oz)	200	30	26	0
Minis	5 (1.5 oz)	190	30	25	0
Mr. Goodbar					
Bar	1 (1.75 oz)	270	27	23	2
Necco					
Banana Splits	4 (1.4 oz)	150	36	21	0
Clark Junior Bar	1 (0.5 oz)	60	10	8	0
Conversation Hearts Tiny	40 (1.4 oz)	160	39	38	0
Double Dipped Peanuts	15 (1.4 oz)	200	25	22	1
Mary Janes	5 (1.4 oz)	160	32	20	0
Mint Juleps	4 (1.4 oz)	150	36	21	0
Nonpareils	10 (1.4 oz)	190	29	23	0
Squirrel Nut Caramel	5 (1.6 oz)	170	37	25	0
Nestle					
Crunch Stix	1 (0.6 oz)	90	12	9	0
Newman's Own					
Organic Chocolate Cups Dark Chocolate Peanut Butter	1 pkg (1.2 oz)	180	18	14	1
Organic Chocolate Cups Milk Chocolate Peanut Butter	1 pkg (1.2 oz)	180	17	14	1
Organic Chocolate Cups Peppermint	1 pkg (1.2 oz)	170	20	18	1
Organic Chocolate Sweet Dark	½ bar (¼ oz)	200	24	20	2
Organic Chocolate Sweet Dark Espresso	½ bar (1.4 oz)	200	20	17	2
Organic Chocolate Sweet Dark Orange	½ bar (1.4 oz)	200	24	20	2
Organic Milk Chocolate	½ bar (1.4 oz)	210	22	20	1
Nutty Ducky's					
Cashew Brittle	4 pieces (1.6 oz)	240	22	13	2
Cashew Brittle Dark Chocolate	2 pieces (1.5 oz)	220	23	16	2
Peanut Brittle	4 pieces (1.6 oz)	230	23	13	4
Peanut Brittle Milk Chocolate	2 pieces (1.5 oz)	220	23	17	2

FOOD	PORTION	CALS	CARB	SUGAR	FIBER
Odense					
Marzipan	2 tbsp (1.4 oz)	170	29	24	0
Pure Fun					
Organic Vegan Barrels Of Fun Root Beer Float	2 (0.5 oz)	60	13	3	0
Organic Vegan Candy Canes	1 (0.5 oz)	62	14	3	1
Organic Vegan Chocolate Meltdowns All Flavors	3 (0.6 oz)	70	16	4	0
Organic Vegan Citrus Slices All Flavors	3 (0.6 oz)	60	15	3	0
Organic Vegan Cotton Candy All Flavors	¼ pkg (0.5 oz)	60	15	15	0
Organic Vegan Jaw Boulders All Flavors	2 (0.5 oz)	58	13	3	0
Organic Vegan Pure Pops All Flavors	3 (0.6 oz)	60	15	3	0
Raisinets					
Candy	3 pkg (1.7 oz)	200	34	29	1
Reese's					
Clusters	3 (1.5 oz)	220	24	21	1
Riesen					
Candy	4 (1.3 oz)	170	28	15	0
Russell Stover					
Assorted	3 pieces (1.4 oz)	170	27	23	1
Private Reserve Triple Chocolate Mousse	3 pieces (1.3 oz)	220	19	15	2
Private Reserve Vanilla Bean Brulee	3 pieces (1.3 oz)	180	19	13	3
Scharffen Berger					
Semisweet 60% Cacao	1 bar (2 oz)	320	32	24	tr
Sencha Naturals					
Green Tea Mints All Flavors	3	5	1	0	0
Shaman Chocolates					
Organic Extra Dark Chocolate 82% Cacao	½ bar (1 oz)	158	7	1	4
Organic Milk Chocolate w/ Macadamia Nuts & Hawaiian Pink Sea Salt	½ bar (1 oz)	91	13	13	2

FOOD	PORTION	CALS	CARB	SUGAR	FIBER
Skittles					
Original Fruit	1 pkg (2.2 oz)	250	56	47	0
Slim-Fast					
Protein Snack Chews Peanut Butter	1 pkg (0.9 oz)	100	12	5	0
Smile Chocolatiers					
Choclatea Ginger Tea Milk Chocolate 37% Cacao	½ bar (1.5 oz)	230	23	21	1
Choclatea Herbal Chai Tea Dark Chocolate 64% Cacao	½ bar (1.5 oz)	220	22	15	5
Choclatea Pistachio Green Tea White Chocolate	½ bar (1.5 oz)	240	22	22	1
Choclatea Pomegranate White Tea Very Dark Chocolate 72% Cacao	½ bar (1.5 oz)	220	16	14	2
Choclatea White Tea Very Dark Chocolate 72% Cacao	½ bar (1.5 oz)	220	22	15	5
Snickers					
Almond	1 (1.8 oz)	230	32	26	2
Bar	1 bar (2.07 oz)	280	35	30	1
Cruncher	1 bar (1.6 oz)	220	28	21	1
Starburst					
Baja California	1 pkg	240	48	34	0
Jellybeans	¼ cup	160	39	30	0
Original Fruit	1 pkg	240	48	34	0
Sour Fruit	1 pkg	240	47	33	0
Sugar Babies					
Candy	30 pieces (1.5 oz)	180	41	32	0
Chocolate	19 pieces (1.4 oz)	180	33	26	0
Sugar Daddy					
Pop	1 lg (1.7 oz)	200	43	29	0
The Chocolate Traveler					
Wedges Dark Chocolate Coffee	4 pieces	130	15	12	2
Wedges Dark Chocolate Mint	4 pieces	130	15	12	2
Wedges Dark Chocolate Orange	4 pieces	120	15	11	2

FOOD	PORTION	CALS	CARB	SUGAR	FIBER
Wedges Dark Chocolate Raspberry	4 pieces	120	15	11	2
Wedges Dark Chocolate Tiramisu	4 pieces	120	15	11	2
Wedges Milk Chocolate	4 pieces	130	15	14	0
Wedges Milk Chocolate Dulce De Leche	4 pieces	120	17	15	tr
Wedges White Chocolate	4 pieces	140	14	14	0
Wedges White Chocolate Creme Brulee	4 pieces	140	14	14	0
Toffifay					
Candy	5 (1.4 oz)	200	25	18	1
Tootsie Roll					
Midgees	6	140	28	20	0
Mini Chews	30 pieces (1.4 oz)	170	27	21	1
Pops	1 (0.6 oz)	60	15	10	0
Pops Caramel Apple	1 (0.6 oz)	60	15	11	0
Twix					
Fun Size	1 (0.6 oz)	80	10	8	0
Peanut Butter	1 bar	280	28	19	2
Vere					
75% Chocolate Gluten Free	1 sm bar	80	6	3	2
Brownie Box Coconut Gluten Free Vegan	3 pieces (1.4 oz)	210	13	6	5
Brownie Box Peanut Butter Gluten Free	3 pieces (1.3 oz)	180	12	6	3
Brownie Box Walnut Gluten Free	3 pieces (1.3 oz)	190	12	6	3
Clusters Chocolate Almond Gluten Free Vegan	2 pieces (1.3 oz)	210	11	3	4
Clusters Chocolate Coconut Gluten Free Vegan	3 pieces (1.7 oz)	280	18	5	6
Clusters Chocolate Rice Gluten Free Vegan	3 pieces (1.3 oz)	170	22	3	3
Clusters Chocolate Seed Gluten Free Vegan	2 pieces (1.3 oz)	210	11	3	4
Wafers Cacao Nibs Gluten Free Vegan	2 (1.1 oz)	170	15	4	4

FOOD	PORTION	CALS	CARB	SUGAR	FIBER
Wafers Espresso Gluten Free Vegan	3 (1.6 oz)	250	21	7	8
Wafers Pink Peppercorn Gluten Free Vegan	3 (1.6 oz)	250	21	7	6
Wafers Spicy Pepita Gluten Free	2 (1.1 oz)	170	14	5	4
Wafers Tamari Almond Gluten Free Vegan	2 (1.2 oz)	170	18	5	5
Werther's					
Caramel Milk Chocolate	6 (1.3 oz)	230	18	17	0
Original	3 (0.5 oz)	60	13	11	0
Original Sugar Free	5 (0.5 oz)	40	14	0	0
Whitman's					
Sampler	3 pieces (1.4 oz)	220	31	26	tr
Yummy Earth					
Organic Lollipops All Flavors	3	70	17	17	0
CANTALOUPE					
dried	3.5 pieces (1.4 oz)	140	34	32	1
fresh cubed	1 cup	57	13	–	1
Del Monte					
Fresh	¼ melon (4.7 oz)	50	12	11	1
CAPERS					
capers	1 tbsp	2	tr	tr	tr
CARAWAY					
seed	1 tbsp	22	3	tr	3
CARDAMOM					
ground	1 tsp	6	1	–	1
CARDOON					
fresh cooked w/o salt	1 serv (3.5 oz)	22	5	–	2
Frieda's					
Cardoon	1 cup	15	4	1	1
Ocean Mist					
Cardone Fresh Shredded	1 cup (6.2 oz)	36	9	0	3

FOOD	PORTION	CALS	CARB	SUGAR	FIBER
CARIBOU					
roasted	3 oz	142	0	0	0
CAROB					
Bob's Red Mill					
Powder Toasted	2 tsp	25	11	7	2
Tree Of Life					
Chips Malt Sweetened	50 (0.5 oz)	70	9	1	1
CARP					
fresh cooked	1 fillet (6 oz)	276	0	0	0
fresh cooked	3 oz	138	0	0	0
fresh raw	3 oz	108	0	0	0
roe salted in olive oil	2 tbsp (1 oz)	40	6	–	0
CARROT JUICE					
Hollywood					
100% Juice	1 can (12 oz)	120	27	14	1
Lakewood					
Organic	6 oz	73	17	8	2
Odwalla					
100% Juice	8 oz	70	15	13	1
CARROTS					
CANNED					
slices low sodium	½ cup	17	4	–	1
Allens					
Tiny Sliced	½ cup	35	8	3	3
Del Monte					
Savory Sides Honey Glazed	½ cup	70	18	12	tr
Tillen Farms					
Crispy Carrots Pickled	5 pieces (1 oz)	30	7	6	1
FRESH					
raw shredded	½ cup	24	6	–	2
Bolthouse Farms					
Matchstix	3 oz	35	9	6	2
Earthbound Farm					
Organic Tops On	1 (2.7 oz)	35	8	5	2
Organic w/ Organic Ranch Dip	1 pkg (2.2 oz)	90	5	3	1
Frieda's					
Gold	⅔ cup (3 oz)	35	9	6	3

FOOD	PORTION	CALS	CARB	SUGAR	FIBER
Grimmway					
Baby	3 oz	38	9	6	2
FROZEN					
Birds Eye					
Steam & Serve Carrots & Cranberries	1 cup	130	20	15	3
C&W					
Whole Baby	⅔ cup	35	7	5	2
Green Giant					
Honey Glazed	1 cup	90	15	11	3
Joy Of Cooking					
Bite Size	½ cup (3.3 oz)	70	12	3	2
CASABA					
cubed	1 cup (6 oz)	46	11	10	2
melon fresh	¼ (14 oz)	115	27	23	4
CASHEW JUICE					
O.N.E.					
Cashew Fruit	1 bottle (11 oz)	140	34	33	1
CASHEWS					
dry roasted w/ salt	18 nuts (1 oz)	160	9	–	1
Arrowhead Mills					
Organic Cashew Butter	2 tbsp	160	9	2	tr
Good Sense					
Jumbo Honey Roasted	¼ cup	170	13	4	1
Jumbo Roasted & Salted	¼ cup	190	9	2	1
Kettle					
Butter Creamy Unsalted	2 tbsp	160	8	0	1
Lance					
Cashews	1 pkg (1.5 oz)	270	11	4	3
Navitas Naturals					
Cashews	1 oz	160	9	2	1
Peeled Snacks					
Nut Picks Cashew Later	1 pkg (1 oz)	180	9	2	tr
Planters					
Chocolate Lovers Milk Chocolate	10 pieces (1.5 oz)	230	20	15	tr
Dry Roasted	19 pieces (1 oz)	160	9	2	tr

FOOD	PORTION	CALS	CARB	SUGAR	FIBER
Organic	23 pieces (1 oz)	170	8	2	1
Sunfood					
Organic	1 oz	164	9	2	1
Tree Of Life					
Cashew Butter Creamy	2 tbsp	180	9	2	1
CASSAVA					
diced cooked w/o fat	1 cup (4.6 oz)	213	51	2	2
root raw	1 (14.3 oz)	653	155	7	7
TAKE-OUT					
fritter crab meat stuffed	1 (4.4 oz)	341	38	7	2
CATFISH					
wolffish atlantic baked	3 oz	105	0	0	0
Simmons					
Farm Raised	4 oz	140	0	0	0
CAULIFLOWER					
flowerets fresh	1 (0.5 oz)	3	1	tr	tr
flowerets fresh cooked w/o salt	3 (2 oz)	12	2	1	1
fresh	1 cup	25	5	2	3
fresh cooked w/o salt	1 cup	29	5	3	3
fresh head small	1 (9.2 oz)	66	14	6	7
frzn cooked w/o salt	1 cup	34	7	2	5
green fresh	1 cup	20	4	2	2
green fresh small head	1 (11.4 oz)	101	20	10	10
pickled	¼ cup	14	3	2	1
pickled chow chow	¼ cup	74	16	15	1
Birds Eye					
Steamfresh Garlic Cauliflower	1 cup (2.4 oz)	40	5	2	1
Green Giant					
Cheese Sauce	½ cup	50	6	2	1
Mann's					
Cauliettes Fresh	1 serv (3 oz)	20	4	2	2
TAKE-OUT					
batter dipped fried	1 cup	178	12	1	2
batter dipped fried	1 piece (0.9 oz)	55	4	tr	1
w/ cheese sauce	1 cup	249	12	6	3

FOOD	PORTION	CALS	CARB	SUGAR	FIBER
CAVIAR					
black or red	2 tbsp	81	1	0	0
CELERY					
fresh	1 lg stalk (2.2 oz)	9	2	1	1
pickled	½ cup	10	2	1	1
raw diced	½ cup	8	2	1	1
seed	1 tsp	1	tr	–	tr
strips	1 cup	17	4	2	2
Dole					
Stalks	2 med (3 oz)	20	5	0	2
Earthbound Farm					
Organic Hearts	2 stalks (3.9 oz)	20	5	0	2
Frieda's					
Celery Root	¾ cup	35	8	2	3
TAKE-OUT					
creamed	½ cup	87	7	4	1
stir fried	½ cup	30	3	2	1
stuffed w/ cheese	1 (5 inch)	38	1	tr	tr
CELERY JUICE					
juice	1 cup	42	9	6	4
CEREAL					
granola	½ cup	285	32	–	6
oatmeal instant as prep w/ water	1 cup (8.2 oz)	138	24		4
oatmeal regular & quick as prep w/ water	¾ cup (6.1 oz)	149	19	–	3
oatmeal regular & quick not prep	⅓ cup (0.9 oz)	104	18	–	3
puffed rice	1 cup	56	13	–	tr
puffed wheat	1 cup	44	10	–	1
shredded mini wheats	1 cup	107	24	–	3
shredded wheat rectangular	1 biscuit (0.8 oz)	85	19	–	2
Alti Plano Gold					
Instant Quinoa Hot Cereal Spiced Apple Raisin	1 pkg	160	35	12	5
Instant Quinoa Organic Hot Cereal Oaxacan Chocolate	1 pkg	170	30	9	5

FOOD	PORTION	CALS	CARB	SUGAR	FIBER
Arrowhead Mills					
Organic Amaranth Flakes	1 cup	140	26	4	3
Organic Kamut Flakes	1 cup	120	25	2	2
Organic Multigrain Flakes	1 cup	170	33	3	3
Organic Nature O's	1 cup	130	25	1	2
Organic Puffed Corn	1 cup	60	12	0	2
Organic Puffed Millet	1 cup	60	11	0	1
Organic Puffed Wheat	1 cup	60	12	0	2
Organic Rice Flakes Sweetened	1 cup	180	40	8	1
Organic Spelt Flakes	1 cup	120	24	3	3
Back To Nature					
Energy Start Hi Protein Crunch	½ cup	170	28	14	3
Heart Basics Organic Apple Cinnamon Harvest	¾ cup	180	45	15	10
Bakery On Main					
Granola Apple Cinnamon Walnut	½ cup (2 oz)	240	29	9	4
Granola Fiber Power Cinnamon Raisin	½ cup (2 oz)	230	40	9	9
Granola Maple Raisin Almond	½ cup (2 oz)	240	30	12	4
Granola Super Fruit & Nut	½ cup (2 oz)	250	29	20	4
Barbara's Bakery					
Alpen No Sugar Added	⅔ cup	200	40	7	4
Organic Breakfast O's Fruit Juice Sweetened	1 cup	120	22	1	3
Organic Brown Rice Crisps Fruit Juice Sweetened	1 cup	120	25	2	1
Organic Corn Flakes Fruit Juice Sweetened	1 cup	110	25	3	1
Organic Wild Puffs	1 cup	100	23	12	tr
Organic Wild Puffs Fruity Punch	1 cup	110	26	9	1
Organic Ultima High Fiber	½ cup	90	24	5	8
Organic Ultima Pomegranate	½ cup	100	24	5	5
Puffins Cinnamon	⅔ cup	100	26	6	6
Puffins Originals	¾ cup (0.9 oz)	90	23	5	5
Shredded Oats Bite Size	1¼ cups (2 oz)	220	46	12	5
Shredded Wheat	2 biscuits (1.4 oz)	140	31	0	5

FOOD	PORTION	CALS	CARB	SUGAR	FIBER
Bob's Red Mill					
Farina Creamy Brown Rice not prep	¼ cup	150	32	0	2
Muesli Old Country	¼ cup	110	21	5	4
Natural Granola No Fat	½ cup	180	35	8	4
Organic Right Stuff Hot Cereal 6 Grain not prep	¼ cup	140	27	0	4
Rolled Oats Gluten Free not prep	½ cup	160	27	1	4
Cascadian Farm					
Organic Clifford Crunch	1 cup	100	25	6	5
Organic Granola Oats & Honey	⅔ cup	230	42	14	3
Chappaqua Crunch					
Original Granola	⅓ cup	115	20	4	3
Simply Granola w/ Raisins	⅓ cup	120	22	6	3
Simply Granola w/ Raspberries	⅓ cup	110	21	4	3
Country Choice Organic					
Multigrain Hot Cereal not prep	½ cup	130	29	0	5
Oats Old Fashioned not prep	½ cup	150	27	1	4
Oats Quick not prep	½ cup	150	27	1	4
Dorset Cereals					
Berries & Cherries	½ cup	150	40	23	3
Simply Delicious Muesli	½ cup	200	37	7	4
Super Cranberry Cherry & Almond	½ cup	200	39	17	4
Earthbound Farm					
Organic Granola Maple Almond	½ cup	260	31	11	4
Enjoy Life					
Allergen Gluten Free Granola Cinnamon	½ cup	160	31	8	5
EnviroKidz					
Organic Orangutan O's	¾ cup	120	26	9	2
Erin Baker's					
Granola Fruit & Nut	½ cup (1.6 oz)	190	27	10	4
Granola Oatmeal Raisin	½ cup (1.6 oz)	180	30	11	4
Granola Ultra Protein Power Crunch	½ cup (1.6 oz)	200	25	6	4
Fantastic					
Oatmeal Big Cup Apple Cinnamon	1 pkg	270	54	17	6

FOOD	PORTION	CALS	CARB	SUGAR	FIBER
Oatmeal Big Cup Maple Raisin 3 Grain	1 pkg	270	60	22	8
Farina					
Original as prep	1 cup	120	22	0	tr
General Mills					
Cheerios Crunch Oat Cluster	¾ cups	100	22	8	2
Cheerios Yogurt Burst Strawberry	¾ cup	120	24	11	2
Chex Whole Grain Chocolate	¾ cup	130	26	8	tr
Curves	¾ cup	100	22	4	2
Fiber One Raisin Bran Clusters	1 cup (2 oz)	170	45	13	11
Total Honey Clusters	¾ cup	170	39	13	3
Total Raisin Bran	1 cup	170	42	19	5
Total Whole Grain	¾ cup (1 oz)	100	23	5	3
Trix	1 cup (1.1 oz)	120	28	12	1
Glucerna					
Crunchy Flakes 'N Raisins	1 bowl (1.6 oz)	140	36	13	6
Crunchy Flakes 'N Strawberries	1 bowl (1.5 oz)	150	37	9	7
Glutino					
Gluten Free Apple Cinnamon	½ cup	120	24	10	1
Gluten Free Honey Nut	½ cup	130	24	8	1
Grandy Oats					
Organic Granola Classic	½ cup	252	27	6	5
Organic Granola Low Fat Cranberry Chew	½ cup	191	41	17	3
Organic Granola Mainely Maple	½ cup	204	31	9	4
Health Valley					
Empower	1 cup	200	42	11	6
Granola Low Fat Tropical Fruit	⅔ cup	180	43	10	6
Heart Wise	1 cup	200	37	11	5
Organic Cherry Lemon Blast Ems	¾ cup	120	25	7	2
Organic Golden Flax	¾ cup	190	38	9	6
Organic Multigrain Apple Cinnamon Square Ems	1¼ cup	210	44	12	8
Organic Oat Bran O's	¾ cup	100	23	14	3
Rice Crunch-Ems	1 cup	110	26	2	2
Hodgson Mill					
Hot Cereal Bulgur Wheat w/ Soy not prep	¼ cup	115	22	0	3

FOOD	PORTION	CALS	CARB	SUGAR	FIBER
Hot Cereal Oat Bran not prep	¼ cup	120	23	0	6
Honest Foods					
Granola Planks Maple Almond Crunch	½ bar (2 oz)	250	37	19	5
Kashi					
7 Whole Grain Flakes	1 cup	180	41	5	6
7 Whole Grain Honey Puffs	1 cup	120	25	6	2
7 Whole Grain Nuggets	½ cup	210	47	3	7
7 Whole Grain Pilaf as prep	½ cup	170	30	0	6
GoLean	1 cup	140	30	6	10
GoLean Crunch!	1 cup	190	36	13	8
GoLean Crunch! Honey Almond Flax	1 cup	200	34	12	8
GoLean Instant Hot Cereal Creamy Truly Vanilla	1 pkg	150	25	6	7
GoLean Instant Hot Cereal Hearty Honey & Cinnamon	1 pkg	150	26	7	5
Good Friends	1 cup	170	43	9	12
Granola Mountain Medley	½ cup	220	37	12	6
Heart To Heart Instant Oatmeal Golden Brown Maple	1 pkg	160	33	12	5
Heart To Heart Instant Oatmeal Raisin Spice	1 pkg	150	33	16	4
Heart To Heart Oat Flakes & Blueberry Clusters	1¼ cups	200	42	12	4
Heart To Heart Toasted Oat	¾ cup	110	25	5	5
Honey Sunshine	¾ cup (1.1 oz)	100	25	6	6
Mighty Bites All Flavors	1 cup	110	23	5	3
Organic Promise Autumn Wheat	1 cup	190	45	7	6
Organic Promise Cinnamon Harvest	1 cup	190	44	9	5
Organic Promise Strawberry Fields	1 cup	120	28	9	1
Vive Probiotic Digestive Wellness	1¼ cups	170	43	10	12
Kellogg's					
All-Bran	½ cup	80	23	6	10
All-Bran Extra Fiber	½ cup	50	20	0	13
Apple Jacks	1 cup	130	30	16	1

FOOD	PORTION	CALS	CARB	SUGAR	FIBER
Caramel Nut Crunch	1 cup	210	41	17	1
Cocoa Krispies	¾ cup	120	27	14	1
Complete Oat Bran Flakes	¾ cup	110	23	6	1
Corn Flakes	1 cup	100	24	2	1
Corn Pops	1 cup	120	28	14	tr
Cracklin' Oat Bran	¾ cup	200	35	15	6
Crispix	1 cup	110	25	3	tr
Froot Loops	1 cup	120	28	15	1
Froot Loops ⅓ Less Sugar	1¼ cups	120	28	10	1
Frosted Flakes	¾ cup	120	28	12	1
Frosted Flakes ⅓ Less Sugar	1 cup	120	28	8	tr
Fruit Harvest	¾ cup	120	25	9	1
Granola Low Fat w/ Raisins	⅔ cup	230	49	18	3
Honey Smacks	¾ cup	100	24	15	1
Mini-Wheat Frosted	5 (1.8 oz)	180	41	10	5
Mueslix Raisins Dates & Almonds	⅔ cup	200	40	17	4
Organic Mini Wheats Frosted	24 pieces	190	44	11	5
Organic Raisin Bran	1 cup	190	46	16	8
Organic Rice Krispies	1¼ cups	120	29	3	0
Product 19	1 cup	100	25	4	1
Raisin Bran	1 cup	190	45	19	7
Rice Krispies	1¼ cups	120	29	3	0
Smart Start Antioxidants	1 cup	190	43	14	3
Smorz	1 cup	120	25	13	tr
Special K	1 cup	110	22	4	tr
Special K Fruit & Yogurt	¾ cup	120	27	11	1
Special K Low Carb Lifestyle Protein Plus	¾ cup	100	14	2	5
Special K Red Berries	1 cup	110	25	10	1
Special K Vanilla Almond	¾ cup	110	25	9	1
Lundberg					
Purely Organic Hot'n Creamy Rice	⅓ cup	190	43	0	3
Malt-O-Meal					
Balance	¾ cup	120	26	6	3
Cinnamon Toasters	¾ cup	130	24	10	1
Colossal Crunch	¾ cup	120	26	13	0
Creamy Hot Wheat not prep	3 tbsp	130	27	0	1
Crispy Rice	1¼ cups	130	29	3	0

FOOD	PORTION	CALS	CARB	SUGAR	FIBER
Frosted Flakes	¾ cup	120	28	12	1
Frosted Mini Spooners	1 cup	190	45	11	6
Honey & Oat Blenders	¾ cup	120	25	6	1
Honey Buzzers	1⅓ cup	110	26	11	1
Instant Oatmeal Apple & Cinnamon	1 pkg	130	27	11	3
Instant Oatmeal Cinnamon & Spice	1 pkg	170	36	16	3
Instant Oatmeal Maple & Brown Sugar	1 pkg	160	33	13	3
Original Hot Wheat not prep	3 tbsp	130	27	0	1
Puffed Rice	1 cup	60	13	0	0
Raisin Bran	1 cup	220	47	21	7
McCann's					
Irish Oatmeal Quick Cooking not prep	½ cup (1.4 oz)	150	26	0	4
Mom's Best Naturals					
Oatmeal Instant	1 pkg	160	33	13	3
Raisin Bran	1 cup	230	49	20	6
Toasted Wheat-fuls	1 cup	200	44	0	7
Toasty O's	1 cup	120	23	4	3
Natural Ovens					
Great Granola	½ cup	250	38	8	3
Nature's Path					
Optimum Organic ReBound	¾ cup	190	35	9	6
Organic Flax Plus Pumpkin Raisin Crunch	¾ cup	200	41	12	9
Organic Smart Bran	⅔ cup	90	24	6	13
Organic Granola Pomegran Plus	½ cup	140	21	7	2
Organic Zen Instant Oatmeal Cranberry Ginger	1 pkg	150	30	11	3
Nature's Plus					
Organic Oatmeal Hemp Plus	1 pkg	160	30	6	4
Newman's Own					
Sweet Enough Honey Flax Flakes	¾ cup	100	24	8	4
Sweet Enough Honey Nut O's	¾ cup	110	22	7	2
Sweet Enough Wheat Puffs	¾ cup	100	22	8	1
Perky's					
Nutty Flax	¾ cup	230	41	41	7

FOOD	PORTION	CALS	CARB	SUGAR	FIBER
PerkyO's Original	¾ cup	120	28	2	3
Post					
100% Bran	1 (0.8 oz)	80	22	7	9
Bran Flakes	1 cup	100	24	5	5
Cocoa Pebbles	¾ cup (1 oz)	110	26	11	3
Golden Crisp	¾ cup (1 oz)	110	25	14	1
Grape Nuts O's	1 cup (1 oz)	120	28	11	2
Grape-Nuts	2 oz	200	47	5	6
Grape-Nuts Trail Mix Crunch	1 cup (1.7 oz)	170	37	9	5
Great Grains Raisins Dates & Pecans	¾ cup (2 oz)	210	40	14	4
Honey Bunches Of Oats	¾ cup	130	25	6	2
Honey Bunches Of Oats Peaches	1 cup	120	26	8	2
Honey Bunches Of Oats Strawberry	¾ cup	120	26	8	2
Honeycomb	1⅓ cups (1 oz)	120	28	10	3
LiveActive Mixed Berry Crunch	1 cup	190	43	12	7
LiveActive Nut Harvest Crunch	1 cup	220	39	8	8
Oreo O's	1 cup	110	22	13	1
Raisin Bran	1 cup (2 oz)	190	46	19	8
Selects Banana Nut Crunch	1 cup (2 oz)	240	44	12	4
Selects Blueberry Morning	2 oz	220	45	16	2
Shredded Wheat Frosted	2 oz	180	43	12	5
Shredded Wheat 'N Bran	2 oz	200	49	1	8
Shredded Wheat Original	2 biscuits (1.6 oz)	160	37	0	6
Shredded Wheat Spoon Size	1 cup	170	40	0	6
Toasties Corn Flakes	1 cup (1 oz)	100	24	2	1
Quaker					
Instant Oatmeal Cinnamon & Spice	1 pkg	170	35	15	3
Instant Oatmeal Cinnamon Roll	1 pkg	160	33	13	3
Instant Oatmeal Crunch Maple & Brown Sugar	1 pkg	190	39	14	3
Instant Oatmeal Crunch Mixed Berry	1 pkg	190	39	16	3
Instant Oatmeal Express Baked Apple	1 pkg	200	42	19	4

FOOD	PORTION	CALS	CARB	SUGAR	FIBER
Instant Oatmeal For Kids Dinosaur Eggs	1 pkg	190	37	14	3
Instant Oatmeal Lower Sugar Maple & Brown Sugar	1 pkg	120	24	4	3
Instant Oatmeal Maple Brown Sugar w/ Pecans	1 pkg	160	30	9	4
Instant Oatmeal Nutrition For Women Golden Brown Sugar	1 pkg	170	32	12	3
Instant Oatmeal Organic Regular	1 pkg	100	19	0	3
Instant Oatmeal Regular	1 pkg	100	19	0	3
Instant Oatmeal Simple Harvest Apples w/ Cinnamon	1 pkg	150	32	12	4
Instant Oatmeal Strawberries & Cream	1 pkg	130	27	12	2
Instant Oatmeal Supreme Apple Raisin	1 pkg	150	32	13	3
Instant Oatmeal Supreme Cinnamon Pecan	1 pkg	180	33	14	3
Instant Oatmeal Take Heart Golden Maple	1 pkg	160	33	9	5
Instant Oatmeal Weight Control Banana Bread	1 pkg	160	29	1	6
Life	¾ cup	120	25	6	2
Life Cinnamon	¾ cup	120	25	8	2
Life Honey Graham	¾ cup	120	25	7	2
Life Vanilla Yogurt Crunch	1¼ cups	210	43	12	4
Oat Bran Hot Cereal not prep	½ cup	150	25	1	6
Old Fashioned Oats not prep	½ cup	150	27	1	4
Quick Oats Sun Country Iron Fortified	1 pkg	150	27	1	4
Ralston					
Corn Flakes	1 cup (1 oz)	100	24	2	tr
Raisin Bran	1 cup	200	47	18	8
Shredded Wheat Frosted Bite Size	1¼ cups	200	47	11	5
Roman Meal					
Cream Of Rye not prep	⅓ cup (1.4 oz)	130	27	2	6
Elements Cranberry Passion	1 cup (1.6 oz)	160	33	9	5
Hot Cereal not prep	⅓ cup (1.3 oz)	120	26	1	6

FOOD	PORTION	CALS	CARB	SUGAR	FIBER
South Beach					
Crunch Strawberry Harvest	1 cup	170	37	9	8
Crunch Vanilla Almond	1 cup	180	35	8	8
Granola Clusters Cherry Almond	1 pkg (1 oz)	130	18	6	6
Granola Clusters Mixed Berry	1 pkg (1 oz)	130	18	6	6
Stark Sisters					
Granola Lo-Fat Raspberry Blueberry	½ cup	230	38	16	4
Granola Nutty Maple	½ cup	250	32	9	4
Granola Original Maple Almond	½ cup	240	33	7	5
Sunbelt					
Granola Low Fat Cinnamon & Raisins	½ cup	250	52	20	3
Udi's					
Granola BanaBerry	¼ cup (1.1 oz)	120	19	5	3
Granola Hawaiian	¼ cup (1.1 oz)	120	19	5	3
Granola Muesli	¼ cup (1.1 oz)	120	18	1	4
Granola Nuggets	¼ cup (1.1 oz)	150	22	6	3
Granola Original	¼ cup (1.1 oz)	130	18	5	2
Uncle Sam					
Original	¾ cup (1.9 oz)	190	38	tr	10
Weetabix					
Organic	2 biscuits (1.2 oz)	120	28	2	4
Organic Crispy Flakes	¾ cup	110	24	4	4
Wheatena					
Toasted Wheat	⅓ cup	160	33	0	5
YogActive					
Probiotic High Fibre Wheat Strawberry Raspberry	⅔ cup	160	29	8	6
Probiotic Kiwi	⅔ cup	120	23	7	1
Probiotic Strawberry	⅔ cup	130	25	7	1
Probiotic Strawberry Dark Chocolate	⅔ cup	130	26	9	2
Zoe's					
Granola Cinnamon Raisin	½ cup	190	32	13	7
Granola Cranberries Currants	½ cup	190	32	14	7
Granola Honey Almond	½ cup	190	32	13	7
O's Cinnamon	¾ cup	120	25	8	5

FOOD	PORTION	CALS	CARB	SUGAR	FIBER
O's Honey	¾ cup	120	25	8	5
O's Natural	¾ cup	120	23	3	tr

CEREAL BARS *(see also ENERGY BARS)*
Aristo
Acai Blueberry Lime	1 (1.3 oz)	130	22	6	3
Pomegranate & Cranberry	1 (1.3 oz)	140	21	6	3

Attune
Wellness Yogurt & Granola Lemon Creme	1 (1.4 oz)	180	24	12	2
Wellness Yogurt & Granola Strawberry Bliss	1 (1.4 oz)	180	24	12	5

Back To Nature
Bakery Squares Banana Walnut	1 (1.1 oz)	130	19	9	2
Chewy Trail Mix Cherry Pecan	1 (1 oz)	120	19	8	2
Fruit & Grain Apple	1 (1.1 oz)	110	20	11	tr

Bakery On Main
Granola Gluten Free Extreme Trail Mix	1 (1.3 oz)	140	23	7	1
Granola Gluten Free Peanut Butter Chocolate Chip	1 (1.2 oz)	140	24	7	1

Barbara's Bakery
Fruit & Yogurt Cherry Apple	1	150	29	15	1
Nature's Choice Blueberry	1 (1.3 oz)	150	29	15	2
Organic Crunchy Granola Cinnamon Crisp	2 (1.5 oz)	190	27	10	3

Cascadian Farm
Organic Chewy Granola Fruit & Nut	1 (1.2 oz)	140	24	11	1

CocoaVia
Dark Chocolate Almond	1 (0.8 oz)	90	13	8	1

Country Choice Organic
Oatmeal Squares Apple Cinnamon	1 (2 oz)	210	41	16	1
Oatmeal Squares Maple	1 (2 oz)	210	41	14	4

Enjoy Life
Allergen Gluten Free Caramel Apple	1 (1 oz)	110	21	8	2

Entenmann's
Multi-Grain Real Strawberry	1 (1.3 oz)	140	26	15	tr

FOOD	PORTION	CALS	CARB	SUGAR	FIBER
EnviroKidz					
Crispy Rice Panda Peanut Butter	1 (1 oz)	110	20	7	tr
Glenny's					
Organic Muesli Raisins & Dates	1 (1.6 oz)	170	34	15	3
Organic Museli Chocolate Chip	1 (1.6 oz)	170	34	15	3
Slim Carb Bars Brownie Cheesecake	1 (1.3 oz)	130	19	2	1
Slim-1 w/ Acai Very Berry Blast	1 (1.1 oz)	100	21	8	2
Slim-1 w/ GreenTea Double Fudge	1 (1.1 oz)	100	20	8	2
Slim-1 w/ Hoodia Peanut Butter Caramel	1 (1.1 oz)	100	20	7	2
Glutino					
Gluten Free Breakfast Bar Apple	1 (1.4 oz)	120	25	17	3
Gluten Free Breakfast Bar Chocolate	1 (¼ oz)	110	25	17	4
Gluten Free Organic Chocolate & Peanut	1 (1 oz)	110	19	8	1
Gluten Free Organic Wildberry	1 (1 oz)	100	21	8	1
Health Valley					
Cafe Creations Cinnamon Danish	1 (1.4 oz)	130	27	17	2
Date Almond Low Fat	1 (1.5 oz)	150	32	15	tr
Granola Chocolate Chip Low Fat	1 (1.5 oz)	160	32	13	1
Granola Moist & Chewy Dutch Apple	1 (1 oz)	100	20	10	tr
Granola Trail Mix Cranberries Nuts & Yogurt Chips	1 (1.2 oz)	140	23	12	1
Organic Fig Cobbler	1 (1.4 oz)	130	26	14	2
Organic Raspberry Tarts	1 (1.4 oz)	150	30	16	tr
Organic Strawberry Cobbler	1 (1.3 oz)	130	26	14	1
Peanut Butter & Grape	1 (1.3 oz)	130	26	16	1
Honest Foods					
Cran Lemon Zest	1 (2.2 oz)	240	35	17	4
Farmer's Trail Mix	1 (2.2 oz)	240	35	17	4
Kashi					
TLC Chewy Granola Honey Almond Flax	1 (1.2 oz)	140	19	5	4
TLC Chewy Trail Mix	1 (1.2 oz)	140	20	5	4

FOOD	PORTION	CALS	CARB	SUGAR	FIBER
TLC Soft Baked Apple Spice	1 (1.2 oz)	110	21	9	3
TLC Soft Baked Blackberry Graham	1 (1.2 oz)	110	21	9	3
TLC Soft Baked Ripe Strawberry	1 (1.2 oz)	110	21	9	3
Kellogg's					
All-Bran Brown Sugar Cinnamon	1	130	27	11	5
All-Bran Oatmeal Raisin	1	120	26	12	5
Crunchy Nut Sweet & Salty Chocolatey Almond	1 (1.1 oz)	160	16	10	2
FiberPlus Antioxidants Chocolate Chip	1 (1.2 oz)	120	26	7	9
FiberPlus Antioxidants Dark Chocolate Almond	1 (1.2 oz)	130	24	7	9
Nutri-Grain Banana Muffin	1	170	30	16	1
Nutri-Grain Yogurt Vanilla	1	140	26	14	tr
Smart Start Healthy Heart Cinnamon	1 (1.4 oz)	150	30	12	2
Snack Bites	1 pkg (0.8 oz)	90	18	7	tr
Special K Chocolatey Drizzle	1 (0.8 oz)	90	17	8	tr
Special K Meal Bar Chocolate Peanut Butter	1 (1.6 oz)	190	23	16	2
Special K Snack Bar Chocolate Peanut	1 (0.9 oz)	110	15	11	1
Special K Strawberry	1 (0.8 oz)	90	18	9	tr
Special K Vanilla Crisp	1 (0.8 oz)	90	17	7	tr
KeriBar					
Vegan Apple Peanut Butter	1 (1.4 oz)	140	21	10	5
Vegan Cherry Almond	1 (1.4 oz)	140	21	10	5
Vegan Strawberry Chocolate Chip	1 (1.4 oz)	130	23	12	5
Kind					
Almond & Coconut	1	193	14	11	4
Almonds & Apricot In Yogurt	1	208	19	17	3
Banana & Oatbran	1	160	23	16	4
Nut Delight	1	203	12	8	3
Walnut & Date	1	150	22	17	3
Kudos					
Granola Chocolate Chip	1 (1 oz)	120	20	11	1
Granola Peanut Butter	1	130	18	10	1

FOOD	PORTION	CALS	CARB	SUGAR	FIBER
Granola w/ M&M's	1	100	17	9	1
Granola w/ Snickers	1	100	16	9	1
Lean Body					
Hi-Protein Granola Peanuts 'N Chocolate	1 (2.8 oz)	340	39	13	4
Natural Ovens					
Great Granola Mixed Fruit	1 (1.4 oz)	150	27	15	2
Nature Valley					
Chewy Granola Blueberry Yogurt	1	140	26	13	1
Chewy Granola Lemon Yogurt	1	140	26	13	1
Chewy Granola Vanilla Yogurt	1	140	26	13	1
Chewy Trail Mix Granola Apple Cinnamon	1	140	259	13	1
Chewy Trail Mix Granola Fruit & Nut	1	140	25	13	2
Chewy Trail Mix Granola Mixed Berry	1	140	26	13	1
Crunchy Granola Apple Crisp	1	104	26	13	1
Crunchy Granola Apple Crisp	1	140	26	13	1
Crunchy Granola Banana Nut	2	190	28	12	2
Crunchy Granola Maple Brown Sugar	2	180	29	11	2
Crunchy Granola Peanut Butter	2	160	30	11	2
Crunchy Granola Roasted Almond	2	190	28	11	2
Heart Healthy Chewy Granola Honey Nut	1	160	28	13	3
Heart Healthy Granola Oatmeal Raisin	1	150	30	14	3
Sweet & Salty Granola Almond	1	160	22	12	2
Sweet & Salty Granola Peanut	1	170	19	11	2
Nutri-Grain					
Nutri-Grain Blueberry	1	140	26	13	tr
Nutri-Grain Mixed Berry	1	140	26	13	tr
Post					
Honey Bunches Of Oats Banana Nut	1 (1.2 oz)	140	24	11	1
Honey Bunches Of Oats Oatmeal Raisin	1 (1.2 oz)	130	25	9	2

FOOD	PORTION	CALS	CARB	SUGAR	FIBER
Quaker					
Breakfast Bar Apple Crisp	1 (1.3 oz)	130	27	9	1
Breakfast Bar Graham Strawberry	1 (1 oz)	120	22	7	1
Breakfast Bar Iced Raspberry	1 (1.3 oz)	130	26	16	1
Breakfast Bites Iced Raspberry	1 pkg (1.3 oz)	130	28	9	3
Breakfast Bites Strawberry	1 pkg (1.3 oz)	130	27	8	2
Chewy Chocolate Chip	1 (0.8 oz)	100	18	7	1
Chewy Cookies & Cream	1 (0.8 oz)	90	18	5	2
Chewy 90 Calorie Cinnamon Sugar	1 (1 oz)	90	19	6	1
Chewy 90 Calorie Honey Nut	1 (0.8 oz)	90	19	6	1
Chewy Dipps Peanut Butter	1 (1 oz)	150	18	12	1
Chewy Low Fat S'mores	1 (1 oz)	110	22	10	1
Crunchy Granola Oats & Berries	1 (1 oz)	130	23	8	1
Oatmeal To Go Oatmeal Raisin	1 (2.1 oz)	220	43	19	5
Oatmeal To Go Raspberry Streusel	1 (2.1 oz)	220	43	19	5
Q-Smart Cranberry Vanilla Almond	1 (1 oz)	120	9	1	2
Trail Mix Cranberry Raisin & Almond	1 (1.2 oz)	150	24	10	1
Revolution Foods					
Jammy Sammy Apple Cinnamon & Oatmeal	1 (1 oz)	100	21	10	1
Organic Jammy Sammy PB & Grape	1 (1 oz)	110	19	10	1
Organic Jammy Sammy PB & Strawberry	1 (1 oz)	110	19	10	1
Rice Krispies					
Treats Original	1 (0.8 oz)	90	17	8	0
Roman Meal					
Whole Grain & Fruit	1 (2 oz)	190	43	21	6
South Beach					
100 Calorie Chocolate Delight	1 (1 oz)	100	18	4	3
100 Calorie Peanut Butter Chocolate Chip	1 (1 oz)	100	18	4	3
100 Calorie Snack Bar Mixed Berry	1 (1 oz)	100	18	5	3
Fiber Fit Granola Mocha	1 (1.2 oz)	120	25	7	9

FOOD	PORTION	CALS	CARB	SUGAR	FIBER
Fiber Fit Granola S'Mores	1 (1.2 oz)	120	25	7	9
High Protein Chocolate	1 (1.2 oz)	140	15	7	3
High Protein Cranberry Almond	1 (1.2 oz)	140	15	7	3
High Protein Maple Nut	1 (1.2 oz)	140	15	7	3
High Protein Peanut Butter	1 (1.2 oz)	140	15	6	3
Wings Of Nature					
Organic Apple Cinnamon	1 (1.2 oz)	119	21	12	3
Organic Cafe Mocha Coffee	1 (1.2 oz)	153	18	9	3
Organic Cappuccino Coffee	1 (1.2 oz)	153	17	9	2
Yotta					
Apple Cinnamon	1 (1.2 oz)	120	25	11	2
Cherry	1 (1.2 oz)	120	26	11	1
Orange	1 (1.2 oz)	120	26	11	2
CHAMPAGNE					
champagne	1 serv (3.5 oz)	84	3	1	0
mimosa	1 serv	117	12	–	tr
punch	1 serv (4 oz)	73	8	6	0

CHEESE *(see also* CHEESE DISHES, CHEESE SUBSTITUTES, COTTAGE CHEESE, CREAM CHEESE, NEUFCHATEL)

FOOD	PORTION	CALS	CARB	SUGAR	FIBER
beaufort	1 oz	115	tr	tr	0
bel paese	1 oz	112	0	0	0
bocconcini smoked	1 oz	90	1	0	0
cacio di roma sheep's milk cheese	1 oz	130	0	0	0
caerphilly	1.4 oz	150	0	–	0
cantal	1 oz	105	tr	tr	0
chabichou	1 oz	95	tr	tr	0
chaource	1 oz	83	tr	tr	0
cheddar reduced fat	1.4 oz	104	0	–	0
cheshire reduced fat	1.4 oz	108	tr	–	0
comte	1 oz	114	tr	tr	0
coulommiers	1 oz	88	tr	tr	0
crottin	1 oz	105	tr	tr	0
derby	1.4 oz	161	0	–	0
edam reduced fat	1.4 oz	92	tr	–	0
frais	1.6 oz	51	3	–	0
gloucester double	1.4 oz	162	0	–	0
goat fresh	1 oz	23	tr	tr	0

FOOD	PORTION	CALS	CARB	SUGAR	FIBER
grana padano parmesan shaved	1 tbsp	20	0	0	0
lancashire	1.4 oz	149	0	–	0
leicester	1.4 oz	160	0	–	0
lymeswold	1.4 oz	170	tr	–	0
maroilles	1 oz	97	tr	tr	0
morbier	1 oz	99	tr	tr	0
mozzarella fresh	1 oz	80	tr	0	0
picodon	1 oz	99	tr	tr	0
pont l'eveque	1 oz	86	tr	tr	0
pyrenees	1 oz	101	tr	tr	0
queso fresco	1 oz	41	1	–	0
queso manchego	1 oz	107	tr	–	0
queso panela	1 oz	74	1	–	0
raclette	1 oz	102	tr	tr	0
reblochon	1 oz	88	tr	tr	0
rouy	1 oz	95	tr	tr	0
saint marcellin	1 oz	94	tr	tr	0
saint nectaire	1 oz	97	tr	tr	0
saint paulin	1 oz	85	tr	tr	0
sainte maure	1 oz	99	tr	tr	0
selles sur cher	1 oz	93	tr	tr	0
stilton blue	1.4 oz	164	0	–	0
stilton white	1.4 oz	145	0	–	0
tome	1 oz	92	tr	tr	0
triple creme	1 oz	113	tr	tr	0
vacherin	1 oz	92	tr	tr	0
wensleydale	1.4 oz	151	0	–	0
whey cheese	1 oz	126	9	0	0
yogurt cheese	1 oz	80	0	0	0
Applegate Farms					
Organic Cheddar Milk	1 slice (0.7 oz)	85	0	0	0
Organic Muenster Kase	1 slice (0.8 oz)	85	0	0	0
Athenos					
Traditional	¼ cup	90	2	0	tr
Traditional Reduced Fat	¼ cup	70	1	0	tr
Bel Gioioso					
Mozzarella Fresh	1 in cube (1 oz)	80	0	0	0
Boar's Head					
American	1 oz	100	1	0	0

FOOD	PORTION	CALS	CARB	SUGAR	FIBER
American 25% Lower Sodium 25% Lower Fat	1 oz	90	1	0	0
ButterKase	1 oz	100	0	0	0
Cheddar Sharp	1 oz	110	tr	0	0
Colby Jack	1 oz	110	0	0	0
Cream Havarti	1 oz	110	0	0	0
Creamy Blue	1 oz	90	0	0	0
Double Gloucester Yellow	1 oz	110	0	0	0
Edam	1 oz	90	0	0	0
Feta	1 oz	60	1	0	0
Gouda	1 oz	110	0	0	0
Lacey Swiss	1 oz	90	0	0	0
Longhorn Colby	1 oz	110	tr	0	0
Monterey Jack	1 oz	100	0	0	0
Mozzarella	1 oz	90	1	0	0
Muenster	1 oz	100	0	0	0
Muenster Low Sodium	1 oz	100	0	0	0
Provolone 42% Lower Sodium	1 oz	100	1	0	0
Provolone Picante Sharp	1 oz	100	1	0	0
Swiss No Salt Added	1 oz	110	tr	0	0
Cabot					
Cheddar	1 oz	110	tr	0	0
Cheddar Horseradish	1 oz	110	1	0	0
Cheddar Tomato Basil	1 oz	110	tr	0	0
Cheddar Light 50% Reduced Fat	1 oz	70	tr	0	0
Cheddar Light 50% Reduced Fat Omega-3	1 oz	70	tr	0	0
Cheddar Light 75% Reduced Fat	1 oz	60	tr	0	0
Cheddar Shake	2 tsp	25	1	1	0
Monterey Jack	1 oz	110	tr	0	0
Pepper Jack 50% Reduced Fat	1 oz	70	tr	0	0
Swiss Slices	1 (1 oz)	110	1	0	0
Connoisseur					
Asiago Spread	1 tbsp	90	2	2	0
Brie Spread	2 tbsp	90	2	2	0
Gorgonzola Spread	1 tbsp	90	2	2	0
Wheel Asiago Pesto	2 tbsp	90	4	4	0
Wheel Swiss Bacon	2 tbsp	90	2	2	0
Cracker Barrel					
Fontina	1 slice (0.7 oz)	80	tr	0	0

FOOD	PORTION	CALS	CARB	SUGAR	FIBER
Sharp Cheddar 2% Milk	1 oz	90	tr	0	0
Crystal Farms					
American Singles	1 slice (0.7 oz)	70	2	1	0
American Singles 2%	1 slice (0.7 oz)	50	2	1	0
American Singles Fat Free	1 slice (0.7 oz)	30	2	2	0
Blue Crumbled	2 tbsp	100	0	0	0
Cheese Curds	8 pieces (1 oz)	110	1	0	0
Cheezoids Sticks	1 piece (0.8 oz)	70	tr	0	0
Danish Havarti	1 oz	110	0	0	0
Deli Slices Muenster	1 slice (0.8 oz)	80	0	0	0
Deli Slices Swiss	1 slice (0.7 oz)	80	0	0	0
Feta Crumbled	¼ cup	90	2	0	tr
Gorgonzola Crumbled	2 tbsp	100	0	0	0
It's So Cheesy Cheddar Aerosol	2 tbsp	90	3	2	0
Little Chunks To Go	1 pkg (0.7 oz)	80	tr	0	0
Marble Jack	1 oz	110	tr	0	0
Parmesan Grated	2 tsp	25	0	0	0
Pepper Jack	1 oz	110	tr	0	0
Ricotta	¼ cup	90	4	2	0
Shredded Mexican 4 Cheese	¼ cup	100	tr	0	0
Shredded Mozzarella	¼ cup	80	tr	0	0
Shredded Pizza Blend	¼ cup	100	tr	0	0
Shredded Sharp Cheddar	¼ cup	110	tr	0	0
Smoked Gouda	1 oz	100	tr	0	0
String	1 piece (1 oz)	80	1	0	0
Dragone					
Mozzarella Whole Milk	1 oz	90	tr	0	0
Parmesan Wedge	1 oz	100	tr	tr	0
Ricotta Part Skim	¼ cup (2.2 oz)	90	4	3	0
Easy Cheese					
American	2 tbsp (1.1 oz)	90	2	1	0
Cheddar	2 tbsp (1.1 oz)	90	2	1	0
Fage					
Feta	1 oz	80	0	0	0
Finlandia					
Muenster	1 slice (1.1 oz)	120	tr	0	0
Swiss Thin Sliced	1 slice (0.5 oz)	55	0	0	0
Fresh Made					
Farmers Cheese Nonfat	2 tbsp	15	1	0	0

FOOD	PORTION	CALS	CARB	SUGAR	FIBER
Friendship					
Farmer	2 tbsp (1 oz)	50	0	0	0
Farmer No Salt Added	2 tbsp (1 oz)	50	0	0	0
Frigo					
Mozzarella Part Skim	1 oz	80	tr	0	0
Parmesan Shredded	¼ cup (1 oz)	100	1	1	tr
Ricotta Whole Milk	¼ cup (2.2 oz)	110	2	2	0
Romano Shredded	¼ cup (1 oz)	100	1	tr	tr
Haolam					
Cheddar Sliced	1 slice (1 oz)	114	1	0	0
Heluva Good Cheese					
Cheddar Extra Sharp	1 oz	110	1	0	0
Horizon Organic					
American	1 slice (0.7 oz)	60	1	1	0
Cheddar	1 oz	110	tr	0	0
Monterey Jack	1 oz	100	0	0	0
Shred Mexican	¼ cup	110	tr	0	0
Shred Parmesan	1 tbsp	20	0	0	0
Slice Provolone	1 slice (0.7 oz)	70	0	0	0
Sticks Colby	1 (1 oz)	110	tr	0	0
String Mozzarella	1 stick (1 oz)	80	tr	0	0
J.L. Kraft					
Spreadable Feta & Spinach	2 tbsp	80	1	tr	0
Kraft					
Cheddar Sharp Shredded 2% Milk	¼ cup	80	tr	0	0
Crumbles Three Cheese	¼ cup (1 oz)	110	tr	0	0
LiveActive 1% Milk Cheddar Cubes	7 (1 oz)	90	tr	0	0
LiveActive 2% Milk Marbled Colby & Monterey Jack	1 stick (1 oz)	90	tr	0	0
LiveActive Cheddar Cheese Sticks	1 (1 oz)	120	0	0	0
LiveActive Colby & Monterey Jack Cubes	7 (1 oz)	110	tr	0	0
LiveActive Mozzarella Sticks	1 (1 oz)	80	tr	0	0
Shredded Mexican Style Cheddar & Monterey Jack	¼ cup	110	1	0	0
Singles American 2%	1 (0.7 oz)	50	2	2	0

FOOD	PORTION	CALS	CARB	SUGAR	FIBER
Land O Lakes					
American	1 slice (0.7 oz)	70	2	1	0
Chedarella	1 oz	110	0	0	0
Cheddar	1 oz	110	0	0	0
Snack 'N Cheese To Go Cheddar Mild	1 serv (0.7 oz)	80	0	0	0
Snack 'N Cheese To Go Cheddar Mild Reduced Fat	1 serv (0.5 oz)	60	0	0	0
Snack 'N Cheese To Go Co-Jack	1 serv (0.7 oz)	80	0	0	0
Snack 'N Cheese To Go Co-Jack Reduced Fat	1 serv (0.7 oz)	60	0	0	0
Swiss	1 oz	110	1	1	0
Lifeway					
Farmer's Kefir	2 tbsp	25	4	1	0
Farmer's Kefir Lite	2 tbsp	25	2	1	0
Sweet Kiss Peach	1 oz	45	6	6	0
Mt Vikos					
Feta Sheep & Goat Milk	1 oz	80	1	0	0
Organic Valley					
Blue Crumbles	1 oz	100	1	0	0
Cheddar Mild	1 oz	110	0	0	0
Feta	1 oz	60	tr	0	0
Monterey Jack Shredded	¼ cup	80	1	0	0
Muenster	1 slice (0.7 oz)	80	0	0	0
Provolone	1 slice (0.7 oz)	70	0	0	0
Swiss	1 oz	110	0	0	0
Polly-O					
Mozzarella Shredded	¼ cup	90	tr	0	0
Rouge Et Noir					
Breakfast	1 oz	90	0	0	0
Brie Garlic	1 oz	90	0	0	0
Brie Pesto	1 oz	90	0	0	0
Brie Tomato Basil	1 oz	90	0	0	0
Brie Triple Creme	1 oz	110	0	0	0
Camembert	1 oz	90	0	0	0
Le Petit Bleu	1 oz	110	0	0	0
Le Petit Chevre	1 oz	90	0	0	0
Marin French Blue	1 oz	110	0	0	0
Marin French Gold	1 oz	110	0	0	0
Schlosskranz	1 oz	85	0	0	0

FOOD	PORTION	CALS	CARB	SUGAR	FIBER
Saladena					
Goat Crumbles	¼ cup	80	tr	0	0
Sap Sago					
Fat Free Cheese Grated	1 tsp	10	0	0	0
Sargento					
4 Cheese Italian Shredded	¼ cup	80	1	0	0
4 Cheese Mexican Reduced Fat Shredded	¼ cup (1 oz)	80	tr	0	0
American Burger	1 slice (0.7 oz)	70	tr	0	0
Bistro Blends Shredded Mozzarella w/ Sun Dried Tomato & Basil	¼ cup	90	1	0	0
Blue Crumbled	¼ cup (1 oz)	100	1	0	0
Cheddar Chipotle Shredded	¼ cup	100	1	0	0
Cheddar Chipotle Sticks	1 (0.7 oz)	80	1	0	0
Cheddar Mild Cubes	7 (1 oz)	120	tr	0	0
Cheddar Mild Shredded Reduced Fat	¼ cup (1 oz)	80	tr	1	0
Cheddar White Vermont Sharp	1 slice (0.7 oz)	80	0	0	0
Cheddar White Vermont Sharp Shredded	¼ cup (1 oz)	110	1	0	0
Cheese Dips Cheddar & Buttery Pretzels	1 pkg (3.8 oz)	360	47	5	2
Cheese Dips Cheddar & Tortilla Chips	1 pkg (3 oz)	320	26	4	1
Colby-Jack Shredded	¼ cup (1 oz)	110	1	0	0
Fancy 6 Cheese Italian Shredded	¼ cup	90	1	0	0
Jarlsberg	1 slice (0.8 oz)	80	tr	0	0
Monterey Jack Shredded	¼ cup (1 oz)	110	1	0	0
Mozzarella Reduced Fat Shredded	¼ cup (1 oz)	80	tr	0	0
Mozzarella Shredded	¼ cup (1 oz)	80	1	0	0
Muenster	1 slice (0.7 oz)	80	0	0	0
Nacho & Taco Shredded	¼ cup (1 oz)	110	1	0	0
Parmesan Grated	2 tsp (5 g)	25	0	0	0
Parmesan Shredded	2 tsp	20	0	0	0
Pepper Jack	1 slice (0.7 oz)	80	0	0	0
Provolone	1 slice (0.7 oz)	70	0	0	0
Provolone Reduced Fat	1 slice (0.7 oz)	50	0	0	0

FOOD	PORTION	CALS	CARB	SUGAR	FIBER
Ricotta Fat Free	¼ cup	50	5	2	0
Ricotta Light	¼ cup	60	3	3	0
Ricotta Whole Milk	¼ cup	90	3	3	0
String	1 piece (1 oz)	80	tr	0	0
String Light	1 piece (0.7 oz)	50	tr	0	0
Swiss Reduced Fat	1 slice (0.7 oz)	80	1	0	0
Swiss Shredded	¼ cup (1 oz)	110	tr	0	0
Swiss Thick Slice	1 slice (1 oz)	110	1	0	0
Swiss Thin Sliced	1 slice (0.6 oz)	70	0	0	0
Smart Balance					
Cheddar Shredded	1 oz	80	tr	0	0
Mozzarella Shredded	1 oz	80	tr	0	0
Sorrento					
Mozzarella Fresh	1 oz	90	0	0	0
Stella					
3 Cheese Italian Shredded	¼ cup	100	1	tr	tr
Asiago Wedge	1 oz	110	tr	tr	0
Gorgonzola Wedge	1 oz	100	tr	0	0
Kasseri Wedge	1 oz	110	tr	tr	0
Weight Watchers					
String Light	1 stick (0.8 oz)	50	tr	0	0
Wholesome Valley					
Organic American	1 slice (0.7 oz)	50	tr	0	0
CHEESE DISHES					
Alexia					
Mozzarella Stix	2 pieces	120	13	tr	tr
Farm Rich					
Cheese Sticks Breaded	2 (2.1 oz)	210	17	0	tr
Mozzarella Bites Breaded	4 (2.2 oz)	150	13	3	1
Original Cheese Bites Breaded	7 (2.1 oz)	180	13	0	tr
Fillo Factory					
Tyropita Cheese Fillo Appetizers	3 (3 oz)	230	19	2	0
Stouffer's					
Welsh Rarebit	¼ pkg (2.5 oz)	140	6	2	0
TAKE-OUT					
fried mozzarella sticks	3 (4.6 oz)	503	20	2	1
souffle	1 serv (7 oz)	504	18	5	1
welsh rarebit	1 slice	228	14	–	1

FOOD	PORTION	CALS	CARB	SUGAR	FIBER
CHEESE SUBSTITUTES					
Playfood					
Cheesey Cheese	1 oz	60	4	0	1
Rice					
American Flavor	1 slice (0.7 oz)	50	tr	0	0
Shreds Mozzarella Flavor	1/3 cup (1 oz)	70	3	0	0
Vegan American Flavor	1 slice (0.7 oz)	45	0	0	0
Sheese					
Blue Style	1 oz	100	3	0	0
Cheddar Style Medium	1 oz	100	3	0	0
Creamy Mexican	2 tbsp	80	2	0	0
Creamy Original	2 tbsp	80	2	0	0
Super Stix					
Mozzarella Flavor	1 (1 oz)	70	0	0	0
Vegan Gourmet					
Cheese Alternative Cheddar	1 oz	50	2	0	2
Cheese Alternative Monterey Jack	1 oz	70	2	0	2
Cheese Alternative Mozzarella	1 oz	70	1	0	1
Cheese Alternative Nacho	1 oz	45	2	0	2
Veggie					
American Flavor	1 slice (0.6 oz)	40	tr	0	0
Grated Parmesan Flavor	2 tsp	15	0	0	0
Pepper Jack Flavor	1 oz	60	2	0	0
Shreds Cheddar Flavor	1 oz	70	0	0	0
Veggy					
Mozzarella Flavor	1 slice (0.7 oz)	40	tr	0	0
CHERRIES					
CANNED					
maraschino	1 (4 g)	7	2	2	tr
maraschino	1/4 cup (1.4 oz)	66	17	16	1
sour in heavy syrup	1/2 cup	116	30	28	1
sour in light syrup	1/2 cup	94	24	–	1
sour water packed	1/2 cup	44	11	9	1
sweet juice pack	1/2 cup	68	17	15	2
sweet pitted in heavy syrup	1/2 cup	105	27	25	2
sweet water pack	1/2 cup	57	15	13	2
Chukar Cherries					
Cherry Jubilee Dessert Sauce	1 tbsp	40	10	8	tr

FOOD	PORTION	CALS	CARB	SUGAR	FIBER
DRIED					
bing unsulfured	¼ cup	130	31	21	2
montmorency tart pitted	⅓ cup	160	36	24	2
tart	½ cup	200	49	41	2
yogurt covered	¼ cup	170	29	22	5
Bob's Red Mill					
Tart	⅓ cup	140	33	18	11
Chukar Cherries					
Bing	3 tbsp	130	33	29	3
Bing Chocolate Covered	3 tbsp (1.4 oz)	180	24	19	2
Cabernet Dark Chocolate Covered	2 tbsp (1.5 oz)	180	26	17	3
Columbia River Tart	⅓ cup	120	36	24	2
Rainier	3 tbsp	130	33	29	3
Totally Tart	⅓ cup	140	33	16	3
De-Lite					
Tart	1 oz	95	23	22	1
Eden					
Montmorency	¼ cup	140	36	31	3
Emily's					
Dark Chocolate Covered	11 (1.4 oz)	180	27	23	2
Frieda's					
Bing	¼ cup (1.4 oz)	120	26	17	3
Tart	⅓ cup (1.4 oz)	150	33	22	2
Good Sense					
Cherries	⅓ cup	145	33	22	2
Peeled Snacks					
Fruit Picks Cherry-Go-Round	1 pkg (1.5 oz)	130	30	24	4
Sunsweet					
Tart & Sweet	¼ cup (1.4 oz)	100	30	22	2
FRESH					
sour	1 cup	52	13	9	2
sour pitted	1 cup	78	19	13	3
sweet	20	86	22	17	3
Rainier					
Sweet Premium Northwest	1 cup	90	22	19	3
FROZEN					
sour unsweetened	½ cup	36	9	7	1
sweet sweetened	½ cup	115	29	26	3

FOOD	PORTION	CALS	CARB	SUGAR	FIBER
CHERRY JUICE					
tart cherry concentrate	1 cup	140	34	27	0
Eden					
Organic Montmorency	8 oz	140	33	25	0
Froose					
Cheerful Cherry	1 box (4.2 oz)	80	19	7	3
HP					
Tart Montmorency Concentrate	1 oz	80	19	15	0
Smart Juice					
Organic 100% Juice Tart Cherry	8 oz	130	32	24	1
Tart Is Smart					
Tart Cherry Concentrate	1 oz	80	19	15	0
CHESTNUTS					
creme de marrons	1 oz	73	18	10	1
ready-to-eat vacuum packed	5 (1 oz)	40	8	0	0
roasted	3 (1 oz)	70	15	3	1
Gefen					
Whole Roasted & Peeled	¼ cup (1.4 oz)	52	11	11	1
CHEWING GUM					
bubble gum	1 block	20	5	5	tr
stick	1 piece	7	2	2	tr
sugarless	1 piece	5	2	0	0
Choward's					
Scented Gum	3 pieces	10	3	3	0
Dubble Bubble					
Gumball	1 piece	10	2	2	0
Orbit					
White Melon Breeze	2 pieces	5	2	0	0
CHICKEN (*see also* CHICKEN DISHES, CHICKEN SUBSTITUTES, DINNER, HOT DOG)					
CANNED					
chicken spread	1 serv (2 oz)	88	2	tr	tr
meat drained	1 can (5 oz)	230	1	0	0
w/ broth	½ can (2.5 oz)	117	0	0	0
Swanson					
Chunk Breast In Water	2 oz	50	1	0	0
Tyson					
Premium Chunk	½ can (2 oz)	60	0	0	0
Premium Chunk Breast	½ can (2 oz)	60	0	0	0

FOOD	PORTION	CALS	CARB	SUGAR	FIBER
Valley Fresh					
Chunk White	2 oz	70	0	0	0
White & Dark Chunk	2 oz	80	0	0	0
FRESH					
back w/ skin roasted bones removed	1 (3.7 oz)	318	0	0	0
back w/o skin roasted bones removed	1 (2.8 oz)	191	0	0	0
breast w/ skin battered fried bones removed	½ breast (4.9 oz)	364	13	0	tr
breast w/ skin roasted bones removed	½ breast (3.4 oz)	193	0	0	0
breast w/ skin stewed bones removed	½ breast (3.9 oz)	202	0	0	0
breast w/o skin fried bones removed	½ breast (3 oz)	161	tr	0	0
breast w/o skin roasted bones removed	½ breast (3 oz)	142	0	0	0
breast w/o skin stewed bones removed	1 (3.3 oz)	143	0	0	0
breast roasted diced	1 cup (5 oz)	231	0	0	0
broiler/fryer w/ skin roasted bones removed	½ (10.5 oz)	715	0	0	0
capon meat & skin roasted bones removed	½ (1.4 lbs)	1459	0	0	0
cornish hen w/ skin roasted	1 (9 oz)	668	0	0	0
cornish hen w/ skin roasted	½ (4.5 oz)	335	0	0	0
cornish hen w/o skin roasted	1 (7.7 oz)	295	0	0	0
cornish hen w/o skin roasted	½ (4 oz)	147	0	0	0
dark meat w/o skin roasted diced	1 cup (5 oz)	287	0	0	0
drumstick w/ skin roasted bones removed	1 (1.8 oz)	112	0	0	0
drumstick w/ skin stewed bones removed	1 (2 oz)	116	0	0	0
drumstick w/o skin fried bones removed	1 (1.5 oz)	82	0	0	0
drumstick w/o skin roasted bones removed	1 (1.5 oz)	76	0	0	0

FOOD	PORTION	CALS	CARB	SUGAR	FIBER
drumstick w/o skin stewed bones removed	1 (1.6 oz)	78	0	0	0
feet cooked	1 (1.2 oz)	73	tr	0	0
ground crumbled fried	3 oz	161	0	0	0
ground patty cooked	1 sm (1.7 oz)	114	0	0	0
ground patty cooked	1 med (2.1 oz)	142	0	0	0
ground patty cooked	1 lg (2.8 oz)	190	0	0	0
meat & skin stewed bones removed	¼ chicken (4.6 oz)	372	0	0	0
neck w/ skin simmered	1 (1.3 oz)	94	0	0	0
roaster meat & skin roasted bones removed	¼ chicken (8.4 oz)	535	0	0	0
skin roasted from ½ chicken	2 oz	254	0	0	0
skin stewed from ½ chicken	2.5 oz	261	0	0	0
tail cooked	1 (1 oz)	84	3	0	tr
thigh w/ skin roasted bones removed	1 (2.2 oz)	153	0	0	0
thigh w/ skin stewed bones removed	1 (2.4 oz)	158	0	0	0
thigh w/o skin roasted bones removed	1 (1.8 oz)	109	0	0	0
thigh w/o skin stewed bones removed	1 (1.9 oz)	107	0	0	0
wing w/ skin roasted bones removed	1 (1.4 oz)	100	0	0	0
wing w/o skin fried bones removed	1 (0.7 oz)	42	0	0	0
wing w/o skin roasted bones removed	1 (0.7 oz)	43	0	0	0
wing w/o skin stewed bones removed	1 (0.8 oz)	43	0	0	0
Tyson					
Breasts Boneless Skinless	4 oz	110	0	0	0
Cornish Hen	1 serv (4 oz)	200	0	0	0
Drumsticks	4 oz	150	0	0	0
Thigh Cutlets Boneless Skinless	4 oz	130	0	0	0
Whole Cut Up	4 oz	220	0	0	0
Wings	4 oz	220	0	0	0
FROZEN					
breast roll roasted	2 oz	75	1	tr	0

FOOD	PORTION	CALS	CARB	SUGAR	FIBER
fajita strips	1 (0.3 oz)	13	tr	0	0
patty cooked	1 (3.5 oz)	287	13	0	tr
Barber					
Buffalo Fingers	1 (3.3 oz)	160	18	0	tr
Nuggets 4 Cheese Stuffed	3 (3 oz)	230	9	1	tr
Nuggets Cheddar & Bacon Stuffed	3 (3 oz)	240	8	1	tr
Potato Chip Sticks	2 pieces (4.5 oz)	350	16	0	tr
Health Is Wealth					
Nuggets	4 (3 oz)	130	11	0	0
Ian's					
Fingers	3 pieces	190	14	1	0
Nuggets	5 pieces	190	14	1	0
Nuggets Allergy Free	5 pieces	190	14	1	0
Patties	1 (3.4 oz)	220	16	1	0
Organic Prairie					
Whole Young Small	4 oz	260	0	0	0
Tyson					
Any'tizers Barbeque Style Wings	3 (3.2 oz)	200	7	7	0
Any'tizers Homestyle Chicken Fries	7 (3.2 oz)	230	19	0	1
Any'tizers Popcorn Chicken	6 (2.8 oz)	220	19	1	1
Breast Pattie	1 (2.6 oz)	180	12	1	1
Cordon Bleu	1 piece (5.9 oz)	380	20	6	1
Diced Strips	1 serv (3 oz)	90	0	0	0
Kiev	1 piece (5.9 oz)	480	19	6	1
Wellshire					
Chicken Bites Dinosaur Shaped Gluten Free	5 pieces	160	15	1	2
READY-TO-EAT					
Applegate Farms					
Organic Roasted	2 oz	60	1	1	0
Boar's Head					
Breast Hickory Smoked	2 oz	60	0	0	0
Breast Oven Roasted	2 oz	60	0	0	0

FOOD	PORTION	CALS	CARB	SUGAR	FIBER
Butterball					
Breast Oven Roasted Thin Sliced	4 slices (2 oz)	50	1	0	0
Healthy Ones					
Oven Roasted 97% Fat Free	4 slices (2 oz)	60	2	tr	0
Oscar Mayer					
Breast Oven Roasted Thin Sliced	⅓ pkg (2 oz)	60	1	1	0
Sara Lee					
Breast Oven Roasted	4 slices (2 oz)	45	0	0	0
Tyson					
Chicken Strips Fajita	1 serv (3 oz)	110	3	0	0
Honey Roasted Breast	2 slices (1.6 oz)	50	3	2	0
Hot Wings Buffalo Style	4	220	1	0	0
Roasted Whole Chicken Lemon Pepper	1 serv (3 oz)	120	1	1	0
Salad Kit Chunk Chicken	1 pkg (3.4 oz)	210	15	3	1
TAKE-OUT					
chicken tenders	4 (2.2 oz)	180	11	1	tr

CHICKEN DISHES
FROZEN

FOOD	PORTION	CALS	CARB	SUGAR	FIBER
Barber					
Broccoli & Cheese Reduced Fat	1 piece (5.5 oz)	250	11	1	tr
Cordon Bleu	1 piece (6 oz)	370	14	1	0
Cordon Bleu Reduced Fat	1 piece (5.5 oz)	260	11	1	0
Creme Brie & Apple	1 piece (6 oz)	350	18	8	tr
Kiev	1 piece (6 oz)	430	15	1	tr
Mashed Potato Stuffed	1 piece (6 oz)	340	21	2	tr
Skinless Breast Stuffed	1 piece (6 oz)	280	24	1	tr
Maple Leaf Farms					
Chicken Breast Stuffed Broccoli & Cheese	1 serv (6 oz)	340	20	2	0
MIX					
Chicken Helper					
Asian Chicken Fried Rice as prep	1 cup	250	22	1	1

FOOD	PORTION	CALS	CARB	SUGAR	FIBER
Classic Creamy Chicken & Noodles as prep	1 cup	280	24	1	tr
Jambalaya as prep	1 cup	280	15	tr	1
REFRIGERATED					
Lunchables					
Chicken Shake-Up	1 pkg	220	29	16	tr
Tyson					
Chicken Breast Medallions In White Wine & Garlic Sauce	1 serv (5 oz)	140	3	0	1
Ventera					
Rollatini w/ Rice Stuffing & Marsala Wine Sauce	1 serv + sauce (6 oz)	230	9	2	0
Wellshire					
Shredded Chicken In BBQ Sauce	¼ cup	70	8	4	0
TAKE-OUT					
arroz con pollo	1 serv (16 oz)	579	62	3	2
barbecued pulled chicken	1 serv (9 oz)	312	37	27	2
boneless breast w/ apple stuffing	1 serv (5 oz)	260	10	2	1
buffalo wing + sauce	2 (1.7 oz)	147	tr	tr	0
cacciatore breast + sauce	1 serv (5.9 oz)	323	9	3	1
cacciatore drumstick + sauce	1 serv (3.2 oz)	172	5	2	1
cacciatore thigh + sauce	1 serv (3.8 oz)	204	6	2	1
cacciatore wing + sauce	1 serv (2.1 oz)	113	3	1	tr
chicharrones de pollo	3 (2.6 oz)	289	14	tr	1
chicken & dumplings	1 cup (8.6 oz)	368	22	1	1
chicken & noodles in cream sauce	1 cup (8 oz)	323	32	5	1
chicken a la king	1 cup (8.5 oz)	465	16	4	1
chicken cordon bleu + sauce	1 roll (8 oz)	504	11	1	1
chicken meatloaf	1 lg slice (5 oz)	243	11	3	1
chicken pie w/ top crust	1 slice (5.6 oz)	472	32	—	1
chicken satay + peanut sauce	2 skewers	239	6	4	1
chicken breast parmigiana	1 serv (5.8 oz)	278	13	3	1
chicken creole w/o rice	1 cup (8.6 oz)	187	8	5	2
chicken kiev breast meat	1 serv (9 oz)	653	11	1	1
creamed chicken	1 cup (8.5 oz)	388	14	8	tr

FOOD	PORTION	CALS	CARB	SUGAR	FIBER
croquette	1 (2.2 oz)	159	8	2	tr
curry	1 cup (8.3 oz)	288	9	5	2
curry breast half + sauce	1 (7 oz)	244	8	4	2
curry drumstick + sauce	1 (3.7 oz)	129	4	2	1
curry thigh + sauce	1 (4.4 oz)	154	5	3	1
curry wing + sauce	1 (2.4 oz)	84	3	1	1
fricassee	1 cup (8.6 oz)	322	8	tr	tr
groundnut stew hkatenkwan	1 serv (15.7 oz)	576	18	3	4
jamaican jerk wings	4 wings (9.9 oz)	709	3	tr	tr
jambalaya w/ sausage & rice	1 cup (8.6 oz)	393	23	2	1
sancocho de pollo dominican chicken stew	1 serv	702	34	4	1
stew	1 cup (8.8 oz)	176	19	4	3
tetrazzini	1 cup (8.6 oz)	369	29	2	2

CHICKEN SUBSTITUTES

Boca
Chik'n Nuggets	1 serv (3 oz)	180	17	2	3
Chik'n Patties	1 (2.5 oz)	160	15	1	2

Chicken Free Chicken
Country Smoked	2 oz	80	5	1	0

Gardenburger
Chik'n Grill	1 (2.5 oz)	100	5	0	5

Health Is Wealth
Chicken-Free Nuggets	3 pieces (2.9 oz)	120	14	0	2

Lightlife
Smart Cutlet Seasoned Chicken	1 (4 oz)	180	11	3	4
Smart Menu Chick'n Nuggets	4 pieces	220	16	1	2
Smart Menu Chick'n Patties	1 patty	160	14	0	2
Smart Menu Chick'n Strips	1 serv (3 oz)	80	5	0	3

Loma Linda
Fried Chik'n w/ Gravy	2 pieces (2.8 oz)	150	5	0	2

Morningstar Farms
Chik'n Roasted Herb	1 pattie (2.2 oz)	110	9	1	2
Meal Starters Chik'n Strips	12 pieces (3 oz)	140	6	1	1

FOOD	PORTION	CALS	CARB	SUGAR	FIBER
Quorn					
Cutlets	1 (3.5 oz)	200	20	2	4
Gruyere Cutlet	1 (4 oz)	260	23	3	3
Naked Cutlet	1 (2.4 oz)	80	5	0	2
Veat					
Chick'n Free Nuggets	1 serv (2.5 oz)	140	5	2	2
Vegetarian Breast	1 (1.8 oz)	90	5	1	tr
Viana					
Veggie Chickin Fillets	1 (3.7 oz)	260	8	5	4
Veggie Chickin Nuggets	3 pieces (2.6 oz)	200	8	1	2
Worthington					
FriChik Original	2 pieces (3.2 oz)	140	3	0	1
Meatless Chicken Style	1 slice (2 oz)	90	2	0	1
Yves					
Meatless Chicken Burger	1 (2.6 oz)	100	5	tr	2
Meatless Smoked Chicken Slices	4 (2.2 oz)	100	5	1	0
CHICKPEAS					
CANNED					
Allens					
Garbanzo Beans	½ cup	120	19	0	8
Eden					
Organic Garbanzo	½ cup	130	23	tr	5
Green Giant					
Garbanzo Beans	½ cup	100	17	2	4
Progresso					
ChickPeas	½ cup	100	17	2	4
DRIED					
Arrowhead Mills					
Organic Dried Chickpeas not prep	¼ cup	160	27	5	8
REFRIGERATED					
Sabra					
Balela Vinaigrette	2 oz	100	11	2	3
Spicy Armenian Salad	2 oz	50	5	2	1

FOOD	PORTION	CALS	CARB	SUGAR	FIBER
CHICORY					
Frieda's					
Belgian Endive	2 cups	115	3	1	3
CHILI					
powder	1 tbsp	24	4	1	3
Ahh!Gourmet					
Wriggly Sambal Chili Sauce Paste	4 tbsp	170	15	11	4
Allergaroo					
Gluten Free Chili Mac	1 pkg (8 oz)	240	50	8	3
Boca					
Chili w/ Ground Burger	1 pkg (9.4 oz)	150	25	6	12
Bush's					
ChiliMagic Chili Starter as prep	1 cup	250	17	5	4
Comfort Care					
Vegetarian White	1 cup (8 oz)	150	26	4	5
Dennison's					
Con Carne	1 cup	350	31	2	11
Fat Free w/ Beans	1 cup	210	29	2	8
Turkey	1 cup	210	29	3	7
Vegetarian	1 cup	190	34	6	9
Fantastic					
3 Bean	1 pkg (8 oz)	180	28	5	5
Vegetarian Mix not prep	¼ cup	100	17	4	4
Health Valley					
Chunky Spicy Vegetarian No Salt Added	1 cup	150	31	5	10
Vegetarian Spicy	1 cup	150	31	5	10
Heinz					
Chili Sauce	1 tbsp (0.6 oz)	20	5	3	0
Lightlife					
Smart Chili	1 pkg	200	34	8	12
McIlhenny					
Original Recipe	½ cup	50	10	5	3
Mimi's Gourmet					
Organic Vegan Gluten Free 3 Bean w/ Rice	1 pkg (11.5 oz)	270	46	9	10
Organic Vegan Gluten Free Black Bean & Corn	1 pkg (10.5 oz)	250	40	9	11

FOOD	PORTION	CALS	CARB	SUGAR	FIBER
Organic Vegan Gluten Free White Bean	1 pkg (10.5 oz)	230	35	11	9
Ro-Tel					
Chili Fixin's	½ cup	35	8	5	3
Spice Hunter					
Powder Blend Salt Free	¼ tsp	0	0	0	0
Stagg					
Chunkero w/ Beans	1 cup	300	26	6	5
Classic w/ Beans	1 cup	330	28	7	5
Ranch House Chicken w/ Beans	1 cup	290	32	6	6
Silverado Beef w/ Beans	1 cup	230	33	7	6
Turkey Ranchero w/ Beans	1 cup	240	31	6	6
Vegetable Garden Four Bean	1 cup	200	37	9	7
Worthington					
Vegetarian	1 cup	280	25	3	8
TAKE-OUT					
chiles rellenos cheese filled	1 (5 oz)	365	8	5	1
chili con carne w/ beans	1 cup	264	22	6	7
chili con carne w/ beans & chicken	1 cup (8.9 oz)	218	19	6	6
con carne w/ beans & rice	1 cup	298	45	2	7
vegetarian con carne	1 cup	272	35	7	11

CHILI PEPPER (see PEPPERS)

CHINESE FOOD (see ASIAN FOOD)

CHIPS (see also SNACKS)

FOOD	PORTION	CALS	CARB	SUGAR	FIBER
apple chips	10 (0.8 oz)	101	16	14	2
banana	1 oz	147	17	10	2
carrot	28 (1 oz)	95	22	11	7
corn	1 oz	147	18	tr	2
plantain	1 oz	158	16	–	1
potato salted	1 oz	155	14	tr	1
potato sticks	1 pkg (1 oz)	148	15	tr	1
potato sticks	½ cup (0.6 oz)	94	10	tr	1
potato unsalted	1 oz	152	15	tr	1
potato unsalted reduced fat	1 oz	138	19	tr	2
soy	1 oz	107	15	1	1
sweet potato	1 oz	141	18	2	1
taro	10 (0.8 oz)	115	16	1	2
tortilla low fat baked	1 oz	118	23	tr	2

FOOD	PORTION	CALS	CARB	SUGAR	FIBER
tortilla low fat unsalted	1 oz	118	23	tr	2
tortilla white corn	1 oz	139	19	tr	2
tortilla yellow corn	1 oz	139	19	tr	1
Athenos					
Pita Chips Original	11 (1 oz)	120	19	tr	0
Boulder Canyon					
Potato 50% Reduced Salt	14 (1 oz)	150	17	0	2
Potato Sour Cream & Chive	14 (1 oz)	150	15	1	2
Potato Spinach & Artichoke	14 (1 oz)	150	17	0	2
Bravos!					
Tortilla Nacho Cheese	1 oz	150	17	tr	1
Brothers-All-Natural					
Potato Crisps Fresh Onion & Fresh Garlic	1 pkg	45	10	0	1
Potato Crisps Original w/ Sea Salt	1 pkg	45	10	0	1
Burger King					
Potato Flame Broiled	16 (1 oz)	150	19	1	1
Potato Ketchup & Fries	16 (1 oz)	150	19	1	1
Butterfield					
Potato Sticks Shoestring	1 pkg (1.7 oz)	250	26	0	3
Cape Cod					
Potato 40% Reduced Fat	19	130	18	tr	1
Potato Beachside BBQ	19	150	17	tr	1
Potato Classic	19	150	17	tr	1
Potato Fresh Garden Herb Reduced Fat	19	130	19	tr	1
Potato Jalapeno & Cheddar	19	140	16	tr	3
Potato No Salt	19	150	14	tr	tr
Potato Robust Russet	19	150	16	tr	1
Potato Salt & Vinegar	19	150	17	tr	1
Potato Sea Salt & Cracked Pepper	19	140	16	tr	1
Tortilla Reduced Carb	10	140	11	0	2
Tortilla Veggie	12	140	18	0	1
Corazonas					
Tortilla Jalapeno Jack	1 oz	140	16	0	3
Tortilla Original	1 oz	140	16	0	3
Tortilla Salsa Picante	1 oz	140	16	0	3

FOOD	PORTION	CALS	CARB	SUGAR	FIBER
Eden					
Brown Rice Chips	25	150	19	0	0
Sea Vegetable Chips	25	140	23	2	0
Vegetable	25	130	24	2	0
Wasabi	25	130	24	2	0
Flat Earth					
Baked Fruit Crisps Apple Cinnamon Grove	14 (1 oz)	130	21	6	2
Baked Fruit Crisps Peach Mango Paradise	14 (1 oz)	130	21	7	1
Baked Fruit Crisps Wild Berry Patch	14 (1 oz)	130	21	6	1
Baked Veggie Crisps Farmland Cheddar	14 (1 oz)	130	19	3	2
Baked Veggie Crisps Garlic & Herb Field	14 (1 oz)	130	19	3	2
Baked Veggie Crisps Tangy Tomato Ranch	14 (1 oz)	130	19	3	2
FoodShouldTasteGood					
Tortilla Buffalo	10 (1 oz)	130	18	1	3
Tortilla Chocolate Gluten Free	1 pkg (1 oz)	140	19	4	3
Tortilla Multigrain Gluten Free	1 pkg (1 oz)	140	18	2	3
Tortilla Sweet Potato Gluten Free	10 (1 oz)	130	18	2	3
French's					
Potato Sticks Barbecue	¾ cup	160	16	2	1
Potato Sticks Cheddar	¾ cup	170	14	tr	tr
Potato Sticks Original	¾ cup	190	16	0	1
Fritos					
Original	32	160	16	0	2
Garden Of Eatin'					
Organic Pita Baked Brown Sugar & Cinnamon	8	120	22	2	1
Organic Tortilla Blue Corn	7	140	18	0	2
Organic Tortilla Blue No Salt Added	16	140	18	0	2
Organic Tortilla White Corn	7	140	19	0	2
Glenny's					
Organic Soy Barbeque	1 oz	110	13	3	3
Organic Soy Creamy Ranch	1 oz	110	12	1	3

FOOD	PORTION	CALS	CARB	SUGAR	FIBER
Soy Crisps Apple Cinnamon	½ pkg (0.6 oz)	70	10	2	2
Soy Crisps Caramel	½ pkg (1.3 oz)	70	9	2	1
Soy Crisps Low Fat Lightly Salted	½ pkg (0.6 oz)	70	9	1	2
Soy Crisps No Salt	½ pkg (0.6 oz)	70	9	1	2
Soy Crisps Salt & Pepper	½ pkg (0.6 oz)	70	9	1	2
Soy Crisps White Cheddar	½ pkg (0.6 oz)	70	9	1	2
Spud Delites Sea Salt	1 pkg (1.1 oz)	100	21	0	1
Veggie Fries	½ pkg (0.6 oz)	70	13	0	0
Zen Health Tortilla Crisps Original	1 oz	110	12	0	tr
Guiltless Gourmet					
Tortilla Blue Corn	18 (1 oz)	120	23	0	2
Tortilla Chili Lime	18 (1 oz)	120	19	0	2
Tortilla Chipotle	18 (1 oz)	123	22	1	2
Tortilla Yellow Corn	18 (1 oz)	120	22	0	2
Tortilla Yellow Corn Unsalted	18 (1 oz)	120	22	1	2
Jay's					
Potato	1 oz	150	14	0	1
Kettle					
Bakes Potato Aged White Cheddar	1 oz	120	20	1	2
Bakes Potato Hickory Honey Barbeque	1 oz	120	21	0	2
Bakes Potato Lightly Salted	1 oz	120	21	0	2
Krinkle Cut Potato Barbeque	1 oz	150	16	1	2
Krinkle Cut Potato Dill & Sour Cream	1 oz	150	16	1	2
Krinkle Cut Potato Lightly Salted	1 oz	150	15	0	2
Krinkle Cut Potato Salt & Fresh Ground Pepper	1 oz	150	16	0	2
Organic Tortilla Blue Corn	1 oz	140	18	0	2
Organic Tortilla Brown Rice & Black Bean w/ Garlic & Onions	1 oz	120	16	0	2
Organic Tortilla Fire Roasted Chili	1 oz	140	18	0	2
Organic Tortilla Five Grain Yellow Corn	1 oz	140	18	0	2

FOOD	PORTION	CALS	CARB	SUGAR	FIBER
Organic Tortilla Lightly Salted Yellow Corn	1 oz	140	19	0	2
Organic Tortilla Little Dippers	1 oz	140	19	0	2
Organic Tortilla Sesame Blue Moons	1 oz	150	18	0	2
Potato Cheddar Beer	1 oz	150	15	2	1
Potato Honey Dijon	1 oz	150	16	1	1
Potato Sea Salt & Vinegar	1 oz	150	16	0	1
Potato Spicy Thai	1 oz	150	15	2	1
Potato Unsalted	1 oz	150	15	0	2
Potato Yogurt & Green Onion	1 oz	150	15	0	1
Lundberg					
Rice Chips Original Sea Salt	1 oz	140	18	0	tr
Rice Chips Sesame Seaweed	1 oz	140	18	0	tr
Rice Chips Wasabi	1 oz	140	18	1	1
Madhouse Munchies					
Potato Sea Salt	16	150	16	0	1
Potato Sea Salt & Vinegar	16	150	16	0	2
Tortilla White	9	140	19	0	1
Mexi-Snax					
Tortilla Multi-Grain Blue	15 (1 oz)	140	17	0	2
Tortilla Pico De Gallo	15 (1 oz)	140	18	0	2
Tortilla Salted	15 (1 oz)	140	18	0	2
Tortilla Tamari	15 (1 oz)	130	17	0	2
Michael Season's					
Potato Kettle Style Reduced Fat	18	130	18	1	1
Potato Reduced Fat	20	140	17	0	1
Potato Reduced Fat Unsalted	20	140	17	0	1
Potato Crisps Thin Baked Low Fat	14	120	23	2	2
Moore's					
Corn Chips	1 oz	160	16	0	1
New York Deli					
Potato Kettle Cooked	1 oz	150	15	0	1
Poore Brothers					
Original	14 (1 oz)	140	15	tr	1
Salt & Vinegar	15 (1 oz)	150	15	1	1
Sweet Maui Onion	14 (1 oz)	140	15	2	1
Popchips					
Corn Hint Of Butter	23 (1 oz)	120	17	0	2

FOOD	PORTION	CALS	CARB	SUGAR	FIBER
Potato Barbeque	19 (1 oz)	120	20	2	1
Potato Original	22 (1 oz)	120	20	0	1
Rice Sea Salt	19 (1 oz)	120	17	0	1
Rice Wasabi	20 (1 oz)	120	17	0	1
Pringles					
Jalapeno	15 (1 oz)	150	14	1	tr
Loaded Baked Potato	15 (1 oz)	150	14	1	tr
Minis Cheddar Cheese	1 pkg	120	12	1	tr
Original	14 (1 oz)	160	14	1	tr
Pizza	15 (1 oz)	150	14	1	tr
Select Cinnnamon Sweet Potato	28 (1 oz)	150	16	3	1
Select Parmesan Garlic	28 (1 oz)	140	15	1	tr
Snack Stacks Original	1 pkg	140	12	0	tr
Revolution Foods					
Organic Popalongs Whole Grains Cheesy Cheese	16 (0.7 oz)	90	14	1	1
Organic Popalongs Whole Grains Original	16 (0.7 oz)	100	15	1	1
Organic Popalongs Whole Grains Simply Cinnamon	16 (0.7 oz)	100	16	3	1
Robert's American Gourmet					
Soy Crisps Country Barbecue	1 oz	130	15	3	3
Salba Smart					
Organic Blue Corn Omega-3 Enriched	1 oz	104	19	0	4
Snyder's Of Hanover					
Kosher Dill	1 oz	140	20	1	4
MultiGrain Sunflower	1 oz	140	20	2	2
MultiGrain Sunflower Southwestern Cheddar	1 oz	140	20	2	2
MultiGrain Tortilla Lightly Salted	1 oz	130	20	2	3
MultiGrain Tortilla Strips Flaxseed Gold	1 oz	140	18	1	2
Organic Veggie Crisps	1 oz	140	18	0	2
Potato Original	1 oz	150	19	0	3
Sweet Potato Baked	1 oz	110	23	4	1
Tortilla White Corn	1 oz	140	23	0	2
Tortilla Pounder Multi-Grain	1 oz	130	20	2	2

FOOD	PORTION	CALS	CARB	SUGAR	FIBER
Solea					
Polenta Corn	1 oz	120	20	1	0
Potato Olive Oil Sea Salt	1 oz	120	14	1	1
Stacy's					
Pita Chips Multigrain	1 pkg	140	17	tr	2
Pita Chips Parmesan Garlic & Herb	1 oz	140	19	1	2
Pita Chips Texarkana Hot	1 oz	130	19	tr	2
Soy Thin Chips Sticky Bun	18 (1 oz)	130	15	3	3
Soy Thin Crisps Simply Cheese	18 (1 oz)	130	13	2	3
SunChips					
Original	1 pkg (1 oz)	140	18	2	2
T.G.I. Friday's					
Potato Cheese Pizza	16 (1 oz)	160	17	1	1
Tater Skins					
Cheddar Bacon	16 (1 oz)	150	19	1	1
Original	16 (1 oz)	150	19	1	1
Terra					
Exotic Vegetable Original	14 (1 oz)	150	16	3	3
Exotic Vegetable Zesty Tomato	14 (1 oz)	150	16	3	3
Kettles Potato Sea Salt & Pepper	15 (1 oz)	140	18	tr	tr
Parsnip Chips	12 (1 oz)	150	13	0	5
Potato Au Natural	18 (1 oz)	150	15	0	2
Potato Blues	1 oz	130	19	0	3
Potato Golds Original	1 oz	130	19	0	0
Potato Potpourri	1 oz	140	17	2	4
Potato Red Bliss	1 oz	140	18	0	2
Potato Frites Sea Salt & Vinegar	1 oz	150	18	7	3
Stix Original Exotic Vegetable	1 oz	150	16	3	3
Sweet Potato	17 (1 oz)	160	15	3	3
Sweets & Beets	16 (1 oz)	150	15	0	1
Taro	1 oz	140	19	1	4
Thunder					
Potato Buffalo Wing w/ Blue Cheese	22 (1 oz)	150	16	tr	tr
Sour Cream & Onion	22 (1 oz)	150	15	tr	tr
Utz					
Pita Natural w/ Sea Salt	1 oz	120	18	1	tr
Potato	20 (1 oz)	150	14	0	1
Potato Baked	1 oz	110	23	2	2

FOOD	PORTION	CALS	CARB	SUGAR	FIBER
Potato BBQ	20 (1 oz)	150	14	1	1
Potato Grandma Kettle	1 oz	140	14	0	1
Potato Homestyle Kettle	1 oz	140	14	0	1
Potato Kettle Classics	20 (1 oz)	150	15	0	1
Potato Mystic Kettle	1 oz	150	15	0	1
Potato Mystic Kettle Reduced Fat	1 oz	130	18	0	1
Potato Natural Lightly Salted Kettle	1 oz	140	15	0	1
Potato No Salt Added	20 (1 oz)	150	14	0	1
Potato Onion & Garlic	1 oz	150	14	tr	1
Potato Ripple	20 (1 oz)	150	14	0	1
Sweet Potato Kettle Classics	20 (1 oz)	150	16	3	2
Tortilla Baked	10	120	23	0	1
Tortilla Organic Yellow Corn	1 oz	140	19	0	2
Vegetable Natural Exotic Medley	1 oz	160	15	2	2
Wise					
Dipsy Doodles Corn Chips	1 oz	160	16	0	1
Potato	1 pkg (1 oz)	150	14	0	1
Potato Lightly Salted	1 oz	150	14	0	1
Potato Ridgies	1 oz	150	14	0	1
Potato Unsalted	1 oz	150	14	0	1
Zapp's					
Potato Cajun Dill	1 oz	150	17	0	1
Potato No Salt	1 oz	150	18	0	1
Potato Original	1 oz	150	17	0	1
Potato Sizzlin Steak	1 oz	150	17	tr	1
Sweet Potato Lightly Salted	1 oz	150	17	6	1

CHITTERLINGS

pork cooked	3 oz	258	0	0	0

CHOCOLATE *(see also* CANDY, CHOCOLATE SPREAD, CHOCOLATE SYRUP, COCOA, HOT CHOCOLATE, ICE CREAM TOPPINGS, MILK DRINKS*)*

baking grated unsweetened	¼ cup	165	10	tr	6
baking liquid unsweetened	1 oz	134	10	0	5
baking squares unsweetened	1 square (1 oz)	145	9	tr	5
mexican baking	1 sq (0.7 oz)	85	15	14	1
E. Guittard					
Chips Cappuccino	30 (0.5 oz)	80	9	9	0

FOOD	PORTION	CALS	CARB	SUGAR	FIBER
Chips Milk Chocolate	12 (0.5 oz)	80	9	9	0
Chips Semisweet	30 (0.5 oz)	70	10	8	tr
M&M's					
Baking Bits Milk Chocolate	1 tbsp	70	10	9	0
Baking Bits Semi-Sweet Chocolate	1 tbsp	70	9	8	1
Sunfood					
Organic Powder	2 tbsp (1 oz)	120	15	0	9
MIX					
Nesquik					
Chocolate Powder	2 tbsp (0.6 oz)	60	14	13	tr
Chocolate Powder No Sugar Added	2 tbsp (0.4 oz)	35	7	3	1

CHOCOLATE MILK (see MILK DRINKS)

CHOCOLATE SPREAD
Love'n Bake

FOOD	PORTION	CALS	CARB	SUGAR	FIBER
Chocolate Schmear	2 tbsp	140	14	11	2

CHOCOLATE SYRUP

FOOD	PORTION	CALS	CARB	SUGAR	FIBER
syrup as prep w/ whole milk	1 cup (9.9 oz)	254	36	32	1
Nesquik					
Calcium Fortified	2 tbsp (1.3 oz)	100	25	23	tr

CHUTNEY

FOOD	PORTION	CALS	CARB	SUGAR	FIBER
apple	1.2 oz	68	18	–	1
coconut	2 oz	87	1	1	3
fresh mint	2 oz	18	3	3	1
mango	¼ cup (2 oz)	227	43	16	10
tomato	1 oz	90	6	6	2
Chukar Cherries					
Curried Cherry	1 tbsp	30	8	7	tr
Patak's					
Major Grey	1 tbsp	60	14	14	0
Mango Hot	1 tbsp	60	14	14	0
Mango Sweet	1 tbsp	60	14	14	0
Robert Rothchild Farm					
Hot Peach & Apple	2 tbsp	45	12	9	tr
School House Kitchen					
Bardshar	1 oz	80	20	19	1

FOOD	PORTION	CALS	CARB	SUGAR	FIBER
Wild Thymes Farm					
Apricot Cranberry Walnut	1 tbsp	16	4	3	tr
Plum Currant Ginger	1 tsp	20	5	4	tr
CILANTRO					
fresh	¼ cup	1	tr	tr	tr
fresh sprigs	5 (5 g)	1	tr	tr	tr
CINNAMON					
cinnamon sugar	1 tsp	16	4	4	tr
ground	1 tsp	6	2	tr	1
sticks	0.5 oz	39	8	0	3
CISCO					
raw	3 oz	84	0	0	0
smoked	1 oz	50	0	0	0
CLAMS					
CANNED					
Brunswick					
Baby	2 oz	50	0	0	0
Bumble Bee					
Baby	¼ cup	50	2	0	0
Chopped Or Minced	¼ cup	25	2	0	0
Smoked	¼ cup	130	1	0	0
Orleans					
Clam Juice	1 tbsp	0	0	0	0
Polar					
Baby	¼ cup	30	3	0	0
FROZEN					
Mrs. Paul's					
Fried	18 (3 oz)	270	29	3	1
CLEMENTINES					
Cuties					
Fresh	2 (6 oz)	80	17	13	4
Disney Garden					
Clementines	1	35	9	7	1
CLOVES					
ground	1 tsp	7	1	tr	1

FOOD	PORTION	CALS	CARB	SUGAR	FIBER
COCOA *(see also HOT CHOCOLATE)*					
cocoa butter	1 tbsp	120	0	0	0
powder unsweetened	1 tbsp	12	3	tr	2
COCONUT					
dried sweetened shredded	¼ cup	116	11	10	1
dried unsweetened	1 oz	187	7	2	5
fresh from 1 coconut	14 oz	1405	60	25	36
fresh shredded	¼ cup	71	3	1	2
Bob's Red Mill					
Shredded	3 tbsp	120	4	1	2
Frieda's					
White	¼ cup (1.4 oz)	140	6	1	4
Let's Do Organic					
Organic Reduced Fat Shredded	1 can (0.5 oz)	70	4	0	2
Shredded	3 tbsp (0.5 oz)	110	4	1	2
Prosperity					
Organic Coconut Flax Butter Garlic & Onion	1 tbsp	140	0	0	0
COCONUT JUICE					
coconut water fresh	½ cup	23	4	3	1
creamed sweetened canned	½ cup	264	39	38	tr
milk canned	½ cup	276	7	4	3
A Taste Of Thai					
Coconut Milk	⅓ cup	140	3	0	0
Lite Coconut Milk	⅓ cup	45	3	0	0
Goya					
Coconut Water	1 can (11.8 oz)	120	29	22	tr
Let's Do Organic					
Creamed	1 oz	220	8	2	6
Milk	¼ cup	100	2	1	0
O.N.E.					
Natural Coconut Water	1 box (11 oz)	60	15	14	0
COD					
atlantic canned	1 can (11 oz)	327	0	0	0
atlantic canned	3 oz	89	0	0	0
atlantic dried	3 oz	246	0	0	0
atlantic fresh cooked	1 fillet (6.3 oz)	189	0	0	0

FOOD	PORTION	CALS	CARB	SUGAR	FIBER
atlantic fresh cooked	3 oz	89	0	0	0
atlantic fresh raw	3 oz	70	0	0	0
pacific fresh baked	3 oz	95	0	0	0
Mrs. Paul's					
Filets Lightly Breaded	1 (4 oz)	220	17	4	1

COFFEE *(see also* COFFEE BEVERAGES, COFFEE SUBSTITUTES*)*
INSTANT

decaffeinated as prep	8 oz	2	0	0	0
decaffeinated powder	1 rounded tsp	4	1	0	0
powder	1 rounded tsp	4	1	0	0
REGULAR					
brewed	8 oz	2	0	0	0
roasted beans	1 oz	64	18	–	2
Flavia					
English Breakfast	1 bag	0	0	0	0
Espresso Roast	1 bag	0	0	0	0
French Roast	1 bag	0	0	0	0
French Vanilla	1 bag	0	0	0	0
Spava					
Calm Decaffeinated	1 cup	0	0	0	0

COFFEE BEVERAGES
Cafe Sepia

House Blend	1 bottle (6.2 oz)	80	15	14	0
Mocha	1 bottle (6.2 oz)	70	14	14	0
Cinnabon					
Lattes All Flavors	1 can (9.5 oz)	190	32	30	1
Click					
Espresso Protein Drink as prep	2 scoops (1.1 oz)	120	12	7	tr
Cool Java					
Cappuccino Dark Roast	1 bottle (11 oz)	190	39	34	0
Cappuccino French Vanilla	1 bottle (11 oz)	190	38	36	0
Cappuccino Mocha	1 bottle (11 oz)	190	38	36	0

FOOD	PORTION	CALS	CARB	SUGAR	FIBER
Frappio					
Iced Coffee Energy Drink	1 can (15 oz)	260	42	38	0
Froid					
Original or French Vanilla	1 bottle (11 oz)	180	34	31	1
Godiva					
Latte French Vanilla	1 bottle (12 oz)	200	36	35	0
Mocha Dark Chocolate	1 bottle (16 oz)	200	37	35	1
Iced 'Spresso					
Ultra Light American Vanilla	1 bottle (9.5 oz)	90	11	8	0
Ultra Light Espresso Latte	1 bottle (9.5 oz)	70	11	8	0
O.N.E.					
Coffee Fruit	1 bottle (11 oz)	107	26	25	1
Shock					
Latte	8 oz	150	28	24	tr
Triple Latte	1 can (8 oz)	125	27	27	0
Triple Mocha	1 can (8 oz)	125	27	27	0
Stomping Grounds					
Latte Caramel not prep	⅓ cup	70	18	17	0
Latte Espresso not prep	⅓ cup	35	9	8	0
Latte Mocha not prep	⅓ cup	60	15	14	0
Latte Vanilla not prep	⅓ cup	60	14	13	0
Tully's Coffee					
Bellaccino All Flavors	1 bottle (9.5 oz)	210	36	34	0
TAKE-OUT					
cafe amaretto w/ alcohol	1 serv	192	15	–	0
cafe brulot w/ alcohol	1 serv	130	16	–	3
coffee con leche	1 cup (6 oz)	104	16	17	0
cuban coffee w/ rum & creme de cacao	1 (9 oz)	112	6	–	0
dutch coffee w/ gin	1 (7 oz)	181	6	5	0
espresso	1 cup (4 oz)	2	0	0	0
french coffee w/ orange liqueur & kahlua	1 (8 oz)	232	24	–	0

FOOD	PORTION	CALS	CARB	SUGAR	FIBER
irish coffee	1 serv (8 oz)	209	5	4	0
italian coffee w/ strega	1 (7 oz)	163	12	10	0
latte w/ skim milk	1 serv (13 oz)	88	12	11	0
latte w/ whole milk	1 serv (14 oz)	143	15	14	0
mocha	1 serv (17 oz)	403	69	54	2
puerto rican coffee w/ rum & kahlua	1 (8 oz)	166	9	—	0
turkish	1 cup (4 oz)	50	12	12	0

COFFEE SUBSTITUTES
Pixie
Mate Latte Chai	½ cup (4 oz)	80	18	17	tr
Mate Latte Dark Roast	½ cup (4 oz)	70	16	13	tr
Mate Latte Mocha	½ cup (4 oz)	70	18	16	0
Mate Latte Original	½ cup (4 oz)	70	17	15	0

COFFEE WHITENERS
Farmland
Nondairy Creamer	2 tbsp	40	2	1	0

Hood
Country Creamer Non Dairy	1 tbsp	20	2	0	0

International Delight
Amaretto	1 tbsp	40	7	6	0
Fat Free Amaretto	1 tbsp	30	7	6	0
Fat Free French Vanilla	1 tbsp	30	7	6	0
Fat Free Irish Creme	1 tbsp	30	7	6	0
French Vanilla	1 tbsp	45	7	6	0
Sugar Free French Vanilla	1 tbsp	20	1	0	0

WildWood
Soymilk Creamer Plain	1 tbsp	15	1	1	0

COLESLAW
Dole
Classic Cole Slaw	1½ cups (3 oz)	25	5	3	2

Fresh Express
3 Color Deli	1½ cups	20	5	3	2
Kit w/ Sweet & Creamy Dressing	3 cups	120	12	10	2
Old Fashioned	2 cups	25	5	3	2

Mann's
Broccoli Cole Slaw w/o Dressing	1 serv (3 oz)	25	5	2	3

FOOD	PORTION	CALS	CARB	SUGAR	FIBER
COLLARDS					
Allens					
Seasoned	½ cup	35	5	1	1
Glory					
Green Fresh	2 cups	25	5	0	3
Seasoned canned	½ cup	35	5	1	2
Sensibly Seasoned canned	½ cup	20	4	1	2
COOKIES					
MIX					
oatmeal	1 (0.6 oz)	74	10	–	tr
King Arthur					
Chocolate Chip Whole Grain not prep	2 tbsp	90	16	10	1
Nature's Path					
Organic Chocolate Chip	⅒ pkg	150	31	16	3
READY-TO-EAT					
australian anzac biscuit	1	98	17	–	1
butter	1 (5 g)	23	3	–	tr
chocolate chip soft-type	1 (0.5 oz)	69	9	–	tr
chocolate w/ creme filling	1 (0.35 oz)	47	7	–	tr
cream cheese	1 (1.1 oz)	141	14	6	tr
digestive biscuits plain	2	141	21	–	1
fortune	1 (0.28 oz)	30	7	–	tr
fudge	1 (0.73 oz)	73	17	–	tr
graham honey	1 (0.24 oz)	30	5	–	tr
hermits	1 (1 oz)	117	18	10	1
jumbles coconut	1 (1 oz)	121	13	7	1
madeleines	1 (0.8 oz)	86	10	5	tr
neapolitan tri-color cookie	1 (0.6 oz)	79	8	5	tr
oatmeal	1 (0.6 oz)	81	12	–	1
oatmeal soft-type	1 (0.5 oz)	61	10	–	tr
oatmeal raisin	1 (0.6 oz)	81	12	–	1
oatmeal raisin soft-type	1 (0.5 oz)	61	10	–	tr
peanut butter soft-type	1 (0.5 oz)	69	9	–	tr
pinenut cookies	1 (1.1 oz)	134	11	8	1
reginette queen's biscuit	1 (0.8 oz)	86	13	4	tr
shortbread pecan	1 (0.49 oz)	79	8	–	tr
spritz	1 (0.4 oz)	42	6	3	tr
toll house original	1 (0.8 oz)	105	13	9	tr
zeppole	1 (0.8 oz)	78	6	4	tr

FOOD	PORTION	CALS	CARB	SUGAR	FIBER
ABC					
Vegan Colossal Chocolate Chip	1 (2.1 oz)	240	41	20	1
Vegan Double Chocolate Decadence	1 (2.1 oz)	240	39	21	2
Vegan Luscious Lemon Poppyseed	1 (2.1 oz)	240	40	17	0
Vegan Mac The Chip	1 (2.1 oz)	250	35	20	3
Vegan Peanut Butter Chocolate Chip	1 (2.1 oz)	240	39	17	1
Vegan Phenomenal Pumpkin Spice	1 (2.1 oz)	220	39	18	3
Archway					
Frosty Lemon	1 (0.9 oz)	110	18	10	0
Arico					
Gluten Free Casein Free Almond Cranberry	1 bar (1.4 oz)	140	22	10	4
Gluten Free Casein Free Double Chocolate	1 (0.9 oz)	100	15	7	3
Gluten Free Casein Free Lemon Ginger	1 (0.9 oz)	90	15	6	3
Gluten Free Casein Free Peanut Butter	1 bar (1.4 oz)	160	19	3	4
Arrowroot					
Biscuit	1 (5 g)	20	4	1	0
Bahlsen					
Hit Minis Chocolate Filled	5 (1.2 oz)	170	23	11	tr
Nuss Dessert	3 (1.1 oz)	170	17	8	0
Barbara's Bakery					
Fig Bars Wheat Free	1	60	13	8	1
Snackimals Wheat Free Oatmeal	10	120	17	6	1
Barnum's					
Animal Crackers	10 (1 oz)	120	22	7	1
Bolands					
Custard Creams	1	62	8	4	tr
Breaktime					
Ginger	4 (1 oz)	130	23	10	0
Oatmeal	4 (1 oz)	130	22	9	tr
Brown & Haley					
Almond Roca	6 (1 oz)	110	19	10	0

FOOD	PORTION	CALS	CARB	SUGAR	FIBER
Buzz Strong's					
Real Coffee	1 (1.2 oz)	150	22	13	1
Cameo					
Sandwich Creme	2 (1 oz)	130	21	10	0
Chips Ahoy!					
Chocolate Chip	1 pkg (1.4 oz)	190	27	13	1
Mini	1 pkg (1.2 oz)	170	24	10	1
Reduced Fat	1 pkg (1.1 oz)	140	23	11	1
Comfort Care					
Cabin Hearth Chocolate Chip	1 (2 oz)	250	38	23	1
Cabin Hearth Oatmeal Peach	1 (2 oz)	200	31	17	3
Cabin Hearth Oatmeal Raisin	1 (2 oz)	200	31	17	3
Country Choice Organic					
Fit Kids Snackin' Grahams Chocolate	18 (1 oz)	110	20	7	2
Oatmeal Chocolate Chip	1 (0.8 oz)	100	15	8	1
Oatmeal Raisin	1 (0.8 oz)	100	16	9	1
Crummy					
Organic Chocolate Chip	1 (2 oz)	240	34	20	0
Organic Lavender Chocolate Chip	1 (2 oz)	240	34	20	0
Dare					
Lemon Creme	1 (0.7 oz)	100	14	7	0
Maple Leaf Creme	1 (0.6 oz)	80	12	6	0
DiCamillo					
Biscotti DiPrato	5 (1 oz)	130	21	12	tr
Divvies					
Chocolate Chip Vegan	1	130	17	11	tr
Oatmeal Raisin Vegan	1	120	17	8	tr
Dove					
Beyond Chocolate Chunk	1 (0.7 oz)	110	13	7	1
Chocolate Walnut Rendezvous	1 (0.7 oz)	110	13	7	1
Milk Chocolate Moment	3 (1.1 oz)	160	20	12	1
Mint Chocolate Serenade	3 (1.1 oz)	160	19	10	1
Earthbound Farm					
Organic Ginger Snaps	2	120	18	8	0
Emily's					
Fortune Dark Chocolate Covered	2 (1.4 oz)	140	23	15	2
Graham Cracker Milk Chocolate Covered	1 (1 oz)	150	17	13	tr

FOOD	PORTION	CALS	CARB	SUGAR	FIBER
Enjoy Life					
Allergen Gluten Free Gingerbread Spice	2 (1 oz)	100	19	10	2
Allergen Gluten Free No Oats Oatmeal	2 (1 oz)	120	21	10	1
Allergen Gluten Free Snickerdoodle	2 (1 oz)	130	21	14	2
Snack Bar Sunbutter Crunch	1 (1 oz)	140	20	4	3
Entenmann's					
Soft Baked Chocolate Chunk	1 (1.3 oz)	190	25	13	0
Erin Baker's					
Breakfast Banana Toasted Flax	1 (3 oz)	300	55	12	6
Breakfast Caramel Apple	1 (3 oz)	290	57	21	6
Breakfast Mocha Cappuccino	1 (3 oz)	300	54	19	6
Breakfast Morning Glory	1 (3 oz)	310	54	17	6
Breakfast Peanut Butter & Jelly	1 (3 oz)	320	52	21	5
Breakfast Vegan Chocolate Chip	1 (3 oz)	310	57	22	6
Organic Breakfast Mini Oatmeal Raisin	1 (1 oz)	100	18	9	2
Organic Breakfast Mini Peanut Butter	1 (1 oz)	110	16	7	2
Fauchon					
Assorted Chocolate	4 (2 oz)	330	34	16	5
Fox's					
Golden Crunch Creams	1	75	9	6	tr
French Meadow Bakery					
Gluten Free Chocolate Chip	1 (1.3 oz)	190	26	0	1
Frieda's					
Asian Almond	2 (1 oz)	170	19	6	0
Gak's Snacks					
Organic Brownie Chip	1 (1 oz)	130	20	11	1
Organic Chocolate Chip	1 (1 oz)	140	21	11	1
Organic Oatmeal	1 (1 oz)	120	19	9	2
Ginger Snaps					
Cookies	4 (1 oz)	120	23	11	0
Girl Scout					
Cafe Cookies	5	150	20	7	1
Lemon Cooler Reduced Fat	5	130	22	10	0

FOOD	PORTION	CALS	CARB	SUGAR	FIBER
Samoas	2	150	19	11	tr
Tagalongs	2	130	13	7	1
Thin Mints	4	140	18	9	tr
Trefoils	4	130	17	5	0
Gluten-Free Pantry					
Gluten Free Buckwheat Raisin	1 (1 oz)	140	21	9	1
Gluten Free Chocolate Chunk	1 (1 oz)	140	19	8	1
Glutino					
Gluten Free Wafers Chocolate	4	160	19	14	3
Gluten Free Wafers Lemon	3	150	24	15	0
Gottena					
Exquisit	5	170	19	6	1
Gourmet Pastries					
Kourabiethes Butter Almond	1 (1.1 oz)	150	15	5	1
Phoenicia Honey & Spice	1 (1.3 oz)	140	20	12	0
Health Valley					
Mini Mint Chocolate Chip	4 (1 oz)	120	16	7	1
Oatmeal Raisin	1 (0.8 oz)	90	14	8	1
Raisin Oatmeal Low Fat	3	110	23	13	1
White Chocolate Chunk	1 (1 oz)	140	17	10	0
Healthy Handfuls					
Organic Crocodile Cookies	1 pkg (1 oz)	130	20	7	7
Organic Koala Krackers	1 pkg (1 oz)	120	21	7	2
Home Free					
Organic Chocolate Chip	1 (1 oz)	140	21	11	1
Organic Oatmeal	1 (1 oz)	120	19	9	2
Honey Maid					
Grahams Honey	1 (1.1 oz)	130	24	8	1
Grahams Honey Low Fat	1 (1.1 oz)	120	25	8	1
Jacob's					
Oat Crumbles Chocolate & Pecan	1	107	13	7	1
Joseph's					
Almond Sugar Free	4	100	13	0	1
Chocolate Chip Sugar Free	4	95	13	0	1
Lemon Sugar Free	4	95	15	0	0
Oatmeal Chocolate Chip w/ Pecans Sugar Free	4	100	14	0	1
Peanut Butter Sugar Free	4	95	14	0	0

FOOD	PORTION	CALS	CARB	SUGAR	FIBER
Kashi					
TLC Happy Trail Mix	1 (1 oz)	130	21	7	4
TLC Oatmeal Raisin Flax	1 (1 oz)	130	20	8	4
TLC Oatmeal Dark Chocolate	1 (1 oz)	130	21	8	3
Keebler					
100 Calorie Pack RightBites Sandies Shortbread	1 pkg (0.7 oz)	100	17	7	tr
Animal Crackers Frosted	8	150	22	13	tr
Chips Deluxe Chocolate Lovers	1	90	10	5	0
Chips Deluxe Coconut	2	150	18	9	1
Chips Deluxe Fudge Stripes	1	100	13	8	tr
Chips Deluxe Original	1 pkg (2 oz)	300	37	18	1
Chocolate Dip & Cookie Sticks	1 pkg (1 oz)	130	18	12	tr
Danish Wedding	4	130	18	10	tr
Dipping Delights Cheesecake	1	90	13	8	0
E.L. Fudge Original	1	90	13	6	tr
Fudge Shoppe Fudge Stripes	3	150	21	10	tr
Fudge Shoppe Grasshoppers	4	140	19	11	tr
Fudge Shoppe Mint Creme Filled	2	160	20	14	tr
Graham Honey	8 (1 oz)	110	22	7	tr
Graham Original	8 (1 oz)	130	22	7	tr
Oatmeal Country Style	2	130	18	8	1
Sandies Drops Butter Pecan	4	140	18	10	tr
Sandies Fudge Drops	4 (1 oz)	140	18	9	tr
Sandies Pecan Shortbread Reduced Fat	1	80	11	4	0
Scooby-Doo Graham Sticks	9	130	21	8	tr
S'mores Snack	1 pkg (0.8 oz)	110	14	10	0
Soft Batch Chocolate Chip	1	80	11	6	tr
Vanilla Wafers	8	140	21	9	tr
Vienna Fingers	2	150	22	10	tr
Vienna Fingers Reduced Fat	2	140	24	12	tr
Khaya					
Krunchi Orange & Chocolate	5 (1.53 oz)	240	29	14	2
Shortbread Grapeseed	13 (1.15 oz)	193	27	6	tr
Shortbread Orange Rooibos	13 (1.15)	259	36	8	tr
La Choy					
Fortune	4 (1 oz)	110	25	9	0

FOOD	PORTION	CALS	CARB	SUGAR	FIBER
Lance					
Oatmeal Creme	1 (2.5 oz)	300	45	26	2
Van-O-Lunch	1 pkg (1.6 oz)	230	34	14	0
Late July					
Organic Sandwich Dark Chocolate	3 (1.2 oz)	150	21	9	2
Organic Sandwich Vanilla Bean w/ Green Tea	2 (0.8)	110	16	8	1
Laura's Wholesome Junk Food					
Anna Banana Split	1	105	13	8	1
Gluten Free Charlotte's Chocolate Chip	2	120	16	8	1
Gluten Free Sally's Raisin	2	110	16	9	tr
Lemon Vanilla	2	120	15	8	1
Oatmeal Chocolate Chip	2	110	14	8	1
Oatmeal Raisin	2	100	11	9	1
Wheat Free X-Treme Chocolate Fudge	2	110	13	7	2
Lean Body					
Cookie Bar Hi-Protein S'Mores	1 (3.2 oz)	360	30	13	2
Lee's					
Dreamy Mallows	2	150	25	16	0
Leibniz					
Butter Biscuits	6	130	23	7	1
Liz Lovely					
Vegan Cowboy	½ cookie (1.3 oz)	190	24	13	2
Vegan Cowgirl	½ cookie (1.5 oz)	210	30	18	0
Vegan Ginger Snapdragons	½ cookie (1.5 oz)	190	29	14	0
Lorna Doone					
Shortbread	4 (1 oz)	140	20	6	0
LU					
Le Chocolatier	3 (1 oz)	150	17	12	1
Le Fondant	4 (1.1 oz)	170	19	9	1
Le Petit Beurre	4 (1.2 oz)	140	28	7	tr
Le Petit Ecolier Milk Chocolate	2 (0.9 oz)	130	17	10	tr
Shortbread	2 (1 oz)	140	16	5	tr

FOOD	PORTION	CALS	CARB	SUGAR	FIBER
M&M's					
Milk Chocolate	1 pkg (1.15 oz)	150	22	11	1
Mallomars					
Cookies	2	120	18	12	1
Miss Meringue					
Chocolatette Strawberry Vanilla	4	130	24	23	1
Chocolettes Crunchy Chocolate	4	110	2	23	21
Classiques Cappuccino	4	110	26	26	0
Classiques Chocolate Chip	4	120	25	24	1
Classiques Dulce De Leche Artisan	4	110	26	26	0
Macaroons Traditional	1 (1.3 oz)	180	20	16	1
Madeleines Traditional	2 (1.2 oz)	160	19	11	0
Minis Vanilla	13 (1.1 oz)	110	27	27	0
Minis Vanilla Sugar Free	13	35	9	6	3
Montana Monster Munchies					
Original	½ (1.4 oz)	177	21	14	2
Raisin	½ (1.4 oz)	172	22	14	2
MoonPie					
Mini All Flavors	1 pkg (1.2 oz)	130	23	11	2
Murray's					
Sugar Free Chocolate Sandwich	3 (1 oz)	130	19	0	1
Sugar Free Chocolate Chip	3 (1.1 oz)	160	20	0	1
Sugar Free Fudge Dipped Grahams	4 (1 oz)	150	19	0	1
Sugar Free Ginger Snap	7 (1.1 oz)	130	23	0	2
Sugar Free Oatmeal	3 (1.1 oz)	140	21	0	3
Sugar Free Shortbread	8 (1 oz)	130	21	0	2
Nabisco					
100 Calorie Barnum's Animal Choco	1 pkg	100	17	6	tr
100 Calorie Pack Alpha-Bits Mini	1 pkg	100	16	6	0
100 Calorie Pack Lorna Doone	1 pkg	100	16	6	0
100 Calorie Pack Teddy Grahams Mini Cinnamon	1 pkg	100	16	4	1
Biscos Sugar Wafers	8 (1 oz)	140	21	14	0
Social Tea	6	140	24	8	1
Nana's					
No Gluten Berry Vanilla	1 bar (1.2 oz)	130	22	7	tr

FOOD	PORTION	CALS	CARB	SUGAR	FIBER
No Gluten Chocolate	1 (3.5 oz)	360	62	20	2
No Gluten Ginger	1 (3.5 oz)	360	64	48	2
No Gluten Nana Banana	1 bar (1.2 oz)	130	23	7	0
No Wheat Oatmeal Raisin	1 (3.5 oz)	280	46	18	6
Vegan Chocolate Chip	1 (4 oz)	320	48	20	6
Vegan Peanut Butter	1 (4 oz)	360	46	18	4
Vegan Sunflower	1 (3.5 oz)	380	60	26	6
Natural Ovens					
Oatmeal Raisin	1 (1.3 oz)	120	20	10	2
Nature's Path					
Organic Signature Lemon Poppyseed	4	130	23	8	tr
Organic Animal Vanilla	9	120	20	8	tr
New York Style					
Biscotti Almond	3 (1 oz)	130	20	12	1
Newman's Own					
Organic Champion Chip Chocolate Chocolate Chip	4	160	20	11	1
Organic Champion Chip Chocolate Chip	4	160	21	11	1
Organic Champion Chip Double Chocolate Mint Chip	4	160	21	11	1
Organic Champion Chip Espresso Chocolate Chip	4	150	21	11	1
Organic Champion Chip Orange Chocolate Chip	4	160	20	11	1
Organic Champion Chip Wheat Free Dairy Free	4	160	21	11	0
Organic Fig Newmans Fat Free	2	120	28	15	1
Organic Fig Newmans Low Fat	2	140	28	15	1
Organic Fig Newmans Wheat Free Dairy Free	2	120	26	12	1
Organic Newman-O's Chocolate Creme	2	130	20	10	1
Organic Newman-O's Ginger-O's	2	120	19	10	0
Organic Newman-O's Mint Creme	2	130	20	10	1
Organic Newman-O's Original	2	130	20	10	1

FOOD	PORTION	CALS	CARB	SUGAR	FIBER
Organic Newman-O's Tops & Bottoms	6	120	21	8	1
Organic Newman-O's Wheat Free Dairy Free	2	130	21	11	0
Newtons					
Fig	2 (1.1 oz)	110	22	12	1
Fig 100% Whole Grain	2 (1.3 oz)	130	26	15	3
Fig Fat Free	2 (1 oz)	90	22	12	1
Raspberry	2 (1 oz)	100	21	13	0
Nilla Wafers					
Cookies	1 oz	140	21	11	0
Reduced Fat	1 oz	110	24	12	0
Nonni's					
Biscotti Cioccolati	1 (0.8 oz)	110	17	9	1
Biscotti Limone	1 (0.8 oz)	110	17	9	0
Biscotti Original	1 (0.7 oz)	90	14	7	0
NutraBalance					
High Fibre	1 (0.7 oz)	90	13	6	3
Nutter Butter					
Bites	1 pkg (1.2 oz)	170	24	10	1
Sandwich Cookie	1 (1 oz)	130	19	8	1
Oreo					
Cakesters	2 (2 oz)	250	36	23	1
Cakesters Mini Golden 100 Calorie Pack	1 pkg (0.8 oz)	100	15	10	0
Double Stuff	1 (1 oz)	140	21	13	1
Mini	1 pkg (1.2 oz)	160	25	14	1
Sandwich Cookie	2 (1.2 oz)	160	25	14	1
Pepperidge Farm					
Chantilly Raspberry	2	120	23	11	tr
Chessmen	3 (0.9 oz)	120	18	5	tr
Dark Chocolate Mint Chocolate Chunk	1	140	16	9	0
Gingerman	4	130	21	11	tr
Medallion Milk Chocolate	5	160	20	11	0
Milano	3	180	21	11	tr
Milano French Vanilla	2	130	18	8	tr
Milano Mint Chocolate Covered	4	130	18	10	1
Milano Sugar Free	3	170	21	0	tr
Nantucket Chocolate Dipped	1	150	20	10	tr

FOOD	PORTION	CALS	CARB	SUGAR	FIBER
Nantucket Dark Chocolate Chunk	1	140	16	9	0
Pirouettes Cappuccino	2	120	18	12	0
Pirouettes Chocolate Mint	2	120	18	14	tr
Sausalito Milk Chocolate Macadamia Nut	1	140	16	9	0
Shortbread	2	140	16	5	tr
Soft Baked Milk Chocolate	1	150	21	11	tr
Soft Baked Oatmeal Cranberry	1	130	22	10	tr
Soft Baked Sugar	1	140	22	11	0
Tahiti	2	170	17	8	2
Verona Apricot Raspberry	3	140	22	10	tr
Pirouette					
Sandwich Vanilla Creamed	3 (1.1 oz)	133	22	7	0
Polar					
Fortune	2	56	12	6	0
Q.bel					
Wafer Rolls Dark Chocolate	1 pkg (0.9 oz)	120	18	13	1
Wafer Rolls Milk Chocolate	1 pkg (0.9 oz)	130	18	13	tr
Quaker					
Breakfast Cookie Oatmeal Raisin	1	180	33	15	5
Right Direction					
Chocolate Chip	1	60	24	12	5
Ruger					
Wafers Vanilla	3 (1 oz)	160	20	15	0
SnackWell's					
Cookie Cakes Chocolate Mint	1 (0.6 oz)	50	12	7	0
Devil's Food Fat Free	1 (0.5 oz)	50	12	7	0
Sugar Free Lemon Creme	2 (1.1 oz)	130	23	0	2
Sugar Free Shortbread	2 (1 oz)	130	21	0	2
Snikiddy					
Cherry Oaties	1 pkg (0.8 oz)	110	17	6	1
South Beach					
Fiber Fit Double Chocolate Chunk	1 pkg (0.8 oz)	100	17	5	5
Fiber Fit Oatmeal Chocolate Chunk	1 pkg (0.8 oz)	100	17	5	5
Wafer Sticke Dark Chocolate Hazelnut Creme	1 pkg	100	10	tr	3

FOOD	PORTION	CALS	CARB	SUGAR	FIBER
Wafer Sticke Dark Chocolate Peanut Butter	1 pkg	100	10	1	3
Stella D'Oro					
100 Calorie Pack Breakfast Treats Original	1 pkg (0.8 oz)	100	19	6	1
Almond Delight	1 (1 oz)	150	18	7	tr
Angelica Goodies	1 (0.7 oz)	90	15	5	0
Anginetti	4 (1.1 oz)	130	25	21	0
Biscotti Almond	1 (0.7 oz)	90	15	8	1
Biscotti French Vanilla	1 (0.7 oz)	90	15	7	0
Breakfast Treats Chocolate	1 (0.9 oz)	110	19	10	tr
Breakfast Treats Original	1 (0.7 oz)	90	14	6	0
Coffee Treats Almond Toast	2 (0.9)	100	20	9	tr
Coffee Treats Angel Wings	3 (1 oz)	160	16	5	0
Coffee Treats Anisette Sponge	2 (0.9 oz)	90	18	8	0
Coffee Treats Anisette Toast	3 (1.2 oz)	130	27	13	tr
Coffee Treats Roman Egg Biscuits	1 (1.1 oz)	130	19	7	0
Egg Jumbo	3 (1.2 oz)	120	25	13	0
Lady Stella	3 (1 oz)	130	19	8	tr
Margherite	2 (1 oz)	130	20	7	0
Swiss Fudge	3 (1.2 oz)	170	22	12	tr
Teddy Grahams					
Chocolate	24 (1.1 oz)	130	22	8	2
Honey	24 (1 oz)	130	23	7	1
Temptations					
Chocolate Alps	1 bar (1.6 oz)	170	28	12	1
Chocolate Mocha	1 bar (1.6 oz)	170	27	11	1
No Gluten Chocolate Rush	1 bar (1.6 oz)	170	25	10	1
Voortman					
Chinese Almond	1 (0.9 oz)	130	16	7	0
Coconut Delight	1 (0.6 oz)	90	10	5	tr
Dutch Creme	1 (0.8 oz)	110	16	8	0
Fudge Swirl	1 (0.6 oz)	80	10	4	0
Gingerboy	1 (0.7 oz)	100	15	7	0
Maple Leaf	1 (0.6 oz)	90	13	7	0
Molasses	1 (1 oz)	110	20	10	tr
Oatmeal Apple	1 (0.7 oz)	90	13	6	1
Peanut Delight	1 (0.9 oz)	130	15	6	tr
Shortbread	1 (0.6 oz)	90	11	4	tr

FOOD	PORTION	CALS	CARB	SUGAR	FIBER
Sugar Free Chocolate Chip	1 (0.7 oz)	80	13	0	0
Sugar Free Lemon Wafers	3 (1 oz)	130	17	0	0
Sugar Free Vanilla Creme	2 (0.7 oz)	100	13	0	0
Sugar Free Wafers Peanut Butter	4 (1 oz)	150	17	0	0
Sugar Free Wafers Vanilla	3 (1 oz)	130	17	0	0
Turnover Blueberry	1 (0.9 oz)	110	18	9	tr
Turnover Cherry	1 (0.9 oz)	110	18	9	tr
Turnover Strawberry	1 (0.9 oz)	110	18	9	tr
Wafer Chocolate Covered	1 (0.7 oz)	100	13	9	0
Wafer Vanilla	3 (1 oz)	140	20	12	0
Wafers Mini Chocolate	5 (1 oz)	130	19	11	0
Walkers					
Shortbread	1	100	11	3	0
Whippet					
Original	2 (1.2 oz)	150	24	16	1
World Of Grains					
Apple Cinnamon	1 pkg	130	21	9	3
Cranberry	1 pkg	130	21	9	3
Multigrain	1 pkg	130	21	6	3
Zwieback					
Toast	1 (8 g)	35	6	1	0
REFRIGERATED					
Pillsbury					
Chocolate Chip	2 (1.3 oz)	170	22	14	tr
Gingerbread	2 (1.1 oz)	170	18	9	0
Oatmeal Chocolate Chip	2 (1.3 oz)	170	23	14	1
Peanut Butter	2 (1 oz)	130	16	9	0
S'Mores	2 (1.3 oz)	160	23	25	tr
Sugar	2 (1.3 oz)	170	22	12	0
TAKE-OUT					
biscotti w/ nuts chocolate dipped	1 (1.3 oz)	117	16	11	1
black & white	1 lg (3 oz)	302	52	31	1
finikia	1 (1.2 oz)	171	16	5	1
koulourakia butter cookie twist	1 (0.9 oz)	113	14	5	tr
linzer tart	1 (2.4 oz)	280	34	12	0
CORIANDER					
leaf dried	1 tsp	2	tr	tr	tr
seed	1 tsp	5	1	—	1

FOOD	PORTION	CALS	CARB	SUGAR	FIBER
CORN					
CANNED					
Del Monte					
Cream Style No Salt Added	½ cup	60	14	7	2
Savory Sides In Butter Sauce	½ cup	90	14	5	tr
Savory Sides Santa Fe	½ cup	70	16	1	1
Green Giant					
Mexicorn	⅓ cup	70	14	4	1
Super Sweet Yellow & White	⅓ cup	60	12	3	1
Orchids					
Whole Young Spears	½ cup (4.6 oz)	25	4	1	2
FROZEN					
Birds Eye					
Steamfresh Singles Super Sweet	1 pkg (3.2 oz)	80	14	6	2
Steamfresh Southwestern	⅔ cup (2.9 oz)	90	16	5	1
Steamfresh Sweet Mini Corn On The Cob	1 (3 oz)	90	19	5	1
C&W					
Cheddar Bacon	½ cup	130	18	9	3
Early Harvest Supersweet Petite	⅔ cup	70	14	6	2
Salsa Corn	1 cup	90	17	7	3
Europe's Best					
Baby Sweet	⅔ cup	50	9	1	2
Glory					
Savory Accents Fried Corn	½ cup	110	24	7	2
Green Giant					
Cream Style	½ cup	110	24	7	2
Nibblers On-The-Cob	1 (2.1 oz)	70	14	2	1
Niblets & Butter Sauce Low Fat	⅔ cup	110	21	5	2
Health Is Wealth					
Creamed	½ pkg (4.5 oz)	110	23	7	1
Pictsweet					
Cut Corn	⅔ cup	100	21	5	1
Roast Works					
Flame Roasted Cob Corn	1 cob (3 oz)	130	25	8	4
Stouffer's					
Souffle	½ pkg (6 oz)	150	22	8	2
TAKE-OUT					
scalloped	1 cup	257	34	11	3

FOOD	PORTION	CALS	CARB	SUGAR	FIBER
CORN CHIPS (see CHIPS)					
CORNISH HEN (see CHICKEN)					
CORNMEAL					
cornmeal mush as prep w/ water	1 cup	223	47	tr	5
cornmeal yellow	½ cup (2.2 oz)	236	52	tr	1
whole grain blue	½ cup (1.9 oz)	201	41	0	5
yellow self-rising	½ cup (3 oz)	296	62	–	5
Indian Head					
Stone Ground	¼ cup	100	20	0	2
Martha White					
White Self Rising	3 tbsp (1.1 oz)	100	22	0	2
Yellow	3 tbsp (1.1 oz)	110	22	0	2
McKenzie's					
Hush Puppies	1 serv (1.9 oz)	190	23	2	2
Quaker					
Quick Grits not prep	¼ cup	130	29	0	2
TAKE-OUT					
corn pone	1 piece (2.1 oz)	128	23	tr	2
fritter puerto rican style	1 (1.4 oz)	109	8	tr	1
harina de maiz con coco	½ cup	383	36	21	4
harina de maize con leche	1 cup	295	51	32	7
hush puppies	1 (0.8 oz)	74	10	tr	1
johnnycake	1 piece (1.7 oz)	134	21	4	2
CORNSTARCH					
cornstarch	1 tbsp (0.3 oz)	34	8	0	tr
cornstarch	¼ cup (1.1 oz)	122	29	0	tr
Bob's Red Mill					
Cornstarch	1 tbsp	30	7	0	0
COTTAGE CHEESE					
creamed large curd	½ cup (4 oz)	110	4	3	0
creamed small curd	½ cup (3.7 oz)	103	4	3	0
dry curd	½ cup (2.5 oz)	52	5	1	0
lowfat 1%	½ cup (4 oz)	81	3	3	0
lowfat 1% lactose reduced	½ cup (4 oz)	84	4	3	1
Axelrod					
Lowfat 1%	½ cup (4 oz)	90	6	4	0

FOOD	PORTION	CALS	CARB	SUGAR	FIBER
Breakstone's					
Fat Free	½ cup	80	8	6	0
LiveActive	1 pkg (4 oz)	90	8	4	3
LiveActive Mixed Berries	1 pkg (4 oz)	120	18	0	3
Cabot					
Cottage Cheese	½ cup	100	4	4	0
No Fat	½ cup	70	5	4	0
Friendship					
1% Lowfat	½ cup	90	3	3	0
1% Lowfat No Salt Added	½ cup	90	4	3	1
1% Lowfat Whipped	½ cup	90	3	3	0
2% Digestive Health	½ cup	90	5	2	3
2% Pot Style	½ cup	90	3	2	0
4% California Style	½ cup	110	3	2	1
Nonfat	½ cup	80	4	4	0
Hood					
4% Fat w/ Pineapple	½ cup	130	15	13	0
Fat Free	½ cup	80	6	5	0
Low Fat	½ cup	90	5	4	0
Low Fat No Salt Added	½ cup	90	6	5	0
Low Fat w/ Peaches	½ cup	110	18	16	0
Horizon Organic					
Lowfat	½ cup	100	4	3	0
Regular	½ cup	120	4	3	0
Knudsen					
LiveActive Pineapple	1 pkg (4 oz)	110	17	0	3
Land O Lakes					
1% Lowfat	½ cup (4 oz)	90	5	3	0
2% Lowfat	½ cup (3.7 oz)	100	5	3	0
Cottage Cheese	½ cup (3.7 oz)	110	5	4	0
Fat Free	½ cup (4 oz)	80	6	4	0
Light N'Lively					
Lowfat	½ cup	80	6	5	0
Nancy's					
Organic Lowfat	½ cup	80	3	3	0
Organic Valley					
Low Fat	½ cup	100	4	tr	0
COUSCOUS					
Hodgson Mill					
Whole Wheat not prep	⅓ cup	210	47	1	5

FOOD	PORTION	CALS	CARB	SUGAR	FIBER
Marrakesh Express					
Mango Salsa as prep	1 cup	190	38	8	1
Mushroom as prep	1 cup	190	39	2	1
Plain as prep	1 cup	270	57	2	2
Near East					
Mediterranean Curry as prep	1 cup	220	40	2	3
Original Plain as prep	1 cup	190	37	1	3
Parmesan as prep	1 cup	220	39	3	2
Toasted Pine Nut as prep	1 cup	230	39	2	2
Wild Mushroom & Herb as prep	1 cup	230	40	1	3
CRAB					
CANNED					
blue	½ cup	67	0	0	0
blue drained	1 can (6.5 oz)	124	0	0	0
Ace Of Diamonds					
Fancy w/ Leg Meat	¼ cup (2 oz)	40	2	1	0
Brunswick					
Crabmeat 15% Leg	2 oz	40	1	1	0
Fancy Lump	2 oz	45	1	0	0
Bumble Bee					
Lump	¼ cup	40	0	0	0
Pink	¼ cup	35	0	0	0
White	¼ cup	40	0	0	0
Polar					
Claw Meat	¼ cup (2 oz)	37	1	1	0
Jumbo Lump Meat	¼ cup (2 oz)	39	0	0	0
FRESH					
alaska king meat only steamed	3 oz	82	0	0	0
blue cooked flaked	1 cup (4 oz)	120	0	0	0
queen steamed	3 oz	98	0	0	0
FROZEN					
Mama Belle's					
Crab Cakes Maryland Style	1 (2 oz)	100	4	1	0
Mrs. Paul's					
Deviled Crab Cakes	1 (3 oz)	220	12	tr	3
TAKE-OUT					
alaska king leg steamed	1 leg (4.7 oz)	130	0	0	0
crab imperial	1 crab (6.8 oz)	289	6	3	0
crab salad	1 serv (5.5 oz)	285	3	1	1
crab thermidor	1 serv (6.4 oz)	456	8	tr	tr

FOOD	PORTION	CALS	CARB	SUGAR	FIBER
deviled	1 serv (4.5 oz)	254	17	6	1
empanada de jueyes	1 (4.4 oz)	341	38	7	2
fried crab puffs	4 (3.2 oz)	323	30	tr	1
kenagi korean crab cooked	1 serv (3 oz)	71	0	0	0
salmorejo de jueyes (in tomato sauce)	1 serv (4.5 oz)	215	3	1	tr
soft-shell breaded & fried	1 med (2.3 oz)	216	11	1	1
taco de jueyes	1 (4.2 oz)	266	18	1	2

CRACKER CRUMBS

FOOD	PORTION	CALS	CARB	SUGAR	FIBER
cracker meal	1 cup	440	93	tr	3
graham-cracker crumbs	1 cup	355	65	26	2
Honey Maid					
Graham Cracker Crumbs	2½ tbsp (0.6 oz)	70	13	4	0
Keebler					
Graham	¼ cup	93	17	4	1
Kellogg's					
Corn Flake Crumbs	6 tbsp (1.2 oz)	120	29	3	tr

CRACKERS

FOOD	PORTION	CALS	CARB	SUGAR	FIBER
melba toast round	1	12	2	tr	tr
oyster cracker	¼ cup	48	8	tr	tr
saltines	1	13	2	tr	tr
water biscuits	3	92	16	–	1
zwieback	1 oz	107	21	–	1
34 Degrees					
Crispbread Sesame	19 (1.1 oz)	140	26	1	1
Athenos					
Pita Chips Whole Wheat	11 (1 oz)	120	18	tr	2
Back To Nature					
Rice Thin Sesame Ginger	16	120	23	0	0
Barbara's Bakery					
Wheatines Original	4	60	11	1	tr
Better Cheddars					
Original	1.1 oz	160	18	0	1
Blue Diamond					
Nut-Thins Almond	16	130	23	0	1
Nut-Thins Hazelnut	16	130	23	0	tr
Nut-Thins Pecan	16	130	23	0	tr

FOOD	PORTION	CALS	CARB	SUGAR	FIBER
Bremner Wafers					
Cracked Wheat	7 (0.5 oz)	70	11	0	0
Original	7 (0.5 oz)	70	11	0	0
Soup & Chili Crackers	50 (0.5 oz)	60	11	0	0
Breton					
Garden Vegetable	4 (0.7 oz)	100	13	1	1
Minis Cheddar Cheese	20 (0.7 oz)	100	13	1	1
Brown Rice Snaps					
Cheddar	6	60	12	tr	tr
Original Tamari Seaweed	9	60	12	0	tr
Unsalted Plain	8	60	13	tr	tr
Cheese Nips					
Cheddar	1 pkg (1.2 oz)	170	22	0	1
Chicken Biskit					
Original	1.1 oz	160	19	2	1
Dare					
Crackers	3 (0.5 oz)	70	9	tr	0
Original	4 (0.7 oz)	90	13	1	1
Reduced Fat & Salt	5 (0.7 oz)	80	16	2	1
Dr. Kracker					
Flatbread Klassic Seed	1 (1 oz)	120	13	0	4
Flatbread Pumpkin Seed Cheddar	1 (1 oz)	120	12	0	4
Flatbread Seeded Spelt	1 (1 oz)	120	12	0	4
Flatbread Seedlander	1 (1 oz)	120	15	2	3
Flatbread Spelt Sunflower Cheddar	1 (1 oz)	120	12	0	4
Krispy Grahams	5 (1 oz)	110	17	6	2
Eden					
Brown Rice	8 (1.1 oz)	120	22	tr	2
Nori Nori Rice	15 (1 oz)	110	24	0	2
Foods Alive					
Golden Flax Maple & Cinnamon	5	150	12	4	8
Golden Flax Mexican Harvest	5	150	10	tr	9
Golden Flax Onion Garlic	5	140	11	1	9
Golden Flax Organic Hemp	5	130	12	tr	11
Golden Flax Regular	5	150	11	0	11
Glutino					
Gluten Free	4 (0.5 oz)	70	12	tr	0
Gluten Free Rusks	2 (0.7 oz)	80	15	1	2

FOOD	PORTION	CALS	CARB	SUGAR	FIBER
GrainsFirst					
Autumn Harvest	7 (1.1 oz)	140	16	2	3
Grissol					
Crispy Baguettes Garden Herb	8 (1 oz)	110	19	2	1
Health Valley					
Organic Bruschetta Vegetable	4	70	10	1	0
Organic Cracked Pepper	4	70	10	1	0
Organic Cracker Stix Garlic Herb	8	70	9	1	tr
Organic Whole Wheat	4	70	9	1	1
Healthy Handfuls					
Lucky Duckies Cheddar Cheese	1 pkg (1 oz)	100	14	0	1
Jacob's					
Table Cracker Bran	1	33	5	tr	tr
Kashi					
TLC Country Cheddar	18 (1 oz)	130	20	1	tr
TLC Honey Sesame	15 (1 oz)	130	22	4	2
TLC Natural Ranch	15 (1 oz)	130	22	4	2
TLC Original 7 Grain	15 (1 oz)	130	22	3	2
TLC Party Mediterranean Bruschetta	4	120	18	3	3
TLC Snack Fire Roasted Vegetable	5	130	21	2	2
Keebler					
Club Multi-Grain	4	70	10	2	tr
Club Original	4	70	9	1	tr
Club Reduced Fat	5	70	12	2	tr
Club Snack Sticks	12	130	19	2	tr
Puffed Original	24	140	20	3	1
Sandwich Cheese & Peanut Butter	1 pkg (1.4 oz)	200	23	4	1
Sandwich Toast & Peanut Butter	1 pkg (1.4 oz)	200	23	4	1
Sandwich Wheat & Cheddar	1 pkg (1.3 oz)	190	23	5	tr
Toasteds Harvest Wheat	16	130	20	3	1
Toasteds Sesame	5	80	10	1	tr
Toasteds Wheat	5	80	10	1	tr
Town House Bistro	2	80	11	1	tr
Town House FlipSides Original	5	70	10	1	tr
Town House Original	5	80	10	1	tr
Town House Reduced Fat	6	60	11	1	tr

FOOD	PORTION	CALS	CARB	SUGAR	FIBER
Town House Reduced Sodium	5	80	10	1.	tr
Town House Toppers	3	70	9	1	0
Wheatables 33% Less Fat	19	140	22	5	1
Wheatables Original	17	140	20	4	1
Zesta Saltine Fat Free	5	60	13	0	tr
Zesta Saltine Original	5	60	11	0	tr
Kellogg's					
All Bran Garlic Herb	18 (1 oz)	120	19	3	5
Kitchen Table Bakers					
Aged Parmesan	3	80	tr	0	0
Everything	3	80	tr	0	0
Garlic	3	80	tr	0	0
Jalapeno	3	80	2	0	1
Lance					
Captain Wafers	4	70	9	1	0
Nekot	1 pkg (1.7 oz)	240	30	13	1
Nipchee	1 pkg (1.4 oz)	190	22	3	1
Peanut Butter On Wheat	1 pkg (1.4 oz)	200	21	4	1
Toastchee	1 pkg (1.5 oz)	220	23	3	2
Toastchee Reduced Fat	1 pkg (1.4 oz)	180	23	2	2
Late July					
Organic Classic Rich	4 (0.5 oz)	70	11	2	0
Organic Classic Saltine	4 (0.5 oz)	60	10	0	0
Mary's Gone Crackers					
Wheat Free Gluten Free Black Pepper	13 (1 oz)	140	21	0	3
Wheat Free Gluten Free Onion	13 (1 oz)	140	21	0	3
Wheat Free Gluten Free Original Seed	13 (1 oz)	140	21	0	3
Milton's					
Multi-Grain	2	70	10	1	0
Nabisco					
Garden Harvest Apple Cinnamon	16 (1 oz)	120	22	6	3
Garden Harvest Banana	16 (1 oz)	120	22	8	3
Garden Harvest Tomato Basil	16 (1 oz)	120	20	2	3
Garden Harvest Vegetable Medley	16 (1 oz)	120	20	2	3
Vegetable Thins	21 (1 oz)	150	20	2	tr
Water Original	4	60	11	0	0

FOOD	PORTION	CALS	CARB	SUGAR	FIBER
Wheat	4	90	12	1	tr
Nature's Path					
Signature Tamari Flax	15	110	18	1	tr
New York Style					
Crispini Seeds & Spice	6	120	19	0	tr
Panetini Original	2	80	10	0	0
Panetini Three Cheese	2	80	9	1	0
Pita Chips Garlic	7	130	17	1	1
Pita Chips Natural Whole Wheat	7	120	17	1	3
Nonni's					
Panetini Roasted Garlic	5 (1 oz)	120	19	1	tr
Panetini Sun Dried Tomato Basil	5 (1 oz)	120	17	1	tr
Orkney					
Oatcakes Thin	4 (1.8 oz)	227	25	tr	3
Pepperidge Farm					
100 Calorie Pack Goldfish Cheddar	1 pkg	100	14	0	1
100 Calorie Pack Goldfish Pretzel	1 pkg	100	18	tr	tr
Goldfish Cinnamon Graham	1 pkg	210	32	13	1
Goldfish Pizza	55	140	20	tr	tr
Goldfish Reduced Sodium Cheddar	60	140	20	tr	tr
Goldfish w/ Whole Grain	55	140	19	tr	2
Snack Sticks Pumpernickel	15	120	24	1	2
Water Crackers	4	60	12	tr	tr
Wheat Crisps Spicy Salsa	16	140	21	6	2
Premium					
Saltine Fat Free	5 (0.5 oz)	60	12	0	0
Saltine Multigrain	5 (0.5 oz)	60	10	0	tr
Saltine Unsalted Tops	5 (0.5 oz)	60	11	0	0
Saltines Low Sodium	5 (0.5 oz)	80	11	0	0
Saltines Original	5 (0.5 oz)	60	11	0	0
Ritz					
Crackers	0.5 oz	80	10	1	0
Low Sodium	0.5 oz	80	10	1	0
Reduced Fat	5 (0.5 oz)	70	11	1	0
Whole Wheat	0.5 oz	70	11	2	1

FOOD	PORTION	CALS	CARB	SUGAR	FIBER
San-J					
Brown Rice Black Sesame	5	140	17	0	1
Brown Rice Sesame	5	130	19	0	1
Brown Rice Tamari	6	170	26	0	1
Sara Lee					
Cracked Pepper Trio	7	130	22	0	tr
English Water	7	130	22	0	tr
Harvest Vegetable	6	140	19	3	tr
Sociables					
Original	0.5 oz	70	9	1	0
South Beach					
Whole Wheat	1 pkg	100	16	2	3
Triscuit					
Deli-Style Rye	1 oz	120	19	0	3
Original	1 oz	120	19	0	3
Reduced Fat	1 oz	120	21	0	3
True North					
Peanut Crunches	¼ cup (1 oz)	150	13	5	4
Pistachio Crisps	12 (1 oz)	140	15	4	2
Utz					
Cheese Peanut Butter	6	200	21	3	2
Vegetable Thins					
Original	21 (1.1 oz)	150	19	2	1
Vinta					
Original	3 (0.7 oz)	100	12	2	1
Wasa					
Crisp'N Light 7 Grain	3	60	13	tr	2
Fiber Rye	1	30	7	0	2
Hearty	1 (0.5 oz)	45	11	0	2
Hearty Rye	1	45	11	0	2
Light Rye	2 (0.6 oz)	60	14	0	3
Sourdough Rye	1	35	9	0	2
Water Crackers					
Original	6 (0.5 oz)	60	11	0	0
Westminster					
Oyster	1 pkg (0.5 oz)	66	11	0	0
Wheat Thins					
100% Whole Grain	1 oz	140	21	3	2
Low Sodium	1.1 oz	150	22	4	1
Original	1.1 oz	150	21	4	1

FOOD	PORTION	CALS	CARB	SUGAR	FIBER
Reduced Fat	1 oz	130	21	3	1
Wheatsworth					
Crackers	5 (0.5 oz)	80	10	1	1
Wisecrackers					
Low Fat Roasted Garlic	10	110	20	3	tr
CRANBERRIES					
cranberry orange relish	¼ cup	118	31	28	2
dried	½ cup	85	23	18	2
fresh chopped	1 cup	13	3	1	1
fresh whole	1 cup	11	3	1	1
sauce	1 slice (2 oz)	86	22	22	1
sauce	¼ cup	109	27	26	1
Chukar Cherries					
North Cove Dried	¼ cup	100	24	22	2
De-Lite					
Dried Sweetened	1 oz	92	23	15	1
Earthbound Farm					
Organic Dried	⅓ cup	130	34	27	2
Eden					
Organic Dried	⅓ cup	140	33	25	2
Emily's					
Milk Chocolate Covered	¼ cup (1.4 oz)	180	24	23	2
Fool					
Cranberry Spread	1 tbsp	30	7	6	1
Frieda's					
Dried	⅓ cup (1.4 oz)	110	28	26	2
Fruitaceuticals					
OmegaCrans Dried	¼ cup	91	22	20	1
Good Sense					
Cranberries 'N More	¼ cup	170	15	3	2
Dried Sweetened	½ cup	130	31	28	4
Mariani					
Dried Sweetened	⅓ cup	130	35	30	2
Newman's Own					
Organic Dried	¼ cup	130	34	31	2
Ocean Spray					
Craisins	⅓ cup	130	33	27	2
Sun-Maid					
Dried Cape Cod	⅓ cup (1.4 oz)	130	33	27	2
Sunsweet					
Dried	⅓ cup (1.5 oz)	140	35	29	2

FOOD	PORTION	CALS	CARB	SUGAR	FIBER
Tree Of Life					
Organic Jellied	¼ cup (2.5 oz)	100	26	17	1
Wild Thymes Farm					
Cranberry Fig Sauce	1 tsp	19	5	4	tr
Original Cranberry Sauce	1 tbsp	21	5	5	tr

CRANBERRY BEANS
Goya

Roman Beans Dried not prep	¼ cup (1.4 oz)	80	24	2	13

CRANBERRY JUICE

cranberry juice cocktail low calorie w/ vitamin C	8 oz	46	11	11	0
cranberry juice cocktail w/ vitamin C	8 oz	137	34	30	0
unsweetened	8 oz	116	31	31	tr
Lakewood					
Organic	6 oz	50	12	8	1
Organic Light	6 oz	45	18	12	1
Nantucket Nectars					
Cranberry Cocktail	8 oz	130	33	32	0

CRAYFISH

cooked	3 oz	97	0	0	0
raw	3 oz	76	0	0	0
raw	8	24	0	0	0

CREAM *(see also WHIPPED TOPPINGS)*

clotted cream	2 tbsp (1 oz)	164	1	–	0
creme fraiche	2 tbsp (1 oz)	100	1	–	0
Cabot					
Whipped	2 tbsp	15	1	1	0
Hood					
Half & Half	2 tbsp	40	1	1	0
Light	1 tbsp	30	tr	tr	0
Simply Smart Fat Free Half & Half	2 tbsp	15	2	2	0
Whipping Cream	1 tbsp	45	tr	1	0
Horizon Organic					
Half & Half	2 tbsp	35	1	1	0
Heavy Whipping	1 tbsp	50	0	0	0

FOOD	PORTION	CALS	CARB	SUGAR	FIBER
Land O Lakes					
Aersol Whipped Light Cream	2 tbsp (0.2 oz)	20	1	1	0
Half & Half	2 tbsp (1.1 oz)	35	1	1	0
Half & Half Fat Free	2 tbsp (1.1 oz)	20	3	2	0
Heavy Whipping	1 tbsp (0.5 oz)	50	0	0	0
Organic Valley					
Half & Half	2 tbsp (1 oz)	40	1	1	0
Straus					
Organic Whipping Cream	1 tbsp (0.5 oz)	52	0	0	0

CREAM CHEESE

FOOD	PORTION	CALS	CARB	SUGAR	FIBER
Boar's Head					
Cream Cheese	2 tbsp (1 oz)	100	2	2	0
Connoisseur					
Wheel Mango Peach	2 tbsp	110	10	5	0
Wheel Wild Blueberry	2 tbsp	100	9	6	0
Crystal Farms					
Regular	1 oz	90	1	tr	0
Tub	2 tbsp	100	2	tr	0
Whipped	2 tbsp	70	1	1	0
Earth Balance					
Brick	2 tbsp	80	2	2	0
Tub	2 tbsp	80	2	2	0
Horizon Organic					
Reduced Fat	2 tbsp	70	2	tr	0
Spreadable	2 tbsp	110	tr	0	0
Lifeway					
Lox & Onion	2 tbsp	80	1	4	0
Vegetable	2 tbsp	80	1	1	0
Whipped	2 tbsp	80	1	1	0
Nancy's					
Organic	2 tbsp	95	2	2	0
Organic Valley					
Cream Cheese	1 oz	100	1	tr	0
Soft	2 tbsp	90	2	2	0
Philadelphia					
1/3 Less Fat	1 oz	70	tr	tr	0
Original	1 oz	100	1	tr	0
Whipped	2 tbsp	60	1	tr	0

FOOD	PORTION	CALS	CARB	SUGAR	FIBER
CREAM CHEESE SUBSTITUTES					
Vegan Gourmet					
Alternative Cream Cheese	2 tbsp (1 oz)	90	3	0	2
WholeSoy & Co.					
Soy Cream Cheese Organic Original & Flavored	2 tbsp	70	3	tr	1
CREAM OF TARTAR					
cream of tartar	1 tsp	8	2	0	0
CREPES					
basic crepe unfilled	1 (7 in)	112	11	2	tr
Ekizian					
Chickpea Crepe	1 (7-in) (1.5 oz)	212	16	3	3
Frieda's					
Ready-To-Use	1 (0.5 oz)	30	5	2	0
CROAKER					
atlantic raw	3 oz	89	0	0	0
CROCODILE					
cooked	3 oz	78	0	0	0
CROISSANT					
apple	1 (2 oz)	145	21	–	1
butter	1 lg (2.4 oz)	272	31	8	2
butter	1 mini (1 oz)	114	13	3	1
cheese	1 (1.5 oz)	174	20	5	1
chocolate	1 (2 oz)	237	25	6	2
Sara Lee					
Croissant	1 (1.5 oz)	170	20	0	1
Petite	2 (2 oz)	230	26	0	1
TAKE-OUT					
w/ egg & sausage	1 (5 oz)	497	31	8	2
w/ egg cheese & bacon	1 (4.1 oz)	385	25	8	1
w/ egg cheese & ham	1 (5.1 oz)	402	25	8	1
w/ egg cheese & sausage	1 (5.6 oz)	539	26	8	1
w/ ham & cheese	1 (4 oz)	338	25	4	1
CROUTONS					
plain	1 cup (1 oz)	122	22	–	2
seasoned	1 cup (1.4 oz)	186	25	–	2

FOOD	PORTION	CALS	CARB	SUGAR	FIBER
Cardini's					
Italian	2 tbsp	30	4	0	0
Edward & Sons					
Organic Lightly Salted	2 tbsp	30	5	0	0
Fresh Gourmet					
Butter & Garlic	7 (7 g)	35	4	0	0
Cheese & Garlic	12 (0.5 oz)	70	9	0	0
Classic Caesar	6 (7 g)	35	4	0	0
Cornbread Sweet Butter	½ cup (1 oz)	110	22	2	1
Fat Free Garlic Caesar	12 (7 g)	30	5	0	0
Italian Seasoned	6 (7 g)	35	4	0	0
Organic Seasoned	5 (7 g)	30	4	0	0
Pepperidge Farm					
Whole Grain Seasoned	6	30	5	tr	tr
Zesty Italian	6	30	5	tr	0
CUCUMBER					
fresh peeled	1 med (7 oz)	24	4	3	1
fresh sliced	1 cup	14	3	2	1
fresh w/ peel sliced	½ cup	34	2	1	tr
Frieda's					
Japanese	⅔ cup	10	2	1	1
Seedless Hothouse	⅔ cup	10	2	1	1
TAKE-OUT					
cucumber & onion salad w/ vinegar	1 cup	52	12	8	1
cucumber raita	1 serv (3.3 oz)	40	3	3	1
cucumber salad w/ oil & vinegar	1 cup	183	11	8	1
cucumber salad w/ sour cream dressing	1 cup	68	3	2	1
kimchee	½ cup (1.8 oz)	36	4	3	tr
tzatziki	½ cup (3.4 oz)	72	4	3	1
CUMIN					
seed	1 tbsp (6 g)	22	3	tr	1
seed	1 tsp (2 g)	8	1	tr	tr
CURRANT JUICE					
CurrantC					
Black Currant Juice	8 oz	130	32	28	0

FOOD	PORTION	CALS	CARB	SUGAR	FIBER
CURRANTS					
Sun-Maid					
Zante	¼ cup (1.4 oz)	120	30	28	2
CURRY					
curry powder	1 tsp	7	1	tr	1
paste	1 tube (6 oz)	465	30	13	12
A Taste Of Thai					
Curry Paste Green	1 tsp	15	1	0	1
Curry Paste Panang	1 tsp	25	2	1	0
Curry Paste Red	1 tsp	20	1	0	0
Curry Paste Yellow	1 tsp	30	1	0	1
Helen's Kitchen					
Indian Curry w/ Tofu Steaks & Rice	1 pkg (9 oz)	300	63	4	5
Patak's					
Curry Paste Biryani	2 tbsp	180	6	0	3
Garam Masala Paste	2 tsp	130	4	1	0
Tandoori Paste	2 tbsp	30	5	2	1
Vegetable Curry w/ Rice Rich Creamy Coconut	1 pkg	400	54	8	5
Vegetable Curry w/ Rice Rich Tomato & Onion	1 pkg (10.5 oz)	290	53	8	5
Vegetable Curry w/ Rice Tangy Lemon & Cilantro	1 pkg	300	54	8	5
Vindaloo Paste	2 tbsp	160	4	0	0
Spice Hunter					
Curry Seasoning Salt Free	¼ tsp	0	0	0	0
TastyBite					
Green Curry Vegetables & Jasmine Rice	1 pkg (12 oz)	320	52	2	2
Yellow Curry Vegetables & Jasmine Rice	1 pkg (12 oz)	380	61	4	3
TAKE-OUT					
beef curry	1 cup	432	14	6	3
beef kurma	1 serv (10 oz)	611	6	3	6
chicken curry ½ breast	1 serv	160	6	3	1
chicken curry boneless	1 serv (6.2 oz)	219	8	4	2
chicken curry leg & thigh	1 serv	180	7	3	1
chickpea curry	1 serv (8.3 oz)	305	23	1	15
lamb curry	1 cup	257	4	1	1

FOOD	PORTION	CALS	CARB	SUGAR	FIBER
pea & potato curry	1 serv (7 oz)	284	19	–	6
potato curry	1 serv (5.5 oz)	791	35	5	14
sambhar dhal curry	1 serv (10 oz)	177	21	–	8

CUSK
fillet baked	3 oz	106	0	0	0

CUSTARD
TAKE-OUT
flan de calabaza	1 piece (3.5 oz)	225	30	22	tr
flan de coco	1 piece (4.2 oz)	340	48	48	tr
tocino del cielo heaven's delight	1 cup	856	156	154	0

DANDELION GREENS
Frieda's
Dandelion Greens, not prep	2 cups	40	8	2	3

DANISH PASTRY
READY-TO-EAT
Entenmann's
Danish Ring Walnut	⅙ ring (2 oz)	260	25	12	2

TAKE-OUT
cheese	1 (2.5 oz)	266	26	5	1
cinnamon	1 (5 oz)	572	63	28	2
fruit	1 (5 oz)	527	68	39	3
lemon	1 (2.5 oz)	263	34	–	1
raisin nut	1 (2.3 oz)	280	30	17	1

DATES
deglet noor chopped	¼ cup (1.3 oz)	104	28	23	3
deglet noor dried	1 (7 g)	20	5	5	1
jujube dried	1 oz	75	19	–	2
medjool	1 (0.8 oz)	66	18	16	2

Bob's Red Mill
Dried Crumbles	⅓ cup	130	33	27	4

Earthbound Farm
Organic Dried	6 (1.4 oz)	120	31	29	3

Frieda's
Medjool	2 to 3 (1.4 oz)	120	31	29	3

SunDate
Fancy Medjool	3 (1.4 oz)	120	31	25	3

FOOD	PORTION	CALS	CARB	SUGAR	FIBER
Sun-Maid					
Pitted	¼ cup (1.4 oz)	110	30	21	4
Sunsweet					
California Pitted	5 to 6 (1.4 oz)	120	30	27	3
Tree Of Life					
Deglet Noor Pitted	5 (1.5 oz)	120	31	28	3
Organic Medjool	5 (1.5 oz)	120	31	28	3

DEER *(see* JERKY, VENISON*)*

DELI MEATS/COLD CUTS *(see also* BEEF, CHICKEN, HAM, MEAT SUBSTITUTES, TURKEY*)*

FOOD	PORTION	CALS	CARB	SUGAR	FIBER
beerwurst beef	2 oz	155	2	0	1
berliner pork & beef	1 slice (0.8 oz)	53	1	1	0
blood sausage	1 slice (0.9 oz)	95	tr	tr	0
bologna beef	1 slice (1 oz)	88	1	0	0
bologna beef low fat	1 slice (1 oz)	57	1	0	0
bologna beef reduced sodium	1 slice (1 oz)	88	1	0	0
bologna beef & pork	1 slice (1 oz)	87	2	1	0
bologna beef & pork low fat	1 slice (1 oz)	64	1	0	0
braunschweiger pork	1 slice (1 oz)	92	1	0	0
corned beef brisket	2 oz	90	0	0	0
dutch brand loaf pork & beef	1 slice (1.3 oz)	104	1	0	tr
headcheese pork	1 slice (1.6 oz)	71	0	0	0
honey loaf pork & beef	1 slice (1 oz)	35	1	0	0
lebanon bologna beef	2 slices (1 oz)	105	tr	0	0
mortadella beef & pork	1 slice (0.5 oz)	47	tr	0	0
olive loaf pork	2 slices (2 oz)	134	5	0	0
pastrami beef	1 slice (1 oz)	41	tr	tr	tr
peppered loaf pork & beef	1 slice (1 oz)	41	1	0	0
pepperoni pork & beef	15 slices (1 oz)	135	1	tr	tr
salami cooked beef & pork	1 slice (0.8 oz)	58	1	0	0
salami hard pork	3 slices (0.9 oz)	14	1	0	0
salami hard pork & beef less sodium	1 slice (1 oz)	113	2	2	tr
sandwich spread pork & beef	¼ cup	141	7	0	tr
summer sausage thuringer cervelat	2 oz	203	2	tr	0
Applegate Farms					
Organic Genoa Salami Sliced	1 oz	100	0	0	0

FOOD	PORTION	CALS	CARB	SUGAR	FIBER
Boar's Head					
Abruzzese Hot & Sweet	1 oz	100	tr	0	0
Bologna 25% Lowered Sodium	2 oz	150	0	0	0
Bologna Beef	2 oz	150	0	0	0
Bologna Garlic	2 oz	150	1	1	0
Bologna Lebanon	2 oz	100	3	3	0
Bologna Pork & Beef	2 oz	150	tr	tr	0
Braunschweiger Lite	2 oz	120	1	0	0
Capocollo Hot & Sweet	1 oz	80	0	0	0
Dutch Loaf	2 oz	150	2	2	0
Liverwurst Smoked	2 oz	170	1	1	0
Mortadella	2 oz	160	0	0	0
Olive Loaf	2 oz	130	tr	tr	0
Pastrami	2 oz	70	1	0	0
Pickle & Pepper Loaf	2 oz	150	2	1	0
Prosciutto	1 oz	60	0	0	0
Salami Beef	2 oz	120	0	0	0
Salami Cooked	2 oz	130	0	0	0
Salami Hard	1 oz	110	tr	0	0
Sopressata Hot & Sweet	1 oz	100	0	0	0
Spiced Ham	2 oz	120	1	0	0
Healthy Ones					
Pastrami 97% Fat Free	4 slices (2 oz)	60	3	0	0
Oscar Mayer					
Salami Beef	3 slices (1.8 oz)	150	1	0	0
Sara Lee					
Corned Beef	1 slice (2 oz)	50	1	0	0
Pastrami	2 slices (1.6 oz)	60	0	0	0
Salami Genoa	4 slices (1 oz)	110	1	0	0
Salami Hard	4 slices (1 oz)	120	0	0	0
Wellshire					
Salami Genoa	1 oz	100	1	0	0
Salami Hard	1 oz	100	1	0	0
Sopressata Sliced	1 oz	100	1	0	0
DILL					
seed	1 tsp	6	1	–	tr
weed dry	1 tbsp	8	2	–	tr

FOOD	PORTION	CALS	CARB	SUGAR	FIBER

DINNER *(see also* ASIAN FOOD, CURRY, PASTA DINNERS, POT PIE, SPANISH FOOD)

Betty Crocker

FOOD	PORTION	CALS	CARB	SUGAR	FIBER
Complete Meals Chicken & Buttermilk Biscuits	⅕ pkg (5.4 oz)	280	37	3	2
Complete Meals Stroganoff	⅕ pkg (5 oz)	200	30	3	1
Birds Eye					
Steamfresh Meals For Two Asian Chicken Vegetable Medley	½ pkg (11.9 oz)	290	36	13	10
Steamfresh Meals For Two Grilled Chicken Marinara	½ pkg (11.9 oz)	360	45	9	4
Steamfresh Meals For Two Sweet & Spicy Chicken	½ pkg (11.9 oz)	370	53	8	4
Voila! Pasta Primavera w/ Chicken	1⅔ cups	250	42	2	7
Voila! Shrimp Scampi	1¾ cups	190	31	4	3
Voila! Southwestern Chicken	2 cups	250	32	7	2
Boston Market					
Glazed Rotisserie Chicken w/ Mashed Potatoes Gravy Vegetables	1 pkg (16 oz)	390	34	6	4
C&W					
Stir Fry Feast Pot Sticker + Sauce	2 cups	200	30	8	4
Stir Fry Feast Ultimate + Sauce	1½ cups	190	25	9	3
Campbell's					
Supper Bakes Cheesy Chicken w/ Pasta	⅙ pkg	170	28	3	1
Supper Bakes Garlic Chicken w/ Pasta	⅙ pkg	220	42	2	2
Supper Bakes Savory Pork Chops w/ Herb Stuffing	⅙ box	160	30	4	1
Supper Bakes Traditional Roast Chicken w/ Stuffing	⅙ pkg	160	29	3	2
Contessa					
Beef Goulash not prep	1¾ cups	210	32	9	3
Chicken Cacciatore not prep	1¾ cups	230	24	5	6
Chicken Alfredo not prep	1¾ cups	330	28	3	2

FOOD	PORTION	CALS	CARB	SUGAR	FIBER
Fantastic					
Ginger Shittake w/ Rice Noodles	1 pkg (7.4 oz)	340	58	3	4
Fillo Factory					
Organic Fillo Pie Eggplant & Red Pepper	1 serv (5 oz)	230	35	5	3
Glory					
Savory Singles Chicken & Dumplings	1 pkg	290	40	1	6
Savory Singles Chicken Smoked Sausage & Rice Casserole	1 pkg	440	49	3	1
Savory Singles Ham & Sausage Jambalaya	1 pkg	400	42	4	2
Savory Singles Turkey & Gravy w/ Cornbread Stuffing	1 pkg	440	49	9	2
Glutino					
Gluten Free Chicken Pomodoro w/ Brown Rice & Vegetables	1 pkg (9.1 oz)	190	33	6	3
Gluten Free Chicken Ranchero w/ Brown Rice	1 pkg (9.1 oz)	180	30	5	4
Golden Cuisine					
Beef Stew	1 pkg	350	32	7	9
Boneless Pork Patty	1 pkg	504	44	25	13
Breaded Baked Fish w/ Rice Pilaf	1 pkg	300	48	6	6
Chicken Cacciatore	1 pkg	417	56	4	10
Chicken & Noodles	1 pkg	331	39	10	8
Chicken Parmesan	1 pkg	430	47	7	14
Chicken w/ Marinara Sauce	1 pkg	329	37	13	15
Meatloaf Patty & Gravy	1 pkg	340	33	9	7
Mesquite Chicken	1 pkg	320	50	18	10
Pot Roast w/ Gravy	1 pkg	343	36	6	10
Salisbury Steak & Mushroom Sauce	1 pkg	350	47	5	7
Swedish Meatballs	1 pkg	440	32	5	9
Turkey Tetrazzini	1 pkg	304	29	5	11
Green Giant					
Create A Meal Stir Fry Sweet & Sour as prep	1 cup	280	36	29	3

FOOD	PORTION	CALS	CARB	SUGAR	FIBER
Skillet Meal Chicken Teriyaki as prep	1½ cups	240	46	8	3
Healthy Choice					
Beef Merlot	1 pkg	240	25	6	6
Beef Pot Roast w/ Gravy	1 pkg (11 oz)	310	45	21	5
Beef Tips Portabello	1 pkg	300	33	14	7
Cafe Steamers Beef Merlot	1 (10 oz)	220	22	6	5
Cafe Steamers Cajun Style Chicken & Shrimp	1 (10.4 oz)	250	36	3	3
Cafe Steamers Chicken Margherita	1 (10 oz)	340	43	8	4
Cafe Steamers Creamy Dill Salmon	1 (9.8 oz)	240	26	1	5
Cafe Steamers Grilled Basil Chicken	1 (10.6 oz)	290	37	3	5
Cafe Steamers Grilled Whiskey Steak	1 (9.4 oz)	250	34	14	6
Chicken Carbonara	1 pkg	290	32	4	2
Chicken Margherita	1 pkg	340	42	11	6
Chicken Parmigiana	1 pkg (11.6 oz)	350	48	16	7
Chicken Breast & Vegetables	1 pkg	260	30	4	6
Chicken Piccata	1 pkg	260	36	5	2
Chicken Tuscany	1 pkg	340	39	4	4
Country Herb Chicken	1 pkg (11.35 oz)	240	34	15	5
Fresh Mixers Southwestern Chicken	1 pkg (7.9 oz)	310	60	3	5
Grilled Chicken Breast & Pasta	1 pkg	250	25	6	4
Lemon Pepper Fish	1 pkg (10.7 oz)	310	53	14	5
Mandarin Chicken	1 pkg (9.1 oz)	240	39	9	5
Oriental Style Chicken	1 pkg	240	28	5	4
Salisbury Steak	1 pkg (12.5 oz)	360	46	19	7
Salisbury Steak w/ Red Skin Mashed Potatoes	1 pkg	200	20	5	4
Slow Roasted Turkey Breast w/ Mashed Potatoes	1 pkg	210	17	1	4
Sweet & Sour Chicken	1 pkg (12 oz)	430	69	29	5
Traditional Turkey Breast	1 pkg	300	42	20	6

FOOD	PORTION	CALS	CARB	SUGAR	FIBER
Ian's					
Chicken Finger Meal Allergen Free	1 pkg (7 oz)	368	56	14	3
Chicken Nugget Meal	1 pkg (8 oz)	440	50	21	2
Fish Stick Meal	1 pkg (8.4 oz)	480	79	23	4
Hamburger Meal	1 pkg (7 oz)	296	45	13	3
Pizza Meal	1 pkg (6.7 oz)	340	60	23	4
Popcorn Turkey Dog Meal Allergen Free	1 pkg (7 oz)	442	67	27	1
Joy Of Cooking					
Braised Beef Tips & Egg Noodles	1 cup (7.7 oz)	220	24	3	1
Roasted Herb Chicken	1 cup (7.7 oz)	170	27	4	3
Kashi					
Black Bean Mango	1 pkg (10 oz)	340	58	11	7
Lemon Rosemary Chicken	1 pkg (10 oz)	330	45	1	5
Lime Cilantro Shrimp	1 pkg (10 oz)	250	33	8	6
Southwest Style Chicken	1 pkg (10 oz)	240	32	3	6
Sweet & Sour Chicken	1 pkg (10 oz)	320	55	25	6
Kid Cuisine					
All Star Chicken Breast Nuggets	1 meal	460	50	7	8
Bug Safari Chicken Breast Nuggets	1 meal	450	58	14	6
Carnival Corn Dog	1 meal	430	68	20	7
Deep Sea Adventure Fish Sticks	1 meal	400	56	16	4
Fiesta Beef Taco Dippers	1 meal	370	44	11	4
Pop Star Popcorn Chicken	1 meal	410	67	22	6
Lean Cuisine					
Cafe Classics Sweet & Sour Chicken	1 pkg (10 oz)	300	51	20	2
Dinnertime Selects Lemon Garlic Shrimp	1 pkg (12 oz)	350	54	3	5
Mon Cuisine					
Vegan Moroccan Couscous	1 pkg (10 oz)	280	46	10	10
Vegan Veal Schnitzel In Sauce	1 pkg (10 oz)	300	38	2	7
Vegetarian Stuffed Cabbage In Tomato Sauce	1 pkg (10 oz)	220	36	8	5
Moosewood					
Organic Vegetarian Moroccan Stew	1 pkg (10 oz)	150	29	11	5

FOOD	PORTION	CALS	CARB	SUGAR	FIBER
Organic Bistro					
Chicken Citron	1 pkg (13.5 oz)	490	53	15	6
Ginger Chicken	1 pkg (13.25 oz)	490	53	15	6
Jamaican Shrimp Cakes	1 pkg (12 oz)	380	55	10	7
Savory Turkey	1 pkg (12 oz)	430	43	5	8
Sockeye Salmon Cakes	1 pkg (12.2 oz)	600	36	7	8
Spiced Chicken Morocco	1 pkg (12.2 oz)	390	46	5	7
Wild Salmon	1 pkg (13.1 oz)	500	41	7	8
Organic Classics					
Chicken Marsala w/ Mashed Potatoes	1 pkg (9.5 oz)	330	31	3	3
Jamaican Style Jerk Chicken w/ Wehani Rice	1 pkg (9.5 oz)	270	37	8	4
Lemon Chicken w/ Wehani Rice	1 pkg (9.5 oz)	320	49	1	3
Seeds Of Change					
Chicken Teriyaki	1 pkg (10 oz)	300	47	11	4
Mushroom Wild Pilaf	1 pkg (11 oz)	350	40	5	5
Seven Grain Pilaf	1 pkg (11 oz)	390	52	7	10
Shady Brook					
Roasted Carved Turkey	1 pkg (18.6 oz)	550	72	22	4
South Beach					
Beef & Broccoli & Asian Style Noodles	1 pkg	320	32	8	9
Caprese Style Chicken w/ Cauliflower & Broccoli	1 pkg	250	12	6	3
Cashew Chicken w/ Sugar Snap Peas	1 pkg	360	31	7	8
Chicken Alfredo A La Roma	1 pkg	270	23	4	8
Chicken Basilico w/ Rotini	1 pkg	280	24	5	7
Chicken Santa Fe Style Rice & Beans	1 pkg (8.9 oz)	340	35	3	4
Garlic Herb Chicken w/ Green Beans Almondine	1 pkg	250	13	3	4

FOOD	PORTION	CALS	CARB	SUGAR	FIBER
Garlic Parmesan Chicken w/ Penne	1 pkg	290	24	3	8
Garlic Sesame Beef w/ Cauliflower Sugar Snap Peas & Peppers	1 pkg	250	19	8	4
Kung Pao Chicken Breast Strips w/ Peppers & Broccoli	1 pkg	300	18	7	5
Meatloaf w/ Gravy	1 pkg (8.9 oz)	210	17	5	4
Orange Beef Slices & Brown Rice In Sauce w/ Broccoli & Carrots	1 pkg	260	27	4	4
Roasted Turkey	1 pkg (9.4 oz)	240	27	2	4
Savory Beef w/ Cheesy Broccoli	1 pkg	240	16	7	3
Szechwan Pork & Asian Noodles In Sauce	1 pkg	270	32	8	9
Stouffer's					
Beef Stew	1 pkg (11 oz)	280	28	4	4
Beef Stroganoff	1 pkg (9.75 oz)	380	34	4	2
Chicken A La King	1 pkg (11.5 oz)	360	44	7	0
Corner Bistro Bourbon Steak Tips	1 pkg (12 oz)	520	56	26	3
Corner Bistro Sesame Chicken	1 pkg (12.63 oz)	510	72	19	5
Country Fried Beef Steak	1 pkg (16 oz)	610	55	12	6
Creamed Chipped Beef	½ pkg (5.5 oz)	140	9	5	0
Fish Filet	1 pkg (9 oz)	400	36	7	4
Fried Chicken Breast	1 pkg (8.88 oz)	360	30	2	2
Green Pepper Steak	1 pkg (10.5 oz)	240	32	5	3
Grilled Chicken Teriyaki	1 pkg (9.38 oz)	300	45	12	3
Grilled Lemon Pepper Chicken	1 pkg (9 oz)	240	24	3	4
Meatloaf	1 pkg (6 oz)	560	40	10	8
Pork Cutlet	1 pkg (10 oz)	370	31	2	3
Roast Pork	1 pkg (9.5 oz)	320	39	18	4
Roast Turkey Breast	1 pkg (16 oz)	390	48	10	6
Salisbury Steak	1 pkg (16 oz)	470	34	9	6

FOOD	PORTION	CALS	CARB	SUGAR	FIBER
Stuffed Pepper	1 pkg (10 oz)	220	22	9	2
Swedish Meatballs	1 pkg (11.5 oz)	560	47	6	3
Swanson					
Chicken & Dumplings	1 cup	230	24	2	2
Chicken A La King	1 can	270	12	2	2
Taste Above					
Meatless Zesty BBQ w/ Veggie Beef & Rice	1 pkg (10 oz)	280	48	18	7
TastyBite					
Beans Masala & Basmati Rice	1 pkg (12 oz)	426	75	5	13
Spinach Dal & Basmati Rice	1 pkg (12 oz)	372	62	4	8
Stir Fry Vegetables & Jasmine Rice	1 pkg (12 oz)	450	67	8	3
Vegetable Supreme & Basmati Rice	1 pkg (12 oz)	317	55	3	11
Yves					
Meatless Santa Fe Beef	1 pkg (10.5 oz)	360	57	12	5
DIP					
spinach sour cream	¼ cup	155	4	1	1
Bravo!					
Salsa	2 tbsp	15	3	2	0
Salsa Con Queso	1 tbsp	25	3	1	0
Cabot					
French Onion	2 tbsp	50	1	0	0
Ranch	2 tbsp	50	1	1	0
Cedarlane					
Organic Five Layer Mexican	2 tbsp	60	4	2	1
Guiltless Gourmet					
Black Bean Mild	2 tbsp (1.1 oz)	40	7	0	2
Health Is Wealth					
Vegetarian Spinach & Artichoke	3 tbsp (1 oz)	30	3	2	0
Kraft					
Green Onion	2 tbsp	60	3	tr	0
LiteHouse					
Avocado	2 tbsp	140	2	1	0
Caramel Low Fat	1 tbsp	110	27	16	0
Caramel Original	2 tbsp	110	25	15	1
Dilly	2 tbsp	150	1	1	0
Fruit Dip Chocolate Yogurt	2 tbsp	110	14	9	0
Fruit Dip Vanilla Yogurt	2 tbsp	60	10	7	0

FOOD	PORTION	CALS	CARB	SUGAR	FIBER
Lite Ranch Veggie	2 tbsp	70	3	1	0
Organic Ranch	2 tbsp	130	2	2	0
Marie's					
French Onion Roasted	2 tbsp	100	2	1	0
Guacamole	2 tbsp	40	3	1	1
Honey Vanilla Cream Fruit Dip	2 tbsp	60	5	3	0
Spinach Parmesan	2 tbsp	90	2	1	0
Naturally Fresh					
Caramel	2 tbsp	100	15	13	0
Chocolate	2 tbsp	70	17	14	0
Cream Cheese Strawberry	2 tbsp	90	14	10	0
Ranch Lite	2 tbsp	80	2	1	0
Ranch Vegetable	2 tbsp	120	2	1	0
Road's End Organics					
Nacho Cheese Gluten Free	2 tbsp	20	3	0	tr
Robert Rothchild Farm					
Artichoke	2 tbsp	60	2	1	tr
Snyder's Of Hanover					
Three Bean	2 tbsp	25	5	1	1
Utz					
Jalapeno Cheddar	2 tbsp	260	2	0	0
Sour Cream & Onion	2 tbsp	60	2	1	0
Wild Thymes Farm					
Indian Vindaloo Curry	1 tbsp	12	1	tr	tr
Indonesian Peanut Sauce	1 tbsp	32	2	1	tr
Wise					
French Onion	2 tbsp	60	3	0	0
Nacho Cheese	2 tbsp	50	3	1	0

DOUGHNUTS

FOOD	PORTION	CALS	CARB	SUGAR	FIBER
chocolate glazed	1 med (1.5 oz)	175	24	13	1
chocolate w/ chocolate icing	1 med (2 oz)	218	26	13	1
creme filled	1 (3 oz)	307	26	12	1
custard filled	1 (2.3 oz)	235	20	9	1
french cruller glazed	1 med (1.4 oz)	169	24	14	1
jelly filled	1 (3 oz)	289	33	18	1
old fashioned plain	1 med (2 oz)	226	25	9	1
oriental okinawan	1 (0.6 oz)	75	10	4	tr
plain chocolate frosted	1 med (1.5 oz)	194	22	11	1
plain glazed	1 med (1.6 oz)	192	23	–	1
whole wheat sugared	1 med (1.6 oz)	162	19	10	1

FOOD	PORTION	CALS	CARB	SUGAR	FIBER
Entenmann's					
Crumb	1	260	36	21	tr
Frosted Devil's Food	1	310	36	25	2
Glazed	1	260	34	20	tr
Glazed Popems	4	220	30	18	0
Mini Frosted	1 (1 oz)	150	13	8	tr
Plain Old Fashion	1	230	25	10	tr
PoP'ettes Chocolate Frosted	3 (2.2 oz)	330	28	16	1
DRINK MIXERS					
McIlhenny					
Bloody Mary Mix as prep	1 cup	70	15	9	2
DRUM					
freshwater fillet baked	5.4 oz	236	0	0	0
freshwater baked	3 oz	130	0	0	0
DUCK					
boneless roasted	½ duck (7.8 oz)	444	0	0	0
boneless w/o skin roasted	3.5 oz	201	0	0	0
boneless w/o skin roasted diced	1 cup (4.9 oz)	281	0	0	0
chinese pressed	1 cup (4.9 oz)	267	26	14	1
chinese pressed	3 oz	162	16	9	1
pekin breast boneless w/ skin roasted	1 (4.2 oz)	242	0	0	0
pekin breast w/o skin broiled	3 oz	133	0	0	0
pekin leg w/ skin w/o bone roasted	1 (3.2 oz)	200	0	0	0
pekin leg w/o skin & bone roasted	1 (2.6 oz)	134	0	0	0
w/ skin & bone roasted	1 serv (6 oz)	583	0	0	0
w/ skin & bone roasted	½ duck (13 oz)	1287	0	0	0
TAKE-OUT					
breast battered & fried bone removed	½ (3.2 oz)	199	6	tr	tr
leg battered & fried bone removed	1 (2.5 oz)	155	5	tr	tr
wing roasted bone removed	1 (1.1 oz)	101	0	0	0

FOOD	PORTION	CALS	CARB	SUGAR	FIBER
DUMPLING					
Health Is Wealth					
Potstickers Vegan	2 (1.6 oz)	90	13	tr	2
Kahiki					
Potstickers Chicken	5 (3.3 oz)	230	24	1	1
Samosas Coconut Curry Chicken	4 (2.8 oz)	170	26	1	1
Pepperidge Farm					
Apple	1	250	32	15	1
Peach	1	320	50	15	4
Traveling Chef					
Potstickers Chicken + Dipping Sauce	5 pieces + 1 tbsp sauce	285	42	11	1
TAKE-OUT					
apple	1 (6.7 oz)	661	83	30	3
cherry	1 (2.7 oz)	238	31	13	1
cornmeal	1 (2.8 oz)	134	20	1	2
fried pork	1 (3.5 oz)	338	25	1	1
fried puerto rican style	1 med (1.1 oz)	117	11	1	tr
gyoza potstickers vegetable	8 (4.9 oz)	210	34	7	5
peach	1 (2.7 oz)	253	33	12	1
piroshki meat filled	1 (3.4 oz)	348	25	tr	1
steamed meat	1 (1.3 oz)	41	4	tr	tr
EDAMAME *(see SOYBEANS)*					
EEL					
fresh cooked	1 fillet (5.6 oz)	375	0	0	0
fresh cooked	3 oz	200	0	0	0
raw	3 oz	156	0	0	0
smoked	3.5 oz	330	0	0	0
EGG *(see also EGG DISHES, EGG SUBSTITUTES)*					
CHICKEN					
hard or soft cooked	1	77	1	1	0
pickled	1	72	1	1	0
poached	1	73	tr	tr	0
sunny side up	2	155	1	1	0
white cooked	1	17	tr	tr	0
yolk cooked	1	55	1	tr	0
Crystal Farms					
In Shell Pasteurized	1	70	1	0	0

FOOD	PORTION	CALS	CARB	SUGAR	FIBER
Peeled Hard Cooked	1	70	1	1	0
Davidson's					
Pasteurized Shell Eggs	1 lg	75	0	0	0
Egg Innovations					
100% Organic Cage Free Large	1 (1.8 oz)	70	1	0	0
Egg-Land's Best					
Extra Large	1 (2 oz)	80	0	0	0
Large	1	70	0	0	0
Eggology					
100% Organic Egg Whites	¼ cup	30	0	0	0
Good Earth Organics					
Organic Instant Whites	1 pkg (0.5 oz)	50	1	1	0
Horizon Organic					
Jumbo	1 (2.2 oz)	90	1	0	0
Organic Valley					
Egg Whites Pasteurized	¼ cup	25	1	0	0
Tree Of Life					
White Large Natural Omega-3	1 (1.8 oz)	70	tr	0	0
OTHER POULTRY					
duck cooked	1 (2.5 oz)	129	1	1	0
duck preserved hard core	1 (1.8 oz)	80	1	0	0
duck preserved soft core	1 (1.8 oz)	80	1	0	0
goose cooked	1 (5 oz)	265	2	1	0
quail canned	1 (0.3 oz)	14	tr	tr	0
quail cooked	1 (0.5 oz)	24	0	0	0
EGG DISHES					
Aunt Jemima					
Eggs & Sausage	1 pkg (6.2 oz)	370	16	3	2
Omelet Ham & Cheese	1 pkg (5.2 oz)	250	17	2	2
Cedarlane					
Zone Omelette Cheese	1 pkg (10.4 oz)	350	31	5	2
Jimmy Dean					
Breakfast Skillets Bacon as prep	1 serv (4.5 oz)	370	14	2	2
Breakfast Skillets Ham as prep	1 serv (4.5 oz)	270	16	1	2
Breakfast Skillets Smoked Sausage as prep	1 serv (4.5 oz)	380	20	1	3
Breakfast Bowls D-Lights Sausage	1 pkg	230	19	1	2
Breakfast Bowls Eggs Potato & Ham	1 pkg	390	23	1	3

FOOD	PORTION	CALS	CARB	SUGAR	FIBER
Breakfast Bowls Eggs Potatoes Sausage & Cheddar Cheese	1 pkg	490	20	1	3
Omelets Ham & Cheese	1 (4.2 oz)	280	4	1	0
Omelets Sausage & Cheese	1 (4.3 oz)	270	5	1	0
TAKE-OUT					
deviled	1 half	62	tr	tr	0
eggs benedict	2	825	26	3	2
omelet cheese	3 eggs	387	6	6	0
omelet mushroom	3 eggs	251	6	4	1
omelet mushroom & onion	3 eggs	294	7	5	1
omelet plain	3 eggs	338	4	4	0
omelet spanish	3 eggs	496	17	11	3
omelet spinach	3 eggs	279	6	4	1
omelet western	3 eggs	355	6	4	tr
salad	½ cup	353	2	1	0
scotch egg	1 (4.2 oz)	301	16	–	2
tortilla de amarillo omelet w/ plantain	3 eggs	536	43	21	3

EGG ROLLS

FOOD	PORTION	CALS	CARB	SUGAR	FIBER
egg roll wrapper fresh	1 (1.1 oz)	93	19	–	1
spring roll deep fried	1 (0.8 oz)	70	7	–	1
Blue Horizon Organic					
Spring Rolls Chinese Shrimp	3 (2.1 oz)	130	16	1	1
Spring Rolls Indian	3 (2.1 oz)	110	15	1	1
Spring Rolls Thai	3 (2.1 oz)	110	16	1	1
Spring Rolls Thai Shrimp	3 (2.1 oz)	130	15	1	1
Frieda's					
Egg Roll Wrappers	2 (1.6 oz)	130	28	1	1
Health Is Wealth					
Spinach	1 (3 oz)	170	18	1	3
Thai Spring Roll	2 (1.6 oz)	90	13	1	1
Kahiki					
Chicken	1 (3 oz)	160	19	2	1
Chipotle Lime Chicken	1 (3 oz)	170	26	3	2
Lemongrass Chicken Stix	3 (2.6 oz)	100	13	3	tr
Pork & Shrimp	1 (3 oz)	140	20	2	1
Vegetable	1 (3 oz)	90	12	2	1
TAKE-OUT					
chicken	1 (3 oz)	140	20	5	4
lobster	1 (4.8 oz)	270	43	4	6

FOOD	PORTION	CALS	CARB	SUGAR	FIBER
lumpia vegetable & shrimp	2 (3 oz)	120	26	1	2
meat & shrimp	1 (4.8 oz)	320	41	3	4
pork & shrimp	1 (5 oz)	300	41	6	7
shrimp	1 (3 oz)	170	24	5	5
spicy pork	1 (3 oz)	200	23	3	3
vegetable	1 (3 oz)	170	28	4	4

EGG SUBSTITUTES
Better'n Eggs
All Whites	¼ cup	30	1	1	0
Ham & Cheese	¼ cup	45	1	0	0
Original	¼ cup (2 oz)	30	1	1	0
Plus	¼ cup	35	1	0	0
Three Cheese	¼ cup	45	1	0	0

Bob's Red Mill
Egg White Dried	2 tsp	15	0	0	0
Vegetarian Egg Replacer	1 tbsp	30	2	1	1

EggPro
Powder	1 tbsp	15	tr	0	0

Fantastic
Tofu Scrambler not prep	1 tbsp	35	7	0	1

Horizon Organic
Liquid Egg	¼ cup	35	1	0	0

Quick Eggs
Fat Free Cholesterol Free	¼ cup	30	1	tr	0

EGGNOG
Farmland
Egg Nog	½ cup	180	23	22	0

Hood
Fat Free Sugar Free	1 cup	110	18	12	0
Golden	½ cup	180	22	20	0
Light	½ cup	140	22	21	0

Horizon Organic
Lowfat	½ cup	140	22	22	0

Organic Valley
Ultra Pasteurized	½ cup	180	18	17	0

Straus
Organic Cream Top	4 oz	160	13	13	0

TAKE-OUT
eggnog	1 cup	306	16	–	0

FOOD	PORTION	CALS	CARB	SUGAR	FIBER
EGGPLANT					
cubed cooked w/ oil	1 cup	133	17	6	5
pickled	½ cup	33	7	3	2
slices grilled	1 (2 oz)	36	5	2	1
Cedarlane					
Eggplant Mediterranean	1 pkg (10 oz)	230	22	7	6
Celentano					
Eggplant Parmigiana	1 serv (7 oz)	330	26	9	5
Frieda's					
Chinese	⅔ cup (3 oz)	20	5	3	2
Japanese Nasu	⅔ cup (3 oz)	20	3	2	2
Peloponnese					
Baba Ganoush	2 tbsp	40	2	0	1
Sabra					
Baba Ghanoush	2 oz	50	4	0	1
TastyBite					
Punjab Eggplant	½ pkg (5 oz)	144	13	4	2
TAKE-OUT					
iman bayildi eggplant w/ onion & tomato	1 serv (15.6 oz)	345	25	6	2
indian eggplant runi	1 serv	180	13	1	1
moussaka	1 serv (9 oz)	372	18	6	5
papoutsaki little shoes	1 serv (15.5 oz)	245	15	1	1
tempura	1 serv (1.5 oz)	118	5	0	1
ELK					
eye of round roasted	3.5 oz	151	1	0	0
ground cooked	3.5 oz	143	0	0	0
Natural Frontier Foods					
Filet	1 (4 oz)	140	0	0	0
ENERGY BARS (see also CEREAL BARS, NUTRITION SUPPLEMENTS)					
Activex					
Organic All Flavors	1 (1.6 oz)	200	17	8	2
Amino Vital					
Fit Apple Pie	1 (1.76 oz)	150	26	2	2
Fit Chocolate Peanut	1 (1.76 oz)	190	25	2	2
Fit Toasted Nut Cranberry	1 (1.76 oz)	180	24	4	2
Attune					
Wellness Chocolate Crisp	1 (0.7 oz)	100	11	8	1

FOOD	PORTION	CALS	CARB	SUGAR	FIBER
Wellness Cool Mint Chocolate	1 (0.7 oz)	100	11	8	1
Balance					
100 Calories Peanut Butter Crisp	1 (1 oz)	100	14	4	5
100 Calories Vanilla Crisp	1 (1 oz)	100	15	5	5
Carbwell Chocolate Fudge	1 (1.8 oz)	190	23	1	2
Gold Chocolate Peanut Butter	1 (1.8 oz)	210	23	14	tr
Gold S'mores Crunch	1 (1.8 oz)	210	23	12	0
Organic Apricot Mango Crisp	1 (1.6 oz)	180	23	11	5
Organic Cranberry Pomegranate Crisp	1 (1.6 oz)	180	23	12	5
Original Almond Brownie	1 (1.8 oz)	200	22	17	2
Original Mocha Crisp	1 (1.8 oz)	200	21	18	tr
Pure Banana Cashew	1 (1.6 oz)	180	23	18	2
Pure Cherry Pecan	1 (1.6 oz)	190	22	18	2
Belly-bar					
Baby Needs Chocolate	1	170	22	12	2
Berry Nutty Cravings	1	170	26	13	2
Mellow Oat	1	180	26	11	2
Boomi Bar					
Almond Protein Plus	1	270	20	15	4
Cashew Almond Delicacy	1	260	23	3	1
Cranberry Apple	1	210	28	18	4
Merry Macadamia	1	220	26	21	3
Pistachio Pineapple	1	200	28	17	3
Bora Bora					
Organic Cranberry Crunch	1 (1.4 oz)	170	18	9	2
Organic Peanut Peanut	1 (1.4 oz)	230	10	5	2
Organic Sesame Raisin	1 (1.4 oz)	170	17	12	3
Clif					
Banana Nut Bread	1 (2.4 oz)	250	43	21	5
Builders Chocolate Mint	1 (2.4 oz)	270	31	20	4
Builders Peanut Butter	1 (2.4 oz)	270	30	20	4
Carrot Cake	1 (2.4 oz)	240	46	21	5
Chocolate Brownie	1 (2.4 oz)	240	45	20	5
Chocolate Chip	1 (2.4 oz)	250	45	21	5
Cool Mint Chocolate	1 (2.4 oz)	250	43	17	5
Crunchy Peanut Butter	1 (2.4 oz)	250	40	18	5
Mojo Mixed Nuts	1 (1.6 oz)	220	21	7	3
Mojo Mountain Mix	1 (1.6 oz)	200	24	12	2

FOOD	PORTION	CALS	CARB	SUGAR	FIBER
Nectar Cinnamon Pecan	1 (1.6 oz)	170	26	19	6
Nectar Lemon Vanilla Cashew	1 (1.6 oz)	180	27	17	6
Oatmeal Raisin Walnut	1 (2.4 oz)	240	43	20	5
ZBar Peanut Butter	1 (1.3 oz)	140	20	11	3
Glucerna					
All Flavors	1 (0.7 oz)	80	12	4	tr
Gnu					
Flavor & Fiber Banana Walnut	1 (1.4 oz)	130	30	8	12
Flavor & Fiber Chocolate Brownie Bar	1 (1.4 oz)	140	32	9	12
Hooah!					
Chocolate Crisp	1 (2.29 oz)	280	40	18	2
JojoBar					
Chocolate Cashew	1 (1.8 oz)	220	18	6	2
Peanut Butter & Jelly	1 (1.8 oz)	220	17	6	3
Kashi					
GoLean Chocolate Almond Toffee	1 (2.7 oz)	290	45	31	6
GoLean Cookies 'N Cream	1 (2.7 oz)	290	50	35	6
GoLean Malted Chocolate Chip	1 (2.7 oz)	290	49	35	6
GoLean Oatmeal Raisin Cookie	1 (2.7 oz)	280	49	33	6
GoLean Peanut Butter & Chocolate	1 (2.7 oz)	290	48	31	6
GoLean Crunchy Chocolate Peanut	1 (1.8 oz)	180	30	13	6
GoLean Roll Caramel Peanut	1 (1.9 oz)	200	29	14	6
GoLean Roll Fudge Sundae	1 (1.9 oz)	190	27	13	6
TLC Chewy Granola Cherry Dark Chocolate	1 (1.2 oz)	120	24	8	4
TLC Crunchy Granola Honey Toasted 7 Grain	1 (1.4 oz)	180	26	7	4
TLC Crunchy Granola Pumpkin Spice	1 (1.4 oz)	180	26	7	4
TLC Crunchy Granola Roasted Almond	1 (1.4 oz)	180	26	7	4
LaraBar					
Jocalat Chocolate	1 (1.7 oz)	190	24	18	5
Lean Body					
Gold Caramel Cookie Twist	1 (2.9 oz)	330	36	10	2

FOOD	PORTION	CALS	CARB	SUGAR	FIBER
Living Harvest					
Organic Hemp Protein Forbidden Fruit	1 (1.6 oz)	170	25	18	4
Luna					
Caramel Nut Brownie	1 (1.7 oz)	190	27	11	4
Chai Tea	1 (1.7 oz)	180	27	9	3
Dulce De Leche	1 (1.7 oz)	180	28	12	3
Iced Oatmeal Raisin	1 (1.7 oz)	180	28	11	3
LemonZest	1 (1.7 oz)	180	26	10	3
Nutz Over Chocolate	1 (1.7 oz)	180	24	8	3
Mommy Munchies					
Chocolate Mint	1 (1.8 oz)	180	32	13	5
Cinnamon Bun	1 (1.8 oz)	180	23	15	5
Mrs. May's					
Trio Blueberry	1 (1.2 oz)	170	15	6	2
Trio Tropical	1 (1.2 oz)	170	14	6	2
Nature's Path					
Optimum Blueberry Flax & Soy	1 (2 oz)	200	37	20	5
Optimum Cranberry Ginger & Soy	1 (2 oz)	200	37	21	5
Optimum Peanut Butter	1 (2 oz)	230	33	14	4
Optimum Pomegran Cherry	1 (2 oz)	230	39	17	4
Nutiva					
Organic Flax & Raisin	1 (1.4 oz)	200	15	8	4
Organic Flaxseed Flax Chocolate	1 (1.4 oz)	200	19	10	5
Organic Original Hempseed	1 (1.4 oz)	210	11	5	5
Odwalla					
Berries GoMega	1	220	41	20	5
Carrot	1	220	43	21	4
Choco-walla	1	240	42	20	5
Cranberry C Monster	1	220	44	21	3
Super Protein	1	230	31	16	4
Superfood	1	230	43	20	3
Oh Mama!					
Chocolate Peanut Butter	1 (1.8 oz)	190	26	13	3
Frosted White Lemon	1 (1.8 oz)	180	28	13	3
Frosted White Raspberry	1 (1.8 oz)	180	26	10	3
Perfect 10					
Bliss Apricot	1 (1.8 oz)	215	29	24	5

FOOD	PORTION	CALS	CARB	SUGAR	FIBER
Bliss Cranberry	1 (1.8 oz)	215	26	20	4
Natural Apricot	1 (1.8 oz)	205	27	20	4
Natural Cranberry	1 (1.8 oz)	164	17	11	4
Natural Lemon	1 (1.8 oz)	210	24	18	5
Prana Bar					
Apricot Goji	1 (1.7 oz)	220	26	16	3
Coconut Acai	1 (1.7 oz)	220	26	18	3
Pear Ginseng	1 (1.7 oz)	220	21	12	4
PureFit					
Almond Crunch	1 (2 oz)	230	25	16	3
Peanut Butter Crunch	1 (2 oz)	240	26	16	2
Sencha Naturals					
Green Tea Bar Lively Lemongrass	1 (2 oz)	220	29	12	3
Green Tea Bar Original	1 (2 oz)	220	29	12	3
Simply Nutrilite					
Sweet & Salty	1 (1.6 oz)	170	27	21	4
Snickers Marathon					
Chewy Chocolate Peanut	1 (1.9 oz)	210	26	15	5
South Beach					
Energy Mix	1 pkg (1 oz)	160	8	3	2
SoyJoy					
Fruit & Soy Bar Mango Coconut	1 (1.1 oz)	140	16	11	3
Fruit & Soy Bar Raisin Almond	1 (1.1 oz)	130	16	11	3
Fruit & Soy Bars Berry	1 (1.1 oz)	130	17	12	3
Think5					
Red Berry	1 (2.5 oz)	240	48	7	3
Red Berry Chocolate Covered	1 (2.8 oz)	290	52	16	3
ThinkPink					
Blueberry Dark Chocolate	1 (2.1 oz)	240	26	0	2
Lemon Burst	1 (2.1 oz)	230	27	0	2
Peanut Butter Caramel	1 (2.1 oz)	230	26	0	1
White Chocolate Raspberry	1 (2.1 oz)	240	28	1	3
Zoe's					
Chocolate Delight	1 (1.7 oz)	190	27	13	5
Chocolate Peanut Butter Bliss	1 (1.7 oz)	200	26	11	5
Heavenly Apple	1 (1.7 oz)	180	28	10	5
Peanut Butter Paradise	1 (1.7 oz)	190	27	8	5

FOOD	PORTION	CALS	CARB	SUGAR	FIBER
ENERGY DRINKS					
1In3Trinity					
Energy Drink	1 can (8.4 oz)	10	3	3	0
Accelerade					
All Flavors	8 oz	80	16	16	0
Bawls					
Guaranexx Sugar Free	1 bottle (10 oz)	0	0	0	0
Boost					
Beauty	1 bottle (12 oz)	220	52	40	tr
High Protein Vanilla	8 oz	240	33	16	0
Youth	1 bottle (12 oz)	200	48	36	tr
Cintron					
Citrus Mango	8 oz	110	27	26	0
Citrus Mango Sugar Free	8 oz	0	0	0	0
Coca-Cola					
Zero	8 oz	1	tr	0	0
Dr. Tim's					
Jungle Juice	1 bottle (4 oz)	20	8	4	0
Ginger Boost					
Ginger Orange	8 oz	110	24	21	1
Gleukos					
Preformance All Flavors	8 oz	70	17	17	0
Guayaki					
Organic Empower Mint	8 oz	38	9	9	tr
Organic Raspberry Revolution	8 oz	50	12	12	tr
Organic Unsweetened	8 oz	15	3	tr	tr
Hiball					
All Flavors	1 bottle (10 oz)	10	0	0	0
Jet Set					
Club Soda	1 can (12 oz)	0	0	0	0
Ginger Ale	1 can (12 oz)	150	37	36	0
Original	1 can (12 oz)	105	29	29	0
Tonic Water	1 can (12 oz)	150	37	36	0
King 888					
Sugar Free	8 oz	0	0	0	0
Liv Naturals					
All Flavors	8 oz	70	16	13	0

FOOD	PORTION	CALS	CARB	SUGAR	FIBER
Marquis Platinum					
Vitality Drink	1 can	30	16	7	1
Mix1					
All Flavors	1 bottle (11 oz)	200	29	22	3
Mr. Re					
Restorative	1 can (11 oz)	80	22	21	0
Odwalla					
Berries GoMega	8 oz	160	34	24	5
Mo' Beta	8 oz	150	37	26	1
Super Protein Original	8 oz	190	35	29	1
Superfood	8 oz	130	30	25	0
Wellness	8 oz	150	33	24	1
Rockstar					
Juiced	8 oz	90	22	21	0
Simply Nutrilite					
Berry Antioxidant	1 can (8.4 oz)	120	29	29	0
Source Burn					
Sugar Free	8 oz	10	0	0	0
T-Fusion					
Energy Tea	8 oz	0	1	0	0
ViB					
Chill-N	1 can (8 oz)	40	10	10	0
Who's Your Daddy					
Sugar Free	8 oz	0	0	0	0
Xcyto					
Sugar Free	1 can (12.5 oz)	10	2	0	0
Youth Juice					
Drink	2 oz	10	3	2	1
Zenergize					
Chill	1 tablet	2	1	0	0
Energy+	1 tablet	2	1	0	0
Hydrate	1 tablet	2	1	0	0
ENGLISH MUFFIN					
READY-TO-EAT					
crumpets	1 (1.5 oz)	80	16	1	tr
whole wheat	1	134	27	–	4
Crystal Farms					
English Muffin	1	130	27	2	1

FOOD	PORTION	CALS	CARB	SUGAR	FIBER
Pepperidge Farm					
100% Whole Wheat	1	140	26	4	3
Original	1	130	25	1	1
Roman Meal					
English Muffin	1 (2.3 oz)	140	29	4	3
Rudi's Organic Bakery					
MultiGrain w/ Flax	1 (2 oz)	130	25	2	2
Whole Grain Wheat	1 (2 oz)	120	23	2	3
Sara Lee					
Heart Healthy Wheat w/ Honey	1	140	28	3	2
Original w/ Whole Grain	1	140	27	2	2
Sun-Maid					
Raisin	1 (2.5 oz)	170	36	13	2
Thomas'					
100 Calories	1	100	24	tr	5
Corn	1	150	29	1	2
Griller Multi Grain	1 (3.2 oz)	210	41	5	3
Griller Onion	1 (3.2 oz)	200	40	2	2
Hearty Grains 100% Whole Wheat	1	120	23	2	3
Hearty Grains Honey Wheat	1	130	27	3	2
Light Multi-Grain	1	100	24	tr	8
Oatmeal & Honey	1	130	25	3	2
Original Whole Grain	1	130	26	1	2
Raisin Cinnamon	1	140	29	8	1
Sandwich Size Original	1	190	38	2	2
FALAFEL					
Near East					
Falafel Patties Vegetarian as prep	2.5	220	18	3	5
Sabra					
Burger	1 (1.8 oz)	90	11	2	3
VeggieLand					
FalafelBurger	1 (4 oz)	190	26	1	8
FAT (see also BUTTER, BUTTER SUBSTITUTES, MARGARINE, OIL)					
bacon grease	1 tbsp	116	0	0	0
beef shortening	1 tbsp	115	0	0	0
beef suet	1 oz	242	0	0	0
chicken	1 tbsp (0.4 oz)	115	0	0	0

FOOD	PORTION	CALS	CARB	SUGAR	FIBER
duck	1 tbsp (0.4 oz)	113	0	0	0
goose	1 tbsp	115	0	0	0
goose	1 oz	257	0	0	0
lamb new zealand	1 oz	182	0	0	0
lard	1 tbsp (0.5 oz)	115	0	0	0
lard	1 cup (7.2 oz)	1849	0	0	0
meat pan drippings	½ tbsp	124	0	0	0
pork raw	1 oz	230	0	0	0
salt pork	1 cube (1 oz)	215	0	0	0
shortening	1 cup	1812	0	0	0
shortening	1 tbsp	113	0	0	0
turkey	1 tbsp	116	0	0	0
ucuhuba butter	1 tbsp	120	0	0	0
whale blubber	1 oz	244	0	0	0
Crisco					
Butter Flavor	1 tbsp	110	0	0	0
Shortening	1 tbsp	110	0	0	0
Earth Balance					
Natural Shortening	1 tbsp	130	0	0	0
Nebraska Land					
Pork Fatback	½ oz	110	0	0	0
Smart Balance					
Shortening	1 tbsp	110	0	0	0

FAVA BEANS

FOOD	PORTION	CALS	CARB	SUGAR	FIBER
fava fresh cooked	½ cup	94	17	2	5
Progresso					
Fava Beans	½ cup (4.6 oz)	100	17	–	5

FENNEL

FOOD	PORTION	CALS	CARB	SUGAR	FIBER
fresh bulb	1 (8.2 oz)	73	17	–	7
fresh sliced	1 cup	27	6	–	3
leaves	1 oz	7	1	–	1
seed	1 tsp	7	1	–	1
stir fried	1 cup	85	9	5	3
Ocean Mist					
Fennel Sweet Anise Sliced Fresh	1 cup	27	6	0	3

FENUGREEK

FOOD	PORTION	CALS	CARB	SUGAR	FIBER
seed	1 tsp	12	2	–	1

FOOD	PORTION	CALS	CARB	SUGAR	FIBER
FIBER					
UniFiber					
Natural Fiber	1 pkg (4 g)	4	tr	–	3
Wellements					
Fiber-Psyll	1 scoop (0.5 oz)	55	14	0	12
FIG JUICE					
Smart Juice					
Organic 100% Juice	8 oz	131	35	29	1
FIGS					
canned in heavy syrup	½ cup	114	30	27	3
canned in light syrup	½ cup	87	23	20	2
canned water pack	½ cup	66	17	15	3
dried cooked	½ cup	139	36	30	5
dried small	1 (1.4 oz)	30	8	7	1
dried whole	1 (8 g)	21	5	4	1
fresh large	1 (2.2 oz)	47	12	10	2
Blue Ribbon					
California Figs	1 pkg (1.5 oz)	120	28	21	5
Figamajigs					
Chocolate Covered Bar	1 bar (1.4 oz)	130	26	19	5
Chocolate Covered Bar w/ Almonds	1 bar (1.4 oz)	150	28	19	4
Hermes					
Organic Adriatic Fig Spread	1 tbsp	60	15	14	0
Nuta Figs					
Mission	¼ cup (1.4 oz)	110	26	20	5
Orchard Choice					
Mission	4–5 (1.4 oz)	110	26	20	5
Sun-Maid					
California Mission	4 (1.5 oz)	120	28	21	5
Calimyrna	3 (1.5 oz)	120	28	21	5
Trucco					
Kalamata	2	100	26	22	4
FISH (see also individual names, FISH SUBSTITUTES, SUSHI)					
CANNED					
Beach Cliff					
Fish Steaks In Louisiana Hot Sauce	1 can (3.7 oz)	160	2	0	0
Fish Steaks In Mustard Sauce	1 can (3.7 oz)	160	2	0	0

FOOD	PORTION	CALS	CARB	SUGAR	FIBER
Fish Steaks In Soybean Oil	1 can (3.7 oz)	200	1	0	0
Fish Steaks w/ Hot Green Chilies	1 can (3.7 oz)	160	1	0	0
Fish Steaks w/ Jalapeno Peppers	1 can (3.7 oz)	130	1	0	0
Brunswick					
Fish Steaks In Louisiana Hot Sauce	1 can (3.7 oz)	160	2	0	0
Fish Steaks In Mustard Sauce	1 can (3.7 oz)	160	2	0	0
Fish Steaks In Soybean Oil	1 can (3.7 oz)	200	1	0	0
Fish Steaks In Spring Water	1 can (3.7 oz)	150	0	0	0
Fish Steaks w/ Hot Tabasco Peppers	1 can (3.7 oz)	220	1	0	0
Seafood Snacks Golden Smoked	1 can (3.2 oz)	170	0	0	0
Seafood Snacks In Lemon & Cracked Pepper	1 can (3.2 oz)	160	0	0	0
Seafood Snacks In Louisiana Hot Sauce	1 can (3.2 oz)	140	2	0	0
Seafood Snacks In Teriyaki Sauce	1 can (3.2 oz)	160	5	4	0
Seafood Snacks In Tomato & Basil Sauce	1 can (3.2 oz)	140	2	1	0
Seafood Snacks Kippered	1 can (3.2 oz)	160	0	0	0
FROZEN					
Dr. Praeger's					
Breaded Fillets	1 (2.1 oz)	100	12	1	0
Fishies	3 (1.5 oz)	90	9	1	0
Gorton's					
Classic Crispy Battered Fillets	2	230	22	3	5
Fillets Beer Battered	2 (3.6 oz)	250	17	4	1
Fillets Potato Crunch	2 (3.6 oz)	240	20	3	2
Fish Sticks Classic Breaded	6	290	19	2	1
Grilled Fillets Cajun Blackened	1 (3.8 oz)	100	1	0	0
Grilled Fillets Lemon Pepper	1 (3.7 oz)	100	1	0	0
Tenders Original Batter	3 pieces (3.6 oz)	230	23	3	2
Ian's					
Fillets	1 (3.4 oz)	260	32	4	2
Fish Stick Allergy Free	5 pieces	190	24	3	1

FOOD	PORTION	CALS	CARB	SUGAR	FIBER
Fish Sticks	5 pieces	190	24	3	1
Van de Kamp's					
Battered Tenders	4 (4 oz)	210	22	5	1
Crisp & Healthy Breaded Fish Sticks	6 (3.6 oz)	140	24	3	1
Crunchy Fillets	2 (3.5 oz)	230	21	2	tr
Sticks	6 (4 oz)	260	26	3	1
TAKE-OUT					
jamaican brown fish stew	1 serv	426	9	–	2
kedgeree	5.6 oz	242	15	–	1
mousse	1 serv (3.5 oz)	185	3	tr	tr
FISH OIL					
cod liver	1 tbsp	123	0	0	0
herring	1 tbsp	123	0	0	0
menhaden	1 tbsp	123	0	0	0
salmon	1 tbsp	123	0	0	0
sardine	1 tbsp	123	0	0	0
shark	1 oz	270	0	0	0
whale beluga	1 oz	252	0	0	0
whale bowhead	1 oz	252	0	0	0
FISH PASTE					
fish paste	2 tsp	15	tr	–	0
FLAXSEED					
Arrowhead Mills					
Organic	3 tbsp (1 oz)	140	9	0	7
Bob's Red Mill					
Flaxseed Meal	2 tbsp	60	4	0	4
Carrington Farms					
Organic Flax Paks	1 pkg (0.4 oz)	50	3	0	3
Flax USA					
Flax Sprinkles	2 tbsp (0.5 oz)	70	4	0	3
Hodgson Mill					
Milled	2 tbsp	60	4	0	4
Natural Ovens					
Flax Complete Supplement	1 tbsp (0.4 oz)	60	4	1	2
Tree Of Life					
Flax Seed	3 tbsp (1 oz)	140	11	0	6

FOOD	PORTION	CALS	CARB	SUGAR	FIBER
FLOUNDER					
FRESH					
cooked	1 fillet (4.5 oz)	148	0	0	0
cooked	3 oz	99	0	0	0
FROZEN					
Mrs. Paul's					
Filets Lightly Breaded	1 (2.7 oz)	150	12	3	1
TAKE-OUT					
stuffed w/ crab	1 piece (7.6 oz)	332	14	2	1
FLOUR					
all-purpose self-rising	½ cup (2.2 oz)	221	46	tr	2
all-purpose unbleached	½ cup (2.2 oz)	228	48	tr	2
arrowroot	½ cup (2.2 oz)	228	56	–	2
bread flour	½ cup (2.4 oz)	247	50	tr	2
buckwheat whole groat	½ cup (2.1 oz)	201	42	2	6
cake	½ cup (2.4 oz)	248	53	tr	1
carob	1 tbsp (0.2 oz)	13	5	3	2
carob	½ cup (1.8 oz)	114	46	25	21
chickpea besan	½ cup (1.6 oz)	178	27	5	5
peanut low fat	½ cup (1.1 oz)	128	9	–	5
potato	½ cup (2.8 oz)	286	66	3	5
rice brown	½ cup (2.8 oz)	287	60	1	4
rice white	½ cup (2.8 oz)	289	63	tr	2
rye dark	½ cup (2.2 oz)	207	44	1	15
rye light	½ cup (1.8 oz)	187	41	1	7
soy lowfat	½ cup (1.5 oz)	165	15	5	7
triticale whole grain	½ cup (2.3 oz)	220	48	–	10
white all-purpose enriched bleached	½ cup (2.2 oz)	228	48	tr	2
whole wheat	½ cup (2.1 oz)	203	44	tr	7
Arrowhead Mills					
Organic Barley	⅓ cup	95	19	0	4
Organic Brown Rice	⅓ cup	130	27	0	2
Organic Kamut	⅓ cup	130	25	0	4
Organic Oat	⅓ cup	120	21	0	3
Organic Rye	¼ cup	110	24	0	4
Organic Spelt	⅓ cup	130	25	0	4
Organic Unbleached White	¼ cup	120	26	0	tr
Organic White Rice	⅓ cup	120	28	0	tr

FOOD	PORTION	CALS	CARB	SUGAR	FIBER
Bob's Red Mill					
Brown Rice	¼ cup	140	31	0	1
Corn	¼ cup	160	22	0	4
Graham	¼ cup	120	21	0	3
Kamut Organic	¼ cup	94	21	0	3
Sorghum Sweet White Gluten Free	¼ cup	120	25	0	3
Spelt	¼ cup	120	22	0	4
Whole Wheat	¼ cup	110	23	1	4
Whole Wheat Hard White Organic	¼ cup	120	24	0	4
Domata Living Flour					
Gluten Free Casein Free	¼ cup	110	26	0	tr
Gold Medal					
All Purpose	¼ cup (1 oz)	100	22	tr	tr
Self Rising	¼ cup (1 oz)	100	23	–	tr
Whole Wheat	¼ cup (1 oz)	100	21	–	3
Wondra	¼ cup (1 oz)	100	23	–	tr
Heckers					
All Purpose Unbleached	¼ cup	100	22	tr	tr
Hodgson Mill					
Best For Bread	¼ cup	100	22	0	1
Buckwheat	¼ cup	100	22	0	3
Oat Bran Flour	¼ cup	110	23	0	3
Kentucky Kernel					
Seasoned Flour	4 tsp	36	8	0	0
King Arthur					
All Purpose	¼ cup	110	22	tr	tr
All Purpose Unbleached	¼ cup	110	22	tr	1
Organic Artisan	¼ cup	110	23	tr	tr
Organic White Whole Wheat	¼ cup	100	18	tr	3
Organic Whole Wheat	½ cup	110	23	0	4
Self-Rising	¼ cup	120	27	0	1
White Whole Wheat	¼ cup	100	18	tr	3
Whole Wheat	¼ cup	110	21	1	4
Lundberg					
Brown Rice	¼ cup	110	26	tr	1
Manitoba Harvest					
Hemp Seed Flour	¼ cup	120	14	tr	12

FOOD	PORTION	CALS	CARB	SUGAR	FIBER
FOOD COLORS					
blue	1 tsp	0	0	0	0
orange	1 tsp	0	0	0	0
red	1 tsp	tr	tr	0	0
yellow	1 tsp	tr	0	0	0
FRENCH FRIES *(see POTATO)*					
FRENCH TOAST					
french toast frzn	1 slice (2 oz)	126	19	–	2
Aunt Jemima					
Cinnamon	2 slices (4 oz)	240	39	6	2
Whole Grain	2 slices (4 oz)	240	39	6	3
Eggo					
Toaster Sticks Original	2	220	36	11	1
Farm Rich					
Original Sticks	5 (4.2 oz)	330	42	10	2
Ian's					
Sticks	5 (3.2 oz)	250	38	5	6
TAKE-OUT					
sticks	5 (4.9 oz)	513	58	–	3
FRUCTOSE					
liquid	1 oz	84	23	23	0
powder	1 tsp (4.2 g)	15	4	4	0
powder	¼ cup (1.7 oz)	180	49	45	0
Bob's Red Mill					
Fructose	1 tsp	15	4	4	0
Tree Of Life					
Fructose	1 tsp (4 g)	15	4	4	0
FRUIT DRINKS *(see also individual names, SMOOTHIES, YOGURT DRINKS)*					
MIX					
Bio Fruit					
Mix	1 scoop (8 g)	42	5	2	1
Crystal Light					
LiveActive On The Go	1 pkg	10	3	0	3
Sugar Free All Flavors as prep	1 serv	5	0	0	0
Luna					
Dragonfruit Kiwi	1 pkg	50	13	11	0
Pomegranate Berry	1 pkg	50	13	10	0

FOOD	PORTION	CALS	CARB	SUGAR	FIBER
South Beach					
Tide Me Over Strawberry Banana	1 pkg	30	6	0	5
Tide Me Over Tropical Breeze	1 pkg	30	6	0	5
Tang					
Orange Pineapple as prep	1 serv (8 oz)	100	24	24	0
Orange Strawberry as prep	1 serv (8 oz)	110	27	27	0
READY-TO-DRINK					
Crayons					
Kiwi Strawberry	1 bottle (12 oz)	130	45	28	4
Outrageous Orange Mango	1 bottle (12 oz)	140	45	28	4
Redder Than Ever Fruitpunch	1 bottle (12 oz)	130	45	28	4
Crystal Light					
Strawberry Kiwi Sugar Free	8 oz	5	0	0	0
Drenchers					
Super Fruit Endurance Grape Apple	8 oz	120	29	27	1
Super Juice Fit N' Lean Heart Healthy Tropical Passion	8 oz	10	2	1	0
Super Juice Fit N' Lean Power Protein Orange Cream	8 oz	20	2	0	0
Super Juice Immunity Fruit & Veggie Berry	8 oz	110	26	22	1
Essn					
Sparkling Blood Orange & Cranberry	1 can (8.4 oz)	160	38	34	tr
Frutzzo					
Organic 100% Juice Pomegranate Passionfruit	1 bottle (12 oz)	140	34	32	0
Organic 100% Juice Pomegranate Acai	1 bottle (12 oz)	140	35	32	0
GoodBelly					
Black Currant Probiotic Drink	8 oz	120	31	27	0
Blueberry Acai Probiotic Drink	1 bottle (2.7 oz)	50	12	9	tr
Cranberry Watermelon Probiotic Drink	8 oz	100	24	21	1

FOOD	PORTION	CALS	CARB	SUGAR	FIBER
Peach Mango Probiotic Drink	1 bottle (2.7 oz)	50	13	9	tr
Strawberry Rosehips Probiotic Drink	1 bottle (2.7 oz)	50	12	9	tr
Hood					
Fruit Punch	1 cup	120	30	28	0
Juicy Juice					
Harvest Surprise Orange Mango	8 oz	130	31	27	1
Kagome					
Burgundy Berry Blossom	8 oz	100	23	22	0
Golden Peach Garden	8 oz	100	25	24	1
Orange Carrot Blossom	8 oz	100	24	19	1
Purple Roots & Fruits	8 oz	130	30	26	1
L&A					
Pineapple Coconut	8 oz	140	28	27	1
Lakewood					
Lean Green	6 oz	90	26	24	2
Organic Acai Amazon Berry	6 oz	95	21	16	3
Land O Lakes					
Juice Cranberry Apple	1 cup (8 oz)	120	30	26	0
Nantucket Nectars					
100% Juice Peach Orange	8 oz	130	32	32	0
100% Juice Pomegranate Cherry	8 oz	120	29	27	0
Kiwi Berry	8 oz	120	29	28	0
Organic Banana Mango Carrot	8 oz	140	32	30	0
Pineapple Orange Guava	8 oz	120	29	29	0
NutraShake					
Fruit Punch Plus Fiber	1 pkg (8 oz)	120	29	24	10
Ocean Spray					
Cran.Raspberry	8 oz	110	28	28	0
Odwalla					
Quenchers AntioxiDance	8 oz	90	23	23	0
Quenchers B Berrier	8 oz	120	30	27	0
OKF					
Sparkling Fresh Guava	1 bottle (8.3 oz)	20	13	1	3
Sparkling Fresh Peach	1 bottle (8.3 oz)	50	12	9	3
Phat Phruit					
Peach Mango	8 oz	40	10	8	0

FOOD	PORTION	CALS	CARB	SUGAR	FIBER
Pineapple Orange	8 oz	40	9	7	0
Sabor Latino					
Nectar Strawberry Banana + Calcium	8 oz	150	37	37	1
Sun Shower					
100% Juice Nectarine Mango	8 oz	93	21	17	2
Sundia					
Tropical Medley	½ cup	70	18	15	2
Tree Ripe					
Organic Fruit Punch	8 oz	150	36	35	0
Tropicana					
Fruit Punch	1 cup	130	32	32	0
Light Fruit Punch	8 oz	10	3	1	0
Orange Tangerine Juice	8 oz	110	25	22	0
Orchard Berry	8 oz	110	27	24	0
Organic Orchard Medley	8 oz	120	29	25	0
Twister Berry Blast	8 oz	120	29	29	0
Twister Citrus Spark	8 oz	120	30	29	0
Twister Fruit Fury	8 oz	120	30	28	0
Twister Light Strawberry Spiral	8 oz	40	10	10	0
V8					
Light Peach Mango	8 oz	50	13	10	0
Splash Berry Blend	8 oz	70	18	18	0
Splash Diet Berry Blend	8 oz	10	3	1	0
Splash Mango Peach	8 oz	80	20	20	0
V-Fusion Pomegranate Blueberry	8 oz	100	25	23	0

FRUIT MIXED *(see also individual names)*
CANNED
Del Monte

FOOD	PORTION	CALS	CARB	SUGAR	FIBER
Carb Clever Fruit Cocktail	½ cup	40	11	10	tr
Dole					
Mixed Fruit Light Syrup	½ cup (4.3 oz)	80	21	20	tr
Tropical Fruit Salad	½ cup	80	20	18	1
Liberty Gold					
Fruit Cocktail In Heavy Syrup	½ cup	90	23	22	1
Polar					
Mixed Fruit Light Syrup	½ cup (4.9 oz)	50	12	11	2

FOOD	PORTION	CALS	CARB	SUGAR	FIBER
DRIED					
Brothers-All-Natural					
Crisps Strawberry Banana	1 pkg (0.42 oz)	45	10	6	2
Fruitaceuticals					
PomaCrans	¼ cup	100	24	18	1
Fun-Yums					
Fresh Crispy Mixed Fruit	1 serv (0.9 oz)	25	18	2	1
Goodniks					
Fruit Medley	¼ cup	110	24	20	2
Mariani					
Berries 'N Cherries	¼ cup	140	38	25	2
Sun-Maid					
Fruit Bits	¼ cup (1.4 oz)	120	29	24	2
Mixed	¼ cup (1.4 oz)	100	26	21	3
Sunsweet					
Berry Blend	¼ cup (1.4 oz)	120	32	24	3
Orchard Mix	¼ cup (1.4 oz)	100	25	14	3
Tropical Mix	⅓ cup	150	33	27	2
FRUIT SNACKS					
Bare Fruit					
Bananas & Cherries	1 pkg (0.6 oz)	55	12	6	2
Funky Monkey					
Bananamon	1 pkg (1 oz)	110	27	21	3
Carnaval Mix	1 pkg (1 oz)	110	26	21	2
Jivealime	1 pkg (1 oz)	110	27	20	2
Purple Funk	1 pkg (1 oz)	120	26	19	3
Jelly Belly					
Fruit Snacks	1 pkg (2.5 oz)	220	58	37	1
Peeled Snacks					
Fruit & Nuts FigSated	⅓ cup	150	20	15	3
Fruit & Nuts Plu-what?	⅓ cup	150	22	13	3
Revolution Foods					
Organic Mashups Berry	1 pkg (3.2 oz)	40	10	8	1
Organic Mashups Tropical	1 pkg (3.2 oz)	60	13	11	1
Sharkies					
Organic Energy Fruit Chews All Flavors	1 pkg (1.8 oz)	170	42	19	1
Stretch Island					
Fruit Leather Bountiful Blueberry	1 pkg (0.5 oz)	45	12	8	1

FOOD	PORTION	CALS	CARB	SUGAR	FIBER
Fruit Leather Harvest Grape	1 pkg (0.5 oz)	45	12	9	1
Fruit Leather Truly Tropical	1 pkg (0.5 oz)	45	11	8	1
Fruit Leather Mango Sunrise	1 pkg (0.5 oz)	45	11	9	1
Organic Smooshed Fruit Apple	1 piece (0.4 oz)	40	10	8	1
Organic Smooshed Fruit Strawberry	1 piece (0.4 oz)	40	10	8	tr
Tahitian Noni					
Soft Chews Raspberry	1 pkg (2 oz)	240	50	44	0
Tropicana					
Fruit Wise Bars All Flavors	1 bar (1.4 oz)	140	36	32	2
Fruit Wise Strips All Flavors	1 strip (0.7 oz)	70	17	15	1
GARLIC					
clove	1	4	1	tr	tr
fresh chopped	1 tbsp	18	4	tr	tr
powder	1 tsp	9	2	1	tr
Dorot					
Crushed Cubes frzn	1 cube (4 g)	7	1	–	tr
Frieda's					
Elephant	1 tbsp	5	1	0	0
Vinegar Marinated	1 oz	30	7	0	0
GEFILTE FISH					
Ungar's					
Gefilte Fish	2 slices (1.8 oz)	83	5	3	0
Lite	2 slices (2.4 oz)	80	5	3	2
No Sugar	2 slices (1.8 oz)	70	3	tr	0
GELATIN					
READY-TO-EAT					
Hunt's					
Snack Pack Juicy Gels Raspberry Mixed Berry	1 serv (3.5 oz)	100	24	22	0
Snack Pack Juicy Gels Strawberry	1 serv (3.5 oz)	100	24	22	0
Snack Pack Juicy Gels Strawberry Orange	1 serv (3.5 oz)	100	24	22	0
Snack Pack Tropical Punch	1 serv (3.5 oz)	100	24	22	0
Jell-O					
Sugar Free Lemon Lime	1 serv (3.2 oz)	10	0	0	0

FOOD	PORTION	CALS	CARB	SUGAR	FIBER
GIBLETS					
capon simmered	1 cup (5 oz)	238	0	0	0
chicken simmered	1 cup (5 oz)	289	1	0	0
GINGER					
ground	1 tsp	6	1	tr	tr
pickled	0.5 oz	5	1	–	tr
preserved	1.5 oz	34	8	7	1
root fresh	5 slices	9	2	tr	tr
root fresh sliced	¼ cup	19	4	tr	1
Eden					
Pickled w/ Shiso Leaves	1 tbsp	20	4	2	tr
Frieda's					
Crystallized	9 pieces (1.1 oz)	100	26	11	0
Galanga Thai Ginger	⅔ cup	60	13	0	2
Tree Of Life					
Crystallized Pieces	7 (1.4 oz)	150	37	33	1
GINSENG					
dried	1 oz	90	20	–	2
fresh	1 oz	28	6	–	tr
GIZZARDS					
chicken simmered	1 cup (5 oz)	212	0	0	0
turkey simmered	1 (3 oz)	103	tr	0	0
GNOCCHI					
Racconto					
Potato Whole Wheat as prep w/o salt	1 cup (5.8 oz)	248	60	tr	8
Vantia					
Gnocchi Whole Wheat	¾ cup	210	46	0	4
GOAT					
roasted	3 oz	122	0	0	0
GOJI BERRIES					
Kopali					
Organic Dark Chocolate Covered	½ pkg (1 oz)	120	18	13	2
Navitas Naturals					
Dried	1 oz	90	18	14	1

FOOD	PORTION	CALS	CARB	SUGAR	FIBER
Sunfood					
Organic	1 oz	90	18	14	3
Superfood Snacks					
Organic Chocolate Goji Treats	3 pieces (1.4 oz)	150	24	12	7
Tree Of Life					
Organic	1 oz	110	25	15	<5
GOJI JUICE					
Arthur's					
Goji Plus	1 bottle (11 oz)	210	49	38	2
Gojilania					
Organic	8 oz	110	23	23	0
GOOSE					
boneless roasted	2.7 oz	231	0	0	0
meat only raw	6.5 oz	298	0	0	0
w/ skin & bone roasted	1 serv (6.6 oz)	573	0	0	0
wild boneless roasted diced	1 cup (4.9 oz)	426	0	0	0
GOOSEBERRIES					
canned in light syrup	1 cup	184	47	–	6
fresh	1 cup	66	15	–	7
Kopali					
Organic Goldenberry	1 pkg (1.8 oz)	150	31	4	18
Navitas Naturals					
Cape Gooseberry Dried	1 oz	80	17	9	3
GRAINS					
Kashi					
7 Whole Grain Pilaf Fiery Fiesta	1 cup (4.9 oz)	210	40	3	7
7 Whole Grain Pilaf Moroccan Curry	1 cup (4.9 oz)	220	42	3	7
7 Whole Grain Pilaf Original	1 cup (4.9 oz)	220	45	1	7
GRAPE JUICE					
bottled unsweetened	1 cup	154	38	38	tr
First Blush					
All Flavors	8 oz	154	38	38	0
Juicy Juice					
Harvest Surprise	8 oz	120	28	27	0
Lakewood					
Organic Concord	6 oz	105	25	23	1

FOOD	PORTION	CALS	CARB	SUGAR	FIBER
Nantucket Nectars					
Grapeade	8 oz	140	33	33	0
Organic Concord Grape	8 oz	130	31	31	0
Tang					
Drink Mix as prep	1 serv (8 oz)	110	28	28	0
Tree Ripe					
Organic 100% Juice	6 oz	120	28	27	0
Tropicana					
Grape	1 bottle (14 oz)	270	67	62	0
Walnut Acres					
Organic	8 oz	120	31	28	0
GRAPE LEAVES					
fresh raw	1 (3 g)	3	1	tr	tr
Sabra					
Stuffed Meatless	1	45	8	0	1
TAKE-OUT					
dolmas w/ beef & rice	1 (0.7 oz)	50	2	1	1
dolmas w/ lamb & rice	1 (0.7 oz)	56	3	1	1
dolmas w/ rice	1 (2 oz)	92	8	2	2
GRAPEFRUIT					
CANNED					
sections juice pack	½ cup (4.4 oz)	46	11	11	1
sections light syrup	½ cup (4.5 oz)	76	20	19	1
sections water pack	½ cup (4.3 oz)	44	11	11	1
FRESH					
pink or red	½ (4.6 oz)	52	13	8	2
sections pink or red	1 cup (8.1 oz)	97	25	16	4
sections white	1 cup (8.1 oz)	76	19	17	3
white	½ (4.1 oz)	39	10	9	1
Ocean Spray					
Sweet Ruby	½ med (5.4 oz)	60	16	10	6
GRAPEFRUIT JUICE					
canned sweetened	1 cup (8.8 oz)	115	28	28	tr
canned unsweetened	1 cup (8.7 oz)	94	22	22	tr
fresh white	1 cup (8.7 oz)	96	23	22	tr
Crystal Light					
Sunrise Sunrise Ruby Red as prep	1 serv (8 oz)	5	0	0	0

FOOD	PORTION	CALS	CARB	SUGAR	FIBER
Odwalla					
100% Juice	8 oz	90	20	16	0
Sundia					
Ruby	½ cup	70	18	14	1
Tropicana					
Sweet	8 oz	130	31	27	0
GRAPES					
muscadine	10–12 (3.5 oz)	76	14	–	3
scuppernongs	10–12 (3.5 oz)	68	12	–	3
seedless red or green	1 cup	110	29	24	1
seedless red or green	20	69	18	15	1
thompson seedless in heavy syrup	½ cup	93	25	24	1
thompson seedless water pack	½ cup	49	13	12	1
with seeds red or green	1 cup	106	28	24	1
with seeds red or green	20	80	21	18	1
Earthbound Farm					
Organic Black	1½ cups	190	24	23	1
Frieda's					
Champagne	½ cup (3 oz)	50	15	14	1
Revolution Foods					
Organic Mashups Grape	1 pkg (3.2 oz)	60	14	12	0
GRAVY					
CANNED					
Campbell's					
Au Jus	¼ cup	5	0	0	0
Chicken	¼ cup	40	3	1	0
Fat Free Beef	¼ cup	15	3	0	0
Fat Free Turkey	¼ cup	20	4	0	0
Mushroom	¼ cup	20	3	1	0
Franco-American					
Fat Free Slow Roast Chicken	¼ cup	20	4	0	0
Slow Roast Chicken	¼ cup	20	3	0	0
Heinz					
Classic Chicken Fat Free	¼ cup	15	3	0	0
Home Style Classic Chicken	¼ cup	25	4	0	0
HomeStyle Roasted Turkey	¼ cup	25	3	0	0

FOOD	PORTION	CALS	CARB	SUGAR	FIBER
FROZEN					
Tofurky					
Giblet & Mushroom	2 tbsp	30	3	2	1
MIX					
Bovril					
Extract	1 heaping tsp	9	tr	–	0
Butterball					
Turkey	¼ cup (2 oz)	30	6	0	0
Road's End Organics					
Savory Herb Cholesterol Free Gluten Free	¼ cup	25	5	0	0
TAKE-OUT					
au jus	1 cup	62	1	tr	tr
giblet gravy	¼ cup	45	3	tr	tr
GREAT NORTHERN BEANS					
CANNED					
Eden					
Organic	½ cup	110	20	1	8
HamBeens					
Great Northerns Dried as prep	½ cup	120	22	1	11
GREEN BEANS					
CANNED					
drained	1 cup	27	6	1	3
Allens					
No Salt	½ cup	15	3	1	2
Del Monte					
Fresh Cut Italian	½ cup	30	6	2	3
Gertie's Finest					
Pickled	1 oz	15	3	3	1
Green Giant					
50% Less Sodium Cut	½ cup	20	4	2	1
Tillen Farms					
Crispy Dilly Beans Pickled	¼ cup	15	3	0	0
FRESH					
cooked w/o salt	1 cup	44	10	2	4
raw	1 cup	34	8	2	4
raw whole beans	10	17	4	1	2

FOOD	PORTION	CALS	CARB	SUGAR	FIBER
Frieda's					
Purple Wax	⅔ cup	25	6	2	3
GreenLine					
Fresh Trimmed	3 oz	25	5	3	2
FROZEN					
cooked	1 cup	38	9	2	4
Birds Eye					
Steamfresh Whole	1 cup (2.9 oz)	35	5	2	2
C&W					
French Cut	1 cup	30	5	2	2
Cascadian Farm					
Organic Petite Whole	1 cup	25	5	1	2
Green Giant					
Green Bean Casserole	⅔ cup	110	8	2	1
Pictsweet					
Cut	⅔ cup	30	5	2	2
TAKE-OUT					
casserole w/ mushroom sauce	1 cup	108	11	3	3
pickled	½ cup	19	4	1	2
GREENS					
Allens					
Seasoned Mixed	½ cup	45	6	2	1
Ready Pac					
Microwave Leafy Greens as prep	½ cup	15	2	1	2
GROUPER					
cooked	1 fillet (7.1 oz)	238	0	0	0
cooked	3 oz	100	0	0	0
raw	3 oz	78	0	0	0
GUAR GUM					
Bob's Red Mill					
Guar Gum	1 tbsp	20	6	0	6
GUAVA					
Frieda's					
Fresh	1 (3 oz)	45	10	5	5
GUINEA HEN					
boneless w/o skin raw	½ hen (9.3 oz)	290	0	0	0
w/ skin raw	½ hen (12 oz)	545	0	0	0

FOOD	PORTION	CALS	CARB	SUGAR	FIBER
HADDOCK					
fresh broiled	4 oz	127	0	0	0
smoked	1 oz	33	0	0	0
Van de Kamp's					
Battered Fillets	2 (3.6 oz)	210	21	5	2
TAKE-OUT					
breaded & fried	4 oz	229	10	1	1
HAGGIS					
scottish haggis	1 serv (6.4 oz)	473	31	3	5
Caledonian Kitchen					
Highland Beef	3 oz	173	12	2	2
Vegetarian	3 oz	190	12	0	3
HALIBUT					
atlantic & pacific cooked	½ fillet (5.6 oz)	223	0	0	0
atlantic & pacific cooked	3 oz	119	0	0	0
atlantic & pacific raw	3 oz	93	0	0	0
greenland baked	3 oz	203	0	0	0
greenland baked	5.6 oz	380	0	0	0
FROZEN					
Van de Kamp's					
Battered Fillets	3 (4 oz)	230	22	3	0
HALVA (see SESAME)					
HAM					
boneless extra lean roasted	3 oz	123	1	0	0
boneless roasted	3 oz	151	0	0	0
deviled	¼ cup	188	1	0	0
ham salad spread	2 tbsp	65	3	0	0
patty grilled	1 patty (2 oz)	205	1	0	0
prosciutto	4 slices (1.3 oz)	72	tr	0	0
sliced	3 slices (2.9 oz)	137	3	0	1
sliced extra lean	3 slices (2.2 oz)	69	2	0	0
westphalian smoked	1 oz	105	0	0	0
whole roasted	3 oz	207	0	0	0

FOOD	PORTION	CALS	CARB	SUGAR	FIBER
Applegate Farms					
Organic Uncured	2 oz	70	1	0	0
Boar's Head					
Black Forest Smoked	2 oz	60	2	2	0
Deluxe	2 oz	60	2	2	0
Deluxe 42% Lowered Sodium	2 oz	60	2	2	0
Fresh Seasoned	2 oz	90	1	1	0
Maple Glazed Honey	2 oz	60	3	3	0
Pepper	2 oz	60	2	1	0
Rosemary & Sundried Tomato	2 oz	70	2	0	0
Virginia Smoked	2 oz	60	2	2	0
Organic Prairie					
Hardwood Smoked Bone In Spiral Sliced	3 oz	110	tr	tr	0
Oscar Mayer					
Virginia Shaved	2 oz	50	1	0	0
Sara Lee					
Bavarian Oven Roasted Honey	2 oz	70	2	2	0
Brown Sugar	2 oz	70	5	4	0
Homestyle Baked	2 oz	60	2	2	0
Virignia Baked	4 slices (1.8 oz)	60	2	1	0
Tyson					
Glazed Ham Maple & Brown Sugar	1 serv (5 oz)	180	18	16	0
Honey Ham	2 slices (1.6 oz)	50	1	1	0
TAKE-OUT					
croquette	1 (2.2 oz)	149	8	2	tr
spam musubi	1 serv (6 oz)	253	42	–	1
thick slice fried	1 (2.2 oz)	140	tr	0	0
HAMBURGER					
Applegate Farms					
Organic Beef Cooked	1 (3 oz)	195	0	0	0
Organic Turkey Burger	1 (4 oz)	190	0	0	0
Hot Pockets					
Cheeseburger	1 (4.5 oz)	310	37	9	2
Ian's					
Mini	2 (4.6 oz)	360	42	5	1
Mini Cheeseburger	2 (5 oz)	420	42	5	1
Kid Cuisine					
Cheeseburger Builder	1 meal	390	58	11	2

FOOD	PORTION	CALS	CARB	SUGAR	FIBER
Lean Pockets					
Cheeseburger	1 (4.5 oz)	280	40	12	3
Oscar Mayer					
Lunchables All-Star Burgers	1 pkg	420	60	38	1
Quaker Maid					
Pure Beef Patties	1 (4 oz)	240	0	0	0
Wellshire					
Beef	1 (4 oz)	260	0	0	0
Turkey Burgers	1 (4 oz)	200	0	0	0
TAKE-OUT					
cheeseburger + condiments	1 reg (4.5 oz)	347	28	5	1
double hamburger + condiments	1 reg (5.8 oz)	384	30	7	2
single patty + condiments	1 reg (4 oz)	299	35	8	2

HAMBURGER SUBSTITUTES (see also MEAT SUBSTITUTES)

FOOD	PORTION	CALS	CARB	SUGAR	FIBER
Boca					
American Flame Grilled	1 (2.5 oz)	90	4	0	3
Cheeseburger	1 (2.5 oz)	100	5	0	3
Grilled Vegetable	1 (2.5 oz)	70	6	0	4
Ground Burger	1 serv (2 oz)	60	6	0	3
Original	1 (2.5 oz)	70	6	0	4
Original Vegan	1 (2.5 oz)	70	6	0	4
Dr. Praeger's					
Veggie Burger Bombay	1 (2.78 oz)	110	13	2	5
Veggie Burger California	1 (2.75 oz)	110	13	1	4
Veggie Burger California Gluten Free	1 (2.75 oz)	120	13	3	4
Fantastic					
Natures Burger Mix not prep	¼ cup	170	30	2	5
Tofu Burger Mix not prep	3 tbsp	80	13	0	1
Gardenburger					
Black Bean Chipotle	1 (2.5 oz)	80	13	1	5
Flamed Grilled	1 (2.5 oz)	90	5	0	4
GardenVegan	1 (2.5 oz)	100	12	0	3
Original	1 (2.5 oz)	100	14	1	5
Portabella	1 (2.5 oz)	90	15	1	5
Lightlife					
Light Burgers	1 (3 oz)	120	11	0	3
Smart Menu Burger	1	80	14	1	2

FOOD	PORTION	CALS	CARB	SUGAR	FIBER
Morningstar Farms					
Classic Burger	1 (2.2 oz)	150	10	2	3
Garden Veggie Patties	1 (2.4 oz)	100	9	1	4
Okara Pattie	1 (2.2 oz)	120	6	tr	3
Vegan Burger	1 (2.5 oz)	100	8	2	5
Sunshine Burgers					
Garden	1 (2.6 oz)	190	14	3	3
Original	1 (2.6 oz)	190	14	3	3
Tofurky					
SuperBurgers Original	1 (3.5 oz)	120	16	0	2
VeggieLand					
Veggie Burger Original	1 (3.5 oz)	132	12	4	7
Veggie Burger Peppadew	1 (5 oz)	210	28	1	4
WildWood					
Organic Original Burgers Tofu-Veggie	1 (3.2 oz)	180	8	1	1
HAZELNUTS					
oil roasted unblanched	1 oz	187	5	–	2
Chukar Cherries					
Chocolate Covered Spiced	3 tbsp (1.4 oz)	228	21	16	2
Kettle					
Butter Creamy Unsalted	2 tbsp	180	5	1	3
Love'n Bake					
Hazelnut Praline	2 tbsp	170	13	10	2
HEART					
beef simmered	3 oz	140	tr	0	0
chicken cooked	1 (3 g)	5	0	0	0
lamb braised	3 oz	157	2	–	0
turkey simmered	½ cup	94	tr	0	0
veal braised	3 oz	158	tr	–	0
Rumba					
Beef	4 oz	130	3	0	0
HEARTS OF PALM					
Native Forest					
Organic	1 oz	15	2	0	1
HEMP					
Living Harvest					
Organic Hemp Nuts	2 tbsp (1 oz)	170	5	1	0

FOOD	PORTION	CALS	CARB	SUGAR	FIBER
Organic Protein Powder	2 scoops (1 oz)	110	9	8	1
Manitoba Harvest					
Hemp Seed Butter	2 tbsp	160	7	1	1
Protein Powder	2 scoops (1 oz)	134	5	1	4
Shelled Seed	2 tbsp	160	7	1	1
Nutiva					
Organic Protein Powder	2 scoops (1 oz)	120	14	0	14
Shelled Hempseed	2 tbsp	110	2	tr	1

HERBAL TEA *(see TEA/HERBAL TEA)*

HERBS/SPICES *(see also individual names)*

FOOD	PORTION	CALS	CARB	SUGAR	FIBER
cajun seasoning	1 tbsp	19	3	–	1
chinese five spice	1 tsp	7	2	–	tr
poultry seasoning	1 tsp	5	1	tr	tr
pumpkin pie spice	1 tsp	6	1	tr	tr
A Taste Of Thai					
Chicken & Rice Seasoning	¼ pkg (6 g)	15	3	3	0
Bragg					
Herb & Spice Seasoning	¼ tsp	0	0	0	0
Chef Paul Prudhomme's					
Magic Blackened Redfish	¼ tsp	0	0	0	0
Magic Fajita	¼ tsp	0	0	0	0
Magic Pork & Veal	¼ tsp	0	0	0	0
Magic Poultry	¼ tsp	0	0	0	0
Eden					
Shake Furikake	½ tsp	5	1	0	1
Emeril's					
Asian Essence	½ tsp	0	0	0	0
Bayou Blast!	½ tsp	0	0	0	0
Chicken Rub	½ tsp	0	0	0	0
Original Essence	½ tsp	0	0	0	0
Steak Rub	½ tsp	0	0	0	0
Mrs. Dash					
Grilling Blend Chicken	¼ tsp	0	0	0	0
Grilling Blend Steak	¼ tsp	0	0	0	0
Original Blend	¼ tsp	0	0	0	0
Tomato Basil Garlic	¼ tsp	0	0	0	0

FOOD	PORTION	CALS	CARB	SUGAR	FIBER
Ortega					
Burrito Seasoning	1½ tsp	20	3	0	tr
Spice Hunter					
All Purpose Blend	¼ tsp	0	0	0	0
Greek Seasoning Salt Free	¼ tsp	0	0	0	0
HERRING					
atlantic baked	4 oz	230	0	0	0
dried salted	1 fillet (1.4 oz)	161	0	0	0
pickled in cream sauce	1 oz	72	2	tr	0
roe	1 tbsp	39	tr	0	0
smoked kippered	1 oz	620	0	0	0
Beach Cliff					
Kippered Snacks	1 can (4 oz)	220	0	0	0
TAKE-OUT					
breaded fried	1 serv (4 oz)	225	9	1	1
HIBISCUS					
flowers dried sweetened	⅓ cup	100	23	21	2
HOMINY					
white canned	1 cup	119	24	3	4
yellow canned	½ cup	115	23	–	4
Allens					
White	½ cup	100	22	1	4
Bush's					
Golden	½ cup	60	13	0	3
HONEY					
honey	¼ cup (3 oz)	258	70	70	tr
orange blossom	1 tbsp	60	17	16	0
Dutch Gold					
Clover	1 tbsp	60	17	16	0
Frieda's					
Honeycomb	½ cup (3 oz)	260	70	70	0
Tree Of Life					
Avocado Honey Raw Unfiltered	1 tbsp (0.7 oz)	60	17	16	0
Wholesome Sweeteners					
Organic Fair Trade Amber	1 tbsp	60	17	16	0
Organic Fair Trade Raw	1 tbsp	60	17	16	0
HONEYDEW					
balls frzn	1 cup (8 oz)	83	21	19	2

FOOD	PORTION	CALS	CARB	SUGAR	FIBER
fresh cut up	1 cup	61	15	14	1
fresh wedge	⅛ melon (4.5 oz)	45	11	10	1
whole fresh	1 (35 oz)	360	91	81	8
HORSE					
roasted	3 oz	149	0	0	0
HORSERADISH					
japanese wasabi	¼ tsp	1	tr	–	0
sauce	1 tbsp	7	2	1	1
Boar's Head					
Horseradish	1 tsp (5 g)	0	0	0	0
Horseradish Sauce Pub Style	1 tsp	15	1	0	0
Horseradish & Beets	1 tsp	0	0	0	0
Gold's					
Horse Radish	1 tsp (5 g)	0	0	0	0
Robert Rothchild Farm					
Sauce	1 tsp	20	1	tr	0
Sara Lee					
Horseradish Sauce	1 tbsp	20	0	0	0
HOT CHOCOLATE					
mix not prep	1 pkg (1 oz)	111	23	18	1
mix w/ no calorie sweetener as prep w/ water	8 oz	72	14	7	2
mix w/ sugar as prep w/ nonfat milk	8 oz	209	30	29	1
mix w/ sugar as prep w/ water	8 oz	138	29	23	1
Nestle					
Hot Cocoa Carb Select Fat Free	1 pkg	25	5	4	tr
Hot Cocoa Milk Chocolate	1 pkg (1 oz)	80	15	13	tr
Starbucks					
Hot Cocoa Mix	1 pkg	130	28	24	2
Swiss Miss					
Cocoa Caramel as prep	1 pkg	120	22	17	tr
Cocoa No Sugar Added as prep	1 pkg	60	10	7	1
Cocoa Rich Creamy as prep	1 pkg	110	22	16	tr
Cocoa w/ Marshmallows as prep	1 pkg	120	24	16	1
Cocoa w/ Marshmallows Fat Free as prep	1 pkg	140	29	21	1

FOOD	PORTION	CALS	CARB	SUGAR	FIBER
French Vanilla as prep	1 pkg	110	24	18	tr
Milk Chocolate as prep	1 pkg	120	23	17	1
TAKE-OUT					
chocolate caliente w/ low fat milk	1 serv (8.4 oz)	221	27	25	1
chocolate caliente w/ whole milk	1 serv (8.4 oz)	276	25	23	1
hot chocolate	1 cup (8.7 oz)	192	30	24	3
mexican hot chocolate	1 cup	173	20	–	1
HOT DOG					
beef	1 (1.5 oz)	149	2	2	0
beef & pork	1 (1.5 oz)	137	1	0	1
beef low fat	1 (2 oz)	133	1	0	0
chicken	1 (1.5 oz)	116	3	0	0
fat free	1 (2 oz)	62	6	0	0
low fat	1 (2 oz)	88	3	0	0
low sodium	1 (2 oz)	180	1	0	0
pork and beef cheese smokie	1 (1.5 oz)	141	1	1	0
turkey	1 (1.5 oz)	102	1	0	0
Applegate Farms					
Natural Beef	1 (1.5 oz)	80	0	0	0
Organic Chicken	1 (1.5 oz)	70	0	0	0
Ball Park					
Franks	1 (2 oz)	180	3	3	0
Franks Beef	1 (2 oz)	180	3	2	0
Franks Bun Size	1 (2 oz)	180	3	3	0
Franks Smoked White Turkey	1 (1.8 oz)	45	5	3	0
Franks Fat Free	1 (1.8 oz)	40	4	2	0
Franks Lite	1 (1.8 oz)	100	3	1	0
Franks Singles Cheese	1 (1.6 oz)	150	2	2	0
Grillmaster Hearty Beef	1	250	3	1	0
Grillmaster Smokehouse	1	210	3	2	0
Boar's Head					
Beef	1 (2 oz)	160	1	0	0
Beef Cocktail	5 (2 oz)	170	0	0	0
Beef Lite	1 (1.6 oz)	90	0	0	0
Pork & Beef	1 (2 oz)	150	0	0	0
Dietz & Watson					
New York Style Beef	1 (2.3 oz)	130	2	2	0

FOOD	PORTION	CALS	CARB	SUGAR	FIBER
Healthy Choice					
Beef Low Fat	1 (1.8 oz)	70	7	2	0
Healthy Ones					
Beef	1 (1.8 oz)	70	7	2	0
Franks	1 (1.8 oz)	70	6	2	0
Ian's					
Popcorn Turkey Corn Dog	5 pieces (3 oz)	237	25	5	0
Organic Prairie					
Beef Uncured	1 (1.5 oz)	120	0	0	0
Chicken Uncured	1 (1.5 oz)	100	1	0	0
Pork Uncured	1 (1.5 oz)	130	0	0	0
Turkey Uncured	1 (1.5 oz)	80	1	0	0
Oscar Mayer					
Beef	1 (1.6 oz)	140	1	1	0
Cheese Dogs	1 (1.6 oz)	140	1	0	0
Corn Dogs	1	210	21	6	1
Smokies	1 (1.8 oz)	150	1	1	0
Wellshire					
Beef Premium	1 (2 oz)	110	0	–	0
Cheese Franks	1 (2 oz)	110	0	0	0
Chicken Franks	1 (1.6 oz)	70	1	1	0
Turkey Franks	1 (1.6 oz)	110	1	1	0
HOT DOG SUBSTITUTES					
Lightlife					
Smart Dogs	1	45	2	1	1
Smart Franks	1 (2 oz)	110	5	2	0
Tofu Pups	1 (1.5 oz)	60	2	0	1
Loma Linda					
Big Franks	1 (1.8 oz)	110	3	0	2
Big Franks Low Fat Vegan	1 (1.8 oz)	80	3	0	2
Morningstar Farms					
Corn Dog Veggie	1 (2.5 oz)	170	22	5	3
Yves					
Meatless Hot Dog	1	50	2	tr	0
Tofu Dogs	1	45	2	0	0
HUMMUS					
Athenos					
Original	2 tbsp	80	5	0	1
Roasted Garlic	2 tbsp	80	5	0	1

FOOD	PORTION	CALS	CARB	SUGAR	FIBER
Roasted Red Pepper	2 tbsp	80	5	0	1
Guiltless Gourmet					
Original	2 tbsp (1.1 oz)	50	8	1	2
Sabra					
Homus	2 oz	110	12	2	3
Homus Spicy	½ cup	171	27	2	5
Tribe					
40 Spices	2 tbsp	50	3	0	1
French Onion	2 tbsp	50	4	0	1
Organic Classic	2 tbsp	50	4	0	1
Organic Roasted Red Peppers	2 tbsp	40	3	0	1
Roasted Eggplant	2 tbsp	35	3	0	1
Scallion	2 tbsp	50	4	0	1
Zesty Lemon	2 tbsp	50	4	0	1
Wholesome Valley					
Organic Classic	2 tbsp (1 oz)	60	5	tr	1
Wild Garden					
Hummus Dip	2 tbsp	35	4	tr	1
WildWood					
Organic Low Fat	2 tbsp	50	6	2	1
Organic Mid-Eastern	2 tbsp	65	6	2	1
TAKE-OUT					
hummus	¼ cup (2.2 oz)	109	12	tr	3

ICE CREAM AND FROZEN DESSERTS *(see also* ICES AND ICE POPS, SHERBET, YOGURT FROZEN*)*

FOOD	PORTION	CALS	CARB	SUGAR	FIBER
freeze dried ice cream chocolate strawberry & vanilla	1 pkg (0.75 oz)	158	24	10	1
Blue Bunny					
Bar Candy Center Crunch	1 (3.2 oz)	370	28	21	1
Bar English Toffee	1 (1.4 oz)	130	12	9	0
Bar Homemade Vanilla	1 (2.3 oz)	190	16	16	0
Bar Orange Dream	1 (2.1 oz)	80	16	14	0
Bar Strawberry Sundae Crunch	1 (2.2 oz)	170	20	13	0
Blendz Peanut Butter Cup	1 (4.4 oz)	270	40	35	tr
Caramel Sundae Bite Size	4 bars (3.1 oz)	340	30	25	1
Chocolate	½ cup	130	17	14	0
Cone Bunny Tracks	1 (4.8 oz)	420	51	36	2
Cone The Champ Chocolate Lovers	1 (3.5 oz)	300	38	28	1
Cone Vanilla Nutty Sundae	1 (3 oz)	250	34	22	1

FOOD	PORTION	CALS	CARB	SUGAR	FIBER
Cups Vanilla & Chocolate	1 (1.7 oz)	100	13	11	0
Mint Chip	½ cup	140	17	14	0
Neapolitan	½ cup	130	16	14	0
Orange Dream	½ cup	130	19	15	0
Premium All Natural Vanilla	½ cup	160	16	16	0
Premium Bunny Tracks	½ cup	190	21	19	tr
Premium Butter Pecan	½ cup	150	15	13	0
Premium Cookies & Cream	½ cup	150	19	15	0
Premium Double Strawberry	½ cup	140	20	18	0
Premium Exquisite Mint	½ cup	170	22	20	0
Premium Rocky Road	½ cup	150	21	16	0
Premium Toasted Almond Fudge	½ cup	160	18	14	tr
Sandwich Big Vanilla	1 (3.7 oz)	260	39	23	0
Sandwich Chips Galore	1 (3.4 oz)	310	40	27	1
Strawberry	½ cup	120	17	14	0
Breyers					
Butter Pecan	½ cup	150	14	14	0
Carb Smart Chocolate	½ cup	90	13	4	4
Carb Smart Fudge Bar	1 (3.5 oz)	100	9	3	1
Carb Smart Vanilla Bar Chocolate Coated	1 (3 oz)	170	9	5	2
CarbSmart Vanilla	½ cup	90	13	4	4
Cherry Vanilla	½ cup	130	8	17	0
Chocolate Crackle	½ cup	160	15	15	0
Chocolate Extra Creamy	½ cup	140	17	15	1
Coffee	½ cup	130	15	15	0
Cookies & Cream	½ cup	150	19	16	0
Double Churn ½ Fat Chocolate Mocha Silk	½ cup	130	19	15	1
Double Churn ½ Fat Creamy Vanilla	½ cup	100	17	13	0
Double Churn ½ Fat Mint Chocolate Chip	½ cup	130	19	15	1
Double Churn ½ Fat Rocky Road	½ cup	130	22	16	1
Double Churn Fat Free Chocolate Fudge Brownie	½ cup	110	25	15	4
Double Churn Fat Free Creamy Vanilla	½ cup	90	21	12	3

FOOD	PORTION	CALS	CARB	SUGAR	FIBER
Double Churn Fat Free French Chocolate	½ cup	90	22	13	4
Double Churn No Sugar Added Vanilla	½ cup	80	14	4	4
Dulce De Leche	½ cup	150	21	19	0
French Vanilla	½ cup	140	14	14	0
Heath English Toffee	½ cup	160	25	20	0
Overload Very Chocolate Cherry	½ cup	120	21	16	1
Overload Waffle Cone	½ cup	130	22	16	0
Peach	½ cup	120	17	16	0
Sandwich Mrs. Fields Brownie	1 (6 oz)	450	64	39	2
Sandwich Mrs. Fields Cookie	1 (3 oz)	190	29	17	0
Sandwich Oreo	1 (3 oz)	170	26	13	1
Snicker	½ cup	170	20	16	0
Strawberry	½ cup	120	15	15	0
Strawberry Cheesecake Sara Lee	½ cup	160	20	17	0
Vanilla Lactose Free	½ cup	130	14	14	0
Vanilla Fudge Brownie	½ cup	150	20	17	1
Bubbies					
Mochi Mango	1 piece (1.3 oz)	110	18	14	0
Celestial Seasonings					
Tea Dreams Cinnamon Apple Spice	½ cup	140	24	6	1
Tea Dreams Vanilla Ginger Spice Chai	½ cup	140	24	5	1
Tea Dreams Bars Chocolate Caramel Chai	1 (2.7 oz)	240	28	17	2
Ciao Bella					
Gelato Chocolate	1 pkg (3.5 oz)	210	22	18	1
Gelato Hazelnut	1 pkg (3.5 oz)	210	21	17	1
Gelato Vanilla	1 pkg (3.5 oz)	184	19	16	0
Dippin' Dots					
Banana Split	½ cup	170	16	14	0
Chocolate	½ cup	165	15	14	0
Fudge Fat Free No Sugar Added	½ cup	92	18	7	0
Horchata	½ cup	170	16	14	0
Java Delight	½ cup	170	16	14	0
Root Beer Float	½ cup	111	20	16	0

FOOD	PORTION	CALS	CARB	SUGAR	FIBER
Vanilla	½ cup	170	16	14	0
Dove					
Beyond Vanilla	½ cup	240	23	20	0
Give In To Mint	½ cup	300	30	24	1
Irresistibly Raspberry	½ cup	240	29	21	1
Milk Chocolate w/ Almonds	1 bar (3.3 oz)	340	28	24	1
Milk Chocolate w/ Vanilla Ice Cream	1 bar (3.3 oz)	330	31	27	1
Miniatures Milk Chocolate w/ Vanilla Ice Cream	5 pieces (3.1 oz)	300	30	27	1
Unconditional Chocolate	½ cup	290	31	27	2
Vanilla w/ A Chocolate Soul	½ cup	290	29	23	1
Edy's					
Carb Benefit Butter Pecan	½ cup	170	13	2	6
Carb Benefit Chocolate	½ cup	150	13	2	7
Carb Benefit Chocolate Chip	½ cup	160	14	2	6
Carb Benefit Mint Chocolate Chip	½ cup	160	14	2	6
Carb Benefit Vanilla Bean	½ cup	140	13	2	6
Eskimo Pie					
Milk Chocolate	1 bar (1.8 oz)	160	12	11	0
Fat Boy					
Casco Nut Sundae On A Stick	1 (3 oz)	310	21	15	2
Casco Nut Sundae On A Stick Cherry Cordial	1 (3 oz)	300	26	20	1
Sandwich Chocolate	1 (3 oz)	210	31	12	1
Sandwich Egg Nog	1 (3 oz)	220	31	18	tr
Sandwich Jr. Vanilla	1 (1.6 oz)	120	17	10	0
Sandwich Vanilla	1 (3 oz)	220	30	17	1
Glace De Vino					
Chocolate Amarretto Cream Sherry	½ cup	180	21	7	0
Raspberry Merlot Cheesecake	½ cup	180	22	6	0
Good Humor					
Bar Chocolate Eclair	1 (3 oz)	160	21	11	1
Bar Cookies & Cream	1 (3 oz)	190	21	14	1
Bar Vanilla Chocolate Coated	1 (4 oz)	260	24	20	1
Bar King Heath	1 (4 oz)	310	31	26	1
Cone King Giant	1 (8 oz)	390	44	30	2
Cone Sundae	1 (4.3 oz)	260	29	18	1

FOOD	PORTION	CALS	CARB	SUGAR	FIBER
King Cone Vanilla	1 (4.6 oz)	250	30	19	1
Sandwich Oreo	1 (4.5 oz)	240	36	19	2
Sandwich Vanilla	1 (3 oz)	130	26	12	2
Sandwich Giant Vanilla	1 (6 oz)	220	43	23	1
Swirlwind	1 (6 oz)	160	31	23	0
GoodBody					
Chocolate Banana	1 bar (3.5 oz)	120	25	19	4
Chocolate Double Dutch	1 bar (3.5 oz)	130	26	21	4
Chocolate Peanut Butter	1 bar (3.5 oz)	180	26	18	5
Vanilla & Raspberry Sorbet	1 bar (3.5 oz)	120	25	20	4
Vanilla & Strawberry Sorbet	1 bar (3.5 oz)	120	25	20	4
Vanilla & Tropical Sorbet	1 bar (3.5 oz)	120	25	20	4
Green & Black's					
Organic Chocolate Covered Chocolate	1 bar (3.5 oz)	214	19	19	2
Organic Chocolate Covered Vanilla	1 bar (3.5 oz)	233	19	18	2
Hawaiian Punch					
Cream Surfers	1 bar	90	16	9	0
Hershey's					
Neapolitan	½ cup	160	18	17	tr
Hood					
Butterscotch Blast	½ cup	160	20	15	0
Chocolate	½ cup	140	17	12	0
Chocolate Eclair	1 bar (2.2 oz)	150	14	8	0
Cookie Dough Delight	½ cup	160	20	14	0
Creamy Coffee	½ cup	140	16	12	0
Fat Free Chocolate Passion	½ cup	100	22	14	0
Fat Free Very Vanilla	½ cup	100	23	14	0
Fudge Twister	½ cup	150	20	15	0
Grasshopper Pie	½ cup	160	22	14	0
Hoodsie Cups	1 (1.7 oz)	100	12	9	0
Light Butter Pecan	½ cup	140	18	11	0
Light Creamy Vanilla	½ cup	110	18	12	0
Low Fat No Sugar Added Vanilla Dream	½ cup	90	20	4	3
Maple Walnut	½ cup	160	17	12	0
No Sugar Added Chocolate Chip	½ cup	100	21	4	3
Nutty Royale	1 cone (2.5 oz)	220	26	18	tr

FOOD	PORTION	CALS	CARB	SUGAR	FIBER
Orange Cream	1 bar (2.2 oz)	90	19	13	0
Sandwich Vanilla	1	180	29	14	tr
Sandwich Vanilla Light	1 (2.2 oz)	160	29	14	tr
Sandwich Vanilla Lowfat	1 (2.8 oz)	80	15	2	2
Spumoni	½ cup	140	17	13	0
Klondike					
Bar Caramel Pretzel	1 (4 oz)	260	30	21	1
Bar Original Vanilla	1 (4.5 oz)	250	22	18	0
Bar Reese's	1 (4 oz)	260	26	21	1
Bar Whitehouse Cherry	1 (4.5 oz)	250	24	20	0
Cone Crunchy Vanilla	1 (4.3 oz)	280	30	20	1
Slim A Bear 100 Calorie Sandwich Vanilla	1 (3 oz)	100	21	10	2
Slim A Bear Bar Vanilla	1 (4 oz)	170	21	7	4
Land O Lakes					
Vanilla	½ cup (2.4 oz)	150	17	16	0
Vanilla Light	½ cup (2.3 oz)	100	17	13	0
M&M's					
Cone	1 (2.8 oz)	250	33	24	1
Sandwich	1 (3 oz)	260	34	24	0
Vanilla Fudge	½ cup	180	20	18	0
Molli Coolz					
Cup Banana Cream Pie	1	120	9	8	1
Cup Chocolate Fusion	1	140	10	7	1
Cup Chocolate Peanut Butter	1	160	12	10	0
Ionz Cotton Candy	1 cup	100	8	5	0
Ionz S'mores	1 cup	110	7	5	1
Rocks Cherry Blue Raz & Lemon	1 cup	80	15	8	0
Rocks Lemon Lime	1 cup	80	15	8	0
Shakers Chocolate	1 (10.2 oz)	250	35	17	5
Natural Choice					
Organic Double Chocolate	½ cup	230	25	23	0
Organic Strawberry	½ cup	210	22	21	0
Organic Vanilla	½ cup	220	22	22	0
No Pudge!					
Giant Strawberry Shortcake 98% Fat Free	1 bar	90	20	12	4
Popsicle					
Creamsicle	1 (2.5 oz)	100	20	12	0

FOOD	PORTION	CALS	CARB	SUGAR	FIBER
Purely Decadent					
Dairy Free Bar Chocolate Coated Vanilla	1 (2.7 oz)	200	26	22	3
Dairy Free Bar Chocolate Coated Vanilla Almond	1 (2.7 oz)	210	28	22	4
Organic Coconut Milk Chocolate	½ cup	150	20	12	6
Organic Coconut Milk Vanilla Bean	½ cup	150	19	12	6
Organic Dairy Free Belgian Chocolate	½ cup	180	30	25	4
Organic Dairy Free Chocolate Obsession	½ cup	210	36	20	5
Organic Dairy Free Gluten Free Cookie Dough	½ cup	230	36	27	5
Organic Dairy Free Mocha Almond Fudge	½ cup	200	32	22	6
Organic Dairy Free Snickerdoodle	½ cup	190	34	20	5
Organic Dairy Free Vanilla	½ cup	170	29	18	6
Rice Dream					
Bar Vanilla Nutty	1 (3.3 oz)	320	27	15	2
Bar Vanilla w/ Chocolate Coating	1 (3 oz)	230	24	16	tr
Carob Almond	½ cup	180	26	2	2
Frozen Pie Chocolate	1 (3.4 oz)	330	40	14	2
Mint Carob Chip	½ cup	170	25	19	0
Strawberry	½ cup	160	25	2	2
Sheer Bliss					
Bar Pomegranate	1 (3.1 oz)	260	24	22	tr
Blissbites	2 (1.1 oz)	100	9	8	0
Blisswich	1 (3.3 oz)	270	39	21	tr
Freedom	½ cup (4 oz)	290	32	29	0
Mediterranean Coffee	½ cup (4 oz)	260	25	23	0
Pomegranate	½ cup (4 oz)	290	32	29	0
Vanilla	½ cup (4 oz)	300	29	27	0
Skinny Cow					
Bar Vanilla Strawberry Sorbet Swirl	1	110	22	17	0
Cone Chocolate w/ Fudge	1	150	28	19	3

FOOD	PORTION	CALS	CARB	SUGAR	FIBER
Cone Vanilla & Caramel	1	150	29	19	3
Fudge Bar	1	100	22	13	4
Sandwich Chocolate Peanut Butter	1	150	30	15	5
Sandwich Strawberry Shortcake	1	140	30	15	3
Sandwich Vanilla	1	140	30	15	3
Sandwich Vanilla No Sugar Added	1	140	30	15	3
SoDelicious					
Dairy Free Sandwich Minis Pomegranate	1 (1.4 oz)	90	18	8	1
Dairy Free Sandwich Mint	1 (2.2 oz)	150	28	13	2
Dairy Free Sandwich Vanilla	1 (2 oz)	150	28	13	2
Dairy Free Sugar Free Chocolate Coated Vanilla Bar	1 (2.2 oz)	150	15	0	6
Dairy Free Sugar Free Fudge Bar	1 (2 oz)	80	12	0	6
Organic Dairy Free Sandwich Neapolitan	1 (2.2 oz)	150	28	13	2
Soy Dream					
Butter Pecan	½ cup	140	17	9	tr
Sandwich Lil' Dreamers Chocolate	1 (1.4 oz)	100	15	8	tr
Vanilla	½ cup	140	18	10	tr
Straus					
Organic Coffee	4 oz	240	19	19	0
Organic Vanilla Bean	4 oz	240	19	19	0
Tofutti					
Cuties Vanilla	1 (1.4 oz)	120	17	9	0
Turkey Hill					
Banana Split	½ cup	150	19	15	1
Choco Mint Chip	½ cup	160	17	13	1
Chocolate All Natural	½ cup	150	18	17	0
Chocolate Marshmallow	½ cup	160	24	18	1
Coconut Cream Pie	½ cup	170	20	20	0
Cookies 'N Cream	½ cup	150	19	13	0
Duetto Cherry	½ cup	120	21	19	0
Duetto Lemon	½ cup	120	21	19	0
Duetto Root Beer	½ cup	120	21	19	0

FOOD	PORTION	CALS	CARB	SUGAR	FIBER
French Vanilla	½ cup	140	16	12	0
Light Banana Split	½ cup	110	19	15	1
Light Dulce De Chocolate	½ cup	120	22	17	1
Light Moose Tracks	½ cup	140	20	15	1
Light Vanilla Bean	½ cup	100	17	13	1
No Sugar Added Cherry Fudge Ripple	½ cup	80	22	5	4
No Sugar Added Vanilla Bean	½ cup	70	19	6	5
Original Vanilla	½ cup	140	16	12	0
Peanut Butter Ripple	½ cup	170	16	11	1
Rocky Road	½ cup	170	23	17	1
Sandwich Chocolate Chunk	1 (3.2 oz)	320	44	29	1
Sandwich Vanilla Bean	1 (2.5 oz)	190	29	15	1
Sandwich Light Vanilla Bean	1 (2.5 oz)	160	32	15	3
Sundae Cone Vanilla Fudge	1 (3.3 oz)	320	35	20	2
Tin Roof Sundae	½ cup	150	19	15	0
Twix					
Ice Cream	½ cup	160	21	17	0
Ice Cream Bar	1 (1.6 oz)	170	19	15	0
Weight Watchers					
English Toffee Crunch	1 bar	110	13	10	2
TAKE-OUT					
gelato chocolate hazelnut	½ cup (5.3 oz)	370	26	21	2
gelato vanilla	½ cup (3 oz)	211	18	18	0
ice cream pie no crust	1 slice (3.4 oz)	218	21	18	1
mud pie	⅛ pie (8 oz)	698	96	64	3
ICE CREAM CONES AND CUPS					
brown sugar cone	1 (10 g)	40	8	3	tr
wafer cone	1	17	3	tr	tr
waffle cone	1 lg	121	23	2	1
Keebler					
Cone Sugar	1	50	10	4	0
Ice Creme Cone	1	15	4	0	0
Waffle Bowl	1	50	10	4	0
Waffle Cone	1	50	10	4	0
ICE CREAM TOPPINGS					
nuts in syrup	2 tbsp	184	24	15	1
Lollipop Tree					
Hot Fudge Sauce	1 tbsp	80	8	7	tr

FOOD	PORTION	CALS	CARB	SUGAR	FIBER
Maple Walnut Cream	2 tbsp	190	22	20	0
Sanders					
Butterscotch Caramel	2 tbsp	90	15	11	0

ICED TEA
MIX
Celestial Seasonings

FOOD	PORTION	CALS	CARB	SUGAR	FIBER
Blueberry Ice	1 cup	0	0	0	0
Crystal Light					
On The Go All Flavors as prep	1 serv	5	0	0	0
Sugar Free All Flavors as prep	1 serv	5	0	0	0
Lipton					
Decaffeinated Lemon Unsweetened as prep	1 serv	0	0	0	0
To Go w/ Honey & Lemon	1 pkg	0	0	0	0
To Go w/ Lemon	1 pkg	0	0	0	0
Unsweetened as prep	1 serv	0	0	0	0

READY-TO-DRINK
Anteadote

FOOD	PORTION	CALS	CARB	SUGAR	FIBER
All Flavors	8 oz	0	0	0	0
Bolthouse Farms					
Perfectly Protein Vanilla Chai Tea w/ Soy	8 oz	160	25	21	0
Cafe Sepia					
Matcha Latte	1 can (8.6 oz)	130	23	21	1
Crystal Light					
Sugar Free Lemon	8 oz	5	0	0	0
Delta Blues					
Tea Punch Black Tea Sumptuous Spearmint	8 oz	90	21	20	0
Enviga					
All Flavors	1 can (12 oz)	5	0	0	0
Hawaiian					
Iced Tea	1 can (11.5 oz)	120	35	35	0
Hood					
Iced Tea	1 cup	100	25	24	0
Ito En					
Apricot	8 oz	60	15	15	0
Green Tea Apple	8 oz	70	18	18	0
Mango	8 oz	50	15	14	0
Sencho Shot	1 can (6.4 oz)	0	0	0	0

FOOD	PORTION	CALS	CARB	SUGAR	FIBER
White Tea Grape	8 oz	60	15	15	0
Lipton					
Diet Green Tea w/ Citrus	8 oz	0	0	0	0
Diet Lemon	8 oz	0	0	0	0
Diet Sweet	8 oz	0	0	0	0
Original Unsweetened	8 oz	0	0	0	0
Nantucket Nectars					
Half & Half	8 oz	90	22	22	0
Original Lemon	8 oz	80	22	21	0
Nestea					
Green Tea Diet Peach	8 oz	0	0	0	0
Sweetened Diet Green Tea	8 oz	0	0	0	0
Old Orchard					
Green Tea w/ Lemon & Honey	8 oz	45	12	12	0
Green Tea w/ Pomegranate	8 oz	45	12	12	0
Osteo					
Fruit Tea All Flavors	1 can (12 oz)	120	32	32	0
Pacific Foods					
Organic Lemon	8 oz	70	17	16	0
Organic Peach	8 oz	70	17	17	0
Organic Raspberry	8 oz	70	18	17	0
Organic Sweetened Black Tea	8 oz	60	16	15	0
Organic Unsweetened Green Tea	8 oz	0	0	0	0
Pixie					
Black Tea Mate Lemon Ginger	8 oz	35	8	6	0
Yerba Mate Authentic	8 oz	30	7	7	0
POM					
Light Tea Pomegranate Hibiscus Green	8 oz	35	16	8	0
Light Tea Pomegranate Orange Blossom	8 oz	35	14	7	0
Light Tea Pomegranate Wildberry White	8 oz	35	16	9	0
SSips					
Diet Green Tea w/ Honey & Ginseng	1 box (7 oz)	0	0	0	0
Lemon	8 oz	100	24	23	0
Sweet Leaf					
Diet Mint & Honey Green Tea	8 oz	0	tr	0	0

FOOD	PORTION	CALS	CARB	SUGAR	FIBER
Lemon & Lime Unsweet	8 oz	0	0	0	0
True Brew					
Cranberry Orange	8 oz	72	18	18	0
Green Tea	8 oz	64	16	16	0
Sweet Tea	8 oz	76	19	19	0
Turkey Hill					
Diet Decaffeinated	8 oz	0	0	0	0
VitaZest					
Green Tea Vitamin Enriched	8 oz	0	0	0	0
Weil For Tea					
Gyokuro	1 can (8.6 oz)	0	0	0	0
Turmeric	1 can (8.6 oz)	0	0	0	0

ICES AND ICE POPS
Blue Bunny

FOOD	PORTION	CALS	CARB	SUGAR	FIBER
Bar Big Fudge	1 (2.7 oz)	110	21	17	0
Chill Cups Double Lemon	1 (4 oz)	100	26	19	0
FrozFruit Creamy Coconut	1 bar (3 oz)	150	14	13	tr
Frozfruit Strawberries & Cream	1 bar (4 oz)	190	27	25	tr
Pop Banana	1 (1.9 oz)	35	9	7	0
Pop Jolly Rancher	1 (4 oz)	120	24	20	0
Pop Root Beer	1 (1.9 oz)	40	10	8	0
The Original Bomb	1 (1.8 oz)	50	11	9	0
Breeze Freeze					
Fruit Granita	1 (8 oz)	120	28	27	tr
Dippin' Dots					
Cherry Berry	½ cup	90	23	12	0
Watermelon	½ cup	90	23	12	0
Hawaiian Punch					
Arctic Surfers	1 pop	50	12	8	0
Hendrie's					
Citrus N' Berry Stix	1 (1.9 oz)	15	3	0	0
Fudge Stix Fat Free	1 bar (1.8 oz)	70	14	11	0
Hood					
Hoodsie Pop	1 (3.3 oz)	60	16	13	0
Luigi's					
Italian Ice Cherry	1 (6 oz)	130	32	25	tr
Italian Ice Lemon Strawberry	1 (6 oz)	120	31	24	tr
Italian Ice No Sugar Added Lemon	1 (6 oz)	60	20	1	0
Italian Ice Pina Colada	1 (6 oz)	130	33	30	0

FOOD	PORTION	CALS	CARB	SUGAR	FIBER
Swirl Blue Ribbon Lemonade	1 (6 oz)	150	39	32	0
Natural Choice					
Organic Vegan Fruit Bars Coconut	1 (2.75 oz)	90	16	15	1
Organic Vegan Fruit Bars Pink Lemonade	1 (2.75 oz)	50	13	13	0
Organic Vegan Grape	1 (2.75 oz)	50	13	13	0
Organic Vegan Sorbet Blueberry	½ cup	110	29	27	tr
Organic Vegan Sorbet Lemon	½ cup	110	30	27	0
Organic Vegan Sorbet Mango	½ cup	110	29	27	1
PickleSickle					
Pop	1 (2 oz)	3	1	0	0
Popsicle					
Creamsicle Pop No Sugar Added	2 (1.65)	45	10	3	2
Creamsicle Pop Sugar Free	2 (1.65 oz)	40	10	0	6
Fudgsicle Bar	1 (2.5 oz)	100	17	14	1
Fudgsicle Pops No Sugar Added	1 (1.65 oz)	40	10	2	2
Pop Ups Orange Burst	1 (2.75 oz)	90	18	10	0
SoDelicious					
Dairy Free Creamy Orange Bar	1 (2.2 oz)	80	18	12	2
Sweet Nothings					
Bar Mango Raspberry	1 (2.6 oz)	100	23	12	0
The Power Of Fruit					
Original Fruit Bar	1 (1.75 oz)	28	7	5	1
Turkey Hill					
Venice Mango	½ cup	100	23	22	0
Venice Pomegranate Blueberry w/ Acai	½ cup	100	25	23	0

JALAPENO (see PEPPERS)

JAM/JELLY/PRESERVES

apple butter	1 tbsp (0.6 oz)	31	8	6	tr
jam all flavors	1 pkg (0.5 oz)	39	10	7	tr
jam all flavors	1 tbsp (0.7 oz)	56	14	10	tr
jam apricot	1 tbsp (0.7 oz)	48	13	9	tr
jam diet all flavors	1 tbsp (0.5 oz)	18	8	5	tr
jelly all flavors	1 tbsp (0.7 oz)	51	13	10	tr
jelly reduced sugar all flavors	1 tbsp (0.7 oz)	34	9	9	tr

FOOD	PORTION	CALS	CARB	SUGAR	FIBER
jelly diet all flavors	1 tbsp (0.7 oz)	25	10	7	1
orange marmalade	1 tbsp (0.7 oz)	49	13	12	tr
preserves all flavors	1 tbsp (0.7 oz)	56	14	10	tr
Chukar Cherries					
Preserve Red Sour Cherry	1 tbsp	40	10	8	tr
Preserves No Sugar Added Cherry Amaretto	1 tbsp	24	18	1	tr
Preserves Vanilla Peach	1 tbsp	28	19	6	tr
Comfort Care					
Country Apple Butter	1 tbsp (1 oz)	40	11	10	1
Eden					
Organic Apple Butter	1 tbsp	20	4	4	1
Organic Butter Apple Cherry	1 tbsp	25	6	5	tr
Organic Cherry Butter	1 tbsp	35	9	8	1
Gedney					
State Fair Preserves Strawberry Rhubarb	1 tbsp	50	12	11	0
Hero					
Swiss Preserves Black Cherry	1 tbsp (0.7 oz)	50	13	10	2
Lollipop Tree					
Butter Pumpkin Maple Pecan	1 tbsp	30	7	6	tr
Jelly Wasabi Lime Pepper	1 tbsp	60	16	15	0
Revolution Foods					
Organic Jelly Grape	1 tbsp (0.7 oz)	60	14	14	0
Organic Preserves Strawberry	1 tbsp (0.7 oz)	60	14	13	0
Robert Rothchild Farm					
Preserves Cherry Acai	1 tbsp	35	9	9	0
Tree Of Life					
Organic Fruit Spread Grape	1 tbsp (0.6 oz)	30	8	7	0
Organic Fruit Spread Peach	1 tbsp (0.6 oz)	30	8	7	0

JAPANESE FOOD *(see* ASIAN FOOD, SUSHI*)*

JELLY *(see* JAM/JELLY/PRESERVES*)*

JELLYFISH

pickled	½ cup (1 oz)	10	0	0	0

JERKY

beef	1 piece (0.7 oz)	82	2	2	tr
pork	1 strip (0.5 oz)	62	2	1	tr
venison	1 strip (0.5 oz)	55	2	2	0

FOOD	PORTION	CALS	CARB	SUGAR	FIBER
Applegate Farms					
Natural Joy Stick	1 (1 oz)	100	0	tr	tr
Dakota Gourmet					
Fruit Jerky Strawberry Kiwi	1	70	16	12	1
Frank's Red Hot					
Chile'N Lime Steak Strips	1 oz	80	2	1	0
Original Beef	1 oz	80	5	4	0
Gary West					
Beef Strips Hickory Smoked	1 oz	70	5	5	0
Buffalo Strips	½ pkg (1 oz)	60	3	2	0
Elk Strips	½ pkg (1 oz)	70	4	2	0
Jack Link's					
Beef Teriyaki	1 oz	80	5	5	0
Organic Prairie					
Beef	1 oz	75	5	3	0
Outpost					
Beef	1 oz	70	4	3	0
Beef Steak	1 pkg (0.9 oz)	60	2	tr	0
Beef Stick	1 (0.4 oz)	60	2	1	0
Pemmican					
Homestyle Tender All Flavors	1 oz	80	3	2	1
Kippered Beef Original	1 pkg (1 oz)	60	2	2	0
Kippered Beef Peppered	1 pkg (1 oz)	60	2	1	0
Kippered Beef Sweet & Hot	1 pkg (1 oz)	70	6	4	0
Kippered Beef Teriyaki	1 pkg (1 oz)	60	2	1	0
Long Lasting Hot & Spicy	1 oz	60	4	3	0
Long Lasting Original	1 oz	60	5	4	0
Long Lasting Peppered	1 oz	60	4	3	0
Long Lasting Teriyaki	1 oz	70	6	4	0
Premium Cut Beef Jerky	1 oz	80	4	2	1
Premium Cut Turkey Peppered	1 oz	70	5	4	0
Premium Cut Turkey Sweet Smoked	1 oz	70	5	4	0
Shredded Beef All Flavors	¼ cup	80	3	2	1
Steak Tips All Flavors	1 oz	70	5	4	0
Slim Jim					
Beef	7 pieces	130	3	tr	0
Beef Jerky Hickory Smoked	1 oz	80	4	3	0
Classic Handipack	1 box	210	3	tr	tr
Giant Caddy Pepperoni	1 pkg	150	3	tr	0

FOOD	PORTION	CALS	CARB	SUGAR	FIBER
Twin Pack Cheese & Pepperoni	1 pkg	150	2	0	1
Tanka					
Natural Buffalo Cranberry Bar	1 (1 oz)	70	7	6	1
Natural Buffalo Cranberry Bite	1 (0.5 oz)	35	3	3	0
Tofurky					
Jurky Original	4 pieces (1 oz)	100	9	3	1
Tony's Smokehouse					
Salmon	1 pkg (0.5 oz)	40	2	1	1
Wellshire					
Matt's Select Pepperoni	1 stick (0.9 oz)	90	1	0	0
Tom Tom Snack Hot n' Spicy Turkey	1 stick (0.8 oz)	50	1	1	0
JICAMA					
fresh	1 sm (12.8 oz)	139	32	7	18
raw sliced	1 cup	46	11	2	6
Frieda's					
Jicama	¾ cup	35	7	0	1
JUTE					
cooked	1 cup	32	6	1	2
KALE					
chopped cooked w/o salt	1 cup	36	7	2	3
fresh cooked w/ fat	1 cup	69	7	2	2
scotch chopped cooked w/o salt	1 cup	36	7	–	2
Allens					
Seasoned	½ cup	35	5	1	1
Glory					
Fresh Greens	1 serv (2.8 oz)	40	8	2	2
Seasoned canned	½ cup	35	5	2	1
KEFIR					
kefir	8 oz	98	12	12	0
Evolve					
Plain	8 oz	120	15	10	5
Strawberry	8 oz	180	31	27	5
Lifeway					
Greek Style	8 oz	202	12	11	0
Nonfat All Fruit Flavors	8 oz	188	33	30	3
Nonfat Plain	8 oz	116	15	12	3

FOOD	PORTION	CALS	CARB	SUGAR	FIBER
Organic Helios All Fruit Flavors	8 oz	160	26	23	2
Organic Helios Plain	8 oz	120	12	10	2
Organic Lowfat All Fruit Flavors	8 oz	160	25	21	3
Organic Lowfat Plain	8 oz	110	12	8	3
Original	8 oz	162	15	12	3
Probugs All Flavors	1 bottle	130	15	13	2
Slim6 All Flavors	8 oz	110	8	6	2
Nancy's					
Organic Lowfat Blackberry	1 cup	180	34	32	2
Organic Lowfat Plain	1 cup	110	14	13	1
Organic Lowfat Raspberry	1 cup	180	35	32	3
KETCHUP					
banana	1 tsp	10	2	2	0
ketchup	1 pkg (0.2 oz)	6	2	–	tr
ketchup	1 tbsp	15	4	3	0
low sodium	1 tbsp	15	4	3	0
Heinz					
Ketchup	1 tbsp	15	4	4	0
Organic	1 tbsp	20	5	4	0
Muir Glen					
Organic	1 tbsp	20	4	3	0
Tree Of Life					
Organic	1 tbsp (0.6 oz)	20	4	4	0
Wholemato					
Organic Agave	1 tbsp	15	3	3	0
KIDNEY					
beef simmered	3 oz	134	0	0	0
lamb braised	3 oz	116	1	–	0
pork braised	3 oz	128	0	0	0
veal braised	3 oz	139	0	0	0
Rumba					
Beef	4 oz	120	2	0	0
KIDNEY BEANS					
canned	½ cup	108	19	2	6
dried cooked w/o salt	½ cup	112	20	tr	6
B&M					
Red Kidney Baked Beans	½ cup (4.6 oz)	200	36	10	6
Bush's					
Light Red	½ cup	110	20	1	7

FOOD	PORTION	CALS	CARB	SUGAR	FIBER
Eden					
Chili Beans	½ cup	130	21	1	7
Organic	½ cup	100	18	tr	10
Organic Cannellini	½ cup	100	17	tr	5
Organic Refried	½ cup	80	15	–	6
Goya					
Dark	½ cup	90	18	2	7
Progresso					
Cannellini	½ cup (4.6 oz)	110	20	2	6
Rienzi					
Red	½ cup	90	18	2	7
Van Camp's					
New Orleans	½ cup	90	19	1	6
KIWI					
fresh	1 med (2.6 oz)	46	11	7	2
fresh	1 lg (3.2 oz)	56	13	8	3
Zespri					
Gold	2 med	80	20	18	2
Green	2 med	100	24	16	4
KIWI JUICE					
Auna					
Kiwifruit Juice	1 bottle (12 oz)	120	33	25	4
KNISH					
TAKE-OUT					
cheese	1 (2.1 oz)	205	19	tr	1
meat	1 (1.8 oz)	174	13	tr	1
potato	1 (2.1 oz)	212	21	tr	1
potato	1 lg (7 oz)	332	49	5	1
KOHLRABI					
raw sliced	1 cup	36	8	4	4
sliced cooked w/o salt	1 cup	48	11	5	2
Frieda's					
Kohlrabi	⅔ cup	25	5	2	3
TAKE-OUT					
creamed	1 cup	150	14	6	1
KRILL					
fresh	1 oz	22	tr	–	0

FOOD	PORTION	CALS	CARB	SUGAR	FIBER
KUMQUATS					
canned in syrup	1	13	3	3	1
fresh	1	13	3	2	1
LAMB					
cubed lean & fat braised	4 oz	253	0	0	0
cubed lean broiled	4 oz	211	0	0	0
ground broiled	4 oz	321	0	0	0
leg roasted	4 oz	213	0	0	0
loin chop lean & fat broiled	1 chop (4 oz)	222	0	0	0
rib chop lean & fat broiled	1 chop (1.6 oz)	165	0	0	0
rib roast baked	4 oz	386	0	0	0
shank lean & fat braised	4 oz	360	0	0	0
shoulder chop lean & fat cooked	1 chop (5.5 oz)	274	0	0	0
shoulder w/ bone braised	4 oz	231	0	0	0
LAMB DISHES					
TAKE-OUT					
keema w/ coconut milk	1 serv (8 oz)	380	18	9	6
moussaka	4 in sq (16 oz)	659	32	10	8
shepherd's pie	1 (21.3 oz)	742	76	9	9
stew w/ potatoes & vegetables	1 cup	260	29	3	4
LECITHIN					
lecithin	1 tbsp	104	0	0	0
Bob's Red Mill					
Lecithin Granules	1 tbsp	60	1	0	0
Tree Of Life					
Granules	1 tbsp (0.3 oz)	55	1	0	0
LEEKS					
cooked	1 (4.4 oz)	38	9	–	1
Frieda's					
Fresh	1 cup	50	12	3	2
LEMON					
fresh	1 med (4 oz)	22	12	–	5
peel	1 tbsp	3	1	tr	1
peel	1 tsp	1	tr	tr	tr
wedge	1 (7 g)	2	1	tr	tr
LEMON CURD					
lemon curd made w/ egg	2 tsp	29	4	–	0

FOOD	PORTION	CALS	CARB	SUGAR	FIBER
Robert Rothchild Farm					
Lemon Curd & Tart Filling	1 tbsp	50	8	7	0
LEMON EXTRACT					
lemon extract	½ tsp	12	0	0	0
LEMON JUICE					
bottled	1 oz	6	2	1	tr
bottled	1 tbsp	3	1	tr	tr
fresh	1 oz	8	3	1	tr
from 1 lemon	1.6 oz	12	4	1	tr
from wedge	6 g	1	1	tr	0
Canarino					
Italian Hot Lemon Beverage as prep	1 cup	0	0	0	0
LEMONADE					
MIX					
Crystal Light					
Lemonade as prep	1 serv	5	0	0	0
On The Go as prep	1 pkg	5	0	0	0
Pink as prep	1 serv	5	0	0	0
READY-TO-DRINK					
Crystal Light					
Sugar Free	8 oz	5	0	0	0
Hood					
Lemonade	1 cup	110	28	28	0
Nantucket Nectars					
Lemondade	8 oz	110	28	28	0
Odwalla					
PomaGrand	8 oz	110	28	27	0
Pure Squeezed	8 oz	120	30	28	0
SSips					
Lemonade	8 oz	110	27	24	0
Tropicana					
Light	1 cup	10	2	1	0
Orchard Style	8 oz	120	31	29	0
Twister Strawberry	8 oz	140	35	34	0
Twister Light	8 oz	50	12	12	0
Uncle Matt's					
Organic	8 oz	120	30	27	0

FOOD	PORTION	CALS	CARB	SUGAR	FIBER
LENTILS					
dried cooked	1 cup	230	40	4	16
Eden					
Organic Green w/ Onion & Bay Leaf	½ cup	90	13	0	4
Near East					
Lentil Pilaf as prep	1 cup	200	36	3	8
Sabra					
Dardara	2 oz	40	5	1	1
TastyBite					
Jodhpur Lentils	½ pkg (5 oz)	106	12	3	7
Madras Lentils	½ pkg (5 oz)	127	14	3	5
TAKE-OUT					
lentil loaf	1 slice (1.6 oz)	83	10	1	3
yemiser selatta ethiopian lentil salad	1 serv (3 oz)	115	11	1	2
LETTUCE (see also SALAD)					
arugula	6 leaves (0.4 oz)	3	tr	tr	tr
arugula shredded	1 cup	5	1	tr	tr
boston	1 head (5.7 oz)	21	4	2	2
boston chopped	6 leaves	7	1	1	1
cornsalad field salad	1 cup (1.9 oz)	7	1	–	1
iceberg	1 lg head (26.5 oz)	106	22	15	9
iceberg	6 med leaves	7	1	1	1
iceberg shredded	1 cup	10	2	1	1
looseleaf outer leaves	6 (5 oz)	22	4	1	2
looseleaf shredded	1 cup	5	1	tr	1
red leaf	6 leaves (3.6 oz)	16	2	tr	1
red leaf shredded	1 cup	4	1	tr	tr
romaine	3 leaves (3 oz)	14	3	1	2
romaine heart	6 leaves (1.3 oz)	6	1	tr	1
romaine shredded	1 cup	8	2	1	1
Andy Boy					
Romaine Hearts	6 leaves (3 oz)	20	3	2	1
Dole					
Classic Romaine	1½ cups (3 oz)	15	4	2	1
Shredded	1½ cups (3 oz)	15	3	2	1

FOOD	PORTION	CALS	CARB	SUGAR	FIBER
Earthbound Farm					
Organic Baby Romaine Salad	2 cups	15	2	0	1
Fresh Express					
5 Lettuce Mix	3 cups	15	1	1	1
Lettuce Trio	2½ cups	15	3	1	1
Organic Baby Arugula	3 cups	20	3	2	1
Organic Hearts Of Romaine	1½ cups	15	2	0	1
Premium Romaine	2 cups	15	3	1	2
Shreds Iceberg	1½ cups	15	3	2	1
Sweet Butter	2½ cups	10	2	1	1
Frieda's					
Limestone	⅔ cup	10	2	1	1
Mann's					
Romaine Hearts	6 leaves (3 oz)	15	3	2	1
Ocean Mist					
Butter Leaf Shredded	1 cup (2 oz)	7	1	1	1
Green Or Green Leaf Shredded	1 cup (1.3 oz)	5	1	0	0
Iceberg	⅙ head (3 oz)	15	3	2	1
Romaine Hearts	6 leaves	20	3	2	1
LILY ROOT					
dried	1 oz	89	21	–	tr
fresh	1 oz	32	8	–	tr
LIMA BEANS					
CANNED					
Allens					
Baby Butter Beans	½ cup	120	22	2	6
Medium Green	½ cup	140	26	0	7
East Texas Fair					
Green	½ cup	120	23	0	8
Hanover					
Butter Beans In Sauce	½ cup	100	18	0	5
DRIED					
cooked	½ cup	150	20	1	5
FROZEN					
C&W					
Baby	½ cup	110	20	2	5
Green Giant					
Baby & Butter Sauce as prep	⅔ cup	100	18	1	5

FOOD	PORTION	CALS	CARB	SUGAR	FIBER
LIME					
fresh	1 (2.4 oz)	20	7	1	1
wedge	1 (8 g)	2	1	tr	tr
True Lime					
Crystallized Lime	1 pkg	0	0	0	0
LIME JUICE					
bottled	1 oz	6	2	tr	tr
fresh	1 oz	8	3	1	tr
from 1 lime	1.1 oz	11	4	1	tr
LING					
blue raw	3.5 oz	83	0	0	0
fresh baked	3 oz	95	0	0	0
fresh fillet baked	5.3 oz	168	0	0	0
LINGCOD					
baked	3 oz	93	0	0	0
fillet baked	5.3 oz	164	0	0	0
LIQUOR/LIQUEUR *(see also* BEER AND ALE, CHAMPAGNE, MALT, WINE)*					
7&7	1 serv	178	19	–	0
alabama slammer	1 serv	103	7	–	tr
amaretto sour	1 serv	295	57	–	4
angel's kiss	1 serv	85	5	–	0
antifreeze	1 serv	177	31	–	tr
apricot sour	1 serv	164	8	–	tr
aquavit	1 oz	65	0	0	0
b 52	1 serv	247	25	–	0
b&b	1 serv	75	0	0	0
bahama breeze	1 serv	70	9	–	tr
bahama mama	1 serv	153	23	–	tr
bailey's & amaretto	1 serv	184	16	–	0
banana colada	1 serv	376	64	–	3
bay breeze	1 serv	173	18	–	tr
bend me over	1 serv	242	32	–	tr
betsy ross	1 serv	206	5	–	0
black devil	1 serv	220	1	–	tr
black russian	1 serv	184	12	–	0
blue whale	1 serv	222	23	–	0
bourbon & soda	1 serv (4 oz)	105	0	0	0
bourbon sour	1 serv	166	8	–	tr

FOOD	PORTION	CALS	CARB	SUGAR	FIBER
brandy sour	1 serv	164	8	—	tr
bushwacker	1 serv	286	27	—	tr
coffee liqueur	1 serv (1.5 oz)	175	24	24	0
cognac	1 oz	67	tr	0	0
cosmopolitan martini	1 serv	126	7	—	tr
creme de menthe	1 serv (1.5 oz)	186	21	21	0
daiquiri	1 serv (2 oz)	112	4	3	tr
daiquiri banana	1 serv	277	32	—	1
dark & stormy	1 serv	64	0	0	0
doctor pepper	1 serv	95	12	—	0
frozen daiquiri pineapple	1 serv	186	28	—	2
frozen tequila screwdriver	1 serv	159	17	—	1
fuzzy navel	1 serv	247	10	—	tr
gin	1 serv (1.5 oz)	110	0	0	0
grasshopper	1 serv	275	26	—	0
happy hawaiian	1 serv	434	60	—	tr
harvey wallbanger	1 serv	198	16	—	tr
head banger	1 serv	165	4	—	0
hot buttered rum	1 serv (8.8 oz)	316	4	4	tr
hot toddy	1 serv	188	13	—	5
hurricane	1 serv	205	19	—	tr
kamikaze	1 serv	136	2	—	0
lynchburg lemonade	1 serv	465	85	—	1
mai tai	1 serv	165	17	—	tr
manhattan	1 serv	171	3	—	tr
margarita	1 serv	173	11	—	0
margarita strawberry	1 serv	106	11	—	1
martini	1 serv (3 oz)	206	2	tr	0
martini apple	1 serv	147	4	—	tr
martini rum	1 serv	131	tr	—	tr
mellow yellow	1 serv	95	4	—	0
mexican grasshopper	1 serv	638	52	—	0
mississippi mud	1 serv	496	46	—	0
mudslide	1 serv	566	46	—	0
narragansett	1 serv	168	2	—	0
nutcracker	1 serv	730	64	—	0
orange crush	1 serv	461	65	—	tr
pain killer	1 serv	277	20	—	tr
peppermint pattie	1 serv	344	37	—	0
pina colada	1 serv (4.5 oz)	245	32	31	tr

FOOD	PORTION	CALS	CARB	SUGAR	FIBER
planter's cocktail	1 serv	105	3	–	tr
presbyterian	1 serv	170	8	–	tr
purple passion	1 serv	215	22	–	0
rob roy	1 serv	171	3	–	tr
rum	1 serv (1.5 oz)	97	0	0	0
rum boogie	1 serv	134	12	–	tr
rum cola	1 serv	209	21	–	tr
rum highball	1 serv	170	11	–	0
rum punch	1 serv	448	88	–	1
rum sour	1 serv	156	8	–	tr
rum swizzle	1 serv	187	15	–	0
rusty nail	1 serv	159	6	–	0
sake	1 serv (1 oz)	39	1	0	0
salty dog	1 serv	210	19	–	tr
scotch & soda	1 serv	104	tr	–	tr
sea breeze	1 serv	207	19	–	tr
sex on the beach	1 serv	190	18	–	tr
slippery nipple	1 serv	142	11	–	0
snake bite	1 serv	362	22	–	0
tequila gimlet	1 serv	150	6	–	1
tequila sour	1 serv	156	8	–	tr
tequila stinger	1 serv	221	14	–	0
vermouth cassis	1 serv	97	5	–	tr
vodka	1 serv (1.5 oz)	97	0	0	0
vodka gimlet	1 serv	150	6	–	1
vodka sour	1 serv	138	3	–	tr
vodka stinger	1 serv	378	28	–	0
whiskey sour	1 serv (3.5 oz)	162	14	14	0
white russian	1 serv	290	17	–	0
zombie	1 serv	235	10	–	tr
LIVER *(see also* PATE)					
beef braised	1 slice (2.4 oz)	130	3	0	0
beef pan-fried	1 slice (2.8 oz)	142	4	0	0
chicken fried	3 oz	146	1	0	0
chicken simmered	3 oz	142	1	0	0
duck raw	1 (1.5 oz)	60	2	–	0
goose raw	1 (3.3 oz)	125	6	–	0
lamb braised	3 oz	187	2	–	0
lamb fried	3 oz	202	3	–	0
turkey simmered	1 liver (2.9 oz)	227	1	0	0

FOOD	PORTION	CALS	CARB	SUGAR	FIBER
veal braised	1 slice (2.8 oz)	154	3	0	0
veal pan fried	1 slice (2.4 oz)	129	3	0	0
Organic Prairie					
Beef	2 oz	80	2	0	0
Rumba					
Beef	4 oz	160	7	0	0
TAKE-OUT					
calves liver w/ onions	1 serv (5 oz)	177	10	2	1

LOGANBERRIES

fresh	½ cup (2.5 oz)	40	9	6	4
frzn thawed	½ cup (2.6 oz)	40	10	6	4

LOQUATS

fresh	1 lg (0.7 oz)	9	2	–	tr
fresh cubed	½ cup (2.6 oz)	35	9	–	1

LOTUS
Eden

Dried Sliced	5 slices (0.3 oz)	35	8	1	2
Frieda's					
Lotus Root Fresh	1 cup	50	15	0	4

LOX *(see SALMON)*

LYCHEES

canned in syrup	1 (0.7 oz)	19	5	5	tr
canned in syrup	½ cup (4.4 oz)	114	29	28	1
dried	1 (2.5 g)	7	2	2	tr
fresh	1 (0.3 oz)	6	2	1	tr
fresh cut up	½ cup (3.3 oz)	63	16	14	1
Frieda's					
Fresh	6 to 8 (3.5 oz)	60	14	13	1
Polar					
Lychee	1	110	27	26	1

MACA ROOT
Navitas Naturals

Powder Gelatinized	1 tsp (5 g)	20	3	1	1
Raw Powder	1 tsp (5 g)	20	4	1	1

MACADAMIA NUTS

dry roasted w/ salt	11 nuts (1 oz)	200	4	2	1

FOOD	PORTION	CALS	CARB	SUGAR	FIBER
Chukar Cherries					
Extra Dark Chocolate Covered	3 tbsp (1.4 oz)	216	14	9	3
Emily's					
Milk Chocolate Covered	4 (1.5 oz)	260	21	18	2
Hawaiian Host					
White Choco	3 pieces (1.4 oz)	230	22	21	0
Mauna Loa					
Maui Onion & Garlic	1 pkg (1.2 oz)	230	5	1	3
MACE					
ground	1 tsp	8	1	–	tr
MACKEREL					
CANNED					
jack	1 can (12.7 oz)	563	0	0	0
jack	1 cup	296	0	0	0
Brunswick					
Jack In Water	2 oz	100	5	0	0
Orleans					
Jack	¼ cup	90	0	0	0
Polar					
Jack	⅓ cup	90	0	0	0
DRIED					
Eden					
Bonito Flakes	2 tbsp	5	0	0	0
FRESH					
atlantic cooked	3 oz	223	0	0	0
atlantic raw	3 oz	174	0	0	0
jack baked	3 oz	171	0	0	0
jack fillet baked	6.2 oz	354	0	0	0
king baked	3 oz	114	0	0	0
king fillet baked	5.4 oz	207	0	0	0
pacific baked	3 oz	171	0	0	0
pacific fillet baked	6.2 oz	354	0	0	0
spanish cooked	1 fillet (5.1 oz)	230	0	0	0
spanish cooked	3 oz	134	0	0	0
spanish raw	3 oz	118	0	0	0
SMOKED					
atlantic	3.5 oz	296	0	0	0

FOOD	PORTION	CALS	CARB	SUGAR	FIBER
MAHI MAHI					
fresh baked	4 oz	192	1	tr	0
MALANGA					
dasheen mashed	1 cup	226	53	1	8
dasheen pieces boiled	1 cup	212	50	1	8
pieces fried	1 cup	304	52	1	8
Frieda's					
Malanga	⅔ cup	90	23	0	2
MALT					
malt liquor	1 bottle (12 oz)	148	13	tr	tr
nonalcoholic	1 bottle (12 oz)	133	29	29	0
MALTED MILK					
chocolate as prep w/ milk	1 cup	179	27	15	1
chocolate flavor powder	3 heaping tsp (0.7 oz)	79	18	5	1
natural flavor as prep w/ milk	1 cup	186	24	22	tr
natural flavor powder	3 heaping tsp (0.7 oz)	87	16	12	tr
MANGO					
dried	1 slice (5 g)	16	4	4	tr
dried	½ cup (1.8 oz)	74	41	38	3
fresh	1 (7.3 oz)	135	35	31	4
fresh sliced	½ cup (3 oz)	54	14	12	2
pickled	1 slice (1 oz)	38	10	9	tr
C&W					
Chunks	¾ cup	90	24	21	3
Kopali					
Organic Dried	1 pkg (1.8 oz)	140	38	34	4
Peeled Snacks					
Fruit Picks Go-Mango-Man-Go	1 pkg (1.4 oz)	120	28	20	2
Polar					
Sliced	3 pieces (5 oz)	100	24	21	2
Sunsweet					
Philippine dried	6 pieces (1.5 oz)	130	30	26	2
Thailand dried	⅓ cup (1.4 oz)	140	34	28	1

FOOD	PORTION	CALS	CARB	SUGAR	FIBER
MANGO JUICE					
nectar canned	1 cup (8.8 oz)	128	33	31	1
GoodBelly					
Mango Probiotic Drink	8 oz	100	25	21	1
MARGARINE					
margarine butter blend	1 tbsp (0.5 oz)	101	tr	0	0
squeeze	1 pkg (0.2 oz)	36	0	0	0
squeeze liquid	1 tbsp (0.5 oz)	102	0	0	0
stick	1 stick (4 oz)	810	1	0	0
stick	1 tbsp (0.5 oz)	100	tr	0	0
tub diet	1 tbsp (0.5 oz)	26	tr	0	0
tub fat free	1 tbsp (0.5 oz)	27	1	0	0
tub light	1 tbsp (0.5 oz)	59	tr	–	0
tub salted	1 tbsp (0.5 oz)	101	tr	0	0
whipped salted	1 tbsp (0.3 oz)	67	tr	0	0
Benecol					
Spread Light	1 tbsp	50	0	0	0
Spread Regular	1 tbsp	70	0	0	0
Brummel & Brown					
Spread w/ Yogurt	1 tbsp	45	0	0	0
Country Crock					
Light	1 tbsp (0.5 oz)	50	0	0	0
Regular	1 tbsp (0.5 oz)	90	0	0	0
Spread w/ Calcium + Vitamin D	1 tbsp (0.5 oz)	50	0	0	0
Crystal Farms					
60/40 Margarine Butter	1 tbsp	100	0	0	0
Margarine	1 tbsp	100	0	0	0
Earth Balance					
Butter Blend Salted	1 tbsp	100	0	0	0
Buttery Spread Original	1 tbsp	100	0	0	0
Buttery Spread Soy Garden	1 tbsp	100	0	0	0
Buttery Sticks Vegan	1 tbsp	100	0	0	0
Land O Lakes					
Soft	1 tbsp (0.5 oz)	100	0	0	0
Stick	1 tbsp (0.5 oz)	100	0	0	0
Move Over Butter					
Spread	1 tbsp	50	0	0	0
Promise					
Buttery Spread	1 tbsp	80	0	0	0
Buttery Spread Activ	1 tbsp	70	0	0	0

FOOD	PORTION	CALS	CARB	SUGAR	FIBER
Fat Free	1 tbsp	5	0	0	0
Light	1 tbsp	45	0	0	0
Light Activ	1 tbsp	45	0	0	0
Smart Balance					
37% Light	1 tbsp	45	0	0	0
67% Light	1 tbsp	80	0	0	0
Omega Plus w/ Flax Oil	1 tbsp	80	0	0	0

MARINADE *(see SAUCE)*

MARJORAM
dried	1 tsp	2	tr	tr	tr

MARLIN
raw	3 oz	110	0	0	0

MARSHMALLOW
chocolate coated	1 (0.4 oz)	41	8	6	tr
coconut coated	1 (0.4 oz)	33	7	5	tr
marshmallow regular	1 (0.3 oz)	23	6	4	0
miniatures	1 cup (1.8 oz)	159	41	29	tr
miniatures	10 (0.3 oz)	22	6	4	0

MATZO
brie	1 piece (0.5 oz)	54	5	3	tr
egg	1 (1 oz)	109	22	–	1
matzo ball	1 med (1.2 oz)	48	6	tr	tr
plain	1 (1 oz)	111	23	–	1
whole wheat	1 (1 oz)	98	22	–	3
Horowitz Margareten					
Egg	1 (1.2 oz)	130	28	2	1
Manischewitz					
Egg & Onion	1 (1 oz)	100	23	2	2
Matzo Ball Mix	2 tbsp	50	11	0	1
Thin Unsalted	1 (0.8 oz)	90	20	1	0
Streit's					
Egg & Onion	1 (1 oz)	100	23	0	1

MAYONNAISE
diet	1 tbsp	36	3	1	0
imitation	1 tbsp	35	2	1	0
mayonnaise	1 tbsp	99	1	tr	0

FOOD	PORTION	CALS	CARB	SUGAR	FIBER
Cains					
All Natural	1 tbsp	100	0	0	0
Light	1 tbsp	50	2	1	0
Hellman's					
Real	1 tbsp	90	0	0	0
Real Canola No Cholesterol	1 tbsp	90	0	0	0
Hollywood					
Canola	1 tbsp	100	0	0	0
Safflower	1 tbsp	100	0	0	0
Kraft					
Mayo	1 tbsp	90	0	0	0
Mayo With Olive Oil	1 tbsp	45	2	tr	0
Miracle Whip					
Light	1 tbsp	25	3	2	0
Original	1 tbsp	40	2	2	0
Smart Balance					
Omega	1 tbsp	120	0	0	0
Vegenaise					
Grapeseed Oil	1 tbsp (0.5 oz)	90	0	0	0
Organic	1 tbsp (0.5 oz)	90	0	0	0
Original	1 tbsp (0.5 oz)	90	0	0	0

MEAT SUBSTITUTES *(see also* BACON SUBSTITUTES, CANADIAN BACON SUBSTITUTES, CHICKEN SUBSTITUTES, HAMBURGER SUBSTITUTES, MEATBALL SUBSTITUTES, SAUSAGE SUBSTITUTES, TURKEY SUBSTITUTES*)*

FOOD	PORTION	CALS	CARB	SUGAR	FIBER
Fantastic					
Sloppy Joe Mix not prep	¼ cup	70	11	3	3
Taco Filling not prep	¼ cup	80	10	1	4
Gardenburger					
BBQ Riblets w/ Sauce	1 serv (5 oz)	240	33	27	5
Health Is Wealth					
Vegetarian Cocktail Franks	3 (2.4 oz)	220	16	0	3
Helen's Kitchen					
GardenSteak Tofu Steak	1 (3 oz)	150	14	1	3
Lightlife					
Bologna	4 slices (2 oz)	60	0	0	2
Gimme Lean Ground Beef	1 serv (2 oz)	50	4	1	2
Smart Cutlet Salisbury Steak	1 (4.5 oz)	130	13	1	6
Smart Deli Country Ham	4 slices (2 oz)	90	5	0	1
Smart Deli Pastrami Style	4 slices (2 oz)	60	1	0	0
Smart Deli Pepperoni Style	13 slices (1 oz)	45	3	1	1

FOOD	PORTION	CALS	CARB	SUGAR	FIBER
Smart Ground Original	⅓ cup (1.9 oz)	80	7	1	3
Smart Ground Taco Burrito	⅓ cup (2 oz)	70	5	1	4
Smart Menu Crumbles	⅓ cup	80	7	1	3
Smart Menu Steak Strips	1 serv (3 oz)	80	5	0	5
Smart Tex Mex	¼ cup	50	6	2	2
Loma Linda					
Dinner Cuts	2 slices (3.2 oz)	90	4	0	2
Swiss Stake	1 piece (3.2 oz)	130	9	tr	3
Morningstar Farms					
Meal Starters Steak Strips	12 pieces (3 oz)	140	5	1	1
Veat					
Gourmet Bites	1 serv (2.5 oz)	90	8	2	1
Vegetarian Fillet	1 (1.8 oz)	170	19	1	1
Viana					
Cowgirl Veggie Steaks	1 (3.7 oz)	260	6	5	4
Veggie Cevapcici	4 pieces (2.8 oz)	240	5	3	3
Veggie Gyros	24 strips (3 oz)	220	5	2	2
Veggie Kebab	½ cup	210	3	2	2
Worthington					
Bolono	3 slices (2 oz)	80	3	1	2
Choplets	2 slices (3.2 oz)	90	4	0	2
Corned Beef Vegetarian	3 slices (2 oz)	140	5	1	0
Dinner Roast	1 slice (3 oz)	180	6	1	3
Multigrain Cutlets	2 slices (3.2 oz)	100	5	0	3
Prime Stakes	1 piece (3.2 oz)	120	7	0	1
Vegetable Skallops	½ cup (3 oz)	90	4	0	3
Wham	2 slices (2 oz)	110	3	2	0
Yves					
Meatless Beef Skewers	1 (2.8 oz)	100	10	5	3
Meatless Bologna	4 slices	60	2	tr	0
Meatless Pepperoni	6 slices	90	4	tr	0

FOOD	PORTION	CALS	CARB	SUGAR	FIBER
Meatless Ground Round Original	⅓ cup	60	5	1	2

MEATBALL SUBSTITUTES

FOOD	PORTION	CALS	CARB	SUGAR	FIBER
meatless	2 (1.3 oz)	71	3	tr	2
Gardenburger					
Mama Mia Meatballs	6 (3 oz)	110	7	0	4
Lightlife					
Smart Menu Meatless Meatballs	5	160	6	1	2
Loma Linda					
Tender Rounds	6 (2.8 oz)	120	6	1	1
VeggieLand					
Veg-T-Balls	3 (3 oz)	113	9	3	5

MEATBALLS

FOOD	PORTION	CALS	CARB	SUGAR	FIBER
beef cocktail	1 (0.2 oz)	18	0	0	0
beef lg	1 (1.5 oz)	111	0	0	0
beef med	1 (1 oz)	74	0	0	0
chicken cocktail	1 (0.2 oz)	12	1	tr	0
chicken lg	1 (1.5 oz)	71	3	1	tr
chicken med	1 (1 oz)	47	2	1	tr
turkey med	1 (1 oz)	47	2	1	tr
Butterball					
Seasoned Italian frzn	6 (3 oz)	170	6	1	1
Honeysuckle White					
Turkey Italian Style frzn	3 (3 oz)	190	6	1	1
Ian's					
Italian	3 (2.2 oz)	145	10	1	1
Mama Lucia					
Homestyle	4	207	8	2	1
Italian Style	4	280	8	1	0
Sausage Beef	8	220	3	0	1
Organic Classics					
Italian Beef	3 (3 oz)	180	5	1	1
Shady Brook					
Italian Beef	3 oz	260	5	1	1
Turkey Meatballs Appetizer Size + Sweet & Sour Sauce	6 + 2 tbsp sauce	235	17	11	tr
Turkey Meatballs Italian Style	3 (3 oz)	190	6	1	tr
Tyson					
Italian Style Chicken	6 (3 oz)	180	6	1	2

FOOD	PORTION	CALS	CARB	SUGAR	FIBER
TAKE-OUT					
albondigas w/ sauce	3 + sauce (5.3 oz)	372	11	3	1
porcupine + tomato sauce	3 + sauce	160	14	3	1
swedish w/ cream sauce	3 + sauce (4.7 oz)	215	9	2	tr
sweet & sour	3 + sauce (4.5 oz)	188	8	1	1
MELON					
sprite	1 (10.6 oz)	110	29	27	1
Frieda's					
Camouflage	1 cup (5 oz)	50	13	7	1
SpriteMelon	1 (10.5 oz)	115	29	27	2
Temptation	1/10 melon (4.7 oz)	55	14	12	1

MEXICAN FOOD (see SALSA, SPANISH FOOD, TORTILLA)

FOOD	PORTION	CALS	CARB	SUGAR	FIBER
MILK					
CANNED					
condensed sweetened	1 cup (10.7 oz)	982	166	166	0
condensed sweetened	1 tbsp (0.7 oz)	61	10	10	0
evaporated nonfat	1 cup (9 oz)	200	29	29	0
evaporated nonfat	1 tbsp (0.5 oz)	12	2	2	1
Borden					
Sweetened Condensed Low Fat	2 tbsp	120	23	23	0
DRIED					
buttermilk	1 tbsp (0.2 oz)	25	3	3	0
buttermilk	1/4 cup (1 oz)	111	14	14	0
nonfat instant	1 pkg (3.2 oz)	326	47	47	0
nonfat instant	1 tbsp (0.6 oz)	61	9	9	0
whole milk	1/4 cup (1.1 oz)	159	12	12	0
Alba					
Instant Non-Fat as prep	1 cup	80	11	11	0
Bob's Red Mill					
Buttermilk Sweet Cream as prep	8 oz	60	7	0	0
Non Fat as prep	8 oz	80	11	11	0
Carnation					
Instant Nonfat as prep	1 cup	80	12	12	0

FOOD	PORTION	CALS	CARB	SUGAR	FIBER
Organic Valley					
Buttermilk	3 tbsp	110	16	12	0
Nonfat	3 tbsp	90	13	12	0
Sanalac					
Powder	¼ cup (0.8 oz)	80	13	12	0
REFRIGERATED					
1%	1 cup (8.6 oz)	102	12	13	0
2%	1 cup (8.6 oz)	122	11	12	0
buttermilk lowfat	1 cup (8.6 oz)	98	12	12	0
fat free	1 cup (8.6 oz)	83	12	12	0
goat	1 cup (8.6 oz)	168	11	11	0
human	1 cup (8.6 oz)	172	17	7	0
whole	1 cup (8.6 oz)	146	11	14	0
Active Lifestyle					
Fat Free w/ Plant Sterols	8 oz	90	13	12	0
Dairy Ease					
Fat Free Lactose Free	1 cup (8 oz)	90	12	12	0
Reduced Fat 2% Lactose Free	1 cup (8 oz)	130	12	12	0
Whole Lactose Free	1 cup (8 oz)	160	11	11	0
Farmland					
Buttermilk	8 oz	160	19	18	0
Fat Free	8 oz	80	12	12	0
Special Request 1% Plus Omega-3	8 oz	130	17	16	0
Special Request Skim Plus	8 oz	110	17	16	0
Special Request Skim Plus 100% Lactose Free	8 oz	110	17	16	0
Whole	8 oz	160	19	18	0
Friendship					
Buttermilk Lowfat	1 cup	120	12	12	0
Hood					
1%	1 cup	110	13	12	0
2%	1 cup	130	13	12	0
Buttermilk Fat Free	1 cup	90	13	12	0
Calorie Countdown 2%	8 oz	90	3	3	0
Calorie Countdown Fat Free	8 oz	45	3	3	0
Fat Free	1 cup	80	13	12	0
Simply Smart 0% Fat	1 cup	90	13	12	0
Simply Smart 1% Fat	1 cup	120	13	12	0
Whole	1 cup	150	12	12	0

FOOD	PORTION	CALS	CARB	SUGAR	FIBER
Horizon Organic					
Fat Free	8 oz	90	12	12	0
Land O Lakes					
1%	1 cup (8 oz)	100	13	13	0
2%	1 cup (8 oz)	120	12	12	0
Skim	1 cup (8 oz)	90	13	13	0
Whole	1 cup (8 oz)	150	12	12	0
Organic Valley					
Fat Free	1 cup	90	13	12	0
Lactose Free Fat Free	1 cup	90	14	13	0
Whole Nonhomogenized	1 cup	150	12	12	0
Straus					
Organic Reduced Fat 2% Cream Top	8 oz	130	13	13	0
SunMilk					
Heart Healthy 1% Sunflower Oil	8 oz	120	15	15	0
Heart Healthy 2% Sunflower Oil	8 oz	120	15	15	0
Turkey Hill					
Cool Moos Whole Milk	8 oz	160	27	26	0
Tuscan					
Whole	8 oz	150	12	11	0
Welsh Farms					
Fat Free	8 oz	80	12	12	0
SHELF-STABLE					
Parmalat					
2% Reduced Fat	8 oz	130	12	12	0
Fat Free	8 oz	80	12	12	0
Lactose Free 2% Reduced Fat	8 oz	130	12	12	0
MILK DRINKS					
chocolate milk	1 cup (8.8 oz)	208	26	24	2
chocolate milk lowfat	1 cup (8.8 oz)	158	26	25	1
Bravo!					
Blenders Creamy Double Chocolate	1 bottle (11 oz)	180	19	16	2
Blenders Creamy French Vanilla	1 bottle (11 oz)	160	20	16	2
Cocio					
Chocolate Milk	8 oz	140	20	17	0

FOOD	PORTION	CALS	CARB	SUGAR	FIBER
CocoaVia					
Indulgence Rice Chocolate	1 bottle (5.65 oz)	150	28	24	3
Dove					
Bravo! Dark Chocolate	1 bottle	310	37	34	2
Bravo! Milk Chocolate	1 bottle	310	36	34	1
Farmland					
Really Really Good! Chocolate Milk	8 oz	160	25	24	0
Hood					
Calorie Countdown Chocolate 2%	8 oz	90	5	3	1
Chocolate Lowfat	1 cup	170	28	26	tr
Chocolate Milk	1 cup	230	31	29	tr
Coffee Lowfat Milk	1 cup	170	28	26	0
Horizon Organic					
Lowfat Chocolate Milk	8 oz	170	27	27	tr
Strawberry	8 oz	200	31	31	0
Land O Lakes					
2% Swiss Chocolate	1 cup (8.4 oz)	190	26	26	tr
Chocolate Skim	1 cup (8 oz)	160	31	28	tr
Strawberry	1 cup (8 oz)	190	22	22	0
Lifeway					
La Fruta All Flavors	8 oz	180	33	33	0
Nesquik					
Chocolate Powder No Sugar Added as prep w/ lowfat milk	1 cup (8 oz)	160	18	3	1
Chocolate Powder as prep w/ lowfat milk	1 cup (8 oz)	180	27	13	tr
Ready-To-Drink Banana	1 cup (8 oz)	200	30	29	0
Ready-To-Drink Chocolate	1 cup (8 oz)	200	32	30	tr
Ready-To-Drink Strawberry	1 cup (8 oz)	200	33	31	0
Ready-To-Drink Vanilla	1 cup (8 oz)	200	30	29	0
Strawberry Powder as prep w/ lowfat milk	1 cup (8 oz)	190	27	15	0
Organic Valley					
Buttermilk Lowfat 1%	1 cup	100	12	12	0
Parmalat					
Chocolate Milk 2% Reduced Fat	1 cup	190	28	27	1

FOOD	PORTION	CALS	CARB	SUGAR	FIBER
Turkey Hill					
Cool Moos 2% Reduced Fat	8 oz	120	12	12	0
Cool Moos Chocolate	8 oz	180	32	30	0
Cool Moos Whole Milk	8 oz	150	12	12	0
MILK SUBSTITUTES					
8th Continent					
Soymilk Chocolate	8 oz	140	23	21	1
Soymilk Original	8 oz	80	8	7	0
Soymilk Vanilla	8 oz	100	11	10	0
Soymilk Fat Free Original	8 oz	60	8	7	0
Soymilk Fat Free Vanilla	8 oz	70	11	10	0
Soymilk Light Chocolate	8 oz	90	13	11	tr
Soymilk Light Original	8 oz	50	2	1	0
Soymilk Light Vanilla	8 oz	60	5	4	0
Almond Breeze					
Chocolate	8 oz	115	22	20	1
Original	8 oz	57	8	7	1
Original Unsweetened	8 oz	40	2	0	1
Vanilla	8 oz	91	16	15	1
Brazsoy					
Condensed Soy Milk	1 serv (0.7 oz)	54	10	9	0
Soy Cream	1 tbsp (0.5 oz)	27	0	0	0
DariFree					
Fat Free as prep	8 oz	70	20	2	0
Fat Free Chocolate as prep	8 oz	110	27	11	tr
EdenBlend					
Organic	8 oz	120	18	8	tr
Edensoy					
Organic Carob	8 oz	170	28	13	tr
Organic Chocolate	8 oz	180	28	14	tr
Organic Original	8 oz	140	14	7	tr
Organic Original Unsweetened	8 oz	120	5	2	tr
Organic Original Light	8 oz	100	15	10	0
Organic Vanilla	8 oz	150	24	16	tr
Organic Vanilla Light	8 oz	110	22	12	0
Lifeway					
SoyTreat All Flavors	8 oz	160	23	22	0
Living Harvest					
Hempmilk Original	1 cup	130	20	15	1
Hempmilk Vanilla	1 cup	130	20	18	1

FOOD	PORTION	CALS	CARB	SUGAR	FIBER
Lundberg					
Organic Drink Rice Original	8 oz	120	22	13	tr
Manitoba Harvest					
Hemp Bliss Chocolate	8 oz	160	17	16	1
Hemp Bliss Original	1 cup	110	7	6	1
Hemp Bliss Vanilla	8 oz	150	14	13	1
Odwalla					
Soymilk Plain	8 oz	110	12	–	3
Soymilk Vanilla Being	8 oz	100	13	10	3
Organic Valley					
Soy Original	1 cup	100	11	6	3
Soy Unsweetened	1 cup	80	3	1	1
Rice Dream					
Carob	8 oz	150	30	26	tr
Heartwise Vanilla	8 oz	140	30	10	3
Horchata	8 oz	130	16	9	2
Original	8 oz	120	24	11	0
Original Enriched	8 oz	120	23	10	0
Vanilla Enriched	8 oz	130	26	12	0
Sno*e					
Tofu as prep	8 oz	80	20	2	0
Tofu Low Fat as prep	8 oz	70	10	1	0
Soy Dream					
Classic Vanilla	8 oz	140	18	10	2
Original Enriched	8 oz	100	8	4	2
WildWood					
Organic Probiotic Soymilk Blueberry	8 oz	190	33	19	4
Organic Probiotic Soymilk Pomegranate	8 oz	180	31	17	4
Organic Soymilk Plain	8 oz	100	8	6	1
Organic Soymilk Unsweetened	8 oz	72	3	2	1
MILKFISH (AWA)					
baked	4 oz	215	0	0	0
MILKSHAKE					
chocolate	1 serv (10.6 oz)	357	63	63	1
malted milk shake	1 serv (10 oz)	402	62	58	1
vanilla	1 (11 oz)	351	56	56	0

FOOD	PORTION	CALS	CARB	SUGAR	FIBER
Buffy's Cool Cow					
Chocolate	1 pkg (8 oz)	150	23	17	tr
Vanilla	1 pkg (8 oz)	150	24	18	0
Lean Body					
Hi-Protein Chocolate Ice Cream	1 (17 oz)	260	9	0	5
Molli Coolz					
Shakers Vanilla as prep w/ skim milk	1 (10.2 oz)	240	30	17	5
Nesquik					
Ready-To-Drink Chocolate	1 cup (8 oz)	170	26	23	tr
MILLET					
cooked	1 cup (6.1 oz)	207	41	–	2
Arrowhead Mills					
Organic Hulled not prep	¼ cup	150	33	0	1
MINERAL WATER (see WATER)					
MISO					
dried	1 oz	86	10	–	1
Eden					
Hacho	1 tbsp	40	4	0	tr
Organic Genmai	1 tbsp	25	3	1	2
Organic Mugi	1 tbsp	25	4	1	tr
Organic Shiro	1 tbsp	30	6	4	tr
Tekka	1 tsp	5	tr	0	0
MOLASSES					
molasses	1 tbsp (0.7 oz)	58	15	11	0
molasses	¼ cup (3 oz)	244	63	47	0
MONKFISH					
baked	3 oz	82	0	0	0
MOOSE					
roasted	4 oz	142	0	0	0
MOUSSE					
TAKE-OUT					
chocolate	½ cup	454	32	30	1
fish timbale	1 cup	329	3	1	0

FOOD	PORTION	CALS	CARB	SUGAR	FIBER
MUFFIN					
MIX					
Glory					
Golden Sweet Corn as prep	1	170	27	7	1
King Arthur					
Cranberry Orange Whole Grain not prep	¼ cup	180	41	20	3
Martha White					
Whole Grain Apple Cinnamon not prep	¼ cup (1.2 oz)	140	24	13	1
Whole Grain Blueberry not prep	¼ cup (1.2 oz)	140	24	13	1
Yellow Corn not prep	¼ cup (1.2 oz)	140	26	6	1
Miracle Muffins					
Banana w/ Splenda as prep	1	86	12	0	7
READY-TO-EAT					
blueberry	1 (2 oz)	158	27	–	2
oat bran wheat free	1 (2 oz)	154	28	–	4
Hostess					
100 Calorie Pack Mini Banana Streusel	1 pkg (1.2 oz)	100	19	7	4
100 Calorie Pack Mini Blueberry Streusel	1 pkg (1.2 oz)	100	20	7	4
VitaMuffin					
AppleBerryBran	1 (2 oz)	100	25	10	5
BlueBran	1 (2 oz)	100	24	13	4
CranBran	1 (2 oz)	100	24	13	4
Sugar Free Low Carb Banana Nut	1 (2 oz)	90	24	0	7
VitaTops Banana Nut	1 (2 oz)	100	19	3	5
VitaTops Dark Chocolate Pomegranate	1 (2 oz)	100	21	11	6
VitaTops Deep Chocolate	1 (2 oz)	100	25	12	6
VitaTops Golden Corn	1 (2 oz)	100	25	9	6
VitaTops MultiBran	1 (2 oz)	100	22	11	5
TAKE-OUT					
corn	1 lg (2.5 oz)	214	32	5	2
raisin bran lowfat	1 (4 oz)	270	61	35	5
MULBERRIES					
fresh	½ cup (2.5 oz)	30	7	6	1

FOOD	PORTION	CALS	CARB	SUGAR	FIBER
fresh	20 (1 oz)	13	3	2	1
Kopali					
Organic Dark Chocolate Covered	½ pkg (1 oz)	140	20	15	2
Organic Dried	1 pkg (1.7 oz)	240	38	22	6
Navitas Naturals					
Dried	1 oz	91	21	12	3
MULLET					
striped cooked	3 oz	127	0	0	0
striped raw	3 oz	99	0	0	0
MUSHROOMS					
CANNED					
caps	8 (1.6 oz)	12	2	1	1
caps pickled	6 (0.8 oz)	5	1	tr	tr
chanterelle	3.5 oz	12	tr	–	6
pickled	1 cup	33	5	2	1
pieces	½ cup	20	2	1	1
Green Giant					
Pieces & Stems	½ cup	25	4	1	1
Polar					
Straw	½ cup	20	4	0	2
Whole Button	½ cup	30	4	1	2
Whole Shiitake	½ cup	30	4	0	tr
Sunny Dell					
Portabella Sliced	½ cup	20	4	0	2
DRIED					
chanterelle	1 oz	25	tr	–	17
shiitake	1 (3.6 g)	11	3	tr	tr
wood ear mok yee	½ cup (0.4 oz)	25	8	–	4
Eden					
Maitake Sliced	10 pieces (0.3 oz)	35	7	0	4
Shiitake	3 (0.4 oz)	35	7	2	5
Shiitake Sliced	3 pieces (0.3 oz)	35	7	2	5
Frieda's					
Chanterelle	2 pieces (4 g)	15	2	0	1
Wood Ear	3 pieces (4 g)	15	2	0	1

FOOD	PORTION	CALS	CARB	SUGAR	FIBER
Ocean Spring					
Fresh Crispy Mixed Mushrooms	1 serv (0.9 oz)	113	18	2	1
FRESH					
brown italian or crimini sliced	1 cup	19	3	1	tr
brown italian or crimini whole	1 (0.7 oz)	5	1	tr	tr
chanterelle	3.5 oz	11	tr	–	6
enoki raw	1 lg (5 g)	2	tr	tr	tr
enoki sliced	1 cup	29	5	tr	2
enoki whole	1 cup	28	5	tr	2
maitake diced	1 cup	26	5	1	2
maitake whole	1 (6.6 g)	2	tr	tr	tr
morel	3.5 oz	9	0	–	7
oyster	1 sm (0.5 oz)	5	1	tr	tr
oyster sliced	1 cup	30	6	1	2
portabella raw	1 cap (3 oz)	22	4	2	1
portabella sliced grilled	1 cup (4.2 oz)	42	6	0	3
raw sliced	½ cup	8	1	1	tr
shiitake cooked	4 (2.5 oz)	40	10	3	2
shiitake pieces cooked	1 cup	81	21	5	3
white	1 (0.6 oz)	4	1	tr	tr
white sliced cooked	1 cup	28	4	0	2
Frieda's					
Enoki	¼ pkg (1 oz)	10	2	1	1
Giorgio					
Mushrooms	3 oz	20	3	1	1
FROZEN					
Alexia					
Mushroom Bites	1 serv (2 oz)	110	16	2	1
Farm Rich					
Breaded	5 (3 oz)	120	23	0	1
TAKE-OUT					
battered fried	1 lg (0.6 oz)	39	3	1	tr
creamed	1 cup	171	15	7	3
stuffed	1 (0.8 oz)	67	6	1	1
MUSKRAT					
roasted	3 oz	199	0	0	0
MUSSELS					
Polar					
Mussels	2 oz	60	tr	0	0

FOOD	PORTION	CALS	CARB	SUGAR	FIBER
MUSTARD					
hot chinese	1 tsp	3	tr	tr	tr
organic yellow	1 tsp	5	0	0	0
seed	1 tsp	15	1	tr	1
yellow prepared	1 tbsp	3	tr	tr	tr
Boar's Head					
Delicatessen Style	1 tsp (5 g)	0	0	0	0
Honey	1 tsp (5 g)	10	2	1	0
Bone Suckin'					
Fat Free Gluten Free	1 tbsp	25	5	4	0
Eden					
Organic Brown	1 tsp	0	tr	0	0
Yellow	1 tsp	0	0	0	0
Emeril's					
Horseradish	1 tbsp	5	0	0	0
French's					
Classic Yellow	1 tsp	0	0	0	0
Horseradish	1 tsp	5	0	0	0
Spicy Brown	1 tsp	5	0	0	0
Hellman's					
Deli	1 tsp	5	tr	–	0
Dijonnaise	1 tsp	5	1	–	0
Honey Mustard	1 tsp	10	2	–	0
Kosciusko					
Spicy Brown	1 tsp	0	0	0	0
Robert Rothchild Farm					
Champagne Garlic	1 tsp	6	1	1	0
Sara Lee					
Country Honey	1 tbsp	10	2	2	0
Cranberry Honey	1 tbsp	10	2	2	0
School House Kitchen					
Sweet Smooth Hot	1 tsp	15	1	1	0
Vivi's					
Classic	1 tbsp (0.5 oz)	15	4	3	0
Sizzlin' Chipotle	1 tbsp (0.5 oz)	15	4	3	0
MUSTARD GREENS					
canned	1 cup	23	3	tr	3
fresh as prep w/ fat	1 cup	50	3	tr	3
fresh chopped boiled w/o salt	1 cup	21	3	tr	3
fresh raw chopped	1 cup	15	3	1	2

FOOD	PORTION	CALS	CARB	SUGAR	FIBER
frozen chopped boiled w/o salt	1 cup	28	5	tr	4
Allen's					
Seasoned	½ cup	45	6	2	1
Glory					
Seasoned canned	½ cup	35	3	1	1
Sylvia's					
Specially Seasoned	½ cup	30	5	2	2
NATTO					
House					
Natto	2 oz	120	5	0	0
NAVY BEANS					
Eden					
Organic	½ cup	110	20	–	7
NECTARINE					
fresh	1 sm (4.5 oz)	57	14	10	2
fresh	1 lg (5.5 oz)	69	16	12	3
fresh sliced	1 cup (5 oz)	63	15	11	2
Sunsweet					
Dried	3 pieces (1.4 oz)	100	25	14	3
NECTARINE JUICE					
Sun Shower					
100% Juice	8 oz	93	21	17	2
NEUFCHATEL					
Organic Valley					
Soft	2 tbsp	70	2	2	0
NONI JUICE					
Lakewood					
Noni Pure Juice	2 oz	8	2	2	0
Tree Of Life					
100% Juice Concentrate	2 tbsp	15	4	3	0
NOODLES					
chow mein	1 cup (1.6 oz)	237	25	–	2
egg cooked	1 cup (5.6 oz)	213	40	–	2
korean acorn noodles not prep	2 oz	195	41	–	tr
rice cooked	1 cup (6.2 oz)	192	44	–	2
spinach/egg cooked	1 cup (5.6 oz)	211	39	–	4

FOOD	PORTION	CALS	CARB	SUGAR	FIBER
A Taste Of Thai					
Rice Wide	2 oz	200	46	0	2
Annie Chun's					
Chow Mein	2 oz	200	39	1	3
Noddle Express Spicy Szechuan	½ pkg	170	29	4	1
Noodle Bowl Teriyaki	1 pkg	310	60	8	2
Noodle Express Chinese Chow Mein	½ pkg	160	27	3	1
Noodle Express Singapore Curry	½ pkg	160	28	3	2
Noodle Express Teriyaki	½ pkg	160	31	5	1
Noodle Express Thai Peanut	½ pkg	200	29	5	1
Rice	2 oz	210	50	0	0
Rice Pad Thai	2 oz	210	50	0	0
Hodgson Mill					
Egg Whole Wheat not prep	2 oz	190	34	0	4
House					
Shirataki Tofu Noodles	2 oz	20	3	0	2
Shirataki Yam Noodles	2 oz	5	1	0	0
La Choy					
Chow Mein Noodles	½ cup (1 oz)	130	19	0	tr
Rice	½ cup	130	21	1	tr
Light 'N Fluffy					
Egg Extra Wide cooked	1½ cups	210	40	2	2
Manischewitz					
Egg Medium	1¼ cups	220	40	2	2
No Yolks					
Dumplings	2 oz	210	41	3	3
NUTMEG					
ground	1 tsp	12	1	1	1
nutmeg butter	1 tbsp	120	0	0	0
NUTRITION SUPPLEMENTS *(see also* CEREAL BARS, ENERGY BARS, ENERGY DRINKS)					
Amino Vital					
Jel All Flavors	1 pkg (4.9 oz)	70	17	16	1
Clif					
Shot Energy Gel All Flavors	1 pkg (1.1 oz)	100	25	8	0
DiabetiTrim					
Shake French Vanilla	1 pkg	90	10	5	4

FOOD	PORTION	CALS	CARB	SUGAR	FIBER
Ensure					
Shake Creamy Milk Chocolate	1 bottle (8 oz)	250	40	22	1
Shake Strawberries & Cream	1 bottle (8 oz)	250	40	23	0
Glucerna					
Shake Creamy Chocolate Delight	1 bottle (8 oz)	200	27	6	5
Shake Homemade Vanilla	1 bottle (8 oz)	200	26	6	5
Slim-Fast					
Optima Ready-To-Drink Creamy Milk Chocolate	1 can (11 oz)	190	25	18	5
NUTS MIXED *(see also individual names)*					
dry roasted w/ peanuts salted	¼ cup	203	9	–	3
dry roasted w/ peanuts w/o salt	¼ cup	203	9	–	3
oil roasted w/o peanuts salted	¼ cup	221	8	2	2
oil roasted w/o peanuts w/o salt	¼ cup	221	8	–	2
Emily's					
Roasted Mixed Nuts	¼ cup (1.3 oz)	230	8	2	2
Good Sense					
Deluxe Mix	¼ cup	180	8	2	2
Organic Trails					
Tamari Roasted Nuts & Seeds	¼ cup	190	10	1	5
Peanut Better					
Mixed Nut Butter Creamy & Crunchy	2 tbsp	190	5	1	3
Planters					
Mixed	30 nuts (1 oz)	170	6	1	2
NUT-rition Energy Mix	¼ cup	180	10	4	3
NUT-rition Heart Healthy Mix	¼ cup	170	5	1	3
True North					
Clusters Pecan Almond Peanut	8 (1 oz)	170	13	5	2
OCA					
Frieda's					
Oca	½ cup	70	15	0	1
OCTOPUS					
dried boiled	3 oz	144	4	0	0
fresh steamed	3 oz	139	4	0	0
smoked	1 oz	40	1	0	0

FOOD	PORTION	CALS	CARB	SUGAR	FIBER
TAKE-OUT					
ensalada de pulpo	1 cup	299	10	4	2
OIL					
almond	1 cup	1927	0	0	0
almond	1 tbsp	120	0	0	0
apricot kernel	1 cup	1927	0	0	0
apricot kernel	1 tbsp	120	0	0	0
avocado	1 cup	1927	0	0	0
avocado	1 tbsp	124	0	0	0
babassu palm	1 tbsp	120	0	0	0
butter oil	1 cup	1795	0	0	0
butter oil	1 tbsp	112	0	0	0
canola	1 cup	1927	0	0	0
canola	1 tbsp	124	0	0	0
coconut	1 tbsp	117	0	0	0
corn	1 cup	1927	0	0	0
corn	1 tbsp	120	0	0	0
cottonseed	1 cup	1927	0	0	0
cottonseed	1 tbsp	120	0	0	0
cupu assu	1 tbsp	120	0	0	0
garlic oil	1 tbsp	150	0	0	0
grapeseed	1 tbsp	120	0	0	0
hazelnut	1 cup	1927	0	0	0
hazelnut	1 tbsp	120	0	0	0
mustard	1 cup	1927	0	0	0
mustard	1 tbsp	124	0	0	0
oat	1 tbsp	120	0	0	0
olive	1 cup	1909	0	0	0
olive	1 tbsp	119	0	0	0
palm	1 cup	1927	0	0	0
palm	1 tbsp	120	0	0	0
palm kernel	1 cup	1879	0	0	0
palm kernel	1 tbsp	117	0	0	0
peanut	1 cup	1909	0	0	0
peanut	1 tbsp	119	0	0	0
peppermint	1 tsp	42	0	0	0
poppyseed	1 tbsp	120	0	0	0
pumpkin seed	1 oz	217	0	0	0
rice bran	1 tbsp	120	0	0	0
safflower	1 cup	1927	0	0	0

FOOD	PORTION	CALS	CARB	SUGAR	FIBER
safflower	1 tbsp	120	0	0	0
sesame	1 tbsp	120	0	0	0
sheanut	1 tbsp	120	0	0	0
soybean	1 cup	1927	0	0	0
soybean	1 tbsp	120	0	0	0
sunflower	1 cup	1927	0	0	0
sunflower	1 tbsp	120	0	0	0
teaseed	1 tbsp	120	0	0	0
tomatoseed	1 tbsp	120	0	0	0
vegetable	1 cup	1927	0	0	0
vegetable	1 tbsp	120	0	0	0
walnut	1 cup	1927	0	0	0
walnut	1 tbsp	120	0	0	0
wheat germ	1 tbsp	120	0	0	0
Asoyia					
Soybean Ultra Low Lin	1 tbsp	129	0	0	0
Bell Plantation					
Extra Virgin Roasted Peanut	1 tbsp	120	0	0	0
Botticelli					
Olive	1 tbsp	120	0	0	0
Bragg					
Olive Extra Virgin	1 tbsp	120	2	2	0
Carapelli					
Grapeseed	1 tbsp	120	0	0	0
Olive Extra Virgin	1 tbsp	120	0	0	0
Crisco					
Cooking Spray Original	⅓ sec spray	0	0	0	0
Frying Oil Blend	1 tbsp	130	0	0	0
Light Olive	1 tbsp	120	0	0	0
Peanut	1 tbsp	120	0	0	0
Pure Vegetable	1 tbsp	120	0	0	0
Eden					
Olive Extra Virgin	1 tbsp	120	0	0	0
Organic Safflower	1 tbsp	120	0	0	0
Organic Soybean	1 tbsp	120	0	0	0
Toasted Sesame	1 tbsp	120	0	0	0
Gourme Mist					
Extra Virgin Olive Cold Pressed	1 sec spray	4	0	0	0
Hollywood					
Canola Enriched	1 tbsp	120	0	0	0

FOOD	PORTION	CALS	CARB	SUGAR	FIBER
Peanut Enriched Gold	1 tbsp	120	0	0	0
Safflower Expeller Pressed	1 tbsp	120	0	0	0
House Of Tsang					
Mongolian Fire	1 tsp	45	0	0	0
Wok Oil	1 tbsp	130	0	0	0
Iowa Natural					
Soybean 1% Linolenic	1 tbsp	129	0	0	0
Kinloch Plantation					
100% Virgin Pecan	1 tbsp	130	0	0	0
Living Harvest					
Organic Hemp Oil	2 tbsp	250	0	0	0
Lucini					
Extra Virgin Premium Select	1 tbsp (0.5 oz)	120	0	0	0
Manitoba Harvest					
Hemp Seed Oil	1 tbsp	126	0	0	0
Martinis					
Kalamata Olive Extra Virgin Cold Pressed	1 tbsp (0.5 oz)	120	0	0	0
Mazola					
Corn	1 tbsp	120	0	0	0
No Stick Spray	⅓ sec spray	0	0	0	0
Right Blend	1 tbsp	120	0	0	0
Vegetable	1 tbsp	120	0	0	0
Monini					
Grapeseed	1 tbsp (0.5 oz)	120	0	0	0
Nutiva					
Organic Coconut Extra Virgin	1 tbsp	120	0	0	0
Organic Hemp Cold Pressed	1 tbsp	120	0	0	0
Nutrium					
Soybean Low Linolenic	1 tbsp	129	0	0	0
Olivo					
Spray Olive Oil 100% Extra Virgin	⅓ sec spray	0	0	0	0
Orville Redenbacher's					
Popping & Topping	1 tbsp	120	0	0	0
Pam					
Organic Canola	⅓ second spray	0	0	0	0
Robert Rothchild Farm					
Basil Infused	1 tbsp	120	0	0	0

FOOD	PORTION	CALS	CARB	SUGAR	FIBER
Smart Balance					
Omega Oil	1 tbsp	120	0	0	0
Tree Of Life					
Almond Expeller Pressed	1 tbsp (0.5 oz)	120	0	0	0
Avocado Expeller Pressed	1 tbsp (0.5 oz)	120	0	0	0
Macadamia Nut Expeller Pressed	1 tbsp (0.5 oz)	120	0	0	0
Organic Coconut Expeller Pressed	1 tbsp	120	0	0	0
Walnut Expeller Pressed	1 tbsp (0.5 oz)	120	0	0	0
Vistive					
Soybean Low Linolenic	1 tbsp	129	0	0	0
Wesson					
Canola	1 tbsp	120	0	0	0
OKRA					
CANNED					
pickled	6 pods (2.3 oz)	18	4	1	2
Allens					
Cut	½ cup	30	6	1	3
Glory					
Cut	½ cup	25	6	2	2
McIlhenny					
Spicy Pickled	1 oz	10	2	1	1
Trappey's					
Creole Gumbo	½ cup	35	6	1	3
FRESH					
cooked w/ salt	8 pods	19	4	2	2
luffa chinese okra cooked	1 cup	39	8	4	4
sliced cooked w/ salt	½ cup	18	4	2	2
FROZEN					
McKenzie's					
Cut	1 serv (3 oz)	25	5	1	3
TAKE-OUT					
batter dipped fried	10 pieces (2.6 oz)	142	12	3	2
OLIVES					
black	2 med (0.3 oz)	8	tr	0	tr
greek	1 (0.5 oz)	16	1	0	tr
green	1 sm (0.2 oz)	8	tr	tr	tr

FOOD	PORTION	CALS	CARB	SUGAR	FIBER
green	2 med (0.2 oz)	10	tr	tr	tr
green	2 lg (0.3 oz)	11	tr	tr	tr
green	2 extra lg (0.5 oz)	19	1	tr	tr
green chopped	¼ cup (1.2 oz)	48	1	tr	1
green olive tapenade	1 tbsp	25	1	1	0
green stuffed	¼ cup (1.3 oz)	47	1	tr	1
green stuffed	2 sm (0.2 oz)	9	tr	tr	tr
green stuffed	2 med (0.3 oz)	10	tr	tr	tr
green stuffed	2 lg (0.3 oz)	12	tr	tr	tr
ripe	2 sm (0.2 oz)	7	tr	0	tr
ripe	2 lg (0.3 oz)	10	1	0	tr
ripe	2 extra lg (0.4 oz)	12	1	0	tr
ripe sliced	¼ cup (1.2 oz)	35	2	0	1
spanish stuffed	5 (0.5 oz)	15	1	0	0
Peloponnese					
Amfissa	3	45	1	0	0
Ionian Green	3	25	1	0	0
Kalamata Pitted	5	45	1	0	0
Kalamata Spread	1 tsp	15	0	0	0
ONION					
CANNED					
cocktail	½ cup	41	9	4	2
Boar's Head					
Sweet Vidalia In Sauce	1 tbsp	10	2	2	0
French's					
Original French Fried	2 tbsp	45	3	0	0
DRIED					
flakes	1 tbsp	17	4	2	1
powder	1 tsp	7	2	1	tr
Bob's Red Mill					
Minced	1 tbsp	40	8	0	1
FRESH					
cooked w/o salt	1 sm (2 oz)	26	6	3	1
cooked w/o salt	1 med (3.3 oz)	41	10	4	1
cooked w/o salt	1 lg (4.5 oz)	56	13	6	2
cooked w/o salt chopped	1 tbsp	7	2	1	tr
raw chopped	1 tbsp	4	1	tr	tr
raw chopped	½ cup	32	7	3	1

FOOD	PORTION	CALS	CARB	SUGAR	FIBER
raw slice	1 (0.5 oz)	6	1	1	tr
raw sliced	½ cup	23	5	2	1
scallions raw	1 med (0.5 oz)	5	1	tr	tr
scallions raw chopped	¼ cup	8	2	1	1
sweet whole raw	1 (11.6 oz)	106	25	17	3
whole raw	1 sm (2.5 oz)	28	7	3	1
whole raw	1 med (4 oz)	44	10	5	2
whole raw	1 lg (5.3 oz)	60	14	6	3
Arrowfarms					
Cipoline	2 (1.1 oz)	20	4	2	5
Bland Farms					
Vidalia Sweet	1 (5 oz)	60	14	5	3
Blue Ribbon					
Yellow	1 med (5.2 oz)	60	14	9	3
Earthbound Farm					
Organic Green Onions	¼ cup	10	2	1	1
Organic Red	1 med (5.2 oz)	60	14	9	3
Frieda's					
Cipoline	3 (3 oz)	30	7	5	2
Maui	⅓ cup (1.1 oz)	10	3	2	1
Pearl	⅔ cup (3 oz)	30	7	5	2
Shallots	1 tbsp (1 oz)	20	5	1	0
Ocean Mist					
Green Onions Chopped	¼ cup	10	2	1	1
OsoSweet					
Onion	1 med (5 oz)	60	14	9	3
FROZEN					
Alexia					
Onion Rings	6 (3 oz)	230	28	3	4
C&W					
Petite Whole	⅔ cup (3 oz)	30	6	3	tr
Farm Rich					
Petals Breaded + Sauce	10 (3 oz)	200	22	3	1
Ian's					
Rings & Strings	5–9 pieces (2.5 oz)	152	16	1	1
TAKE-OUT					
creamed	1 cup	187	22	10	2
fried	½ cup	57	3	tr	1

FOOD	PORTION	CALS	CARB	SUGAR	FIBER
OPOSSUM					
roasted	3 oz	188	0	0	0
ORANGE					
FRESH					
california valencia	1 (4.2 oz)	59	14	–	3
california valencia sections	½ cup (3.2 oz)	44	11	–	2
florida	1 (5.3 oz)	69	17	14	4
florida sections	½ cup (3.2 oz)	43	11	8	2
navel	1 (4.9 oz)	69	18	12	3
navel sections	1 cup (5.8 oz)	81	21	14	4
peel	1 tbsp (0.2 oz)	3	1	tr	1
Darling					
Mandarine	1 med (3.8 oz)	50	13	9	3
Frieda's					
Cara Cara	1 med (5 oz)	70	16	12	3
Mandarin Delite	1 cup (5 oz)	60	16	12	3
Mandarin Page	1 cup (5 oz)	60	12	12	3
Mandarin Pixie	1 cup (5 oz)	60	16	12	3
Mandarin Satsuma	1 (5 oz)	60	16	12	3
Melogold	½ (6 oz)	50	13	10	2
Seville	1 (3 oz)	40	10	8	2
ORANGE JUICE					
chilled	1 cup (8.7 oz)	112	26	21	1
fresh	1 cup (8.7 oz)	112	26	21	1
Crystal Light					
Sunrise Sunrise Sugar Free Mix as prep	1 serv	5	0	0	0
Florida's Natural					
Calcium & Vitamin D	8 oz	110	26	22	0
Hood					
100% Juice	1 cup	120	30	30	0
Land O Lakes					
Juice	1 cup (8 oz)	110	25	23	0
Juice w/ Calcium	1 cup (8 oz)	120	29	28	0
NutraBalance					
Fortified	1 pkg (4 oz)	60	17	–	4
Odwalla					
100% Juice	8 oz	110	25	24	0

FOOD	PORTION	CALS	CARB	SUGAR	FIBER
Organic Valley					
W/ Calcium	1 cup	110	26	26	0
Tang					
Orange Drink as prep	1 serv	90	23	23	0
Sugar Free Orange as prep	1 serv (8 oz)	5	0	0	0
Tree Ripe					
100% Juice + Calcium & Vitamins	8 oz	120	29	28	0
Organic 100% Juice	6 oz	90	22	21	0
Tropicana					
Antioxidant Advantage	8 oz	110	26	22	0
Calcium + Vitamin D	8 oz	110	26	22	0
Fiber	8 oz	120	29	22	3
Healthy Heart	8 oz	120	26	22	0
Healthy Kids	8 oz	110	26	22	0
Light 'n Healthy w/ Calcium	8 oz	50	13	10	0
Light 'n Healthy w/ Pulp	8 oz	50	13	10	0
No Pulp	8 oz	110	26	22	0
Orangeade	8 oz	111	33	30	0
Organic	8 oz	120	28	22	0
Uncle Matt's					
Organic 100% Juice Pulp Free	8 oz	110	26	22	0
Organic 100% Juice w/ Pulp	8 oz	110	26	22	0
TAKE-OUT					
orange julius	1 cup (9.2 oz)	212	39	35	tr

OREGANO

crumbled	1 tsp	3	1	tr	tr
ground	1 tsp	6	1	tr	1

ORGAN MEATS *(see BRAINS, GIBLETS, GIZZARDS, HEART, KIDNEY, LIVER, SWEETBREAD)*

OSTRICH

cooked	4 oz	195	0	0	0
cooked diced	1 cup (4.7 oz)	215	0	0	0
Natural Frontier Foods					
Filets	1 (4 oz)	130	0	0	0
Ground Lean	4 oz	130	0	0	0

OYSTERS

canned eastern	1 cup	112	6	0	0

FOOD	PORTION	CALS	CARB	SUGAR	FIBER
eastern sauteed	6 med	76	3	0	0
smoked	6	33	2	0	0
Brunswick					
Smoked	1 can (3 oz)	140	7	0	1
Bumble Bee					
Smoked	¼ cup	120	6	0	0
Whole	¼ cup	70	3	0	0
Polar					
Whole	¼ cup	70	4	0	0
Whole Smoked	⅓ cup	95	4	0	0
TAKE-OUT					
fritter	1 (1.4 oz)	121	12	tr	tr
oysters rockefeller	1 cup	302	22	2	4
stew	1 cup	208	11	9	0
PANCAKE/WAFFLE SYRUP					
lite	¼ cup	98	27	20	0
pancake syrup	1 pkg (2 oz)	156	41	38	0
pancake syrup	¼ cup	209	55	50	0
Aunt Jemina					
Butter Lite	¼ cup (2.1 oz)	100	26	25	1
Hungry Jack					
Lite	¼ cup	100	24	23	0
Original	¼ cup	210	52	31	0
Naturally Fresh					
Maple Mountain Sugar Free	2 tbsp	0	0	0	0
Wholesome Sweeteners					
Organic	¼ cup	240	60	60	0
PANCAKES					
FROZEN					
Aunt Jemima					
Buttermilk	3 (3 oz)	210	40	8	2
Buttermilk Low Fat	3 (3 oz)	210	40	7	2
Whole Grain	3 (3 oz)	230	38	5	3
Dr. Praeger's					
Broccoli	1 (2 oz)	80	9	1	2
Potato	1 (2.2 oz)	100	13	1	3
Eggo					
Buttermilk	3	280	44	11	1
Minis	11	260	42	10	1

FOOD	PORTION	CALS	CARB	SUGAR	FIBER
Golden					
Potato Latkes	1 (1.3 oz)	70	10	2	1
Ian's					
Blueberry	1 (1.3 oz)	100	19	7	1
Pancake	1 (1.3 oz)	100	19	7	1
Inland Valley					
Potato	1 (2 oz)	120	12	tr	2
Jimmy Dean					
Breakfast Bowls Pancake & Sausage Links	1 pkg	710	93	34	3
Griddle Cake Sandwich Sausage Egg & Cheese	1 (4 oz)	370	32	13	1
Original Pancakes & Sausage On A Stick	1 (2.5 oz)	110	21	8	0
McCain					
Homestyle BabyCakes	4 pieces (2.6 oz)	150	17	0	2
Pillsbury					
Blueberry	3 (4 oz)	230	46	14	2
Buttermilk	3 (4 oz)	240	47	13	2
Original	3 (4 oz)	250	49	14	2
Ratner's					
Potato Latkes	1 (1.5 oz)	80	15	tr	tr
MIX					
Arrowhead Mills					
Gluten Free Pancake & Waffle as prep	2 (5 in)	240	42	1	0
Batter Blaster					
Organic Original Pancake & Waffle Batter not prep	¼ cup (2 oz)	112	23	7	2
Don's Chuck Wagon					
Buckwheat Mix not prep	⅓ cup	160	33	2	1
Hodgson Mill					
Buckwheat not prep	⅓ cup	140	28	1	3
Whole Wheat Buttermilk not prep	⅓ cup	120	28	2	4
Hungry Jack					
Buttermilk Pancake & Waffle not prep	⅓ cup	150	31	7	tr
Easy Pack Blueberry not prep	½ cup	200	40	12	1

FOOD	PORTION	CALS	CARB	SUGAR	FIBER
Pancake & Waffle Extra Light & Fluffy not prep	⅓ cup	150	30	5	tr
Potato not prep	2 tbsp	70	15	0	1
King Arthur					
Multi-Grain Buttermilk not prep	6 tbsp	160	31	2	5
TAKE-OUT					
buckwheat	1 (7 in)	142	19	4	2
norwegian lefse	1 (9 in) (2.7 oz)	163	27	2	2
plain	1 (7 in)	183	35	10	1
potato	1 (1.3 oz)	70	8	tr	1
whole wheat	1 (7 in)	183	23	5	3

PANCREAS *(see SWEETBREAD)*

PANINI *(see SANDWICHES)*

PAPAYA

FOOD	PORTION	CALS	CARB	SUGAR	FIBER
canned in syrup	½ cup (2.3 oz)	50	13	11	1
dried	1 strip (0.8 oz)	59	15	9	3
fresh	1 sm (5.3 oz)	59	15	9	3
fresh	1 lg (13.3 oz)	148	37	22	7
fresh cubed	1 cup (4.9 oz)	55	14	8	3
green cooked	½ cup (2.3 oz)	18	5	3	1
Frieda's					
Mexican	1 cup (5 oz)	50	14	8	3

PAPAYA JUICE

FOOD	PORTION	CALS	CARB	SUGAR	FIBER
nectar	1 cup (8.8 oz)	142	36	35	2
Lakewood					
Red	8 oz	80	20	16	2
Yellow	8 oz	105	26	22	2
Langers					
Papaya Delight 100% Juice	8 oz	130	32	29	1

PAPRIKA

FOOD	PORTION	CALS	CARB	SUGAR	FIBER
dried	1 tsp	1	tr	0	tr
Bob's Red Mill					
Hungarian	½ tsp	11	2	0	1

PARSLEY

FOOD	PORTION	CALS	CARB	SUGAR	FIBER
dried	1 tbsp	4	1	tr	1

FOOD	PORTION	CALS	CARB	SUGAR	FIBER
freeze dried	1 tbsp	1	tr	–	tr
fresh chopped	1 tbsp	1	tr	tr	tr
fresh chopped	¼ cup	5	1	tr	1
fresh sprigs	5 (1.8 oz)	18	3	tr	2
Frieda's					
Parsley Root	⅔ cup	10	2	0	1

PARSNIPS

fresh sliced cooked w/o salt	½ cup (2.7 oz)	55	13	4	3
whole cooked	1 (5.6 oz)	114	27	8	6
Frieda's					
Sliced	1 cup	100	24	6	7
TAKE-OUT					
creamed	1 cup (8 oz)	237	31	10	5

PASSION FRUIT

fresh	1 (0.6 oz)	17	4	2	2
fresh cut up	½ cup (4.1 oz)	114	28	13	12

PASSION FRUIT JUICE

nectar	1 cup (8.8 oz)	168	44	43	tr
yellow lilikoi	1 cup (8.7 oz)	138	35	34	1

PASTA *(see also NOODLES, PASTA DINNERS, PASTA SALAD)*

DRY

corn cooked	1 cup (4.9 oz)	176	39	–	7
elbows cooked	1 cup (4.9 oz)	197	40	–	2
shells small cooked	1 cup (4 oz)	162	33	–	2
spaghetti cooked	1 cup (4.9 oz)	197	40	–	2
spirals cooked	1 cup (4.7 oz)	189	38	–	2
vegetable cooked	1 cup (4.7 oz)	172	36	–	6
whole wheat all shapes cooked	1 cup	174	37	–	4
Amish Natural					
Fettuccine	2 oz	201	41	5	2
Fettuccine Fiber Rich	2 oz	200	42	3	11
Fettuccine Whole Wheat	2 oz	210	41	2	7
Annie Chun's					
Soba Noodles	2 oz	200	39	1	3
Barilla					
Plus Rotini not prep	2 oz	210	38	2	4
DeBoles					
Angel Hair Rice Pasta	¼ pkg (2 oz)	210	46	0	tr

FOOD	PORTION	CALS	CARB	SUGAR	FIBER
Elbow Corn Pasta Wheat Free	1/6 pkg (2 oz)	200	43	0	5
Fettuccine	1/4 pkg (2 oz)	210	41	2	1
Organic Angel Hair Whole Wheat	1/4 pkg (2 oz)	210	42	2	5
Organic Eggless Ribbon	1 cup (2 oz)	210	43	2	1
Organic Fettucine Spinach	1/4 pkg (2 oz)	210	43	1	3
Organic Lasagna	1/4 pkg (2.5 oz)	260	54	2	1
Organic Rigatoni Whole Wheat	1 cup (2 oz)	210	42	2	5
Rigatoni	1/4 pkg (2 oz)	210	41	2	1
DeCecco					
Spaghetti w/ Spinach	1/8 pkg (2 oz)	200	41	1	2
Dreamfields					
Lasagna not prep	2 pieces (2 oz)	190	42	1	5
Rotini not prep	2/3 cup (2 oz)	190	42	1	5
Eden					
Bifun Pasta not prep	2 oz	200	44	0	0
Harusame Pasta not prep	2 oz	190	47	0	0
Kudzu	2 oz	200	48	0	2
Organic Gemelli Spelt & Buckwheat not prep	1/2 cup (2 oz)	210	41	2	4
Organic Ribbons Artichoke not prep	1/2 cup (2 oz)	210	40	1	2
Organic Rigatoni Kamut & Buckwheat not prep	1/2 cup (2 oz)	200	39	3	5
Organic Spaghetti 100% Whole Wheat not prep	2 oz	210	40	2	6
Organic Spirals Kamut Vegetable not prep	1/2 cup (2 oz)	210	40	3	6
Organic Spirals Flax Rice not prep	1/2 cup (2 oz)	200	40	0	4
Organic Spirals Rye not prep	1/2 cup (2 oz)	200	44	1	8
Organic Spirals Spinach not prep	1/2 cup (2 oz)	210	41	2	5
Organic Udon not prep	1/4 pkg	200	38	1	3
Organic Udon Spelt not prep	1/4 pkg	200	39	tr	2
Organic Vegetable Alphabets not prep	1/2 cup (2 oz)	210	40	1	4
Organic Vegetable Shells not prep	1/2 cup (2 oz)	210	40	1	4

FOOD	PORTION	CALS	CARB	SUGAR	FIBER
Organic Ziti Rigati Spelt not prep	½ cup (2 oz)	210	41	1	5
Soba Japanese 100% Buckwheat not prep	2 oz	200	43	2	3
Soba Japanese Lotus Root not prep	2 oz	190	37	2	4
Soba Japanese Mugwort not prep	2 oz	190	37	2	2
Soba Japanese Wild Yam not prep	2 oz	190	37	2	2
Udon Japanese Brown Rice not prep	2 oz	190	38	2	2
Udon Japanese not prep	2 oz	190	37	5	3
Gillian's					
Penne Brown Rice Pasta Wheat Gluten Egg Free	2 oz	200	43	0	2
Hodgson Mill					
Lasagne Whole Wheat not prep	2 oz	190	41	0	6
Organic Fettuccine Whole Wheat w/ Milled Flax Seed not prep	2 oz	200	40	0	6
Pasta Ribbons Whole Wheat not prep	2 oz	190	34	0	5
Spaghetti Whole Wheat not prep	2 oz	190	41	0	6
Veggie Bows not prep	2 oz	200	41	0	1
Wagon Wheels Veggie not prep	2 oz	200	41	0	1
LifeStream					
Organic All Shapes	2 oz	208	36	3	8
Lundberg					
Organic Spaghetti Brown Rice	2 oz	210	44	3	3
Maddy's					
Gluten Free not prep	4 oz	310	66	4	2
Mueller's					
Elbow Macaroni not prep	½ cup	210	41	2	2
Multi Grain Rotini not prep	1 cup (2 oz)	190	40	4	5
Notta Pasta					
Rice Pasta All Shapes	2 oz	200	48	0	2
Ronzoni					
Elbows not prep	½ cup (2 oz)	210	42	2	2

FOOD	PORTION	CALS	CARB	SUGAR	FIBER
Healthy Harvest Multigrain Spaghetti	½ pkg (2 oz)	190	40	1	5
Healthy Harvest Whole Wheat Blend Spaghetti	½ pkg (2 oz)	180	42	1	6
Smart Pasta not prep	2 oz	180	43	1	8
Wacky Mac					
Veggie All Shapes	2 oz	200	41	0	1
REFRIGERATED					
Buitoni					
Ravioli Four Cheese 100% Whole Wheat	1¼ cups	320	42	2	5
Tortellini Spinach Cheese	1 cup	320	49	4	3
Tortelloni Chicken & Prosciutto	1 cup	320	46	2	2
Tortelloni Mozzarella & Herb	1 cup	330	47	3	2
Tortelloni Portabello Mushroom & Cheese	1 cup	290	49	3	3
Pasta Prima					
Ravioli Spinach & Mozzarella	1 cup	200	29	0	4
Ravioli Sun Dried Tomato & Mozzarella	1 cup	200	29	1	3
PASTA DINNERS *(see also PASTA SALAD)*					
CANNED					
Chef Boyardee					
99% Fat Free Beef Ravioli	1 cup	170	33	6	2
Beef Ravioli	1 cup	240	35	5	3
Beefaroni	1 cup	260	33	5	3
Mini Ravioli	1 cup	250	35	5	3
Mini-Bites Spaghetti & Meatballs	1 cup	250	30	7	3
Spaghetti & Meat Balls	1 cup (9 oz)	270	32	8	2
SpaghettiOs					
A to Z's w/ Meatballs	1 cup	260	33	12	3
A to Z's w/ Sliced Franks	1 cup	230	32	9	2
Mini Beef Ravioli In Meat Sauce	1 cup	260	43	14	5
Pasta	1 cup	180	37	13	3
Plus Calcium	1 cup	170	35	13	3
FROZEN					
4Real					
Mac+Cheese	1 pkg (8 oz)	230	33	1	2
Meat Sauce w/ Beef Ravioli	1 pkg (8 oz)	190	32	5	2

FOOD	PORTION	CALS	CARB	SUGAR	FIBER
Spaghetti Rings	1 pkg (8 oz)	180	37	5	2
Bertolli					
Meatballs Pomodoro & Penne	1 serv (12 oz)	600	54	8	6
Birds Eye					
Steamfresh Meals For Two Shrimp Alfredo	½ pkg (11.9 oz)	420	55	7	4
Steamfresh Meals For Two Shrimp Pasta Primavera	½ pkg (11.9 oz)	450	39	6	3
Blue Horizon Organic					
Penne Alfredo w/ Shrimp	½ pkg (9.9 oz)	430	39	0	2
Penne Alla Vodka w/ Shrimp	½ pkg (9.9 oz)	270	38	0	3
Pesto Farfalle w/ Shrimp	½ pkg (9.9 oz)	280	38	0	3
Scampi Rotini w/ Shrimp	½ pkg (9.9 oz)	410	44	0	4
Boca					
Lasagna Meatless	1 pkg (9.4 oz)	290	42	8	5
Cedarlane					
Zone Chicken & Vegetables Pasta & Ginger	1 pkg (10 oz)	340	35	2	3
Zone Lasagna Vegetable	1 pkg (10.9 oz)	310	33	12	5
Celentano					
Cheese Ravioli	4 (4.3 oz)	230	36	0	2
Contessa					
Ravioli Portobello	6 (6.7 oz)	360	39	4	2
Glory					
Macaroni & Cheese	1 pkg	480	47	10	1
Glutino					
Gluten Free Duo Mushroom Penne	1 pkg (10.5 oz)	380	73	1	5
Gluten Free Macaroni & Cheese	1 pkg (8.8 oz)	430	44	5	2
Gluten Free Penne Alfredo	1 pkg (9.1 oz)	340	48	2	3
Golden Cuisine					
Cheese Manicotti	1 pkg	360	43	11	6
Spaghetti & Meatballs	1 pkg	490	51	16	12
Tuna Casserole	1 pkg	386	53	7	8
Green Giant					
Skillet Meal Chicken & Cheesy Pasta as prep	1¼ cups	270	42	7	4
Healthy Choice					
Creamy Garlic Shrimp w/ Bow Tie Pasta	1 pkg (11.5 oz)	280	44	16	5

FOOD	PORTION	CALS	CARB	SUGAR	FIBER
Fettuccini Alfredo Chicken	1 pkg	290	32	3	3
Lasagna Bake	1 pkg	270	38	13	4
Macaroni & Cheese	1 pkg	290	44	5	5
Manicotti	1 pkg	280	44	16	4
Rigatoni w/ Broccoli & Chicken	1 pkg	270	29	4	5
Spaghetti w/ Meat Sauce	1 pkg	310	48	8	7
Helen's Kitchen					
Farfalle & Basil Pasta w/ Tofu Steaks	1 pkg (9 oz)	320	70	5	5
Joy Of Cooking					
Al Dente Cavatappi Bolognese	1 cup (7.7 oz)	280	29	5	2
Best Loved Macaroni & Cheese	1 cup (5.4 oz)	280	36	4	1
Cheese Ravioli Pomodoro	1 cup (7.7 oz)	250	34	5	3
Creamy Fettuccine Carbonara	1 cup (7.5 oz)	330	31	3	3
Kashi					
Chicken Pasta Pomodoro	1 pkg (10 oz)	280	38	5	6
Kid Cuisine					
Cheese Blaster Mac & Cheese	1 meal	380	58	11	5
Twist & Twirl Spaghetti w/ Mini Meatballs	1 meal	460	66	23	6
Marie Callender's					
Meat Lasagna	1 cup	240	24	9	2
Michelina's					
Lasagna w/ Meat Sauce	1 pkg (9 oz)	340	40	6	3
Milton's					
Lasagna Vegetable w/ Multi-Grain Pasta	1 cup (8 oz)	340	30	7	5
Mon Cuisine					
Vegetarian Spaghetti & Meatballs	1 pkg (10 oz)	360	54	8	9
Moosewood					
Organic Vegetarian Broccoli & Pasta Parmesan	1 pkg (10 oz)	380	52	7	4
Organic Vegetarian Farfalle & Spinach Pesto Sauce	1 pkg (10 oz)	370	56	6	4
Organic Vegetarian Spicy Penne Puttanesca	1 pkg (10 oz)	300	45	5	2
New York Ravioli					
Jolie Kid Shapes Ravioli Cheese	1 cup	330	47	5	4

FOOD	PORTION	CALS	CARB	SUGAR	FIBER
Jolie Kid Shapes Ravioli Cheese & Broccoli	1 cup	340	53	2	2
Ravioli Four Cheese	1 cup	360	58	2	2
Ravioli Tomato Basil & Mozzarella	1 cup	340	64	3	2
Organic Bistro					
Pasta Puttanesca	1 pkg (12.15 oz)	330	57	6	9
Organic Classics					
Cajun Chicken Tetrazzine w/ Penne Pasta	1 pkg (10 oz)	370	43	4	3
Chicken Cacciatore w/ Penne Pasta	1 pkg (10 oz)	270	37	5	3
Macaroni & Meat Sauce	1 pkg (10 oz)	340	49	9	3
Plum Organics					
Bowtie Pasta	1 pkg (6.9 oz)	230	37	2	3
Cheese Filled Spinach Tortellini	1 pkg (6.9 oz)	190	37	6	3
Putney Pasta					
Tortellini Tri-Color Three Cheese	1 cup	340	51	–	1
Seeds Of Change					
Chicken Fettuccine Alfredo	1 pkg (10 oz)	340	40	5	3
Lasagna Creamy Spinach	1 pkg (11 oz)	370	36	4	7
Lasagna Vegetable	1 pkg (11 oz)	310	41	9	5
Penne Marinara	1 pkg (11 oz)	290	44	11	5
South Beach					
Penne & Chicken In Roasted Red Pepper Sauce w/ Broccoli	1 pkg	290	26	5	8
Stouffer's					
Cheesy Spaghetti Bake	1 pkg (12 oz)	460	39	6	4
Chicken Parmigiana	1 pkg (13.13 oz)	460	56	9	4
Escalloped Chicken & Noodles	1 pkg (8 oz)	330	28	4	2
Homestyle Chicken & Noodles	1 pkg (12 oz)	340	33	10	3
Italian Sausage Stuffed Rigatoni	1 pkg (9.13 oz)	380	46	8	2
Lasagna Bake w/ Meat Sauce	1 pkg (11.5 oz)	380	47	10	5
Lasagna Vegetable	1 pkg (10.5 oz)	390	40	9	4
Macaroni & Beef	1 pkg (11.5 oz)	330	38	12	4
Macaroni & Cheese	1 cup (6 oz)	350	34	2	2
Manicotti Cheese	1 pkg (9 oz)	360	41	8	2

FOOD	PORTION	CALS	CARB	SUGAR	FIBER
Shrimp Scampi	1 pkg (14 oz)	410	57	5	6
Tuna Noodle Casserole	1 pkg (10 oz)	350	35	8	2
Turkey Tettrazini	1 pkg (10 oz)	380	32	6	1
Taste Above					
Meatless Thai Peanut Coconut Sauce w/ Veggie Chicken & Vermicelli	1 pkg (10 oz)	320	22	3	8
Meatless Tuscan Marinara Sauce w/ Veggie Chicken & Penne Pasta	1 pkg (10 oz)	320	22	3	8
Weight Watchers					
Smart Ones Lasagna w/ Meat Sauce	1 pkg (10.5 oz)	300	43	8	5
Yves					
Meatless Lasagna	1 pkg (10.5 oz)	300	51	9	4
MIX					
A Taste Of Thai					
Coconut Ginger	1 cup	280	5	2	1
Pad Thai For Two	½ pkg	345	89	8	4
Peanut Noodles as prep	1 cup	330	53	11	1
Red Curry Noodles as prep	1 cup	280	51	6	2
Carapelli					
Penne Alfredo as prep	1 cup	240	47	6	4
Spirals Creamy Tomato as prep	1 cup	240	49	8	4
DeBoles					
Organic Macaroni & Cheese Whole Wheat as prep	1 cup	410	60	6	9
Pasta & Cheese as prep	1 cup	420	60	5	6
Rice Shells & Cheddar as prep	½ cup	260	57	0	1
Hamburger Helper					
Cheesy Jambalaya as prep	1 cup	330	30	2	1
Knorr					
Pasta & Sauce Jalapeno Jack as prep	1 cup	230	45	4	2
Pasta Sides w/ Whole Grains Alfredo as prep	⅔ cup	300	42	2	4
Kraft					
Bistro Deluxe Sundried Tomato Parmesan as prep	1 cup	300	40	3	3

FOOD	PORTION	CALS	CARB	SUGAR	FIBER
La Bella Vita					
Chicken & Lemon Borsellini as prep	1 cup	270	39	1	2
Near East					
Basil & Herb as prep	1 cup	240	42	1	3
Spicy Tomato as prep	1 cup	230	38	2	3
Pasta Roni					
Angel Hair w/ Herbs as prep	1 cup	310	41	6	2
Chicken as prep	1 cup	300	39	4	2
Chicken Quesadilla as prep	1 cup	310	40	6	2
Fettuccine Alfredo as prep	1 cup	450	47	6	2
Nature's Way Mushrooms In Cream Sauce as prep	1 cup	280	39	8	2
Sour Cream & Chives as prep	1 cup	310	38	4	2
Stroganoff as prep	1 cup	350	47	7	2
Road's End Organics					
Mac & Cheese Dairy Free Gluten Free as prep	1 cup	310	63	0	5
Shells & Cheese as prep	1 cup	330	66	5	7
REFRIGERATED					
Country Crock					
Elbow Macaroni & Cheese	1 cup (8 oz)	370	40	6	1
Four Cheese Pasta	1 cup (8 oz)	380	41	7	2
SHELF-STABLE					
Allergaroo					
Gluten Free Spaghetti	1 pkg (8 oz)	220	49	9	3
Gluten Free Spyglass Noodles	1 pkg (8 oz)	230	49	9	3
Betty Crocker					
Bowl Appetit! Cheddar Broccoli Pasta	1 bowl (2.8 oz)	330	49	7	2
Bowl Appetit! Garlic Parmesan Pasta	1 bowl (2.8 oz)	320	50	5	1
Healthy Choice					
Fresh Mixers Ziti & Meat Sauce	1 pkg (6.9 oz)	340	56	10	8
TastyBite					
Peanut Sauce w/ Noodles	1 pkg (10 oz)	530	104	40	12
TAKE-OUT					
bami goreng indonesian noodle dish	1 cup	170	25	4	4
lasagna meatless	1 piece (9 oz)	356	46	8	3

FOOD	PORTION	CALS	CARB	SUGAR	FIBER
lasagna w/ meat	1 piece (8 oz)	362	37	6	3
lasagna w/ vegetables	1 serv (9 oz)	315	41	8	4
macaroni & cheese w/ ham	1 cup	542	41	7	3
manicotti cheese filled w/ marinara sauce	1 (5 oz)	229	22	3	1
manicotti cheese filled w/ meat sauce	1 (5 oz)	239	20	1	3
pasta w/ pesto sauce	1 cup	370	27	1	2
ravioli cheese & spinach filled w/ cream sauce	1 cup	362	38	5	2
ravioli cheese w/ tomato sauce	1 cup	335	38	4	2
ravioli meat filled w/ marinara sauce	1 cup	372	36	5	3
spaghetti w/ red clam sauce	1 cup	285	41	3	3
spaghetti w/ sauce & meatballs	2 cups	670	80	15	12
spaghetti w/ white clam sauce	1 cup	456	43	1	3
tortellini cheese w/ tomato sauce	1 cup	332	38	4	2
tortellini meat filled w/ marinara sauce	1 cup	281	33	3	2
tortellini spinach filled w/ marinara sauce	1 cup	238	32	3	2

PASTA SALAD
MIX
Dole

Veggie Pasta Salads Broccoli Ranch	1½ cups	230	25	4	2
Veggie Pasta Salads Cheddar Bacon Ranch	1½ cups	370	35	5	3
Veggie Pasta Salads Garden Vegetable	1½ cups	240	25	4	2
Veggie Pasta Salads Italian Herb	1½ cups	270	33	4	2

TAKE-OUT

pasta salad w/ crab vegetables mayonnaise	1 cup	317	33	2	2
tortellini salad cheese filled w/ vinaigrette dressing	1 cup	333	30	1	1

FOOD	PORTION	CALS	CARB	SUGAR	FIBER
PATE					
chicken liver canned	1 tbsp	26	1	0	0
mushroom anchovy pate	1 can (2.25 oz)	130	7	1	1
pork pate	1 oz	107	1	1	0
pork pate en croute	1 oz	91	3	tr	tr
shrimp	1 can (2.25 oz)	140	7	1	0
Patchwork					
All Flavors	2 oz	270	5	0	0
PEACH					
CANNED					
halves in light syrup	1 half (3.4 oz)	53	14	13	1
halves juice pack	1 half (3.4 oz)	43	11	10	1
in heavy syrup	½ cup (2.6 oz)	85	22	20	2
peach sauce	½ cup	120	32	31	1
pickled	½ cup (4.2 oz)	143	35	34	1
pickled whole	1 (3.1 oz)	104	26	25	1
slices juice pack	½ cup (4.4 oz)	55	14	13	2
slices light syrup	½ cup (4.4 oz)	68	18	17	2
slices water pack	½ cup (4.3 oz)	29	7	6	2
spiced in heavy syrup	½ cup (4.2 oz)	91	24	23	2
Del Monte					
Carb Clever Sliced	½ cup	30	7	6	1
Sliced Light Syrup Raspberry Flavor	½ cup	80	20	19	tr
Liberty Gold					
Sliced Cling In Heavy Syrup	½ cup	100	24	23	1
Polar					
White	½ cup	70	17	16	1
S&W					
Yellow Cling In Heavy Syrup	½ cup	100	24	23	1
DRIED					
halves	1 (0.5 oz)	31	8	5	1
halves	½ cup (2.8 oz)	191	49	33	7
halves cooked w/o sugar	½ cup (4.5 oz)	99	25	22	4
Mrs. May's					
Fruit Chips	1 pkg	35	8	7	1
FRESH					
peach	1 med (5.3 oz)	58	14	13	2
peach	1 lg (6.1 oz)	68	17	15	3
sliced	½ cup (2.7 oz)	30	8	6	1

FOOD	PORTION	CALS	CARB	SUGAR	FIBER
FROZEN					
C&W					
Ulimate Sliced	¾ cup	50	13	9	2
PEACH JUICE					
nectar	1 cup (8.7 oz)	134	35	33	2
Froose					
Playful Peach	1 box (4.2 oz)	80	19	7	3
PEANUT BUTTER					
chunky w/o salt	1 cup	1520	56	–	17
chunky w/o salt	2 tbsp	188	7	–	2
smooth	1 cup	1517	53	–	15
smooth	2 tbsp	188	7	–	2
smooth w/o salt	1 cup	1517	53	–	15
smooth w/o salt	2 tbsp	188	7	–	2.
Arrowhead Mills					
Organic Creamy	2 tbsp	190	6	1	2
Organic Honey Sweetened Creamy	2 tbsp	190	7	2	2
Organic Natural Crunchy	2 tbsp	190	6	1	2
Barney Butter					
Crunchy	2 tbsp	180	7	3	3
Smooth	2 tbsp	180	8	3	3
Better'n Peanut Butter					
Creamy	2 tbsp (1.1 oz)	100	13	2	2
Low Sodium	2 tbsp (1.1 oz)	100	13	2	2
Chet's					
Chocolate	2 tbsp	180	10	4	2
Roasted Nut	2 tbsp	180	9	4	2
Cream-Nut					
Natural	2 tbsp	190	6	1	2
Earth Balance					
Creamy or Chunky	1 tbsp	190	7	2	3
Jif					
Creamy	2 tbsp	190	7	3	2
Creamy To Go	1 pkg (2.25 oz)	270	15	7	4
Extra Crunchy	2 tbsp	190	7	3	2
Peanut Butter & Honey	2 tbsp	190	11	7	2
Reduced Fat Creamy	2 tbsp	190	15	4	2

FOOD	PORTION	CALS	CARB	SUGAR	FIBER
Reduced Fat Crunchy	2 tbsp	190	15	4	2
Simply	2 tbsp	190	6	2	2
Justin's					
Organic Cinnamon	2 tbsp (1.1 oz)	180	8	2	3
Organic Classic	2 tbsp (1.1 oz)	150	7	1	2
Kettle					
Organic Unsalted	2 tbsp	170	5	2	2
PB2					
Powdered Chocolate	2 tbsp	52	6	4	1
Powdered Chocolate Chip	2 tbsp	53	3	2	tr
Peanut Better					
Cinnamon Currant	2 tbsp	180	9	5	3
Deep Chocolate	2 tbsp	170	11	8	2
Hickory Smoked	2 tbsp	190	5	1	3
Onion Parsley	2 tbsp	180	6	1	3
Peanut Praline	2 tbsp	180	8	4	3
Rosemary Garlic	2 tbsp	180	7	2	3
Spicy Southwestern	2 tbsp	190	5	1	3
Sweet Molasses	2 tbsp	180	8	4	2
Thai Ginger & Red Pepper	2 tbsp	180	7	2	3
Vanilla Cranberry	2 tbsp	170	9	6	2
Reese's					
Creamy	2 tbsp	200	8	3	2
Revolution Foods					
Organic Creamy & Crunchy	1 tbsp (1.1 oz)	200	5	2	2
Smart Balance					
Chunky Omega	2 tbsp	200	6	1	2
Teddies					
Old Fashioned	2 tbsp	190	7	1	3
Wonder					
Peanut Spread	2 tbsp	100	13	2	0
Peanut Spread Low Sodium	2 tbsp	100	13	2	0
PEANUT BUTTER SUBSTITUTES					
NoNuts					
Golden Peabutter	1 tbsp	93	6	–	1
PEANUTS					
chocolate coated	1	21	2	2	tr
chocolate coated	¼ cup	193	18	14	2
cooked w/ salt	½ cup	286	19	2	8

FOOD	PORTION	CALS	CARB	SUGAR	FIBER
dry roasted w/ salt	28 (1 oz)	164	6	2	1
dry roasted w/ salt	1 oz	166	6	1	2
dry roasted w/o salt	¼ cup	214	8	2	3
dry roasted w/o salt	28 (1 oz)	164	6	1	2
honey roasted	¼ cup	191	8	5	3
sugar coated	¼ cup	203	18	16	2
yogurt coated	¼ cup	230	18	15	2
A Taste Of Thai					
Spicy Peanut Bake	¼ pkg	45	7	5	1
Lance					
Salted	1 pkg (1.1 oz)	200	6	0	4
Nuts Are Good					
Buffalo	1 oz	120	16	12	2
Pina Colada	1 oz	130	16	14	1
Raspberry	1 oz	130	16	14	1
Vanilla Rum	1 oz	130	17	14	1
Planters					
Cocktail	1 oz	170	6	1	2
Dry Roasted	1 oz	170	5	2	2
Sunfood					
Organic Wild Jungle	1 oz	174	5	1	2
True North					
Clusters	6 (1 oz)	170	9	5	2

PEAR
CANNED

FOOD	PORTION	CALS	CARB	SUGAR	FIBER
halves in heavy syrup	1 (1.7 oz)	36	9	8	1
halves in heavy syrup	½ cup (3.5 oz)	74	19	17	3
halves in light syrup	1 (2.7 oz)	43	12	9	1
halves juice pack	1 (2.7 oz)	38	10	7	1
halves juice pack	½ cup (4.4 oz)	62	16	12	2
halves water pack	1 (2.7 oz)	22	6	5	1
halves water pack	½ cup (4.2 oz)	35	10	7	2
Del Monte					
Carb Clever Sliced	½ cup	40	10	9	1
Liberty Gold					
Bartlett In Heavy Syrup	½ cup (4.5 oz)	90	23	22	2
S&W					
Halves In Lightly Sweetened Juice	½ cup	80	21	17	2

FOOD	PORTION	CALS	CARB	SUGAR	FIBER
DRIED					
halves	1 (0.6 oz)	47	13	11	1
halves	½ cup (3.2 oz)	236	63	56	7
halves	5 (3 oz)	229	61	54	7
halves cooked w/o sugar	½ cup (4.5 oz)	162	43	35	8
Bare Fruit					
Organic	1 pkg (0.6 oz)	46	12	9	2
Brothers-All-Natural					
Crisps Asian Pear	1 pkg (0.35 oz)	40	9	7	1
FRESH					
asian	1 med (4.3 oz)	51	13	9	4
asian	1 lg (9.6 oz)	116	30	19	10
pear	1 sm (5.2 oz)	86	23	15	5
pear	1 med (6.2 oz)	103	28	17	6
pear	1 lg (8.1 oz)	133	36	23	7
sliced w/ skin	1 cup (4.9 oz)	81	22	14	4
PEAR JUICE					
nectar canned	1 cup (8.8 oz)	150	39	38	2
Froose					
Perfect Pear	1 box (4.2 oz)	80	18	5	3
PEAS					
CANNED					
Del Monte					
Sweet No Salt Added	½ cup	60	11	6	4
Green Giant					
50% Less Sodium Young Tender Sweet	½ cup	60	11	4	3
Young Tender Sweet	½ cup	60	12	5	3
Le Sueur					
50% Less Sodium Young Tender	½ cup	60	11	4	3
Tillen Farms					
Crispy Snapper Pickled	¼ cup	15	3	1	1
DRIED					
Arrowhead Mills					
Organic Green Split not prep	¼ cup	160	24	1	4
HamPeas					
Green Split Peas as prep	½ cup	120	21	1	4

FOOD	PORTION	CALS	CARB	SUGAR	FIBER
Jack Rabbit					
Green Split	¼ cup (1.6 oz)	110	27	1	11
Snapea Crisps					
Baked Original	22 (1 oz)	70	14	tr	2
Tree Of Life					
Wasabi Peas	¼ cup (1.1 oz)	120	17	5	2
FRESH					
Frieda's					
Snow Peas	1 cup	35	6	3	2
Sugar Snap	⅔ cup (3 oz)	35	6	3	2
Mann's					
Snow Peas	1 serv (3 oz)	35	6	3	2
FROZEN					
Birds Eye					
Steamfresh Garlic Baby Peas & Mushrooms	¾ cup	80	12	4	3
Steamfresh Singles Sweet Peas	1 pkg (3.2 oz)	70	13	4	4
C&W					
Alfredo	½ cup	110	11	5	4
Early Harvest Petite No Salt Added	⅔ cup	70	12	4	4
Sugar Snap	⅔ cup	40	7	3	2
Green Giant					
Early June No Sauce	⅔ cup	50	11	3	4
SHELF-STABLE					
TastyBite					
Agra Peas & Greens	½ pkg (5 oz)	138	9	2	4
PECANS					
candied	1 oz	190	10	4	5
halves dry roasted w/ salt	20 (1 oz)	200	4	1	3
halves dried	1 cup	721	20	–	7
Emerald					
Glazed Pecan Pie	¼ cup	150	12	10	1
Emily's					
Roasted & Salted	¼ cup (1 oz)	210	4	1	3
PECTIN					
liquid	1 oz	3	1	0	1
powder	1 pkg (1.75 oz)	162	45	–	4

FOOD	PORTION	CALS	CARB	SUGAR	FIBER
PEPPER					
black	1 tsp	5	1	tr	1
cayenne	1 tsp	6	1	tr	1
white	1 tsp	7	2	–	1
PEPPERMINT					
fresh chopped	2 tbsp	2	tr	–	tr
PEPPERS					
CANNED					
chili green	1 cup (5.5 oz)	29	6	–	2
chili pepper paste	1 tbsp	6	1	–	1
B&G					
Sweet Fried	1 oz	25	2	0	1
Gedney					
Hot & Sweet Jalapeno Peppers	¼ cup	30	5	5	0
Hot Banana Pepper Rings	¼ cup	10	1	0	0
Gertie's Finest					
Piquillo	1 oz	10	2	1	tr
Las Palmas					
Diced Green Chiles	2 tbsp	5	1	0	1
Jalapenos Sliced	3 tbsp	10	2	1	0
Pace					
Green Chiles Diced	2 tbsp	10	2	tr	tr
Tillen Farms					
Bell Peppers Pickled Sweet	¼ cup	25	6	5	0
DRIED					
ancho	1 tsp	3	1	–	tr
casabel	1 tsp	3	1	–	tr
chipotle smoked	1 tsp	3	1	–	tr
guajillo	1 tsp	3	1	–	tr
mulato	1 tsp	3	1	–	tr
pasilla	1 tsp	3	1	–	tr
Frieda's					
California Chili	2 tbsp	15	2	1	0
FRESH					
green	1 (2.6 oz)	20	5	–	1
green chopped	½ cup	13	3	–	1
habanero	1 tsp	9	2	–	1
red chopped	½ cup	13	3	–	1
serrano chopped	1 cup (3.7 oz)	34	7	4	4

FOOD	PORTION	CALS	CARB	SUGAR	FIBER
Frieda's					
Peppadew	⅓ cup	40	32	29	3
FROZEN					
C&W					
Strips	¾ cup	25	4	3	1
Roast Works					
Flame Roasted Red	1 serv (3 oz)	45	7	3	3
PERCH					
FRESH					
cooked	1 fillet (1.6 oz)	54	0	0	0
cooked	3 oz	99	0	0	0
ocean perch atlantic cooked	1 fillet (1.8 oz)	60	0	0	0
ocean perch atlantic cooked	3 oz	103	0	0	0
ocean perch atlantic raw	3 oz	80	0	0	0
raw	3 oz	77	0	0	0
red raw	3.5 oz	114	0	0	0
PERSIMMONS					
dried japanese	1 (1.2 oz)	93	25	–	5
fresh	1 (6 oz)	118	31	21	6
Frieda's					
Dried Fuyu	⅓ cup (1.4 oz)	140	35	27	3
PHEASANT					
breast boneless cooked	½ (4.4 oz)	312	0	0	0
cooked diced	1 cup	332	0	0	0
drumstick & thigh cooked	1 (2.6 oz)	184	0	0	0
PHYLLO					
sheet	1 (0.7 oz)	57	10	tr	tr
Fillo Factory					
Kataifi Shredded Fillo	1 (2 oz)	180	35	1	4
Organic	2 sheets (1.5 oz)	130	27	0	1
Organic Whole Wheat	2 sheets (1.8 oz)	140	30	0	2
Shells Large	1 (0.7 oz)	80	13	0	0
PICANTE *(see* SALSA*)*					
PICKLES					
bread & butter	6 slices	39	9	4	1

FOOD	PORTION	CALS	CARB	SUGAR	FIBER
dill	1 lg (4.7 oz)	24	6	5	2
dill low sodium	1 med (2.3 oz)	12	3	–	1
dill sliced	6 slices	7	2	1	1
sweet gherkin	1 (1.2 oz)	41	11	5	tr
tsukemono japanese pickles sliced	¼ cup	10	2	1	1
B&G					
Kosher Dill	⅓ pickle (1 oz)	0	0	0	0
Sour	½ pickle (1 oz)	0	0	0	0
Claussen					
Kosher Dills Halves	1 (1 oz)	5	1	0	0
Gedney					
Baby Dills	3 (1 oz)	5	1	0	0
Organic Baby Dills	2 (1 oz)	5	1	0	0
Tree Of Life					
Organic Sweet Bread & Butter Chips	4 (1 oz)	30	8	7	0

PIE *(see also PIE CRUST, PIE FILLING)*

FROZEN

Edwards

FOOD	PORTION	CALS	CARB	SUGAR	FIBER
Pie Slices Chocolate Creme	1 slice (2.7 oz)	290	30	21	tr
Pie Slices Key Lime	1 slice (3.2 oz)	330	42	33	0
Mrs. Smith's					
Bake & Serve No Sugar Added Apple	1 slice (4.6 oz)	310	40	7	4
Blueberry Crumb	1 slice (4.2 oz)	320	48	23	2
Cherry	1 slice (4.6 oz)	330	44	17	1
Cinnabon Apple Crumb	1 slice (4.6 oz)	350	49	23	2
Classic Cream Key Lime	1 slice (4.2 oz)	410	56	44	1
Coconut Custard	1 slice (4.4 oz)	300	31	15	1
Deep Dish Berry Burst	1 slice (4.2 oz)	340	51	28	3
Dutch Apple Crumb	1 slice (4.6 oz)	370	52	22	2
Pumpkin Custard	1 slice (4.6 oz)	300	38	18	2
Soda Shoppe Boston Cream	1 slice (2.7 oz)	220	32	21	0
Soda Shoppe Chocolate Cream	1 slice (4.6 oz)	350	47	27	1
Soda Shoppe Lemon Meringue	1 slice (4.2 oz)	300	51	31	0
Sara Lee					
Apple	1 slice (4.6 oz)	340	46	26	1
Cherry	1 slice (4.6 oz)	320	44	16	0
Coconut Cream	1 slice (4.8 oz)	330	42	37	2

FOOD	PORTION	CALS	CARB	SUGAR	FIBER
Dulce de Leche Caramel Swirl	1 slice (4.4 oz)	400	37	20	2
French Silk	1 slice (4.8 oz)	340	51	34	2
Key West Lime	1 slice (4.2 oz)	400	41	30	2
Lemon Meringue	1 slice (5 oz)	220	41	37	1
Mince	1 slice (4.6 oz)	370	55	26	2
Pumpkin	1 slice (4.6 oz)	260	37	18	2
Southern Pecan	1 slice (4.2 oz)	520	70	28	3
Southern Sweet Potato	1 slice (4.6 oz)	280	45	26	2
READY-TO-EAT					
Entenmann's					
Peach Raspberry Melba	⅛ pie (2.6 oz)	250	40	22	tr
SNACK					
Lance					
Pecan	1 (3 oz)	350	46	35	3
Lifestream					
Pie Oh-My Apple	1 (3.5 oz)	280	43	16	2
Lifestream					
Pie Oh-My Pineapple	1 (3.5 oz)	280	45	16	2
TAKE-OUT					
apple one crust	1 slice (5.3 oz)	363	59	36	2
apple tart	1 (4.2 oz)	370	48	20	1
apple two crust	1 slice (5.3 oz)	356	51	23	2
apricot tart	1 (4.2 oz)	356	48	20	2
apricot two crust	1 slice (5.3 oz)	417	59	28	3
banana cream	1 slice (5.1 oz)	387	47	17	1
blackberry one crust	1 slice (4.4 oz)	341	44	18	4
blackberry two crust	1 slice (5.3 oz)	394	54	24	5
blueberry one crust	1 slice (4.8 oz)	292	45	23	3
blueberry tart	1 (4.2 oz)	346	47	21	2
blueberry two crust	1 slice (5.3 oz)	348	52	15	2
cherry one crust	1 slice (4.8 oz)	312	50	30	2
cherry two crust	1 slice (5.3 oz)	390	60	21	1
chess	1 slice (3 oz)	365	48	37	1
chocolate cream	1 slice (5 oz)	380	50	29	2
coconut creme	1 slice (5 oz)	429	54	52	2
custard	1 slice (4.8 oz)	286	28	16	2
grasshopper	1 slice (3.5 oz)	341	33	23	1
key lime	1 slice (5 oz)	420	71	28	tr
lemon meringue	1 slice (4.8 oz)	367	65	33	2
lemon meringue tart	1 (4.1 oz)	298	41	22	1

FOOD	PORTION	CALS	CARB	SUGAR	FIBER
mince two crust	1 slice (5.3 oz)	434	72	42	4
peach two crust	1 slice (5.3 oz)	334	49	9	1
pear two crust	1 slice (5.3 oz)	400	57	27	3
pecan	1 slice (4 oz)	456	65	32	4
pineapple two crust	1 slice (5.3 oz)	394	55	23	2
plum two crust	1 slice (5.3 oz)	441	61	29	2
prune one crust	1 slice (5.3 oz)	450	77	55	2
pumpkin	1 slice (5.4 oz)	323	42	21	4
raisin tart	1 (4.2 oz)	348	49	21	2
raisin two crust	1 slice (5.3 oz)	376	55	26	2
raspberry one crust	1 slice (4.8 oz)	330	52	29	6
raspberry two crust	1 slice (5.3 oz)	422	58	25	5
rhubarb two crust	1 slice (5.3 oz)	444	55	16	2
shoo-fly	1 slice (4 oz)	404	69	39	1
strawberry rhubarb two crust	1 slice (5.3 oz)	422	53	18	2
strawberry two crust	1 slice (6 oz)	386	58	29	3
sweet potato	1 piece (5.4 oz)	276	32	13	2

PIE CRUST

FOOD	PORTION	CALS	CARB	SUGAR	FIBER
baked	⅙ crust (1 oz)	147	14	1	tr
chocolate wafer	⅛ crust (1.2 oz)	177	19	8	1
chocolate wafer tart shell	1 (0.8 oz)	111	12	5	tr
deep dish frzn	⅛ crust (1.8 oz)	266	27	–	1
graham cracker	⅙ crust (1.2 oz)	172	23	13	1
graham cracker tart shell	1 (0.8 oz)	109	14	8	tr
puff pastry shell	1 (1.4 oz)	223	18	tr	1
tart shell	1 (1 oz)	149	14	1	tr
Honey Maid					
Graham Cracker Crumbs as prep	⅛ pie	160	18	4	0
Keebler					
Graham Reduced Fat	⅛ pie (0.7 oz)	100	15	6	tr
Ready Crust Chocolate	⅛ pie (0.7 oz)	100	14	6	tr
Ready Crust Graham	1/10 pie (0.9 oz)	130	18	7	tr
Ready Crust Shortbread	⅛ pie (0.7 oz)	110	14	6	0
Mrs. Smith's					
Deep Dish Shell frzn	1 slice (1 oz)	130	14	2	0

FOOD	PORTION	CALS	CARB	SUGAR	FIBER
Nilla Wafers					
Pie Crust	⅙ (1 oz)	140	18	10	0
Pepperidge Farm					
Puff Pastry Sheets frzn	⅙ sheet	170	14	1	tr
Puff Pastry Shell frzn	1	190	16	2	tr
Pillsbury					
Crusts Just Unroll	⅛ (1 oz)	110	12	0	0
Deep Dish frzn	⅛ (0.7 oz)	90	11	1	0
Pet Ritz frzn	⅛ (0.6 oz)	80	9	1	0
PIE FILLING					
apple	1 cup	155	41	34	2
blueberry	1 cup	474	116	99	7
cherry	1 cup	317	76	66	2
lemon	1 cup	923	185	166	1
Chukar Cherries					
Triple Cherry	½ cup	190	47	39	2
Comstock					
Blueberry	⅓ cup	100	24	17	1
Country Cherry Original	⅓ cup (3.1 oz)	90	23	19	1
Farmer's Market					
Organic Pumpkin Pie Mix	½ cup	100	25	20	2
PIEROGI					
potato	1 (1.3 oz)	70	11	tr	1
Mrs. T's					
Potato & 4 Cheese Blend	3 (4.2 oz)	230	36	2	1
Potato & Cheddar	3 (4.2 oz)	180	34	1	1
PIGNOLIA (see PINE NUTS)					
PIG'S FEET					
cooked	1	201	0	0	0
pickled	1	177	tr	tr	0
Hormel					
Pigs Feet	2 oz	80	0	0	0
PIKE					
northern cooked	½ fillet (5.4 oz)	176	0	0	0
northern cooked	3 oz	96	0	0	0
northern raw	3 oz	75	0	0	0
walleye baked	3 oz	101	0	0	0
walleye fillet baked	4.4 oz	147	0	0	0

FOOD	PORTION	CALS	CARB	SUGAR	FIBER
PINE NUTS					
Frieda's					
Pine Nuts	¼ cup	150	4	0	1
Good Sense					
Pignolias	¼ cup	190	9	0	4
PINEAPPLE					
CANNED					
Gefen					
Chunks In Juice	½ cup (4.9 oz)	80	19	17	1
Liberty Gold					
Chunks In Natural Juice	½ cup (4.7 oz)	80	21	19	2
Crushed No Sugar Added	½ cup	80	21	19	2
Slices Natural Juice	½ cup	80	21	19	1
DRIED					
Brothers-All-Natural					
Crisps	1 pkg (0.53 oz)	60	14	11	1
Kopali					
Organic	1 pkg (1.7 oz)	170	43	36	2
Mrs. May's					
Fruit Chips	1 pkg	35	8	7	1
Sunsweet					
Pineapples	⅓ cup (1.4 oz)	130	34	31	1
FRESH					
slice	1 slice	42	10	–	1
Frieda's					
Zululand Queen	1 cup (5 oz)	70	17	16	2
FROZEN					
Europe's Best					
Aloha Gold	1 cup	70	20	14	2
Roast Works					
Flame Roasted	1 serv (3 oz)	80	22	18	1
PINEAPPLE JUICE					
Sundia					
Purely	½ cup	60	15	19	1
PINTO BEANS					
dried cooked	1 cup	245	45	1	15
Arrowhead Mills					
Organic Dried not prep	¼ cup	150	27	2	10

FOOD	PORTION	CALS	CARB	SUGAR	FIBER
Eden					
Organic Spicy	½ cup	120	24	2	7
Organic Spicy Refried	½ cup	90	19	1	7
HamBeens					
Dried as prep	½ cup	120	22	1	6
Tree Of Life					
Organic	½ cup (4.6 oz)	120	23	2	<9
TAKE-OUT					
stewed w/ viandas	1 cup	222	27	2	6
PISTACHIOS					
dry roasted w/ salt	49 nuts (1 oz)	161	8	2	3
dry roasted w/o salt	49 nuts (1 oz)	162	8	2	3
in shells	½ cup	165	8	2	3
Love'n Bake					
Pistachio Paste	2 tbsp	160	14	10	2
True North					
Sea Salted In Shells	½ cup	170	7	2	4
Wonderful					
Roasted & Salted In Shells	½ cup	170	8	2	3
PIZZA *(see also PIZZA CRUST)*					
4Real					
Cheese	1 (4.2 oz)	220	38	2	5
Cheesy Pizza Quesadilla	1 (2.5 oz)	160	15	1	1
Turkey Pepperoni	1 (4.2 oz)	220	38	2	5
Alexia					
Pizza Snack Sweet Italian Sausage Roasted Peppers & Parmesan	6 pieces (3 oz)	210	23	2	1
Pizza Snacks Pesto Chicken w/ Fresh Mozzarella	6 pieces (3 oz)	220	23	2	1
Boca					
Supreme w/ Rising Crust Sausage & Pepperoni	⅓ pkg (4.3 oz)	280	38	5	3
Cedarlane					
Zone Cheese	1 (6.5 oz)	380	39	4	6
Celeste					
4 Cheese	1 (5.7 oz)	360	38	4	2
Dr. Praeger's					
Bagel Pizza	1 (2 oz)	120	17	2	2

FOOD	PORTION	CALS	CARB	SUGAR	FIBER
Ellio's					
All Cheesy	1 slice	160	23	2	1
Cheese	1 slice	150	23	5	1
Microwave Single Slice	1 slice	360	53	7	4
Pepperoni	1 slice	160	20	tr	1
Farm Rich					
Slices Pepperoni	2 (3.5 oz)	280	22	6	1
Glutino					
Gluten Free Duo Cheese	1 (6.1 oz)	420	68	0	2
Gluten Free Spinach & Feta	1 (6.1 oz)	430	62	0	4
Health Is Wealth					
Vegetarian Mini Pizza Bagels	4 (3.1 oz)	150	28	4	3
Hot Pockets					
Croissant Five Cheese	1 (4.5 oz)	350	35	10	2
Croissant Pepperoni	1 (4.5 oz)	380	32	7	2
Sausage	1 (4.5 oz)	330	36	6	2
Ian's					
Cheese	1 slice (1.5 oz)	100	14	2	1
Jeno's					
Crisp 'N Tasty Cheese	1 pie (6.8 oz)	440	47	5	2
Crisp 'N Tasty Pepperoni	1 (6.7 oz)	490	50	5	2
Crisp 'N Tasty Supreme	1 (7.2 oz)	490	49	5	2
Kid Cuisine					
Cheese Pizza Painter	1 meal	320	53	25	5
Dip & Dunk Cheese Pizza Strips	1 meal	510	74	27	9
Primo Pepperoni Pizza	1 meal	400	71	30	6
Lean Pockets					
Pepperoni	1 (4.5 oz)	260	35	9	3
Sausage & Pepperoni	1 (4.5 oz)	280	39	10	2
Lunchables					
Maxed Deep Dish	1 pkg	510	77	35	2
Mini Pizza	1 pkg	480	72	36	4
Pepperoni Sausage	1 pkg	440	68	35	3
Mr. P's					
Cheese	1 pie (6.5 oz)	410	58	6	5
Red Baron					
Classic Crust 4 Cheese	1 pie (8.6 oz)	740	62	6	3
Deep Dish Single Pepperoni	1 pizza	460	41	3	2
French Bread Supreme	1 pie (5.8 oz)	370	43	3	2

FOOD	PORTION	CALS	CARB	SUGAR	FIBER
South Beach					
Deluxe w/ Wheat Crust	1 pie	340	37	5	10
Four Cheese w/ Wheat Crust	1 pie	340	36	4	10
Grilled Chicken & Vegetable w/ Wheat Crust	1 pie	330	37	4	10
Pepperoni w/ Wheat Crust	1 pie	350	36	4	9
Stouffer's					
Corner Bistro Flatbread Chicken Bacon & Spinach	1 pkg (9.13 oz)	640	65	5	3
Corner Bistro Flatbread Margherita	1 pkg (9.13 oz)	540	65	7	4
Corner Bistro Flatbread Shrimp & Roasted Garlic	1 pkg (9.33 oz)	600	75	5	5
French Bread Grilled Vegetable	1 pkg (11.63 oz)	340	44	5	4
French Bread Sausage	1 pkg (4.2 oz)	420	43	5	4
French Bread Sausage & Pepperoni	1 pkg (4.2 oz)	460	42	5	4
French Bread White Pizza	1 pkg (10.13 oz)	470	44	3	4
Tony's					
Pizza For One Cheese	1 (6.5 oz)	500	58	5	3
Totino's					
Crisp Crust Canadian Bacon	½ pie (5.1 oz)	320	34	4	1
Crisp Crust Combination	½ pie (5.3 oz)	380	34	3	1
Crisp Crust Pepperoni Trio	½ pie (5 oz)	370	33	4	1
Crisp Crust Three Meat	½ pie (5.2 oz)	350	34	3	1
Pizza Rolls Combination	6 (3 oz)	220	24	2	1
Pizza Rolls Supreme	6 (3 oz)	210	25	3	2
Pizza Rolls Mega Ultimate Combination	3 (3.3 oz)	200	25	3	1
TAKE-OUT					
cheese	⅛ of 16 in pie	423	46	5	3
cheese	16 in pie	3384	372	44	23
cheese deep dish individual	1 (5.5 oz)	460	47	4	2
cheese & vegetables	⅛ of 16 in pie	428	55	5	3
ground beef	16 in pie	3753	392	25	20
ham & pineapple	⅛ of 16 in pie	439	55	7	3
no cheese	⅛ of 16 in pie	262	43	3	2
pepperoni	⅛ of 16 in pie	469	49	3	3

FOOD	PORTION	CALS	CARB	SUGAR	FIBER
white pizza	⅛ of 16 in pie	484	61	1	2
PIZZA CRUST					
crust	1 slice (1.7 oz)	130	25	1	1
whole wheat	⅛ crust	140	27	0	1
Boboli					
100% Whole Wheat	⅕ crust (2 oz)	150	27	2	5
Original	⅛ crust (1.8 oz)	140	24	1	1
Thin Crust	⅕ crust (2 oz)	170	28	1	1
Martha White					
Mix not prep	¼ pkg	160	32	2	1
Pillsbury					
Classic	⅙ crust (2.3 oz)	160	31	4	tr
PLANTAINS					
cooked mashed	1 cup	232	62	28	5
sliced cooked	1 cup	179	48	22	4
Grab Em Snacks					
Chips Black Pepper	1 oz	150	19	tr	2
TAKE-OUT					
mofongo	1 serv	320	71	31	5
ripe fried	1 serv (2.8 oz)	214	38	–	4
sweet baked w/ ice cream	1 serv	285	57	35	3
PLUM JUICE					
Nantucket Nectars					
Red Plum	8 oz	120	30	30	0
Sunsweet					
PlumSmart Light	8 oz	60	15	11	3
PLUMS					
canned in heavy syrup	1 cup	163	42	39	3
canned purple juice pack	1 cup	146	38	35	2
canned purple water pack	1 cup	102	27	25	2
dried japanese	1	9	2	1	tr
fresh	1	30	8	7	1
pickled	1	34	9	9	tr
Eden					
Umeboshi Plum Paste	1 tsp	5	0	0	0
Umeboshi Plums	1 (8 g)	5	1	0	0

FOOD	PORTION	CALS	CARB	SUGAR	FIBER
Oregon					
Whole In Heavy Syrup	½ cup (4.6 oz)	100	25	19	2
POLENTA					
Bob's Red Mill					
Corn Grits Polenta not prep	¼ cup	130	27	0	2
Frieda's					
Organic	2 slices (3.5 oz)	70	15	1	1
POLLACK					
altantic fillet baked	5.3 oz	178	0	0	0
atlantic baked	3 oz	100	0	0	0
POMEGRANATE					
fresh	1 (5.4 oz)	105	26	26	1
POMEGRANATE JUICE					
Arthur's					
Pom Plus	1 bottle (11 oz)	220	54	33	1
Frutzzo					
Organic 100% Juice	1 bottle (12 oz)	130	32	29	0
Odwalla					
PomaGrand 100% Juice	8 oz	160	40	31	0
Smart Juice					
Organic 100% Juice	8 oz	149	37	33	1
Tart Is Smart					
Concentrate	0.5 oz	37	9	9	0
POMPANO					
smoked	2 oz	109	0	0	0
steamed or poached	4 oz	156	0	0	0
TAKE-OUT					
battered & fried	4 oz	304	8	tr	tr
breaded & fried	4 oz	242	10	1	1
POPCORN *(see also POPCORN CAKES)*					
caramel coated	1 cup (1.2 oz)	152	28	14	2
caramel coated w/ peanuts	⅔ cup (1 oz)	114	23	11	1
oil popped	1 cup (0.4 oz)	55	6	tr	1
Cape Cod					
White Cheddar	2⅓ cups	170	13	2	2
Dale & Thomas					
Caramel	½ cup	75	17	15	0

FOOD	PORTION	CALS	CARB	SUGAR	FIBER
Hall Of Fame Kettlecorn	½ cup	34	6	6	1
North Country Cheddar	½ cup	73	7	1	1
Peanut Butter & White Chocolate Drizzlecorn	½ cup	115	15	12	1
Purepopped Natural	½ cup	26	3	0	1
Sweet Georgia Pecan	½ cup	96	18	10	1
Toffee Crunch Drizzlecorn	½ cup	107	15	11	1
Divvies					
Caramel Corn Vegan	½ cup	80	14	10	tr
Jay's					
Caramel	¾ cup	110	26	17	1
Ok-Ke-Doke Cheese	1 oz	160	13	1	2
Jolly Time					
American's Best Yellow	5 cups	90	23	tr	9
Butter Licious Light	5 cups	130	22	0	4
Crispy'n White Light	5 cups	125	20	0	7
Healthy Pop Caramel Apple	5 cups	110	23	tr	6
Healthy Pop Minis	4 cups	90	23	tr	8
Mallow Magic	2.5 cups	180	15	5	3
The Big Cheez	3.5 cups	140	17	tr	6
Lance					
White Cheddar	1 pkg (0.7 oz)	100	8	1	2
LesserEvil					
Black&White	1 cup	120	25	16	1
KettleCorn	1 cup	120	25	14	2
MaplePecan	1 cup	120	25	14	3
PeanutButter & Choco	1 cup	120	24	15	1
SinNamon	1 cup	120	24	14	2
Mrs. Fields					
Clusters Butter Toffee Crunch	⅔ cup	170	31	20	3
Newman's Own					
Microwave 94% Fat Free	3½ cups	110	20	0	4
Microwave Butter	3½ cups	130	18	0	3
Microwave Butter Boom	3½ cups	130	18	0	3
Microwave Light Butter	3½ cups	120	19	0	4
Microwave Low Sodium Butter	3½ cups	130	18	0	3
Microwave Natural	3½ cups	130	18	0	3
Organic Pop's Corn Butter	3½ cups	160	17	0	1
Organic Pop's Corn No Butter No Salt 94% Fat Free	3½ cups	120	21	0	1

FOOD	PORTION	CALS	CARB	SUGAR	FIBER
Oogie's					
Romano & Pesto	1 oz	138	16	0	3
Smoked Gouda	1 oz	132	14	0	3
Spicy Chipotle & Lime	1 oz	143	17	0	3
White Cheddar	1 oz	142	17	0	3
Orville Redenbacher's					
Hot Air	1 cup	15	3	0	1
Kernel Original	1 cup	15	3	0	1
Microwave Butter Light	1 cup	20	3	0	1
Microwave Kettle Korn Sweet	1 cup	35	3	0	1
Microwave Movie Theater Butter Light	1 cup	20	3	0	1
Microwave Movie Theater Extra Butter	1 cup	35	3	0	1
Microwave Natural Light	1 cup	20	3	0	1
Microwave Pour Over Butter	1 cup	40	3	0	1
Microwave Pour Over Cheddar	1 cup	50	6	0	1
Microwave Regular Butter	1 cup	35	3	0	1
Microwave Regular Corn On The Cob	1 cup	35	3	0	1
Microwave Regular Natural	1 cup	15	3	0	1
Microwave Regular Old Fashioned Butter	1 cup	35	3	0	1
Microwave Regular Tender White	1 cup	40	3	0	1
Microwave Smart Pop Butter	1 cup	15	3	0	1
Microwave Smart Pop Kettle Korn	1 cup	20	3	0	1
Microwave Smart Pop Movie Theater Butter	1 cup	20	3	0	1
Microwave Sweet Caramel	1 cup	90	15	4	4
Microwave Sweet Cinnabon	1 cup	50	6	1	tr
Microwave Sweet Honey Butter	1 cup	35	3	0	1
Microwave Sweet 'N Buttery	1 cup	40	3	0	1
Microwave Ultimate Butter	1 cup	30	3	0	1
White	1 cup	15	3	0	1
Poppycock					
Cashew Lovers	½ cup (1.1 oz)	148	21	12	tr
Original	½ cup (1.1 oz)	160	20	13	1
Pecan Delight	½ cup (1.1 oz)	150	20	13	0

FOOD	PORTION	CALS	CARB	SUGAR	FIBER
Smart Balance					
Light as prep	4 cups	120	18	0	4
Low Fat as prep	5 cups	120	24	0	5
Movie Style as prep	3.5 cups	170	18	0	3
Snyder's Of Hanover					
Butter	⅝ oz	100	6	0	1
Tree Of Life					
Organic Lightly Salted	4 cups	100	21	0	5
Utz					
Butter	2 cups	170	13	tr	2
Cheese	2 cups	160	14	1	3
Puff'n Corn Original Hulless	2 cups	150	11	0	0
Wise					
Butter	1 pkg (0.5 oz)	80	7	0	1
Hot Cheese	1 oz	150	14	3	2
POPCORN CAKES					
Orville Redenbacher's					
Butter	2	60	14	0	2
Caramel	1	40	10	3	tr
Chocolate	1	45	10	4	tr
Mini Butter	8	60	12	0	1
Mini Caramel	7	50	13	4	1
Mini Peanut Caramel Crunch	6	60	12	4	1
Mini Peanut Crunch	6	60	12	4	2
Mini Sour Cream & Onion	8	60	12	0	2
White Cheddar	2	60	13	0	2
POPPY SEEDS					
poppy seeds	1 tbsp	47	2	1	1
Bob's Red Mill					
Poppy Seeds	3 tbsp	170	6	0	3
Love'n Bake					
Poppy Seed Filling	2 tbsp	120	18	16	tr
PORGY					
fresh	3 oz	77	0	0	0
PORK (see also HAM, JERKY, PORK DISHES)					
FRESH					
boneless loin lean & fat roasted	3.5 oz	195	0	0	0

FOOD	PORTION	CALS	CARB	SUGAR	FIBER
center loin chop bone in broiled	1 (3 oz)	178	0	0	0
center rib chop lean & fat bone in broiled	1 (3 oz)	189	0	0	0
country style ribs bone in lean & fat braised	3.5 oz	288	0	0	0
dehydrated oriental style	1 cup (0.8 oz)	135	tr	0	0
fresh ham rump half lean & fat roasted	4 oz	278	0	0	0
fresh ham shank half lean & fat roasted	4 oz	319	0	0	0
fresh ham whole lean & fat roasted	4 oz	302	0	0	0
ground cooked	4 oz	328	0	0	0
ham hock cooked	1	167	0	0	0
shoulder chop bone in braised	1 (3 oz)	229	0	0	0
sirloin roast lean & fat bone in roasted	4 oz	231	0	0	0
spareribs bone in roasted	3 oz	304	0	0	0
tail simmered	3 oz	336	0	0	0
tenderloin roast boneless lean & fat roasted	4 oz	145	0	0	0
top loin chop boneless lean & fat broiled	1 (3.5 oz)	195	0	0	0
Hormel					
Extra Lean Boneless Tenderloin	4 oz	120	0	0	0
Organic Prairie					
Chop	1 (3.3 oz)	220	0	0	0
Ground	4 oz	300	0	0	0
Smithfield					
Boneless Smoked Pork Chop	3 oz	110	4	3	0
Smoked Pork Chop	3 oz	100	2	2	0
Tyson					
Baby Back Ribs Buffalo	4 oz	300	4	1	0
Ground Reduced Fat	4 oz	260	0	0	0
Half Loin Boneless	4 oz	190	0	0	0
Loin Chops Bone-In Center Cut	4 oz	190	0	0	0
Spareribs	4 oz	290	0	0	0
Stew Meat	4 oz	130	0	0	0

FOOD	PORTION	CALS	CARB	SUGAR	FIBER
READY-TO-EAT					
Sara Lee					
Oven Roasted	2 oz	70	1	0	0
TAKE-OUT					
chicharrones pork cracklings fried	1 cup	492	1	0	0
chop breaded & fried	1 med (3.4 oz)	304	13	1	1
chop breaded & fried	1 lg (5 oz)	441	19	2	1
chop stewed	1 lg (4.6 oz)	315	0	0	0
PORK DISHES					
A La Carte Gourmet					
Pork Loin w/ Cream Spinach Feta Stuffing	1 serv (5 oz)	200	8	3	tr
Hormel					
Extra Lean Apple Bourbon	1 serv (4 oz)	140	5	5	0
Morton's Of Omaha					
Tender Pork Roast w/ Gravy & Vegetables	1 serv (5 oz)	210	10	2	1
Tyson					
Roast Pork w/ Vegetables	1 serv (4 oz)	190	18	0	2
Wellshire					
Baby Back Ribs w/ Sauce	2 ribs (5 oz)	260	5	4	0
Shredded Pork In BBQ Sauce	¼ cup	90	9	6	0
TAKE-OUT					
kalua pork	1 cup (7 oz)	497	1	–	0
spareribs barbecued w/ sauce	2 med (2.8 oz)	248	3	1	tr
PORK RINDS (see SNACKS)					
POT PIE					
Hot Pockets					
Pot Pie Express Chicken	1 (4.5 oz)	330	34	8	2
Ian's					
Chicken	1 pkg (9.4 oz)	510	50	2	2
Mon Cuisine					
Vegan	1 pkg (9 oz)	650	60	6	8
Pepperidge Farm					
Chili Beans & Cornbread	1 cup	360	40	11	3
Reduced Fat Roasted White Meat Chicken	1 cup	470	56	9	0
Roasted White Meat Chicken	1 cup	510	43	7	3

FOOD	PORTION	CALS	CARB	SUGAR	FIBER
Stouffer's					
Chicken White Meat	1 pkg (10 oz)	660	62	14	2
TAKE-OUT					
beef	1 (14.6 oz)	938	72	4	5
chicken	1 (14.6 oz)	897	69	5	6
ham	1 serv (11 oz)	752	58	3	4
oyster	1 serv (11.5 oz)	817	67	6	3
puerto rican pastelon de carne	1 piece (5 oz)	666	35	1	2
st. stephen's day pie	1 serv (16.7 oz)	549	38	5	6
tuna	1 (27 oz)	1715	126	10	10
vegetarian w/ meat substitute	1 (8 oz)	511	39	3	5
POTATO *(see also CHIPS, KNISH, PANCAKES)*					
CANNED					
Butterfield					
Whole White	3.5 pieces (5.8 oz)	90	20	0	2
Del Monte					
Savory Sides Au Gratin	½ cup	80	13	1	1
Sunshine					
Whole White	3 pieces (5.9 oz)	90	20	0	2
FRESH					
Frieda's					
Fingerling	4 (5 oz)	100	25	3	3
Green Giant					
Red Potatoes	1 med (5 oz)	100	26	3	3
FROZEN					
Alexia					
Hashed Brown	1 serv (3 oz)	80	17	2	2
Mashed Red w/ Garlic & Parmesan	½ cup	150	20	1	2
Mashed Yukon Gold & Sea Salt	½ cup	150	20	1	2
Oven Crinkles Classic	1 serv (3 oz)	120	19	1	3
Oven Crinkles Salt & Pepper	1 serv (3 oz)	120	19	0	3
Oven Fries Garlic	12 pieces	140	20	0	2
Oven Reds	1 serv (3 oz)	120	19	0	2
Waffle Fries	8 pieces	150	24	0	3
Yukon Gold Fries w/ Sea Salt	1 serv (3 oz)	130	22	0	2

FOOD	PORTION	CALS	CARB	SUGAR	FIBER
Cascadian Farm					
Organic Country Style	¾ cup	50	12	0	1
Organic Hash Browns	1 cup	60	14	0	1
Funster					
BBQ Lite	14 pieces (3 oz)	140	25	tr	<2
Cheddar	14 pieces (3 oz)	135	25	tr	<2
Original	14 pieces (3 oz)	135	25	tr	2
Green Giant					
Roasted Potatoes w/ Garlic & Herb Sauce as prep	½ cup	90	15	1	1
Health Is Wealth					
Twice Baked Cheddar Cheese	1 (5 oz)	200	25	2	2
Vegetarian Potato Skins	2 (2.7 oz)	110	8	0	1
Ian's					
Alphatots	1 serv (3.5 oz)	156	23	1	1
Inland Valley					
Crinkle Cuts	15 pieces (3 oz)	150	25	tr	2
Crisscut Fries	13 pieces (3 oz)	160	22	tr	2
Curly QQQ's	1⅓ cups (3 oz)	180	25	tr	2
Fajita Fries	17 pieces (3 oz)	170	22	1	2
French Fries	15 pieces (3 oz)	130	21	tr	2
Hash Browns	⅔ cup	70	16	tr	2
Home Browns	1 patty (2.2 oz)	130	15	tr	2
Mashed Homestyle	⅔ cup	160	22	2	3
Simply Shreds	1 cup	70	15	tr	2
Stix	5 pieces (3 oz)	170	19	tr	2
Stuffed Spudz w/ Cheese	5 pieces	210	20	tr	2
Tater Babies	8 pieces (3 oz)	130	19	tr	2
Tater Puffs	10 pieces	160	20	tr	2
Twice Baked	1 (5.2 oz)	230	23	3	2
Twice Baked Sour Cream Bacon & Chives	1 (5.2 oz)	240	36	2	3
Twice Baked Triple Cheese	1 (5.2 oz)	250	33	3	3
Joy Of Cooking					
Elegant Scalloped	1 cup (8 oz)	300	21	2	2

FOOD	PORTION	CALS	CARB	SUGAR	FIBER
Red Skin Mashed	1 cup (4.2 oz)	160	17	2	2
Larry's					
Mashed Broccoli & Cheddar Cheese	1 serv (5 oz)	180	22	7	2
Mashed Cheddar Cheese	1 serv (5 oz)	190	25	8	2
Mashed Old Fashioned Butter	1 serv (5 oz)	190	25	9	2
Mashed Sour Cream & Chives	1 serv (5 oz)	180	25	8	2
Mashed Sweet Potatoes	1 serv (4 oz)	140	27	11	2
McCain					
French Fries Crinkle Cut	18 pieces (3 oz)	130	21	0	2
Mash-Bites	1 serv (3 oz)	50	24	2	1
Roasters All American	1 serv (3 oz)	120	21	2	tr
Roasters Grilled Garlic & Onion	1 serv (3 oz)	120	22	1	2
Seasoned Wedges Skin On	1 serv (3 oz)	120	17	tr	2
Shoestring French Fries	45 pieces (3 oz)	140	21	0	2
Smiles	6 pieces (3 oz)	160	24	tr	2
Steak Fries	8 pieces (3 oz)	120	21	0	2
Tasti Tater	1 serv (3 oz)	160	20	tr	3
Oh Boy!					
Stuffed w/ Onion Sour Cream & Chives	1 (5 oz)	110	22	0	2
Roast Works					
Roasted Wedges Rosemary Redskin	1 serv (3 oz)	110	17	1	2
Roasted Wedges Seasoned	1 serv (3 oz)	100	18	0	1
Roasted Wedges Yukon Gold	1 serv (3 oz)	110	18	1	1
MIX					
Betty Crocker					
Au Gratin as prep	⅔ cup	150	24	0	1
Cheddar & Bacon as prep	⅔ cup	120	21	1	1
Cheesy Scalloped as prep	½ cup	120	21	1	1
Julienne as prep	⅔ cup	140	20	1	1
Mashed Four Cheese as prep	½ cup	170	21	1	1
Mashed Sour Cream & Chives as prep	½ cup	170	21	1	1
Scalloped as prep	½ cup	130	20	1	1
Seasoned Skillets Hash Browns as prep	½ cup	120	19	0	2

FOOD	PORTION	CALS	CARB	SUGAR	FIBER
Hungry Jack					
Casserole Potatoes Au Gratin as prep	½ cup	100	21	1	2
Casserole Potatoes Creamy Scalloped as prep	½ cup	150	21	1	2
Casserole Potatoes Four Cheese as prep	½ cup	150	21	1	2
Easy Mash'd Cheesy Homestyle not prep	¼ cup	150	17	1	2
Easy Mash'd Creamy Butter not prep	¼ cup	150	17	1	2
Easy Mash'd Premium Homestyle not prep	¼ cup	150	17	1	2
Original Mashed not prep	⅓ cup	80	19	0	1
REFRIGERATED					
Country Crock					
Homestyle Mashed	⅔ cup (5 oz)	180	23	1	2
Loaded Mashed	⅔ cup (5 oz)	200	22	2	2
Diner's Choice					
Mashed	⅔ cup	110	15	3	3
Reser's					
Potato Express Red Skinned Mashed	½ cup	140	22	1	2
Simply Potatoes					
Diced w/ Onion	⅔ cup	60	13	0	1
Homestyle Slices	⅔ cup	70	16	0	1
Mashed	⅔ cup	170	17	0	1
Mashed Sweet Potatoes	⅔ cup	160	33	18	2
Red Potato Wedges	½ cup	50	10	2	2
Shredded Hash Browns	½ cup	50	12	0	tr
SHELF-STABLE					
TastyBite					
Bombay Potatoes	½ pkg (5 oz)	105	13	2	3
TAKE-OUT					
indian yogurt potatoes	1 serv	315	52	–	0
potato dumpling	3.5 oz	334	74	–	3
red new boiled	5 sm (5 oz)	120	27	3	2
POTATO STARCH					
Bob's Red Mill					
Potato Starch	1 tbsp	40	10	0	0

FOOD	PORTION	CALS	CARB	SUGAR	FIBER
POUT					
ocean baked	3 oz	86	0	0	0
ocean fillet baked	4.8 oz	139	0	0	0
PRETZELS					
chocolate covered	1 (0.4 oz)	47	8	2	tr
soft	1 lg (5 oz)	483	99	tr	2
twists salted	10 (2.1 oz)	229	48	–	2
twists w/o salt	10 (2.1 oz)	229	48	1	2
yogurt covered	1 (4 g)	19	3	1	tr
yogurt covered	1 cup (3 oz)	391	61	30	1
Braids					
Honey Wheat	7 (1 oz)	110	23	4	1
Mini Knots	17 (1 oz)	110	23	tr	tr
Cape Cod					
Pretzels	25	130	27	tr	tr
Combos					
Cheddar Cheese Cracker	1 pkg (1.7 oz)	240	31	7	1
Nacho Cheese	1 pkg (1.7 oz)	230	34	9	1
Pizzeria Pretzel	1 pkg (1.7 oz)	230	35	7	1
Glenny's					
Organic Original Salted	8 (1 oz)	110	23	1	1
Organic Sourdough	6 (1 oz)	110	23	1	1
Glutino					
Gluten Free All Shapes	44 (1.4 oz)	190	28	tr	0
Goodniks					
Yogurt Pretzels	15	180	28	15	0
Handi-Snack					
Mister Salty Pretzels 'N Cheese	1 pkg	90	12	1	0
Healthy Handfuls					
Python Pretzels	1 box (1.5 oz)	170	36	0	1
New York Style					
Pretzel Flatz Original Salt	12	110	23	0	1
Newman's Own					
Organic Bavarian Sour Dough	1	90	19	1	1
Organic Hi Protein	22	120	22	1	4
Organic Salt & Pepper Rounds	8	100	24	1	1
Organic Salt & Pepper Thins	10	120	24	1	tr
Organic Salted Nuggets	20	120	25	1	2
Organic Salted Rods	4	120	25	1	2
Organic Salted Rounds	8	110	24	1	tr

FOOD	PORTION	CALS	CARB	SUGAR	FIBER
Organic Salted Sticks	13	110	24	1	1
Organic Salted Thins	10	110	24	1	1
Organic Spelt	20	120	23	0	4
Organic Unsalted Rounds	8	110	24	1	tr
Quinlan					
Low Fat Mini	1 oz	110	23	tr	tr
Rold Gold					
Braided Twists	1 oz	110	22	tr	1
Braided Twists Honey Wheat	1 oz	110	23	3	1
Dipped Twists Fudge Coated	1 oz	140	18	11	2
Mini Sticks Honey Mustard & Onion	1 oz	140	19	2	1
Pretzel Waves Cheddar	1 oz	130	20	tr	1
Pretzel Waves Dark Chocolate Drizzle	1 oz	130	20	6	2
Pretzel Waves Vanilla Yogurt Drizzle	1 oz	130	21	8	tr
Sourdough Hard	1	100	21	tr	1
Sticks Classic	1 oz	100	23	1	1
Tiny Twists	1 oz	100	23	tr	1
Salba Smart					
Omega-3 Enriched	1 oz	110	21	1	1
Snyder's Of Hanover					
100 Calorie Pack Snaps	1 pkg (0.9 oz)	100	22	tr	tr
100 Calorie Pack Stick	1 pkg (0.9 oz)	100	20	tr	tr
Dips Milk Chocolate	1 oz	140	19	11	tr
Dips Special Dark Chocolate	1 oz	140	22	8	2
Mini Unsalted	1 oz	110	25	tr	tr
MultiGrain Sticks Lightly Salted	1 oz	120	23	2	3
MultiGrain Twists	1 oz	120	22	2	2
Nibblers Sourdough	1 oz	120	25	tr	tr
Old Tyme	1 oz	120	24	tr	1
Organic Honey Wheat	1 oz	130	24	4	1
Organic Oat Bran	1 oz	120	25	3	2
Pieces Garlic Bread	1 oz	140	18	0	1
Pieces Honey Mustard & Onions	1 oz	140	18	3	tr
Pieces Hot Buffalo Wing	1 oz	140	17	0	tr
Pretzel Sandwich Peanut Butter	1 oz	140	16	2	tr
Rods	1 oz	120	24	tr	1

FOOD	PORTION	CALS	CARB	SUGAR	FIBER
Snaps	1 oz	120	25	tr	1
Sourdough Unsalted	1 oz	100	22	0	1
Sticks 12 Multi Grain	1 oz	130	22	3	3
Superpretzel					
Mozzarella	2 (1.8 oz)	130	20	0	1
Pretzelfils Pizza	2 (1.8 oz)	130	22	1	1
Soft	1 (2.25 oz)	160	34	1	1
Soft Bites	5 (1.9 oz)	150	32	1	1
Softstix	2 (1.8 oz)	130	22	1	1
Tom Sturgis					
Little Cheesers	17 (1 oz)	120	22	tr	2
Little Ones	17 (1 oz)	110	22	tr	tr
Utz					
Braided Twists Baked Honey Wheat	1 oz	110	23	4	1
Chocolate Covered	6 (1.1 oz)	140	22	11	tr
Hard	1	90	18	tr	tr
Special	1 oz	110	21	tr	1
Special Multigrain	1 oz	110	21	1	2
Sticks Organic Whole Grain	1 oz	120	22	1	3
Wise					
Fat Free Sticks	1 oz	100	23	tr	tr
Low Fat Honey Wheat Braided Twists	1 oz	110	24	3	1
PRUNE JUICE					
jarred	1 cup	182	45	42	3
L&A					
100% Juice	8 oz	180	41	23	3
Lakewood					
Organic	8 oz	165	40	16	3
Langers					
Plus 100% Juice	8 oz	180	41	23	1
Old Orchard					
Healthy Balance	8 oz	70	12	9	5
Sunsweet					
100% Juice	8 oz	180	43	18	3
PlumSmart	8 oz	160	39	27	3
Tree Of Life					
Organic 100% Juice	8 oz	180	43	23	2

FOOD	PORTION	CALS	CARB	SUGAR	FIBER
PRUNES					
cooked w/o sugar	½ cup	133	35	31	4
dried	1	20	5	3	1
Earthbound Farm					
Organic Dried Plums	5	110	25	18	3
Love'n Bake					
Prune Lekvar	2 tbsp	90	21	17	1
Newman's Own					
Organic	½ cup	110	26	13	2
Sunsweet					
Pitted Dried	5	100	24	12	3
PUDDING					
MIX					
Uncle Ben's					
Rice Pudding Cinnamon & Raisins as prep	½ cup	160	37	15	1
Rice Pudding French Vanilla as prep	½ cup	120	28	10	1
READY-TO-EAT					
Hunt's					
Dessert Favorites Banana Cream Pie	1 serv (3.5 oz)	140	20	13	0
Dessert Favorites Chocolate Brownie	1 serv (3.5 oz)	190	28	22	0
Dessert Favorites Chocolate Mud Pie	1 serv (3.5 oz)	170	25	20	0
Dessert Favorites Chocolate Peanut Butter Pie	1 serv (3.5 oz)	190	27	21	0
Dessert Favorites Dulce De Leche Caramel Cream	1 serv (3.5 oz)	140	23	17	0
Dessert Favorites Lemon Meringue Pie	1 serv (3.5 oz)	130	26	21	0
Snack Pack Butterscotch	1 serv (3.5 oz)	130	20	15	0
Snack Pack Chocolate	1 serv (3.5 oz)	104	22	17	0
Snack Pack Chocolate Fudge	1 serv (3.5 oz)	150	23	16	0
Snack Pack Chocolate Marshmallow	1 serv (3.5 oz)	130	21	16	0
Snack Pack Fat Free Chocolate	1 serv (3.5 oz)	90	20	15	0
Snack Pack Fat Free Vanilla	1 serv (3.5 oz)	80	19	13	0
Snack Pack Lemon	1 serv (3.5 oz)	120	23	20	0

FOOD	PORTION	CALS	CARB	SUGAR	FIBER
Snack Pack Swirl Chocolate Caramel	1 serv (3.5 oz)	140	22	17	0
Snack Pack Swirl S'mores	1 serv (3.5 oz)	140	21	17	0
Snack Pack Tapioca	1 serv (3.5 oz)	130	20	14	0
Snack Pack Vanilla	1 serv (3.5 oz)	130	21	18	0
Jell-O					
100 Calorie Pack Fat Free Chocolate Vanilla Swirl	1 pkg (4 oz)	100	23	17	tr
100 Calorie Pack Fat Free Tapioca	1 pkg (4 oz)	100	23	17	0
Sugar Free Dulce De Leche	1 pkg (3.7 oz)	60	13	0	0
Vanilla	1 serv (4 oz)	110	23	18	0
Kozy Shack					
Black Forest	1 pkg (4 oz)	120	22	18	1
Tapioca	1 pkg (4 oz)	130	23	17	0
Swiss Miss					
Chocolate	1 pkg	150	27	22	0
Low Fat Chocolate	1 pkg	130	26	19	0
Pie Lovers Banana Cream	1 pkg	130	23	17	0
Pie Lovers Lemon Meringue	1 pkg	140	28	21	0
Swirl Chocolate Vanilla	1 pkg	140	27	20	0
TAKE-OUT					
blancmange	1 serv (4.7 oz)	154	25	–	tr
bread w/ raisins	1 cup	306	47	29	2
coconut	1 cup	291	45	38	2
corn	1 cup	328	43	17	4
indian pudding	½ cup	156	25	16	1
noodle pudding kugel	1 cup	297	44	15	2
plum pudding	1 slice (1.5 oz)	125	20	12	1
queen of puddings	1 serv (4.4 oz)	266	41	–	tr
rice pudding	1 cup	302	60	37	1
sweet potato	½ cup	107	19	7	3
tapioca	1 cup	236	35	31	0
yorkshire	1 serv (3 oz)	177	22	–	tr
PUFFERFISH					
raw	3 oz	72	0	0	0
PUMPKIN					
Farmer's Market					
Organic Puree	½ cup	50	10	4	4

FOOD	PORTION	CALS	CARB	SUGAR	FIBER
Tree Of Life					
Organic Puree	½ cup (4.3 oz)	50	10	4	4
TAKE-OUT					
indian sago	1 serv (2.3 oz)	75	6	3	3
PUMPKIN SEEDS					
Eden					
Dry Roasted & Salted	¼ cup	200	5	–	5
Good Sense					
Roasted & Salted	½ cup	160	3	0	1
Mrs. May's					
Pumpkin Crunch	1 oz	164	8	4	1
Tree Of Life					
Seeds Roasted & Salted	¼ cup (2 oz)	300	8	1	4
QUAIL					
cooked bone removed	1 (2.7 oz)	177	0	0	0
QUICHE					
Mrs. Smith's					
Pour-A-Quiche Bacon & Onion	1 serv (4.3 oz)	230	6	4	0
TAKE-OUT					
cheese	⅛ (9 in) pie	566	27	1	1
lorraine	⅛ (9 in) pie	568	27	1	1
mushroom	1 slice (3 oz)	256	17	–	1
spinach	⅛ (9 in) pie	342	17	1	1
QUINOA					
cooked	1 cup (6.5 oz)	222	39	–	5
quinoa not prep	¼ cup (1.5 oz)	156	27	–	3
Alti Plano Gold					
Natural	1 pkg	170	30	9	5
Ancient Harvest Quinoa					
Flakes not prep	¼ cup	159	28	1	3
Organic Inca Red not prep	¼ cup	163	29	5	4
Organic Traditional not prep	¼ cup	172	31	3	3
Eden					
Quinoa not prep	¼ cup	180	29	2	11
Seeds Of Change					
French Herb Quinoa Blend as prep	1 cup	290	56	7	3

FOOD	PORTION	CALS	CARB	SUGAR	FIBER
RABBIT					
domestic w/o bone roasted	3 oz	167	0	0	0
wild w/o bone stewed	3 oz	147	0	0	0
RACCOON					
roasted	3 oz	217	0	0	0
RADISHES					
Eden					
Daikon Dried Shredded	2 tbsp	45	9	6	3
Frieda's					
Black	¾ cup	15	3	2	1
Chinese Lo Bok	⅔ cup	25	5	3	2
Daikon	½ cup	15	1	0	0
Korean Moo	⅔ cup	15	3	2	1
TAKE-OUT					
moo namul saengche korean salad	1 serv (3.7 oz)	34	8	6	2
RAISINS					
cinnamon coated	¼ cup	108	29	21	1
cooked	¼ cup	162	42	35	1
golden seedless	¼ cup	109	29	21	1
jumbo golden	¼ cup	130	31	29	2
milk chocolate coated	¼ cup	176	31	28	2
milk chocolate coated	28 (1 oz)	109	19	17	1
seedless	55 (1 oz)	86	23	17	1
sultanas	1 oz	88	23	–	2
Amazin' Raisin					
All Flavors	1 pkg (1 oz)	84	22	20	2
Bob's Red Mill					
Unsulfured	⅓ cup	130	31	26	3
Earthbound Farm					
Organic Jumbo Flame Seedless	¼ cup	120	32	30	2
Emily's					
Milk Chocolate Covered	29 (1.4 oz)	180	26	24	2
Fool					
Cinnamon Raisin Spread	1 tbsp	20	5	4	1
Godiva					
Milk Chocolate Covered	1 pkg (1.2 oz)	150	21	20	1
Goodniks					
Yogurt Raisins	3 tbsp	145	23	17	1

FOOD	PORTION	CALS	CARB	SUGAR	FIBER
Newman's Own					
Organic	¼ cup	130	26	13	2
Revolution Foods					
Organic	1 pkg (1.2 oz)	100	28	21	1
Sun-Maid					
Chocolate Covered	30 (1.4 oz)	170	26	25	1
Golden	¼ cup (1.4 oz)	130	31	29	2
Jumbo	¼ cup (1.4 oz)	130	31	29	2
Seedless	¼ cup (1.4 oz)	130	31	29	2
Snack Box	1 (1 oz)	90	22	20	2
Sunsweet					
Red Flame	¼ cup	130	31	29	2
RAMBUTAN					
canned in syrup	1 (0.3 oz)	7	2	–	tr
canned in syrup	1 cup (4.3 oz)	123	31	–	1
puerto rican fresh	5 (1.6 oz)	34	8	8	tr
Polar					
In Syrup	½ cup	68	17	14	tr
RASPBERRIES					
black fresh	1 cup	70	16	6	9
canned in heavy syrup	½ cup	116	30	26	4
canned water pack	1 cup	43	10	4	5
fresh	1 cup	64	15	5	8
fresh	1 pt	162	37	14	20
frzn sweetened	1 cup	129	33	27	6
frzn unsweetened	1 cup	65	15	6	8
C&W					
Ultimate Red	¾ cup	70	15	9	7
Cascadian Farm					
Organic frzn	1¼ cup	60	17	6	6
Europe's Best					
Raspberries frzn	¾ cup	60	13	7	2
Frieda's					
Dried	⅓ cup (1.4 oz)	145	36	25	6
Oregon					
In Heavy Syrup	½ cup	120	30	22	5
RASPBERRY JUICE					
Crystal Light					
Raspberry Ice Sugar Free	8 oz	5	0	0	0

FOOD	PORTION	CALS	CARB	SUGAR	FIBER
RED BEANS					
Allens					
Red Beans	½ cup	100	19	1	9
RELISH					
piccalilli	1.4 oz	13	2	–	1
tomato	¼ cup (2.8 oz)	119	28	26	1
Cascadian Farm					
Organic Sweet Relish	1 tbsp (0.5 oz)	15	4	4	0
Claussen					
Sweet Pickle	1 tbsp (0.5 oz)	15	3	2	0
Frieda's					
Kim Chee	¼ cup	15	2	0	1
Gedney					
Hot Dog	1 tbsp	18	4	3	0
Organic Sweet	1 tbsp	15	4	3	0
Patak's					
Brinjal Eggplant Sweet Spicy	1 tbsp	70	8	6	1
Garlic	1 tbsp	45	4	3	0
Lime Mild	1 tbsp	30	0	0	0
Mango Mild	1 tbsp	40	1	1	0
Peloponnese					
Sun Dried Tomato	1 tbsp	25	2	1	0
Tree Of Life					
Organic Sweet Pickle	1 tbsp (0.5)	15	4	3	0
RICE (see also RICE CAKES, WILD RICE)					
brown long grain cooked	1 cup (6.8 oz)	216	45	–	4
brown medium grain cooked	1 cup (6.8 oz)	218	46	–	4
glutinous cooked	1 cup (6.1 oz)	169	37	–	2
white long grain cooked	1 cup (5.5 oz)	205	45	–	1
white long grain instant cooked	1 cup (5.8 oz)	162	35	–	1
white medium grain cooked	1 cup (6.5 oz)	242	53	–	1
A Taste Of Thai					
Coconut Garlic Basil as prep	¾ cup	160	35	2	0
Coconut Ginger as prep	¾ cup	190	42	2	2
Jasmine not prep	¼ cup	160	36	0	0
Yellow Curry as prep	¾ cup	180	38	2	0
Arrowhead Mills					
Organic Brown Basmati not prep	¼ cup	140	31	1	2

FOOD	PORTION	CALS	CARB	SUGAR	FIBER
Organic Long Grain Brown not prep	¼ cup	160	32	0	1
Betty Crocker					
Bowl Appetit! Teriyaki Rice	1 bowl (2.5 oz)	260	54	6	2
Carolina					
Saffron Yellow Mix not prep	1 serv	190	43	1	1
Country Crock					
Cheddar Broccoli Rice	1 cup (7 oz)	270	35	3	1
Fantastic					
Arborio not prep	¼ cup	160	36	0	tr
Basmati not prep	¼ cup	160	36	0	tr
Jasmine not prep	¼ cup	160	36	0	tr
Green Giant					
Rice Pilaf	1 pkg (9.9 oz)	200	40	3	3
White & Wild & Green Beans	1 pkg (9.9 oz)	260	48	3	3
Knorr					
Asian Side Dish Chicken Fried Rice as prep	1 cup	240	48	2	1
Rice Sides Rice Medley as prep	1 cup	250	45	3	1
Rice Sides Sesame Chicken w/ Whole Grains as prep	⅔ cup	300	51	6	3
Lundberg					
Eco-Farmed Black Japonica not prep	¼ cup	170	38	1	3
Eco-Farmed California Brown Basmati not prep	¼ cup	160	34	1	2
Eco-Farmed White California Arborio not prep	¼ cup	160	43	0	1
Organic Brown Golden Rose not prep	¼ cup	160	34	0	1
Organic Rice Sensations Ginger Miso not prep	½ cup	116	24	1	1
Organic Risotto Porcini Mushroom not prep	½ cup	143	35	1	1
Organic White Sushi Rice no prep	¼ cup	150	36	0	1
Organic Wild Blend not prep	¼ cup	150	35	0	3
RiceXpress Chicken Herb	½ pkg (4.4 oz)	250	47	2	6
RiceXpress Santa Fe Grill	½ pkg (4.4 oz)	260	50	2	3

FOOD	PORTION	CALS	CARB	SUGAR	FIBER
Risotto Butternut Squash not prep	½ cup	143	31	2	1
Marrakesh Express					
Pilaf Tomato & Basil as prep	1 cup	190	41	3	0
Risotto Parmesan as prep	1 cup	200	42	2	1
Minute					
Boil-In-Bag White as prep	1 cup	180	41	0	1
Brown as prep	1 cup	150	34	0	2
Ready To Serve Brown	1 pkg (4.4 oz)	170	28	0	2
Ready To Serve White	1 pkg (4.4 oz)	190	34	0	0
Ready To Serve Yellow	1 pkg (4.4 oz)	190	35	0	1
White as prep	1 cup	200	45	0	0
Near East					
Long Grain & Wild Original as prep	1 cup	220	43	0	2
Pilaf Curry as prep	1 cup	220	44	0	2
Pilaf Original as prep	1 cup	220	43	0	1
Pilaf Sesame Ginger as prep	1 cup	270	55	6	1
Pilaf Spanish Rice as prep	1 cup	310	54	2	2
Whole Grains Brown Rice as prep	1 cup	210	41	1	3
Nueva Cocina					
Arroz A La Mexicana	1 cup	190	41	2	2
Arroz Con Pollo	1 cup	150	35	1	1
Gallo Pinto	⅓ pkg	220	47	1	3
Moros Y Cristianos	⅓ pkg	220	47	tr	3
Paella	⅕ pkg	160	35	1	1
Patak's					
Basmati	1 pkg	430	87	1	2
Coconut	1 pkg	500	87	5	4
Yellow	1 pkg	440	89	6	2
Rice A Roni					
Beef as prep	1 cup	310	51	3	2
Chicken as prep	1 cup	310	51	2	2
Express Asian Fried	1 cup	280	51	2	2
Fried Rice as prep	1 cup	320	49	4	2
Garden Vegetable as prep	1 cup	270	41	3	2
Long Grain & Wild as prep	1 cup	250	43	1	1
Lower Sodium Chicken as prep	1 cup	270	51	1	2
Parmesan Chicken as prep	1 cup	370	51	5	3

FOOD	PORTION	CALS	CARB	SUGAR	FIBER
Red Beans & Rice as prep	1 cup	290	51	3	5
Savory Whole Grain Blends Spanish as prep	1 cup	250	42	4	3
Spanish as prep	1 cup	260	44	6	2
Rice Select					
Royal Blend w/ Lentils	1 serv	130	28	–	1
Royal Blend w/ Red Beans	1 serv	130	27	–	2
Texmati Brown	1 serv	170	35	–	2
Texmati Light Brown	1 serv	170	33	–	1
Seeds Of Change					
Moroccan Lentil Rice Pilaf as prep	1 cup	180	38	3	3
Tuscan Rice & Beans as prep	1 cup	180	40	3	2
Success					
Boil-In-Bag Brown as prep	1 cup	150	33	0	2
Boil-In-Bag Jasmine as prep	¾ cup	150	36	0	0
Boil-In-Bag White as prep	1 cup	190	43	0	1
Ready To Serve Brown	1 cup	170	28	0	2
Ready To Serve White	1 pkg	190	34	0	0
Ready To Serve Yellow Rice Mix	1 pkg	190	35	1	1
Whole Grain Herb Roasted Chicken as prep	1 cup	290	43	1	3
Whole Grain Multigrain Pilaf as prep	1 cup	230	43	1	3
Whole Grain Portobello Mushroom as prep	1 cup	220	45	2	3
TastyBite					
Pilaf Multigrain	½ pkg (5 oz)	200	33	3	4
Pilaf Tandoori	½ pkg (5 oz)	183	37	3	1
Uncle Ben's					
Boil-In-Bag	1 cup	190	44	0	1
Country Inn Chicken & Broccoli as prep	1 cup	190	42	1	1
Country Inn Chicken & Vegetables as prep	1 cup	200	41	1	1
Country Inn Mexican Fiesta as prep	1 cup	200	42	0	1
Country Inn Oriental Fried as prep	1 cup	200	42	1	1

FOOD	PORTION	CALS	CARB	SUGAR	FIBER
Country Inn Three Cheese as prep	1 cup	200	40	4	1
Country Inn Wheat as prep	1 cup	200	43	1	1
Fast & Natural	1 cup	190	42	0	2
Flavorful Four Cheese as prep	1 cup	190	43	0	1
Flavorful Garlic & Butter as prep	1 cup	200	44	0	tr
Flavorful Lemon & Herb as prep	1 cup	200	45	1	tr
Flavorful Spanish as prep	1 cup	200	45	2	tr
Instant as prep	1 cup	190	43	0	1
Long Grain & Wild Herb Roasted Chicken as prep	1 cup	190	39	1	3
Long Grain & Wild Original as prep	1 cup	200	42	1	1
Long Grain & Wild Roasted Garlic as prep	1 cup	200	42	0	1
Long Grain & Wild Sun-Dried Tomato Florentine as prep	1 cup	180	39	1	3
Ready Rice Long Grain & Wild as prep	1 cup	240	44	1	1
Ready Rice Original as prep	1 cup	230	44	0	1
Ready Rice Roasted Chicken as prep	1 cup	230	44	0	1
Ready Rice Teriyaki as prep	1 cup	190	51	2	1
Ready Rice Whole Grain Brown	1 cup	220	41	0	1
White Original as prep	1 cup	170	38	0	0
Zatarain's					
Black Beans & Rice as prep	1 cup	230	47	0	6
Caribbean Rice Mix as prep	1 cup	160	34	0	1
Yellow as prep	½ cup	110	23	0	0
TAKE-OUT					
coconut rice	1 serv	500	30	–	2
dirty rice w/ chicken giblets	1 cup (6.9 oz)	291	38	tr	1
nasi goreng indonesian rice & vegetables	1 cup (4.9 oz)	130	28	1	1
pea palau rice & peas fried in ghee	1 serv	144	21	1	2
risotto	1 serv (6.6 oz)	426	65	–	3

FOOD	PORTION	CALS	CARB	SUGAR	FIBER
RICE CAKES (see also POPCORN CAKES)					
Hain					
Mini Munchies Apple Cinnamon	9 (0.5 oz)	60	14	2	tr
Lundberg					
Eco-Farmed Apple Cinnamon	1 (0.7 oz)	80	18	2	tr
Eco-Farmed Brown Rice Salt Free	1 (0.7 oz)	70	14	0	tr
Eco-Farmed Toasted Sesame	1 (0.7 oz)	70	15	0	1
Organic Caramel Corn	1 (0.7 oz)	80	18	2	1
Organic Green Tea w/ Lemon	1 (0.7 oz)	80	17	2	1
Organic Mochi Sweet	1 (0.7 oz)	70	15	0	tr
Mr. Krispers					
Baked Rice Krisps Barbecue	37	110	21	3	1
Baked Rice Krisps Nacho	37	120	21	3	1
Baked Rice Krisps Sea Salt & Pepper	37	110	20	2	1
Baked Rice Krisps Sour Cream & Onion	37	110	19	2	1
Quaker					
Mini Delights Chocolatey Drizzle	1 pkg (0.7 oz)	90	14	6	1
Riceworks					
Sweet Chili	10 (1 oz)	140	19	tr	1
Wasabi	10 (1 oz)	140	19	tr	1
ROCKFISH					
pacific cooked	1 fillet (5.2 oz)	180	0	0	0
pacific cooked	3 oz	103	0	0	0
pacific raw	3 oz	80	0	0	0
ROE (see also individual fish names)					
ROLL					
FROZEN					
Alexia					
Ciabatta	1 (1.5 oz)	100	19	1	1
French	1 (1.5 oz)	100	20	1	1
Three Cheese Focaccia	1 (1.5 oz)	110	19	1	tr
Whole Grain	1 (1.5 oz)	90	19	1	3

FOOD	PORTION	CALS	CARB	SUGAR	FIBER
Eggo					
Toaster Swirlz Cinnamon Roll Minis	4 (1.6 oz)	120	20	6	tr
Joy Of Cooking					
Ciabatta Olive Oil Rosemary	1 (1.7 oz)	120	21	0	1
French Baguettes Mini	1 (1.6 oz)	100	20	0	1
Pillsbury					
Dinner Rolls Crusty Sourdough	1 (1.2 oz)	90	17	0	tr
Dinner Rolls Crusty French	1 (1.2 oz)	90	15	1	tr
Dinner Rolls Whole Wheat	1 (1.2 oz)	90	17	2	3
Sara Lee					
Deluxe Cinnamon Rolls w/ Icing	1 (2.7 oz)	320	41	21	1
READY-TO-EAT					
bialy	1 (2.2 oz)	138	32	–	1
brioche sweet roll	1 (3.5 oz)	410	41	5	3
cheese	1 (2.3 oz)	238	29	–	1
cinnamon raisin	1 (2.1 oz)	223	31	19	1
dinner	1 (1 oz)	78	14	2	1
egg	1 (1.2 oz)	107	18	2	1
french	1 (1.3 oz)	105	19	tr	1
garlic	1 (1.5 oz)	133	22	2	1
hamburger or hot dog	1 (1.5 oz)	120	21	3	1
hamburger or hot dog multi grain	1 (1.5 oz)	113	19	3	2
hamburger or hot dog reduced calorie	1 (1.5 oz)	84	18	2	3
hamburger or hot dog whole wheat	1 (1.5 oz)	114	22	4	3
hard	1 (2 oz)	167	30	1	1
hoagie or submarine roll whole wheat	1 (4.7 oz)	359	69	11	10
hot cross bun	1	202	38	–	1
mexican bolillo	1 (4.1 oz)	305	60	tr	2
oat bran	1 (1.2 oz)	78	13	2	1
oatmeal	1 (1.3 oz)	103	17	2	1
pumpernickel	1 (1.3 oz)	100	19	tr	2
rye	1 med (1.3 oz)	103	19	tr	2
sourdough	1 (1.6 oz)	130	25	1	1
wheat	1 (1 oz)	76	13	tr	1
whole wheat	1 med (1.3 oz)	96	18	3	3

FOOD	PORTION	CALS	CARB	SUGAR	FIBER
Ecce Panis					
Focaccia	1 (3.2 oz)	260	49	tr	2
Mrs Baird's					
Home Bake	1 (1 oz)	80	13	2	tr
Natural Ovens					
Better Wheat Buns	1 (2.2 oz)	170	30	5	4
Nature's Own					
100% Whole Grain Sugar Free	1 (1.9 oz)	110	23	0	4
Butter Buns	1 (1.7 oz)	120	23	2	1
Pepperidge Farm					
Hamburger 100% Whole Wheat	1	120	18	3	2
Hoagie Soft w/ Sesame Seeds	1	210	35	3	2
Hot & Crusty Sourdough	1	100	21	tr	1
Hot Dog	1	140	26	4	tr
Hot Dog Whole Grain White	1	110	21	2	2
Parker House Dinner	1	80	14	2	tr
Premium Wheat	1	220	36	6	1
Sandwich Buns Sesame Seeds	1 (1.6 oz)	130	22	3	1
Rudi's Organic Bakery					
100% Whole Wheat	1 (2.3 oz)	160	29	3	5
Hot Dog Spelt	1 (2 oz)	140	28	3	2
Hot Dog Wheat	1 (2 oz)	150	28	4	2
Hot Dog White	1 (2 oz)	150	28	4	tr
S. Rosen's					
Brat & Sausage Rolls	1 (2.1 oz)	160	28	2	1
Klassic Kaiser	1 (2.6 oz)	230	46	7	1
Sara Lee					
Hamburger Bun Classic	1 (2.6 oz)	200	37	5	1
Hamburger Bun Classic Wheat	1 (2.6 oz)	200	38	6	3
Heart Healthy Hamburger Bun Wheat	1 (2.6 oz)	190	37	6	3
Hot Dog Gourmet	1 (1.5 oz)	120	23	4	tr
Stroehmann					
Hot Dog Wheat	1 (1.8 oz)	140	25	5	2
Weight Watchers					
Sandwich Wheat	1 (2 oz)	140	28	2	5
REFRIGERATED					
crescent	1 (1 oz)	78	14	2	1
Pillsbury					
Crescent Big & Buttery	1 (1.7 oz)	170	20	4	tr

FOOD	PORTION	CALS	CARB	SUGAR	FIBER
Crescent Butter Flake	1 (1 oz)	110	11	2	0
Crescent Original	1 (1 oz)	110	11	2	0
Crescent Reduced Fat	1 (1 oz)	90	12	2	0
ROSEMARY					
dried	1 tsp	4	1	–	1
fresh	1 tbsp	1	tr	–	tr
ROUGHY					
orange baked	3 oz	75	0	0	0
RUBS *(see HERBS/SPICES)*					
RUTABAGA					
cooked mashed	1 cup	94	21	14	4
cubed cooked	1 cup	66	14	10	3
Glory					
Cut Fresh	1 cup	50	11	8	4
Sunshine					
Diced	½ cup	30	7	2	1
SABLEFISH					
baked	3 oz	213	0	0	0
fillet baked	5.3 oz	378	0	0	0
smoked	1 oz	72	0	0	0
smoked	3 oz	218	0	0	0
SAFFRON					
dried	1 tsp	2	tr	–	tr
SAGE					
ground	1 tsp	2	tr	tr	tr
SALAD *(see also SALAD TOPPINGS)*					
Dole					
American Blend	1½ cups	15	3	2	1
Baby Spinach Salad	1½ cups (3 oz)	20	3	0	2
Butter & Red Leaf	1½ cups (3 oz)	10	3	1	1
Classic Iceberg	1½ cups (3 oz)	15	4	2	1
Classic Romaine	1½ cups (3 oz)	15	4	2	1
European Blend	1½ cups (3 oz)	15	3	2	1
Field Greens	1½ cups (3 oz)	15	4	2	2
French Blend	1½ cups (3 oz)	15	4	2	2
Greener Selection	1½ cups (3 oz)	15	3	2	1

FOOD	PORTION	CALS	CARB	SUGAR	FIBER
Hearts Delight	1½ cups (3 oz)	15	3	2	1
Italian Blend	1½ cups (3 oz)	15	3	2	1
Kits Asian Crunch	1½ cups (3.5 oz)	120	12	5	2
Kits Bacon Lettuce Toss	1½ cups (3.5 oz)	130	8	3	1
Kits Caesar	1½ cups (3 oz)	170	8	2	2
Kits Caesar Light	1½ cups (3 oz)	100	8	2	1
Kits Romano	1½ cups (3 oz)	150	9	2	2
Kits Spring Garden	1½ cups (3.5 oz)	140	11	6	2
Kits Sunflower Ranch	1½ cups (3 oz)	160	5	3	2
Mediterranean Blend	1½ cups	15	3	0	2
Very Veggie Blend	1½ cups (3 oz)	20	4	3	1
Earthbound Farm					
Organic Baby Arugula Salad	2 cups	20	3	2	1
Organic Baby Lettuce Salad	2 cups	15	3	0	1
Organic Baby Spinach Salad	2 cups	10	7	0	7
Organic Fresh Herb Salad	2 cups	15	4	0	2
Organic Mixed Baby Greens	2 cups	15	4	0	2
Fresh Express					
50/50 Mix	3 cups	10	5	2	4
Caesar Lite w/ Dressing as prep	2½ cups	100	8	2	2
Caesar w/ Dressing as prep	2½ cups	150	8	2	2
Fancy Field Greens	3 cups	20	3	1	2
Gourmet Cafe Caribbean Chicken as prep	1 pkg (3.5 oz)	120	14	8	1
Gourmet Cafe Chicken Caesar w/ Crostini as prep	1 pkg (3.5 oz)	150	5	1	1
Gourmet Cafe Chopped Turkey Chef as prep	1 pkg (3.5 oz)	120	7	4	tr
Gourmet Cafe Orchard Harvest as prep	1 pkg (3.5 oz)	230	13	9	2
Gourmet Cafe Tuscon Pesto Chicken as prep	1 pkg (3.5 oz)	130	6	3	1
Gourmet Cafe Waldorf Chicken as prep	1 pkg (3.5 oz)	190	19	14	2
More Carrots American	1½ cups	15	3	2	1
Organic Italian	2½ cups	15	3	2	1

FOOD	PORTION	CALS	CARB	SUGAR	FIBER
Original Iceberg Garden With Zip	1½ cups	15	3	2	4
Pacifica! Veggie Supreme w/ Dressing as prep	3 cups	220	18	14	2
Spring Mix	3 cups	15	3	1	2
Sweet Baby Greens	3 cups	10	2	1	1
Veggie Lover's	2 cups	20	4	2	1
Mann's					
Rainbow	3 oz	25	5	2	2
TAKE-OUT					
7-layer salad	2 cups	557	15	8	3
caesar	4 cups	734	28	6	7
cobb w/ dressing	4 cups	645	23	9	11
greek w/ dressing	4 cups	424	14	8	4
mixed salad greens shredded	1 cup	9	2	tr	1
somen w/ lettuce egg fish pork	2 cups	550	57	4	4
spinach w/o dressing	4 cups	429	45	5	6
tossed w/ avocado w/o dressing	2 cups	90	9	4	5
tossed w/ chicken w/o dressing	3 cups	194	5	3	2
tossed w/ egg w/o dressing	2 cups	93	6	4	2
tossed w/ seafood w/o dressing	3 cups	120	8	5	3
tossed w/ shrimp & egg w/o dressing	3 cups	185	5	3	2
tossed w/o dressing	2 cups	22	5	3	2
waldorf	1 cup	242	15	10	3
wilted lettuce w/ bacon dressing	1 cup	99	3	1	1

SALAD DRESSING *(see also SALAD TOPPINGS)*
MIX
A Taste Of Thai

Peanut Dressing as prep	2 tbsp	40	7	5	1

READY-TO-EAT
Bernstein's

Chunky Blue Cheese	2 tbsp	120	2	1	0
Creamy Caesar	2 tbsp	120	1	0	0
Italian Restaurant Recipe	2 tbsp	120	1	0	0

FOOD	PORTION	CALS	CARB	SUGAR	FIBER
Light Fantastic Roasted Garlic Balsamic	2 tbsp	45	3	2	0
Red Wine & Garlic Italian	2 tbsp	110	2	1	0
Bragg					
Ginger & Sesame	2 tbsp	150	2	2	0
Organic Vinaigrette	2 tbsp	150	3	2	0
Cains					
Caesar Creamy	2 tbsp	170	1	0	0
Caesar Fat Free	2 tbsp	30	6	2	0
Caesar Light	2 tbsp	70	5	2	0
Chianti Vinaigrette	2 tbsp	130	5	3	0
Creamy Dill Cucumber Fat Free	2 tbsp	35	8	3	0
French	2 tbsp	120	6	4	0
French Light	2 tbsp	80	10	6	0
Greek	2 tbsp	160	2	2	0
Italian Fat Free	2 tbsp	15	4	2	0
Ranch	2 tbsp	180	1	1	0
Ranch Light	2 tbsp	80	6	2	0
David Burke					
Flavor Spray Ranch	2 sprays	0	0	0	0
Follow Your Heart					
Lemon Herb	2 tbsp (1 oz)	100	1	0	0
Sesame Miso	2 tbsp (1 oz)	64	3	2	0
Thousand Island	2 tbsp (1 oz)	80	3	0	tr
Gotta Luv It					
Chipotle Lime	2 tbsp	110	3	2	0
Raspberry Balsamic Vinaigrette	2 tbsp	150	6	5	0
Sweet & Tangy Italian	2 tbsp	140	2	2	0
Ken's					
Bacon Ranch	2 tbsp	140	2	2	0
Caesar	2 tbsp	170	1	1	0
Country French w/ Vermont Honey	2 tbsp	150	10	9	0
Fat Free Italian	2 tbsp	25	5	4	0
Fat Free Raspberry Pecan	2 tbsp	50	12	10	0
Honey Mustard	2 tbsp	130	7	6	0
Italian w/ Aged Romano	2 tbsp	110	11	1	0
Lite Chunky Blue Cheese	2 tbsp	80	4	1	0
Lite Italian	2 tbsp	50	2	1	0
Lite Ranch	2 tbsp	80	6	2	0

FOOD	PORTION	CALS	CARB	SUGAR	FIBER
Lite Red Wine Vinegar & Olive Oil	2 tbsp	50	2	2	0
Lite Vinaigrette Balsamic & Basil	2 tbsp	50	3	2	0
Red Wine Vinegar & Olive Oil	2 tbsp	120	2	2	0
Russian	2 tbsp	140	52	3	0
Thousand Island	2 tbsp	140	4	3	0
Kraft					
Free French	2 tbsp	50	11	2	0
Free Ranch	2 tbsp	50	11	2	1
Free Thousand Island	2 tbsp	45	10	5	0
Honey Dijon	2 tbsp	100	6	5	0
Italian Creamy	2 tbsp	100	2	2	0
Light Done Right Caesar	2 tbsp	60	3	1	0
Light Done Right Red Wine Vinaigrette	2 tbsp	45	3	2	0
Ranch Garlic	2 tbsp	120	3	2	0
Special Collection Classic Italian Vinaigrette	2 tbsp	60	5	2	0
Special Collection Parmesan Romano	2 tbsp	140	2	1	0
Special Collection Tangy Tomato Bacon	2 tbsp	100	10	9	0
Thousand Island w/ Bacon	2 tbsp	100	7	6	0
LiteHouse					
Bleu Cheese Bacon	2 tbsp	150	1	1	0
Organic Vinaigrette Raspberry Lime	2 tbsp	40	5	5	0
Ranch Homestyle	2 tbsp	120	2	1	0
Ranch Lite	2 tbsp	70	2	2	0
Sesame Ginger	2 tbsp	35	8	7	0
Spinach Salad	2 tbsp	50	11	7	0
Vinaigrette Huckleberry	2 tbsp	20	4	4	0
Vinaigrette Lite Honey Dijon	2 tbsp	130	3	2	0
Marie's					
Blue Cheese Lite Chunky	2 tbsp	80	7	1	4
Blue Cheese Vinaigrette	2 tbsp	120	4	4	0
Caesar	2 tbsp	170	1	0	0
Coleslaw	2 tbsp	120	8	7	0
Creamy Ranch	2 tbsp	170	1	1	0

FOOD	PORTION	CALS	CARB	SUGAR	FIBER
Red Wine Vinaigrette	2 tbsp	60	6	5	0
Sesame Ginger	2 tbsp	70	7	6	0
Milo's					
Gorgonzola Pear Riesling	2 tbsp	70	2	1	0
Pomegranate Port	2 tbsp	90	6	6	0
Naturally Fresh					
Balasamic Vinaigrette	2 tbsp	10	2	1	0
Bleu Cheese	2 tbsp	170	1	0	0
Bleu Cheese Bacon	2 tbsp	170	1	0	0
Bleu Cheese Lite	2 tbsp	100	1	1	0
Buffalo Ranch	2 tbsp	110	4	3	0
Classic Oriental	2 tbsp	100	9	8	0
Ginger	2 tbsp	70	1	0	0
Greek Feta	2 tbsp	100	1	0	0
Honey French	2 tbsp	100	5	5	0
Honey Mustard	2 tbsp	140	5	4	0
Orange Miso	2 tbsp	100	4	3	0
Ranch Classic	2 tbsp	150	1	1	0
Ranch Lite	2 tbsp	80	2	1	0
Slaw	2 tbsp	90	6	6	0
Newman's Own					
Balsamic Vinaigrette	2 tbsp	90	3	1	0
Caesar	2 tbsp	150	1	1	0
Creamy Caesar	2 tbsp	150	1	1	0
Family Recipe Italian	2 tbsp	120	1	1	0
Lighten Up Balsamic Vinaigrette	2 tbsp	45	2	1	0
Lighten Up Caesar	2 tbsp	70	3	2	0
Lighten Up Honey Mustard	2 tbsp	70	7	5	0
Lighten Up Italian	2 tbsp	60	0	0	0
Lighten Up Low Fat Sesame Ginger	2 tbsp	35	5	4	0
Lighten Up Raspberry & Walnut	2 tbsp	70	7	5	0
Olive Oil & Vinegar	2 tbsp	150	1	1	0
Parmesan & Roasted Garlic	2 tbsp	110	2	1	0
Ranch	2 tbsp	140	2	2	0
Two Thousand Island	2 tbsp	140	4	3	0
School House Kitchen					
Balsamic Vinaigrette Basico	2 tbsp	160	3	2	0
Seeds Of Change					
Vinaigrette Balsamic	2 tbsp	60	6	3	0

FOOD	PORTION	CALS	CARB	SUGAR	FIBER
Vinaigrette Greek Feta	2 tbsp	60	5	2	0
Vinaigrette Roasted Garlic	2 tbsp	60	6	3	0
Vinaigrette Sweet Basil	2 tbsp	60	6	2	0
Sonoma					
Creamy Tomato Bacon	2 tbsp	150	3	2	0
South Beach					
Balsamic Vinaigrette	2 tbsp	50	4	2	0
Italian	2 tbsp	60	3	2	0
Ranch	2 tbsp	70	2	0	0
Soy Vay					
Cha-Cha Chinese Chicken	3 tbsp	190	11	9	0
Vino De Milo					
Gorgonzola Pear Riesling	2 tbsp	80	2	1	0
Pomegranate Port	2 tbsp	90	5	5	0
Wild Thymes Farm					
Salad Refreshers Black Currant	1 tbsp	36	3	3	tr
Salad Refreshers Meyer Lemon	1 tbsp	35	3	3	tr
Salad Refreshers Morello Cherry	1 tbsp	34	3	2	tr
Salad Refreshers Pomegrante	1 tbsp	33	3	2	0
Vinaigrette Mandarin Orange Basil	1 tbsp	43	2	1	tr
Vinaigrette Raspberry Pear	1 tbsp	43	1	1	tr
Vinaigrette Roasted Apple Shallot	1 tbsp	42	2	1	tr
Vinaigrette Toasted Sesame Wasabi	1 tbsp	42	1	1	tr
Wishbone					
Blue Cheese w/ Gorgonzola	2 tbsp	140	1	tr	0
Caesar w/ Aged Romano	2 tbsp	80	3	2	0
Classic Ranch Extra Thick	2 tbsp	140	2	1	0
Creamy Caesar	2 tbsp	170	1	tr	0
Creamy Italian	2 tbsp	110	4	2	0
Deluxe French	2 tbsp	50	8	6	tr
Fat Free Chunky Blue Cheese	2 tbsp	35	7	3	tr
Fat Free Italian	2 tbsp	20	4	3	0
Fat Free Ranch	2 tbsp	30	7	3	tr
Five Cheese Italian	2 tbsp	120	6	2	0
Italian	2 tbsp	90	3	3	0
Just 2 Good Blue Cheese	2 tbsp	45	6	2	0

FOOD	PORTION	CALS	CARB	SUGAR	FIBER
Just 2 Good Creamy Caesar	2 tbsp	50	7	2	0
Just 2 Good Deluxe French	2 tbsp	50	8	6	tr
Just 2 Good Italian	2 tbsp	35	4	4	0
Just 2 Good Ranch	2 tbsp	40	5	2	0
Just 2 Good Thousand Island	2 tbsp	50	9	5	0
Just 2 Good Western	2 tbsp	70	13	12	0
Light Ranch Extra Thick	2 tbsp	70	2	1	0
Light Vinaigrette Asian Sesame	2 tbsp	70	6	5	0
Light Vinaigrette Raspberry Walnut	2 tbsp	80	7	5	0
Ranch	2 tbsp	160	1	tr	0
Russian	2 tbsp	110	14	6	0
Salad Spritzers Balsamic Breeze	10 sprays	10	1	1	0
Salad Spritzers Italian	10 sprays	10	1	1	0
Salad Spritzers Red Wine Mist	10 sprays	10	1	1	0
Thousand Island	2 tbsp	130	6	6	0
Vinaigrette Berry	2 tbsp	50	2	2	0
Vinaigrette Lemon Garlic & Herb	2 tbsp	70	5	3	0
Vinaigrette Olive Oil	2 tbsp	60	4	3	0
Western	2 tbsp	160	12	11	0

SALAD TOPPINGS
Fresh Gourmet
Tortilla Strips Lightly Salted	2 tbsp	35	5	0	0
Wonton Strips Wasabi Ranch	2 tbsp	35	4	0	0

Naturally Fresh
Fruit & Nut Mix	½ tbsp	45	2	1	1
Glazed Almond & Pecan Pieces	½ tbsp	40	3	2	1

Salad Pizazz!
Asian Medley	1 tbsp	40	2	2	tr
Cherry Cranberry Pecano	1 tbsp	35	4	3	tr
Honey-Toasted Delites	1 tbsp	40	2	2	1
Orange Cranberry Almondine	1 tbsp	35	4	3	tr
Raspberry Cranberry Walnut Frisco	1 tbsp	30	4	3	0
Tomato 'N Bacon Parmesano	1 tbsp	30	3	1	tr
Tomato Pinenut Tuscano	1 tbsp	130	2	1	tr

FOOD	PORTION	CALS	CARB	SUGAR	FIBER
SALBA					
Salba Smart					
Ground	2 tbsp	65	5	–	4
Whole Grain	1 tbsp	65	5	–	4
SALMON					
CANNED					
w/ bone	½ cup	106	0	0	0
Bumble Bee					
Blueback	¼ cup	110	0	0	0
Keta	¼ cup	90	0	0	0
Pink	¼ cup	90	0	0	0
Red	¼ cup	110	0	0	0
Skinless & Boneless	¼ cup	50	0	0	0
Smoked Fillets In Oil	⅓ cup	150	0	0	0
Polar					
Pink	¼ cup	90	0	0	0
Sockeye Red	¼ cup	110	0	0	0
FRESH					
atlantic farmed baked	4 oz	233	0	0	0
coho wild poached	4 oz	209	0	0	0
pink baked	4 oz	169	0	0	0
sockeye baked	4 oz	245	0	0	0
FROZEN					
Dr. Praeger's					
Salmon Cakes	1 (2.9 oz)	190	15	0	3
SMOKED					
lox	1 oz	33	0	0	0
TAKE-OUT					
guisado salmon stew	1 serv (7.4 oz)	320	18	3	3
roulette w/ spinach stuffing	1 serv (4 oz)	160	10	0	tr
salmon cake	1 (4.2 oz)	264	14	1	1
salmon loaf	1 slice (3.7 oz)	206	9	2	tr
SALSA					
black bean & corn	2 tbsp	15	3	1	tr
citrus	2 tbsp (1 oz)	10	2	2	0
peach	2 tbsp	15	4	4	0
tomatoless corn & chile	2 tbsp	45	10	6	tr
Bone Suckin'					
Fat Free Gluten Free	2 tbsp	40	10	8	0

FOOD	PORTION	CALS	CARB	SUGAR	FIBER
Cape Cod					
Medium & Mild	2 tbsp	15	3	1	1
Chi-Chi's					
Fiesta Mild	2 tbsp	10	2	2	0
Chukar Cherries					
Peach Cherry	1 tbsp	13	3	2	tr
Dei Fratelli					
Casera Mild	2 tbsp (1.1 oz)	5	2	1	0
Emeril's					
Original Recipe	2 tbsp	10	3	2	0
Muir Glen					
Organic Medium	2 tbsp	10	3	1	0
Newman's Own					
Bandito Pineapple	2 tbsp	15	3	3	1
Bandito Mild	2 tbsp	10	2	1	1
Bandito Peach	2 tbsp	25	6	5	tr
Bandito Roasted Garlic	2 tbsp	10	2	1	1
Ortega					
Garden Style Mild	2 tbsp	10	2	1	tr
Pace					
Black Bean & Corn	2 tbsp	25	5	2	1
Organic Picante	2 tbsp	10	2	2	tr
Thick & Chunky	2 tbsp	10	2	2	tr
Robert Rothchild Farm					
Tomatillo & Pepper	2 tbsp	20	5	2	tr
Salba Smart					
Organic Omega-3 Enriched	2 tbsp	12	2	0	1
Seeds Of Change					
Black Bean & Tomato Mild	2 tbsp	15	3	1	tr
Garlic & Cilantro Mild	2 tbsp	15	2	1	tr
Snyder's Of Hanover					
Sweet	2 tbsp	20	5	4	0
Utz					
Sweet	2 tbsp	10	2	1	tr
Walnut Acres					
Organic Fiesta Cilantro	2 tbsp	10	2	2	0
Organic Sweet Southwestern Peach	2 tbsp	20	5	4	0

FOOD	PORTION	CALS	CARB	SUGAR	FIBER
SALSIFY					
Frieda's					
Salsify	¾ cup	70	16	2	3
SALT SUBSTITUTES					
gomasio sesame salt	2 tsp	34	2	–	1
AlsoSalt					
Butter Flavored	¼ tsp	1	0	0	0
Garlic Flavored	¼ tsp	1	0	0	0
Original	¼ tsp	1	0	0	0
Chef Paul Prudhomme's					
Magic Salt Free Seasoning	¼ tsp	0	0	0	0
Eden					
Organic Seaweed Gomasio Sesame Salt	1 tsp	15	tr	0	0
Organic Gomasio Sesame Salt	1 tsp	15	tr	0	0
French's					
No Salt	¼ cup	0	0	0	0
Nu-Salt					
Salt Substitute	1 pkg (1 g)	0	0	0	0
SALT/SEASONED SALT					
kosher	¼ tsp	0	0	0	0
salt	1 dash (0.4 g)	0	0	0	0
salt	1 tbsp (0.6 oz)	0	0	0	0
salt	1 tsp (6 g)	0	0	0	0
sea salt coarse	1 tsp	0	0	0	0
sea salt fine	¼ tsp	0	0	0	0
BaconSalt					
Original	¼ tsp	0	0	0	0
Peppered	¼ tsp	0	0	0	0
Bob's Red Mill					
Garlic Salt Blend	¼ tsp	0	0	0	0
Sea Salt	¼ tsp	0	0	0	0
Eden					
French Celtic Salt	¼ tsp	0	0	0	0
Portuguese Coast Salt	¼ tsp	0	0	0	0
Maine Coast					
Sea Salt w/ Sea Veg	¼ tsp	0	0	0	0
Morton					
Iodized	¼ tsp	0	0	0	0

FOOD	PORTION	CALS	CARB	SUGAR	FIBER
Ocean's Flavor					
Natural Sea Salt	¼ tsp	0	0	0	0
Spice Hunter					
Celery Salt	¼ tsp	0	0	0	0
Garlic Salt	¼ tsp	0	0	0	0

SANDWICHES

FOOD	PORTION	CALS	CARB	SUGAR	FIBER
Alexia					
Panini Tuscan Four Cheese w/ Roasted Tomato & Basil	1 pkg (6 oz)	380	42	5	6
Panini Tuscan Grilled Chicken w/ Mozzarella	1 pkg (6 oz)	400	37	2	5
Panini Tuscan Grilled Steak w/ Mushrooms & Onions	1 pkg (6 oz)	370	43	9	5
Panini Tuscan Smoked Chicken w/ Fire Roasted Vegetables & Parmesan	1 pkg (6 oz)	410	37	3	5
Aunt Jemima					
Biscuit Sausage Egg & Cheese	1 (4 oz)	340	27	2	1
Croissant Sausage Egg & Cheese	1 (4 oz)	350	22	3	1
Griddlecake Sausage Egg & Cheese	1 (4.4 oz)	350	30	11	tr
Aunt Trudy's					
Classic Samosa Fillo Pocket	1 (5 oz)	280	43	1	3
Fillo Pocket Cheese & Tomato	1 (5 oz)	320	36	1	2
Fillo Pocket Mediterranean Olive & Veggies	1 (5 oz)	270	41	1	2
Organic Fillo Pocket Roasted Sweet Potato	1 (5 oz)	310	45	0	4
Cedarlane					
Wrap Low Fat Couscous & Vegetable Veggie	1 (6 oz)	220	36	2	3
Fillo Factory					
Organic Fillo Pocket Asian Vegetable	1 (5 oz)	240	34	2	3
Gardenburger					
Pizza Wrap 100% Meatless Margherita	1 (4.7 oz)	240	34	3	5
Wrap Black Bean Chipotle	1 (4.7 oz)	240	32	2	6

FOOD	PORTION	CALS	CARB	SUGAR	FIBER
Guiltless Gourmet					
Wrap Black Bean Chipotle	1 (5.7 oz)	270	51	6	7
Wrap California Veggie	1 (5.7 oz)	300	53	2	6
Wrap Mediterranean Spinach	1 (5.7 oz)	270	45	4	4
Hot Pockets					
Bacon Egg & Cheese	1 (2.2 oz)	160	17	4	1
Barbecue Beef	1 (4.5 oz)	310	42	11	1
Biscuit Sausage Egg & Cheese	1 (4.5 oz)	270	32	7	2
Calzone Four Meat & Four Cheese	½ (4.2 oz)	300	35	13	2
Calzone Pepperoni & Three Cheese	½ (4.2 oz)	330	39	14	2
Chicken Melt	1 (4.5 oz)	300	36	8	1
Croissant Chicken Parmesan	1 (4.5 oz)	340	41	10	3
Croissant Turkey Bacon Club	1 (4.5 oz)	320	34	10	1
Ham & Cheese	1 (4.5 oz)	290	36	9	1
Meatballs & Mozzarella	1 (4.5 oz)	300	36	7	2
Philly Steak & Cheese	1 (4.5 oz)	270	34	6	2
Steak Fajita	1 (4.5 oz)	280	33	8	2
Turkey & Ham w/ Cheese	1 (4.5 oz)	280	35	8	1
Ian's					
Mini Chicken Patty	2 (5.3 oz)	368	54	6	1
Jimmy Dean					
Bagel Sausage Egg & Cheese	1 (4.8 oz)	380	34	3	1
Biscuit Sausage Egg & Cheese	1 (4.5 oz)	440	27	5	1
Croissant Sausage Egg & Cheese	1 (4.5 oz)	430	30	6	1
D-Lights Croissants Turkey Sausage Egg White & Cheese	1 (4.8 oz)	300	31	4	4
D-Lights Honey Wheat Muffin Canadian Bacon Egg White & Cheese	1 (4.5 oz)	230	30	3	2
Muffin Sausage Egg & Cheese	1 (4.6 oz)	350	28	3	1
Lean Pockets					
Bacon Egg & Cheese	1 (2.2 oz)	150	18	3	1
Barbecue Beef	1 (4.5 oz)	290	46	11	2
Chicken Cheddar & Broccoli	1 (4.5 oz)	260	40	11	2
Chicken Fajita	1 (4.5 oz)	240	35	6	3
Chicken Parmesan	1 (4.5 oz)	290	45	5	3
Ham & Cheese	1 (4.5 oz)	270	39	11	2

FOOD	PORTION	CALS	CARB	SUGAR	FIBER
Meatballs & Mozzarella	1 (4.5 oz)	260	35	9	4
Philly Steak & Cheese	1 (4.5 oz)	270	38	8	1
Sausage Egg & Cheese	1 (2.2 oz)	140	18	6	1
Steak Fajita	1 (4.5 oz)	250	36	8	4
Three Cheese & Chicken Quesadilla	1 (4.5 oz)	260	34	6	3
Turkey & Ham w/ Cheddar	1 (4.5 oz)	280	40	9	2
Turkey Broccoli & Cheese	1 (4.5 oz)	270	39	12	2
Lunchables					
Chicken Dunks	1 pkg	310	52	35	0
Stackers Ham & American	1 pkg	430	56	36	tr
Stackers Turkey & American	1 pkg	420	55	39	tr
Madalena's Masterpiece					
Calzone Artichoke Parmesan	1 (10 oz)	570	51	6	2
Calzone Grilled Chicken	1 (10 oz)	520	43	5	1
Calzone Sausage Pepperoni	1 (10 oz)	640	48	6	tr
Panini Garlic Chicken	1 (8 oz)	450	42	5	2
Panini Honey Ham	1 (8 oz)	520	46	7	tr
Panini Turkey Pesto	1 (8 oz)	500	43	4	0
Panini Veggie	1 (8 oz)	480	43	5	1
Quesabake Mexican Sausage	1 (7 oz)	510	48	2	2
Quesabake Roasted Veggie	1 (7 oz)	460	47	tr	1
Oscar Mayer					
Deli Creations Honey Ham & Swiss	1 pkg (6.8 oz)	440	51	15	4
Deli Creations Steakhouse Cheddar	1 pkg (7.1 oz)	450	50	14	3
Deli Creations Turkey & Cheddar Dijon	1 pkg (6.7 oz)	430	48	12	5
PBJammerz					
Peanut Butter & Jelly All Flavors	1 (2 oz)	220	22	10	3
Pillsbury					
Toaster Scrambles Cheese Egg & Bacon	1 (1.6 oz)	180	15	1	0
Toaster Scrambles Cheese Egg & Sausage	1 (1.6 oz)	180	15	1	0
South Beach					
Breakfast Wraps All American	1 serv (4.6 oz)	200	26	2	15
Breakfast Wraps Denver	1 serv (4.6 oz)	180	27	3	15

FOOD	PORTION	CALS	CARB	SUGAR	FIBER
Wrap Kit Deli Ham & Turkey	1 pkg	220	23	0	15
Wrap Kit Grilled Chicken Caesar	1 pkg	230	23	1	14
Wrap Kit Southwestern Style Chicken	1 pkg	250	26	2	15
Wrap Kit Turkey & Bacon Club	1 pkg	250	24	1	15
Stouffer's					
Corner Bistro Panini Philly Style Steak & Cheese	1 pkg (6 oz)	340	33	3	3
Corner Bistro Panini Southwestern Chicken	1 pkg (6 oz)	360	31	2	3
Van's					
Breakfast In A Pocket Sandwich Ham Egg & Cheese	1 (4.5 oz)	370	30	3	tr
Breakfast In A Pocket Sandwich Veggie Egg & Cheese	1 (4.5 oz)	340	31	3	1
Breakfast Panini Huevos Rancheros	1 (4.5 oz)	270	33	2	5
Breakfast Panini Sausage Egg & Cheese	1 (4.5 oz)	290	28	1	3
TAKE-OUT					
bacon & egg	1 (6.2 oz)	388	28	4	1
bacon lettuce & tomato w/ mayo	1 (5.8 oz)	344	35	5	3
beef barbecue w/ bun	1 (6.7 oz)	417	42	6	2
calzone beef & cheese	1 (14 oz)	1476	131	1	6
calzone cheese	1 (15 oz)	1632	117	2	5
chicken salad	1 (5 oz)	333	28	3	2
crab cake w/ bun	1	308	36	4	2
crispy chicken fillet w/ lettuce tomato & mayo	1 (7.7 oz)	537	49	tr	3
croque monsieur	1 (12.4 oz)	765	43	9	2
egg salad	1 (5.6 oz)	485	28	3	1
french dip w/ roll	1 (6.8 oz)	357	34	4	1
fried egg	1 (3.4 oz)	226	26	3	1
grilled cheese	1 (2.9 oz)	290	28	4	1
gyro	1 (13.7 oz)	593	74	8	4
ham & egg	1 (4.4 oz)	272	27	3	2
ham w/ cheese lettuce & mayo	1 (5.4 oz)	369	32	4	2
hot turkey w/ gravy	1	389	32	2	2

FOOD	PORTION	CALS	CARB	SUGAR	FIBER
peanut butter & banana	1	617	43	11	4
peanut butter & jelly	1 (3.3 oz)	327	42	12	3
reuben w/ sauerkraut & cheese	1 (6.4 oz)	463	30	7	4
roast beef w/ gravy	1 (7.8 oz)	386	30	2	2
sloppy joe pork on bun	1 (6.5 oz)	318	34	6	2
tuna melt	1 (5.3 oz)	350	30	6	1
tuna salad w/ lettuce	1 (5.9 oz)	289	37	6	2
turkey w/ mayo	1 (5 oz)	329	26	2	1

SARDINES
CANNED

FOOD	PORTION	CALS	CARB	SUGAR	FIBER
atlantic in oil w/ bone	1 can (3.2 oz)	192	0	0	0
atlantic in oil w/ bone	2	50	0	0	0
pacific in tomato sauce w/ bone	1	68	0	0	0
pacific in tomato sauce w/ bone	1 can (13 oz)	658	0	0	0
Beach Cliff					
In Louisiana Hot Sauce	1 can (3.7 oz)	150	2	0	0
In Mustard Sauce	1 can (3.7 oz)	150	2	0	0
In Olive Oil	1 can (3.7 oz)	200	0	0	0
In Tomato Sauce	1 can (3.7 oz)	140	2	1	0
In Water	1 can (3.7 oz)	150	0	0	0
Small In Soybean Oil	1 can (3.7 oz)	200	1	0	0
W/ Hot Green Chilies	1 can (3.7 oz)	180	1	0	0
Brunswick					
In Louisiana Hot Sauce	1 can (3.7 oz)	150	2	0	0
In Mustard Sauce	1 can (3.7 oz)	150	2	0	0
In Soybean Oil	1 can (3.7 oz)	110	1	0	0
In Spring Water	1 can (3.7 oz)	150	0	0	0
In Tomato Sauce	1 can (3.7 oz)	150	3	2	0
W/ Hot Tabasco Peppers	1 can (3.7 oz)	110	0	0	0
Bumble Bee					
In Hot Sauce	¼ cup	90	0	0	0
In Mustard	¼ cup	70	1	1	1
In Oil	1 can (3.7 oz)	130	0	0	0
In Water	1 can (3.7 oz)	120	0	0	0
King Oscar					
In Olive Oil	1 can (3.75 oz)	150	0	0	0
Polar					
In Mustard	1 can (4.5 oz)	170	10	1	0
In Tomato Sauce	1 can (4.5 oz)	120	5	tr	0
In Water	1 can (3 oz)	100	tr	tr	0

FOOD	PORTION	CALS	CARB	SUGAR	FIBER
FRESH					
raw	3.5 oz	135	0	0	0
SAUCE (see also BARBECUE SAUCE, GRAVY, SPAGHETTI SAUCE)					
adobo fresco	2 tbsp	81	7	tr	1
enchilada sauce green	¼ cup	46	3	2	1
enchilada sauce red	¼ cup	79	2	1	1
fish sauce chinese	1 tbsp	9	tr	–	0
fish sauce vietnamese nuoc mam	1 tbsp	6	1	–	0
hoisin	1 tbsp	35	7	–	tr
morroccan tagine	½ cup (4 oz)	70	10	10	1
oyster	1 tbsp	8	2	–	0
plum sauce	0.5 oz	42	10	10	0
satay peanut sauce	1 oz	77	3	3	1
A Taste Of Thai					
Chili Sauce Garlic Pepper	1 tsp	10	2	2	0
Chili Sauce Sweet Red	1 tsp	10	2	2	0
Pad Thai Sauce Mix	2 tbsp	90	20	16	1
Peanut Satay	2 tbsp	80	9	5	1
Peanut Sauce Mix	¼ pkg	45	7	5	1
Ahh!Gourmet					
Perky Savory Coffee Sauce	4 tbsp	71	17	15	tr
Ritzy Kumquat Plum Sauce	4 tbsp	98	24	21	1
Spicy Garlicky Sweet Sauce Paste	4 tbsp	101	16	13	2
Spicy Ginger Soy Sauce Paste	4 tbsp	137	15	13	2
Annie Chun's					
Marinade & Dressing Lemongrass Herb	1 tbsp	25	4	3	0
Noodle Sauce & Dressing Sesame Cilantro	1 tbsp	60	4	4	0
Shiitake Mushroom	1 tbsp	15	3	2	0
Asian Creations					
Marvelous Mango	¼ cup	20	6	5	0
Pad Thai Pizzazz	2 oz	110	14	9	tr
Peanut Passion	¼ cup	130	12	7	1
Bear-Man					
Sap-Happy Golden Bear	2 tbsp	60	20	17	0
Boar's Head					
Ham Glaze Sugar & Spice	2 tbsp	120	30	29	0

FOOD	PORTION	CALS	CARB	SUGAR	FIBER
Bone Suckin'					
Hiccuppin' Hot	1 tsp	10	2	2	0
Yaki Stir Fry	1 tbsp	30	7	6	0
Cains					
Tartar	2 tbsp	160	2	1	0
China Pride					
Duck Sauce Sweet & Pungent	2 tbsp	80	19	11	1
Dei Fratelli					
Sloppy Joe Sauce	¼ cup (2.2 oz)	35	9	5	1
Emeril's					
Kicked Up Red Sauce	1 tsp	0	0	0	0
Fage					
Tzatziki	2 tbsp	30	2	2	0
Frank's					
Buffalo Wing Sauce	1 tbsp	5	0	0	0
RedHot Chile & Lime Sauce	1 tsp	0	0	0	0
RedHot Original Cayenne Pepper Sauce	1 tsp	0	0	0	0
RedHot X-tra Hot	1 tsp	0	0	0	0
French's					
Worchestershire	1 tsp	0	1	0	0
Good Clean Food					
Simmer Sauce Balsamic Mushroom	⅜ cup (3 oz)	100	9	4	tr
Simmer Sauce Cacciatore	⅜ cup (3 oz)	70	7	4	2
Simmer Sauce Creole	⅜ cup (3 oz)	45	7	4	1
Simmer Sauce French Tarragon	⅜ cup (3 oz)	90	8	2	tr
Simmer Sauce Mediterranean	⅜ cup (3 oz)	50	6	2	1
House Of Tsang					
General Tsao	1 tsp	45	10	7	0
Hoisin	1 tsp	15	4	3	0
Kobe Steak Grill	1 tbsp	50	2	2	0
Korean Teriyaki Stir Fry	1 tbsp	35	5	4	0
Peanut Sauce Bangkok Padang	1 tbsp	45	4	3	0
Spicy Brown Bean	1 tbsp	15	3	2	0
Sweet & Sour	1 tbsp	35	8	7	0
Sweet Ginger Sesame	1 tbsp	40	8	7	0
Thai Peanut	1 tbsp	50	4	4	0
Ken's					
Marinade Herb & Garlic	1 tbsp	20	3	2	0

FOOD	PORTION	CALS	CARB	SUGAR	FIBER
Marinade Lemon & Pepper	1 tbsp	10	2	1	0
Marinade Teriyaki	1 tbsp	20	4	3	0
La Choy					
Sweet & Sour	2 tbsp (1.2 oz)	60	14	11	0
Teriyaki	1 tbsp (0.6 oz)	40	10	8	0
Las Palmas					
Enchilada Green	¼ cup	25	3	1	0
Enchilada Mild	¼ cup	20	2	0	1
Red Chili	¼ cup	20	2	0	1
Latino Chef					
Chimichurri Sun Dried Tomato	2 tbsp	120	8	5	2
Lollipop Tree					
Grilling & Glazing Chipotle	1 tbsp	50	14	13	0
Grilling & Glazing Mango Garlic	2 tbsp	60	14	13	0
Manwich					
Sloppy Joe Original	¼ cup (2.2 oz)	30	7	5	1
Milo's					
Simmer Sauce Bombay Cabernet	3 oz	35	7	3	1
Nando's					
Curry Coconut	¼ cup	71	6	3	1
Fresh Lemon	¼ cup	61	5	2	0
Marinade Lime & Cilantro	1 tbsp	27	2	1	0
Marinade Sundried Tomato	1 tbsp	15	1	1	0
Roasted Red	¼ cup	70	7	4	1
Sweet Apricot	¼ cup	51	12	7	0
Naturally Fresh					
Seafood Cocktail	2 tbsp	25	5	5	0
Tartar Sauce	2 tbsp	130	2	2	0
Newman's Own					
Fra Diavolo	½ cup	70	10	4	3
Steak Sauce	1 tbsp	20	4	1	0
Old El Paso					
Enchilada Mild	¼ cup	25	4	1	0
Ortega					
Enchilada	¼ cup	15	4	tr	tr
Pace					
Taco Sauce Green	1 tbsp	5	1	1	0
Taco Sauce Red	2 tbsp	10	2	1	0

FOOD	PORTION	CALS	CARB	SUGAR	FIBER
Patak's					
Dopiaza	½ cup	90	11	8	0
Jalfrezi Sweet Peppers & Coconut	½ cup	140	15	10	1
Korma Rich Creamy Coconut	½ cup	240	13	9	1
Rogan Josh Spicy Tomato & Cardamon	½ cup	90	12	6	2
Tikka Masala Tangy Lemon & Cilantro	½ cup	120	12	6	1
Road's End Organics					
Alfredo Style Dairy Free Gluten Free	⅓ pkg	35	5	0	1
Cheddar Style Dairy Free	⅓ pkg	35	6	0	1
Robert Rothchild Farm					
Anne Mae's Smoky Sweet Chipotle	2 tbsp	35	9	8	0
Simply Boulder					
Coconut Peanut	2 tbsp (1 oz)	90	6	5	0
Lemon Pesto	2 tbsp (1 oz)	50	3	2	0
Zesty Pineapple	2 tbsp (1 oz)	45	7	5	0
South Beach					
Steak Sauce	1 tbsp	5	1	1	0
Soy Vay					
Hoisin Garlic Asian Glaze & Marinade	1 tbsp	40	7	7	0
Veri Veri Teriyaki	1 tbsp	35	6	5	0
Tabasco					
Pepper Sauce	1 tsp	0	0	0	0
The Wizard's					
Organic Worcestershire Vegetarian Wheat Free	1 tsp	0	1	tr	0
Wild Thymes Farm					
Marinade Hawaiian Teryaki	1 tbsp	19	3	2	tr
Marinade Korean Ginger Scallion	1 tbsp	20	3	2	tr
Marinade New Orleans Creole	1 tbsp	11	3	1	tr
WildWood					
Aioli	1 tbsp	80	0	0	0
Pesto Basil & Pine Nuts	¼ cup	230	2	0	1

FOOD	PORTION	CALS	CARB	SUGAR	FIBER
Wingers					
Hotter Than Hot	1 tsp	0	0	0	0
Zatarain's					
Cocktail	¼ cup	70	17	13	0
Etouffee Base as prep	½ cup	35	7	0	1
TAKE-OUT					
cucumber yogurt sauce	1½ tbsp	20	3	—	0
SAUERKRAUT					
Ba-Tampte					
Kosher	2 tbsp (1 oz)	5	1	0	1
Boar's Head					
Sauerkraut	2 tbsp (1 oz)	5	1	0	tr
Dei Fratelli					
Sauerkraut	2 tbsp (1 oz)	5	1	0	tr
Eden					
Organic	½ cup	25	4	1	3
Gedney					
Sauerkraut	½ cup	15	3	0	0
Tree Of Life					
Organic	½ cup (3.6 oz)	15	3	0	<3
SAUSAGE					
beef & pork	1 link (2.3 oz)	196	1	0	0
beef & pork w/ cheddar cheese	1 link (2.7 oz)	228	2	tr	0
bierwurst	3.5 oz	258	0	0	0
blutwurst uncooked	3.5 oz	424	0	0	0
bockwurst	3.5 oz	276	0	0	0
bratwurst chicken cooked	1 (3 oz)	148	0	0	0
bratwurst pork cooked	1 link (2.5 oz)	226	2	2	0
bratwurst pork & beef	1 link (2.5 oz)	226	2	2	0
chipolata	3.5 oz	342	1	1	0
chorizo	1 link (2.1 oz)	273	1	0	0
fleischwurst	3.5 oz	305	0	0	0
free range chicken breakfast	2 links (2.7 oz)	110	1	1	0
gelbwurst uncooked	3.5 oz	363	0	0	0
italian pork cooked	1 (2.4 oz)	230	3	1	1
jagdwurst	3.5 oz	211	0	0	0
knockwurst pork & beef	1 (2.5 oz)	221	2	0	0
mettwurst uncooked	3.5 oz	483	0	0	0
plockwurst uncooked	3.5 oz	312	0	0	0

FOOD	PORTION	CALS	CARB	SUGAR	FIBER
polish kielbasa	2 oz	127	2	0	0
pork cooked	2 links (1.7 oz)	163	0	0	0
regensburger uncooked	3.5 oz	354	0	0	0
turkey italian smoked	1 (2 oz)	88	3	2	1
vienna canned	1 can (4 oz)	260	3	0	0
vienna canned	1 link (0.5 oz)	37	tr	0	0
weisswurst uncooked	3.5 oz	305	0	0	0
zungenwurst (tongue)	3.5 oz	285	0	0	0
Applegate Farms					
Organic Andouille	1 (3 oz)	120	3	1	1
Organic Spinach & Feta	1 (3 oz)	120	2	0	0
Armour					
Sizzle & Serve Turkey	3 (1.8 oz)	130	2	1	0
Banquet					
Brown 'N Serve Lite Maple	3 (2 oz)	130	4	2	0
Brown 'N Serve Lite Original	3 (2.1 oz)	120	2	1	0
Boar's Head					
Bratwurst	1 (4 oz)	300	0	0	0
Hot Smoked	1 (3.2 oz)	250	1	0	0
Kielbasa	2 oz	120	0	0	0
Knockwurst Beef	1 (4 oz)	310	1	0	0
Butterball					
Breakfast Turkey	3 (3 oz)	130	0	0	0
Polska Kielbasa Turkey	2 oz	100	4	1	0
Healthy Ones					
Smoked	2 oz	80	6	2	0
Honeysuckle White					
Turkey Roll Mild Italian	2.5 oz	100	1	0	0
Jimmy Dean					
Fully Cooked Original Links	3 (2.4 oz)	240	1	1	0
Fully Cooked Original Patties	2 (2.4 oz)	240	1	2	0
Fully Cooked Turkey Links	3 (2.4 oz)	120	1	1	0
Fully Cooked Turkey Patties	2 (2.4 oz)	120	1	1	0
Original Links	3 (2 oz)	170	1	1	0
Original Patties cooked	2 (2.4 oz)	240	1	0	0
Pork All Natural cooked	2 oz	190	1	1	0
Pork Light cooked	2 oz	140	1	0	0
Johnsonville					
Original Summer	1 (2 oz)	170	1	0	0
Smoked Turkey	1 (3 oz)	110	4	2	0

FOOD	PORTION	CALS	CARB	SUGAR	FIBER
Libby's					
Vienna Sausage BBQ	3	140	4	2	1
Organic Prairie					
Bratwurst Pork	1 (3 oz)	210	1	0	0
Shady Brook					
Turkey Breakfast	1 (2.3 oz)	80	0	0	0
Wampler					
Bratwurst as prep	1 (2.5 oz)	230	0	0	0
Breakfast Links as prep	2 (1.2 oz)	130	0	0	0
Breakfast Patties as prep	1 (1.1 oz)	120	0	0	0
Italian as prep	1 (2.5 oz)	230	0	0	0
Wellshire					
Andouille	1 link (3 oz)	197	4	0	0
Andouille Turkey	2 oz	59	1	1	0
Chorizo	1 piece (2 oz)	130	2	0	0
Chorizo Dried	1 oz	100	1	0	0
Italian Turkey Mild	1 link (2 oz)	70	1	0	0
Kielbasa Polska	1 piece (2 oz)	130	2	0	0
Kielbasa Turkey	1 piece (2 oz)	59	1	1	0
Turkey Maple Breakfast	1 link (2 oz)	70	1	0	0

SAUSAGE DISHES
TAKE-OUT

sausage roll	1 (2.3 oz)	311	22	–	1

SAUSAGE SUBSTITUTES

meatless	1 link (0.9 oz)	64	2	0	1
meatless	1 patty (1.3 oz)	98	4	0	1
Boca					
Bratwurst	1 (2.5 oz)	140	6	1	1
Breakfast Links	2 (1.6 oz)	70	5	2	2
Breakfast Patties	1 (1.3 oz)	60	5	1	2
Italian	1 (2.5 oz)	130	6	2	1
Gardenburger					
Veggie Breakfast	1 patty (1.5 oz)	45	3	0	2
Lightlife					
Gimme Lean	2 oz	50	4	1	2
Smart Brats	1 (2 oz)	120	5	0	1
Smart Links Breakfast	2 (2 oz)	100	8	2	4
Smart Links Italian	1 (2 oz)	120	7	2	3
Smart Menu Breakfast Patty	1	45	3	0	1

FOOD	PORTION	CALS	CARB	SUGAR	FIBER
Morningstar Farms					
Breakfast Patties	1 (1.3 oz)	80	4	tr	1
Tofurky					
Turkey Beerbrats	1 (3.5 oz)	280	8	1	5
Turkey Breakfast Links	1 (1.6 oz)	130	6	1	4
Turkey Italian Sweet	1 (3.5 oz)	280	12	3	8
Turkey Kielbasa	1 (3.5 oz)	240	12	2	8
Worthington					
Saucettes Breakfast Links	1 (1.3 oz)	90	1	0	1
Yves					
Veggie Brats Classic	1 (3.3 oz)	160	5	2	1
SAVORY					
ground	1 tsp	4	1	–	tr
SCALLOP					
Mrs. Paul's					
Fried	13 (3.7 oz)	260	28	3	tr
SCONE					
King Arthur					
English Cream Tea Scone not prep	⅓ cup	180	38	10	tr
TAKE-OUT					
blueberry	1 (3 oz)	270	41	7	2
cheese	1 (3.5 oz)	364	44	–	2
orange poppy	1 (3 oz)	260	47	12	2
plain	1 (3.5 oz)	362	54	–	2
raisin	1 (3 oz)	270	43	12	2
SCUP					
fresh baked	3 oz	115	0	0	0
SEA BASS (see BASS)					
SEA CUCUMBER					
dried	1 oz	74	1	–	0
fresh	1 oz	20	tr	–	0
SEA TROUT (see TROUT)					
SEA URCHIN					
canned	1 oz	39	3	–	0
fresh	1 oz	36	3	–	tr

FOOD	PORTION	CALS	CARB	SUGAR	FIBER
roe paste	1 tbsp	19	3	–	0
SEAWEED					
hijiki dried	1 tbsp	9	2	–	1
nori sheet dried	1 (8 x 8 in)	5	1	–	1
seahair dried	1 tbsp	13	3	–	tr
Eden					
Agar Agar Bars	1 bar (7 g)	25	5	0	5
Agar Agar Flakes	1 tbsp	0	1	0	1
Arame Wild	½ cup	30	7	0	7
Hiziki Wild	½ cup	30	6	0	6
Kombu Wild	½ piece (3.3 g)	5	1	0	1
Nori Sheets	1 (2.5 g)	10	0	0	0
Organic Dulse Flakes	1 tsp	3	0	0	0
SEITAN (see WHEAT)					
SEMOLINA					
dry	1 cup (5.9 oz)	601	122	–	7
SESAME					
sesame butter	1 tbsp	95	4	–	1
Arrowhead Mills					
Organic Seeds	¼ cup	210	3	0	1
Organic Tahini	2 tbsp	190	3	1	tr
Mrs. May's					
Black Sesame Crunch	1 oz	165	14	5	4
Peloponnese					
Tahini	1 tbsp	100	2	0	1
Sabra					
Tahini Sauce Taratore	1 oz	80	1	0	0
Tree Of Life					
Organic Sesame Tahini	2 tbsp	108	8	–	5
Seeds	¼ cup (1.3 oz)	210	8	0	3
SHAD					
american baked	3 oz	214	0	0	0
cooked	1 oz	55	1	tr	0
SHALLOTS (see ONION)					
SHARK					
raw	3 oz	111	0	0	0

FOOD	PORTION	CALS	CARB	SUGAR	FIBER
SHEEPSHEAD FISH					
cooked	1 fillet (6.5 oz)	234	0	0	0
cooked	3 oz	107	0	0	0
raw	3 oz	92	0	0	0
SHELLFISH (see individual names, SHELLFISH SUBSTITUTES)					
SHELLFISH SUBSTITUTES					
crab imitation	1 cup (4.4 oz)	144	16	0	tr
TAKE-OUT					
crab salad	1 cup	395	21	1	1
SHERBET					
Blue Bunny					
Cool Tubes Orange Sherbet	1 (3 oz)	110	24	20	0
Lime	½ cup	110	25	20	0
Rainbow	½ cup	110	25	20	0
Raspberry	½ cup	110	26	20	0
Ciao Bella					
Mango	1 pkg (3.5 oz)	100	25	24	1
Raspberry	1 pkg (3.5 oz)	110	28	25	2
Dippin' Dots					
Lemon Lime	½ cup	97	22	19	0
Hola Fruta					
Bar Pomegranate & Blueberry	1 (2.5 oz)	100	22	14	0
Mango	½ cup	130	31	20	0
Margarita	½ cup	140	30	21	0
Peach	½ cup	130	30	19	0
Pomegranate	½ cup	140	32	21	0
Hood					
Orange Burst	½ cup	120	27	20	0
Land O Lakes					
Orange	½ cup (3.2 oz)	130	28	27	1
Turkey Hill					
Fruit Rainbow	½ cup	120	26	17	0
Orange Grove	½ cup	120	26	18	0
SHRIMP					
CANNED					
canned	1 can (6 oz)	136	1	0	0
chinese shrimp paste	1 tbsp	46	10	8	tr

FOOD	PORTION	CALS	CARB	SUGAR	FIBER
Bumble Bee					
Broken Shrimp	¼ cup	40	0	1	0
Medium Or Large Or Jumbo	¼ cup	40	0	1	0
Small	¼ cup	40	0	1	0
Tiny	¼ cup	40	0	1	0
Polar					
Tiny Peeled	¼ cup (2 oz)	44	1	1	0
DRIED					
dried	10	15	tr	0	0
FRESH					
broiled	6 med	46	tr	0	0
steamed	6 med	41	tr	0	0
FROZEN					
Blue Horizon Organic					
Garlic Shrimp	1 serv (3.5 oz)	160	21	0	1
Panko Shrimp	1 serv (3.5 oz)	160	22	0	1
Popcorn Shrimp	1 serv (3.5 oz)	160	21	0	1
Tempura Shrimp	1 serv (3.5 oz)	160	21	0	1
Contessa					
Orange Shrimp	11 to 13 (6 oz)	250	33	12	5
Ragin' Cajun	8 to 10 (4 oz)	170	9	0	3
Shrimp Scampi	8 to 10 (4 oz)	290	4	1	2
Gorton's					
Popcorn Crunchy Golden	20 (3.2 oz)	240	24	2	0
Temptations Breaded Butterfly	5 (3.5 oz)	250	27	4	4
Mrs. Paul's					
Butterfly	7 (4 oz)	250	27	3	1
Van de Kamp's					
Battered	6 (4 oz)	200	22	tr	1
Breaded Popcorn	20 (4 oz)	260	30	3	2
TAKE-OUT					
breaded & fried	6 med (2.3 oz)	162	8	tr	tr
cocktail w/ sauce	4 shrimp	87	7	4	2
curried	1 cup	295	14	8	tr
jambalaya	1 cup	309	28	2	1
scampi	1 cup	310	1	tr	0
shrimp newburg	1 serv (6.4 oz)	456	8	tr	tr
shrimp salad	¾ cup	212	4	1	1
shrimp w/ crab stuffing	5	158	5	tr	tr

FOOD	PORTION	CALS	CARB	SUGAR	FIBER
SMELT					
rainbow cooked	3 oz	106	0	0	0
rainbow raw	3 oz	83	0	0	0
SMOOTHIES (see also FRUIT DRINKS, YOGURT DRINKS)					
8th Continent					
Refresher Orange Pineapple Banana	8 oz	150	30	29	0
Refresher Strawberry Banana	8 oz	150	30	29	0
Arthur's					
Carrot Energizer	1 bottle (11 oz)	200	47	37	3
Green Energy	1 bottle (11 oz)	230	53	39	3
Bolthouse Farms					
Green Goodness	8 oz	140	33	27	1
Mango Lemonade	8 oz	120	30	30	tr
Passion Fruit Apple Carrot Juice	8 oz	120	29	28	2
C&W					
Berry Blend	½ cup	90	15	11	2
Peach	½ cup	80	15	12	1
E4B					
100% Fruit Puree Blueberry Raspberry	4 oz	70	18	14	3
100% Fruit Puree Kiwi	4 oz	70	16	13	1
100% Fruit Puree Mango	4 oz	70	18	16	1
100% Fruit Puree Pear Caramel	4 oz	70	18	16	1
100% Fruit Puree Strawberry Banana	4 oz	70	18	16	1
Horizon Organic					
Tropical Punch	1 bottle (6.2 oz)	120	25	23	1
Jammin' Juice					
Mambo Mango	6 oz	92	25	24	1
Jammin' Nectars					
C-Beta Carrot	6 oz	96	23	21	1
Ginger Party	6 oz	6	19	17	1
Guanabana Limbo	6 oz	78	20	18	2
Pure Passion	6 oz	78	20	18	1
Razz-Ade	6 oz	89	21	20	1

FOOD	PORTION	CALS	CARB	SUGAR	FIBER
Kidz Dream					
Orange Cream	1 box	120	21	17	tr
LightFull					
Satiety Smoothie Cafe Latte	1 (11 oz)	90	39	10	5
Satiety Smoothie Chocolate Fudge	1 (11 oz)	90	39	10	6
Satiety Smoothie Peaches & Cream	1 (11 oz)	100	41	13	6
Satiety Smoothie Strawberries & Cream	1 (11 oz)	90	40	10	6
Luna					
Berry Pomegranate	1 pkg	140	30	12	2
Orange Blossom	1 pkg	130	30	12	3
Vanilla Macadamia	1 pkg	150	28	8	3
Nutiva					
Organic HempShake Amazon Acai not prep	4 tbsp	100	15	3	8
Organic HempShake Chocolate not prep	4 tbsp	80	19	7	12
Odwalla					
Bluberry B Monster	8 oz	140	33	27	0
Citrus C Monster	8 oz	150	36	27	0
Mango Tango	8 oz	150	34	30	0
Sambazon					
Acai Amazon Cherry	8 oz	156	16	15	1
Acai Mango Banana	8 oz	190	38	29	3
Acai Mango Uprising	8 oz	190	38	29	3
Acai Protein Warrior Chocolate	8 oz	215	33	27	3
Acai Protein Warrior Vanilla	8 oz	215	33	27	3
Acai Shaman's Immunity	8 oz	90	24	22	1
Acai Soy Energy	8 oz	210	25	19	4
Acai Strawberry Sensation	8 oz	210	42	37	2
Acai Supergreens Revolution	8 oz	200	40	29	3
Organic Acai	1 bottle	155	31	22	2
Smooze					
Mango + Coconut	1 box (8.5 oz)	250	33	33	0
Passion Fruit + Coconut	1 box (8.5 oz)	225	33	28	3
Pineapple + Coconut	1 box (8.5 oz)	200	33	23	0

FOOD	PORTION	CALS	CARB	SUGAR	FIBER
Tropicana					
Fruit Smoothie Mixed Berry	1 bottle (11 oz)	220	54	44	2
Fruit Smoothie Tropical Fruit	1 bottle (11 oz)	220	53	42	1
V8					
Splash Tropical Colada	8 oz	100	21	18	1
WholeSoy & Co.					
Organic Soy Peach	8 oz	210	34	29	0
Organic Soy Raspberry	8 oz	210	35	30	0
Organic Soy Strawberry	8 oz	210	34	29	0
SNACKS					
cheese puffs	1 oz	122	21	2	3
pork skins	1 oz	154	0	0	0
Carole's					
Soycrunch Cinnamon & Raisins	½ cup	110	19	12	2
Soycrunch Original	½ cup	120	16	10	2
Soycrunch Toffee	½ cup	110	15	13	2
Cheetos					
Crunchy	1 pkg (1.25 oz)	200	19	1	1
Cheez It					
Right Bites Party Mix	1 pkg (0.74 oz)	100	15	tr	tr
Garden Of Eatin'					
Organic Baked Cheese Puffs	32 pieces	150	15	1	1
Organic Baked Chunchitos	35 pieces	140	18	1	1
Good Sense					
Snack Mix Cajun Corn 'N Sesame	¼ cup	150	17	0	2
Lance					
Cheese Puffs	9 (1 oz)	170	13	1	0
Gold-N-Chees	1 oz	150	17	0	tr
Medora Snacks					
Corners Sea Salt	1 oz	130	22	0	0
Pucci Garlic	1 oz	120	17	2	1
Pucci Tomato Basil	1 oz	120	17	2	1
Sotos Cheese Olive Oil & Lemon	1 oz	120	19	3	2
Michael Season's					
Cheese Puffs & Curls	1½ cups	180	13	3	2

FOOD	PORTION	CALS	CARB	SUGAR	FIBER
Robert's American Gourmet					
Booty Barbeque	1 oz	130	20	1	1
Booty Pirate's	1 oz	130	18	0	1
Booty Veggie	1 oz	130	17	1	1
Smart Puffs	1 oz	130	17	1	0
Tings	1 oz	160	17	0	0
Snikiddy					
Puffs Grilled Cheese	1 pkg (0.6 oz)	80	10	0	1
Puffs Rockin' Ranch	1 pkg (0.6 oz)	83	11	0	1
Snyder's Of Hanover					
CheddAirs	1 oz	130	20	0	tr
MultiGrain Cheese Puffs	1 oz	130	19	2	2
T.G.I. Friday's					
Mozzarella Sticks	20 (1 oz)	150	14	1	1
Tumaro's					
Organic Krispy Crunchy Puffs Cheddar	22	120	21	tr	1
Organic Krispy Crunchy Puffs Natural Corn	22	120	23	0	1
Organic Krispy Crunchy Puffs Ranch & Herb	22	130	20	2	tr
Organic Krispy Crunchy Puffs Tangy BBQ	22	120	21	2	tr
Utz					
Cheese Balls	50 (1 oz)	150	16	tr	tr
Cheese Curls	18 (1 oz)	150	16	tr	tr
Onion Rings	41 (1 oz)	130	20	2	0
Party Mix	1 oz	150	19	tr	1
Pork Cracklins	0.5 oz	90	0	0	0
Pork Rinds Original	0.5 oz	80	0	0	0
Wise					
Cheez Doodles Crunchy	1 pkg (1 oz)	150	17	1	0
Cheez Doodles Crunchy Reduced Fat	1 oz	130	20	2	tr
Cheez Doodles Puffed	1 pkg (0.7 oz)	110	13	1	0
Doodle O's	1 oz	160	14	2	0
Onion Rings	1 oz	140	20	0	0
Pork Rinds Original	1 oz	90	0	0	0

FOOD	PORTION	CALS	CARB	SUGAR	FIBER
SNAIL					
TAKE-OUT					
escargot cooked	5	25	1	–	0
SNAKE					
fresh	3 oz	78	3	–	0
SNAPPER					
cooked	1 fillet (6 oz)	217	0	0	0
cooked	3 oz	109	0	0	0
raw	3 oz	85	0	0	0
SODA					
club	12 oz	0	0	0	0
shirley temple	1 serv	159	41	–	0
Barq's					
Diet French Vanilla Creme	8 oz	1	tr	tr	0
Diet Red Creme	8 oz	4	0	0	0
Diet Root Beer	8 oz	1	tr	tr	0
Floatz	8 oz	127	34	34	0
French Vanilla Creme	8 oz	112	30	30	0
Red Creme	8 oz	115	31	31	0
Root Beer	8 oz	111	30	30	0
Carver's					
Ginger Ale	8 oz	94	24	24	0
Coca-Cola					
Classic	8 oz	97	27	27	0
W/ Lime	8 oz	98	27	27	0
Coke					
Cherry	8 oz	104	28	28	0
Diet	8 oz	1	tr	0	0
Diet Cherry	8 oz	1	tr	tr	0
Diet Plus	8 oz	0	0	0	0
Diet Vanilla	8 oz	1	tr	tr	0
Diet w/ Lime	8 oz	2	tr	tr	0
Vanilla	8 oz	100	28	28	0
Fanta					
Apple	8 oz	121	33	33	0
Citrus	8 oz	91	25	25	0
Orange	8 oz	111	35	35	0
Fresca					
Soda	8 oz	2	tr	tr	0

FOOD	PORTION	CALS	CARB	SUGAR	FIBER
Hiball					
Club	1 bottle (10 oz)	5	0	0	0
Inca Kola					
Diet	8 oz	1	tr	tr	0
Soda	8 oz	96	26	26	0
Jones Soda					
Blue Bubble Gum	1 bottle (12 oz)	190	48	48	0
Cream	1 bottle (12 oz)	190	48	48	0
Crushed Melon	1 bottle (12 oz)	190	48	48	0
FuFu Berry	1 bottle (12 oz)	190	46	46	0
Green Apple	1 bottle (12 oz)	180	46	46	0
Orange Cream	1 bottle (12 oz)	180	46	46	0
Lucozade					
Soda	7 oz	136	36	–	0
Manzana Mia					
Soda	8 oz	99	27	27	0
Mello Yellow					
Diet	8 oz	3	tr	tr	0
Soda	8 oz	118	32	32	0
Mr. Pibb					
Diet	8 oz	1	tr	tr	0
Northern Neck					
Diet Ginger Ale	8 oz	4	0	0	0
Ginger Ale	8 oz	94	24	24	0
Oogave Natural					
All Flavors	8 oz	68	17	17	0
Pibb					
Zero	8 oz	2	tr	tr	0
Polar					
Seltzer All Flavors	8 oz	0	0	0	0
Vichy Water	8 oz	0	0	0	0
Red Flash					
Soda	8 oz	105	28	28	0

FOOD	PORTION	CALS	CARB	SUGAR	FIBER
Reed's					
Ginger Brew Original	1 bottle (12 oz)	145	37	37	0
Sex Kola					
Diet All Flavors	1 bottle (12 oz)	0	0	0	0
Sprite					
Diet Zero	8 oz	0	0	0	0
Soda	8 oz	96	26	26	0
Stirrings					
Ginger Ale	8 oz	120	31	30	0
Tava					
Sparkling Brazilian Samba	8 oz	0	0	0	0
Sparkling Mediterranean Fiesta	8 oz	0	0	0	0
Windy City					
Root Beer	1 bottle (12 oz)	170	43	43	0
SOLE					
cooked	1 fillet (4.5 oz)	148	0	0	0
cooked	3 oz	99	0	0	0
lemon raw	3.5 oz	85	0	0	0
SOUFFLE					
Heavenly Souffle					
Chocolate	1 (2.6 oz)	262	29	26	0
TAKE-OUT					
cheese	1 cup	194	6	3	tr
chicken	1 cup (5.6 oz)	278	9	4	tr
corn	1 cup	257	34	11	3
lime chilled	1 cup	388	48	45	2
seafood	1 cup	245	9	4	tr
spinach	1 cup	124	7	3	1
SOUP					
CANNED					
Allens					
Chicken Broth	1 cup	10	1	1	0
Butterball					
Chicken Broth 99% Fat Free	1 cup	10	2	0	0

FOOD	PORTION	CALS	CARB	SUGAR	FIBER
Campbell's					
25% Less Sodium Chicken Noodle as prep	1 cup	60	8	1	1
25% Less Sodium Cream of Mushroom as prep	1 cup	110	8	1	2
98% Fat Free Cream Of Broccoli as prep	1 cup	70	10	1	2
98% Fat Free Cream Of Celery as prep	1 cup	60	8	1	1
98% Fat Free Cream Of Chicken as prep	1 cup	70	10	1	1
Cheddar Cheese as prep	1 cup	110	12	2	1
Chicken & Stars as prep	1 cup	70	11	1	1
Chicken Alphabet as prep	1 cup	70	12	1	1
Chicken Noodle O's as prep	1 cup	90	15	2	1
Chunky Beef and Country Vegetables	1 cup	150	21	4	4
Chunky Chicken Mushroom Chowder	1 cup	210	19	3	3
Chunky Grilled Chicken w/ Vegetables & Pasta	1 cup	100	15	2	2
Chunky Hearty Vegetable w/ Pasta	1 cup	120	23	7	4
Chunky New England Clam Chowder	1 cup	210	25	2	5
Chunky Roadhouse Beef & Bean Chili	1 cup	230	25	11	8
Chunky Sirloin Burger w/ Country Vegetables	1 cup	180	20	4	4
Curly Noodle as prep	1 cup	80	11	1	1
Double Noodle Chicken as prep	1 cup	110	20	1	1
Goldfish Pasta Meatball as prep	1 cup	90	11	1	1
Healthy Request Chicken Noodle as prep	1 cup	60	8	1	1
Healthy Request Chicken Rice as prep	1 cup	70	13	1	1
Healthy Request Cream Of Chicken as prep	1 cup	80	12	2	1
Healthy Request Italian Style Wedding	1 cup	120	15	3	2

FOOD	PORTION	CALS	CARB	SUGAR	FIBER
Healthy Request Minestrone as prep	1 cup	80	15	4	3
Healthy Request Tomato as prep	1 cup	90	10	10	1
Low Sodium Chicken Broth	1 can	25	1	1	0
Mega Noodle as prep	1 cup	90	15	1	1
Microwavable Bowl Chicken Noodle	1 cup	70	10	0	tr
Microwavable Bowl Vegetable	1 cup	110	22	7	3
Select Beef w/ Roasted Barley	1 cup	130	22	4	2
Select Blended Red Pepper Black Bean	1 cup	110	21	9	4
Select Chicken With Egg Noodles	1 cup	90	12	2	2
Select Harvest Tomato w/ Basil	1 cup	80	18	10	1
Select Honey Roasted Chicken w/ Golden Potatoes	1 cup	110	19	3	3
Select Italian Sausage w/ Pasta & Pepperoni	1 cup	150	18	4	2
Select Italian Style Wedding	1 cup	110	15	5	2
Select Mexican Chicken Tortilla	1 cup	130	19	3	3
Select Potato Broccoli Cheese	1 cup	120	18	2	4
Select Savory Chicken & Long Grain Rice	1 cup	90	15	3	1
Select Split Pea w/ Roasted Ham	1 cup	160	29	5	5
Select Vegetable Beef	1 cup	110	16	2	3
Select Harvest Chicken w/ Egg Noodles	1 cup	120	12	2	1
Select Harvest Light Savory Chicken w/ Vegetables	1 cup	80	15	3	4
Select Harvest Light Southwestern Style Vegetable	1 cup	50	13	4	3
Soup At Hand 25% Less Sodium Chicken w/ Mini Noodles	1 pkg (10.75 oz)	80	11	2	2
Soup At Hand Creamy Chicken	1 pkg (10.75 oz)	130	13	1	4
Soup At Hand Italian Style Wedding	1 pkg (10.75 oz)	90	10	3	2

FOOD	PORTION	CALS	CARB	SUGAR	FIBER
Soup At Hand Vegetable Medley	1 pkg (10.75 oz)	100	19	9	4
Soup At Hand Velvety Potato	1 pkg (10.75 oz)	160	21	5	4
V8 Garden Broccoli	1 cup	80	15	6	3
V8 Golden Butternut Squash	1 cup	140	28	6	3
V8 Sweet Red Pepper	1 cup	120	22	10	4
V8 Tomato Herb	1 cup	90	19	14	3
College Inn					
Chicken Broth Light & Fat Free	1 cup	5	0	0	0
Comfort Care					
Hearty Beef Barley	1 cup (8 oz)	190	23	9	4
Savory Chicken	1 cup (8 oz)	200	25	9	5
Tomato Cheddar Jack	1 cup (8 oz)	90	13	7	5
Gold's					
Borscht Unsalted	1 cup	70	13	11	tr
Hungarian Cabbage	6 oz	70	18	14	2
Health Valley					
Beef Broth Fat Free	1 cup	10	0	0	0
Chicken Broth Fat Free	1 cup	20	0	0	0
Chicken Broth Fat Free No Salt Added	1 cup	35	0	0	0
Chicken Broth Low Fat	1 cup	35	0	0	0
Clam Chowder Manhattan	1 cup	90	13	5	1
Clam Chowder New England	1 cup	110	15	5	0
Corn & Vegetable Fat Free	1 cup	70	17	8	7
Garden Vegetable Fat Free	1 cup	80	18	6	4
Lentil & Carrot Fat Free	1 cup	100	25	7	7
Organic Black Bean	1 cup	130	25	7	5
Organic Cream Of Mushroom	1 cup	90	11	0	0
Organic Minestrone	1 cup	100	20	3	5
Organic Minestrone No Salt Added	1 cup	70	17	5	3
Organic Mushroom Barley	1 cup	70	17	4	3
Organic Mushroom Barley No Salt Added	1 cup	70	17	4	3
Organic Split Pea No Salt Added	1 cup	110	23	5	8
Organic Tomato	1 cup	80	18	14	1
Organic Tomato No Salt Added	1 cup	80	18	14	1

FOOD	PORTION	CALS	CARB	SUGAR	FIBER
Tomato Vegetable Fat Free	1 cup	80	17	9	5
Vegetable Broth Fat Free	1 cup	20	5	1	0
Healthy Choice					
Bean & Ham	1 cup	180	29	4	10
Chicken & Dumplings	1 cup	140	21	2	3
Chicken w/ Rice	1 cup	90	14	tr	2
Country Vegetable	1 cup (8.6 oz)	110	19	4	4
Old Fashioned Chicken Noodle	1 cup	100	13	1	2
Vegetable Beef	1 cup	130	22	5	4
Zesty Gumbo	1 cup	100	16	2	4
Imagine					
Organic Creamy Butternut Squash	1 cup	90	18	7	2
Organic Creamy Chicken	1 cup	70	12	1	1
Organic Creamy Sweet Corn	1 cup	120	20	9	3
Organic Sweet Potato	1 cup	110	23	2	1
Organic Bistro Cuban Black Bean Bisque	1 cup	170	30	4	6
Organic Broth Beef	1 cup	20	1	1	0
Organic Broth Free Range Chicken	1 cup	10	1	0	0
Organic Broth Vegetable	8 oz	20	2	2	0
Lucini					
Roman Tomato Cream	1 cup (8.6 oz)	170	18	10	4
Umbrian Lentil	1 cup (8.6 oz)	160	23	6	9
Muir Glen					
Organic Garden Vegetable	1 cup	80	16	5	3
Organic Southwest Black Bean	1 cup	140	27	4	8
Original SoupMan					
Italian Wedding	1 cup	120	18	4	4
New England Clam Chowder	1 cup	290	16	1	1
Organic Butternut Squash	1 cup	250	33	12	3
Tomato Basil	1 cup	140	18	11	4
Turkey Chili	1 cup	210	18	4	5
Progresso					
40% Less Sodium Italian Style Wedding	1 cup (8.7 oz)	90	11	2	1
50% Less Sodium Garden Vegetable	1 cup (8.8 oz)	100	22	4	3

FOOD	PORTION	CALS	CARB	SUGAR	FIBER
50% Less Sodium Zesty Chicken Gumbo	1 cup (8.7 oz)	110	18	2	2
Light Beef Pot Roast	1 cup (8.4 oz)	80	12	4	2
Light Chicken Vegetable Rotini	1 cup (8.3 oz)	70	10	2	2
Light Italian Style Vegetable	1 cup (8.6 oz)	60	12	3	4
Light Savory Vegetable Barley	1 cup (8.5 oz)	60	14	3	4
Light Vegetable	1 cup (8.4 oz)	60	14	4	4
Light Vegetable & Noodle	1 cup (8.7 oz)	60	12	2	4
Rich & Hearty Beef Pot Roast	1 cup (8.7 oz)	120	20	4	2
Rich & Hearty Chicken & Homestyle Noodles	1 cup (8.6 oz)	100	14	1	1
Rich & Hearty Chicken Pot Pie	1 cup (8.6 oz)	170	21	3	2
Rich & Hearty Savory Beef Barley Vegetable	1 cup (8.6 oz)	130	22	4	3
Rich & Hearty Sirloin Steak & Vegetables	1 cup	130	21	5	2
Rich & Hearty Slow Cooked Vegetable Beef	1 cup (8.6 oz)	120	20	6	3
Rich & Hearty Steak & Roasted Russet Potatoes	1 cup (8.6 oz)	140	23	3	2
Traditional Beef & Vegetable	1 cup (8.7 oz)	120	18	4	2
Traditional Beef Barley	1 cup (8.5 oz)	120	20	3	4
Traditional Chickarina	1 cup (8.3 oz)	120	12	1	2
Traditional Chicken & Sausage Gumbo	1 cup (8.7 oz)	130	18	2	1
Traditional Chicken & Wild Rice	1 cup (8.4 oz)	100	15	1	1
Traditional Chicken Noodle	1 cup (8.3 oz)	100	12	1	1
Traditional Homestyle Chicken	1 cup (8.4 oz)	100	14	1	1
Traditional Italian Style Wedding	1 cup (8.4 oz)	100	12	1	1
Traditional Manhattan Clam Chowder	1 cup (8.4 oz)	100	17	4	2
Traditional New England Clam Chowder	1 cup (8.4 oz)	110	20	2	2
Traditional Potato Broccoli & Cheese	1 cup (8.8 oz)	180	18	2	2
Traditional Split Pea w/ Ham	1 cup (8.5 oz)	140	24	3	4
Traditional Turkey Noodle	1 cup (8.4 oz)	80	12	1	1
Vegetable Classics Creamy Mushroom	1 cup (8.1 oz)	130	9	2	1

FOOD	PORTION	CALS	CARB	SUGAR	FIBER
Vegetable Classics French Onion	1 cup (8 oz)	50	8	3	tr
Vegetable Classics Hearty Black Bean w/ Bacon	1 cup (8.5 oz)	160	29	3	8
Vegetable Classics Hearty Tomato	1 cup (8.6 oz)	110	23	9	3
Vegetable Classics Lentil	1 cup (8.5 oz)	150	28	1	5
Vegetable Classics Vegetable	1 cup (8.4 oz)	80	16	3	2
Rienzi					
Chicken & Rice	1 cup	110	17	2	2
Italian Wedding Bell	1 cup	130	12	2	tr
Snow's					
Clam Chowder	1 cup (8.4 oz)	200	13	3	1
Swanson					
100% Fat Free Lower Sodium Beef Broth	1 cup	15	1	0	0
Organic Beef Broth	1 cup	15	1	0	0
Organic Chicken Broth	1 cup	15	1	1	0
Organic Vegetable Broth	1 cup	15	3	2	0
FROZEN					
Kettle Cuisine					
Angus Beef Steak Chili w/ Beans Gluten Free Dairy Free	1 pkg (10 oz)	250	17	9	4
Chicken w/ Rice Noodles Gluten Free	1 pkg (10 oz)	140	12	3	1
New England Clam Chowder Gluten Free	1 pkg (10 oz)	330	26	6	1
Roasted Vegetable Gluten Free Dairy Free	1 pkg (10 oz)	140	19	4	5
Tabatchnick					
Barley Mushroom	1 serv (7.5 oz)	80	17	1	3
Chicken w/ Dumplings	1 serv (7.5 oz)	150	19	1	tr
Cream Of Broccoli	1 serv (7.5 oz)	130	18	8	2
Macaroni & Cheese	1 serv (7.5 oz)	250	34	4	tr
Minestrone	1 serv (7.5 oz)	100	18	3	4
No Salt Pea	1 serv (7.5 oz)	140	34	0	14
Old Fashioned Potato	1 serv (7.5 oz)	100	21	2	2
Southwest Bean	1 serv (7.5 oz)	220	35	4	9
Split Pea	1 serv (7.5 oz)	140	34	0	13
Vegetable	1 serv (7.5 oz)	90	17	3	4

FOOD	PORTION	CALS	CARB	SUGAR	FIBER
Vegetarian Chili	1 serv (7.5 oz)	180	28	3	8
Wild Rice	1 serv (7.5 oz)	80	16	1	1
MIX					
A Taste Of Thai					
Coconut Ginger	2 tsp	15	2	2	0
Annie Chun's					
Noodle Bowl Chicken Noodle	1 pkg	260	52	1	2
Noodle Bowl Hot & Sour	1 pkg	280	55	1	2
Noodle Bowl Korean Kimchi	½ pkg	140	28	0	1
Noodle Bowl Miso	1 pkg	230	45	1	2
Noodle Bowl Thai Tom Yum	½ pkg	150	30	2	1
Noodle Bowl Udon	1 pkg	220	45	3	1
Edward & Sons					
Bouillon Cubes Not-Beef	½ cube	20	1	tr	0
Bouillon Cubes Not-Chicken	½ cube	15	1	0	0
Veggie Low Sodium	½ cup	20	1	1	0
Fantastic					
Noodle Bowl Hot & Sour as prep	2 cups	138	22	1	1
Noodle Bowl Miso w/ Tofu as prep	1 cup	100	19	2	tr
Noodle Bowl Sesame Miso as prep	2 cups	90	17	1	tr
Noodle Bowl Spring Vegetable as prep	2 cups	90	19	1	tr
Noodle Soup Spicy Thai as prep	2 cups	110	22	3	1
Noodle Soup Cup Vegetarian Chicken as prep	1 cup	90	19	0	1
Soup Cup Italian Tomato as prep	2 cups	130	26	5	2
Soup Cup Mandarin Broccoli as prep	2 cups	110	20	1	2
HamBeens					
15 Bean as prep	½ cup	120	20	1	9
15 Bean Beef as prep	½ cup	120	20	1	9
15 Bean Chicken as prep	½ cup	120	20	1	9
15 Bean Soup Cajun as prep	½ cup	120	20	1	9
Spanish American Black Bean as prep	½ cup	120	22	1	8

FOOD	PORTION	CALS	CARB	SUGAR	FIBER
Health Valley					
Chicken Noodles w/ Vegetables	1 cup	110	24	1	3
Creamy Potato w/ Broccoli Fat Free	1 cup	80	17	2	3
Leahey Gardens					
No Beef Noodle	1½ cups	89	16	tr	6
No Chicken Noodle	1½ cups	94	16	tr	6
Manischewitz					
Lentil as prep	1 cup	150	29	2	12
Matzo Ball Soup	1 cup	40	9	3	1
Southwestern Black Bean as prep	1 cup	90	16	2	4
Split Pea w/ Barley as prep	1 cup	110	21	2	3
Vegetable & Pasta as prep	1 cup	90	17	1	2
Miso-Cup					
Golden Vegetable as prep	1 cup	30	3	1	tr
Japanese Restaurant Style as prep	1 cup	60	7	tr	tr
Organic Traditional w/ Tofu as prep	1 cup	35	4	tr	tr
Reduced Sodium as prep	1 cup	25	3	tr	tr
Savory Seaweed as prep	1 cup	30	3	1	tr
Nissin					
Chicken Vegetable as prep	1 pkg	290	38	2	2
White Cheddar as prep	1 pkg	290	38	1	2
Nueva Cocina					
Frijoles Negros Con Chipotle Chile	1 cup	140	27	2	9
Sopa De Calabaza	1 cup	180	25	7	1
Sopa De Frijoles Colorados	1 cup	140	27	2	7
Sopa De Frijoles Negros	1 cup	140	27	2	9
Sopa De Maiz	1 cup	150	28	13	2
Sopa De Tortilla	1 cup	140	34	5	2
San-J					
Miso Dark	1 pkg	40	3	–	1
Miso Mild	1 pkg	45	5	1	1
Streit's					
Matzo Ball as prep	1 cup	50	12	4	0
Uncle Ben's					
Black Bean & Rice as prep	1 cup	150	28	2	7

FOOD	PORTION	CALS	CARB	SUGAR	FIBER
Broccoli Cheese & Rice as prep	1 cup	110	19	2	1
REFRIGERATED					
Moosewood					
Organic Creamy Potato & Corn Chowder	1 cup (8.4 oz)	170	28	5	3
Organic Hungarian Vegetable Noodle	1 cup (8.4 oz)	80	13	4	2
Organic Savannah Sweet Potato Bisque	1 cup (8.4 oz)	200	20	6	2
Organic Texas Two Bean Chili	1 cup (8.4 oz)	200	34	9	8
Organic Tuscan White Bean & Vegetable	1 cup (8.4 oz)	130	24	5	5
Organic Classics					
French Onion w/ Croutons	1 cup	140	17	8	2
Seafood Chowder	1 cup	160	17	4	1
TAKE-OUT					
ban mien fish head	1 serv (10 oz)	277	27	2	4
bird's nest	1 cup (8.6 oz)	112	8	1	0
broccoli cheese	1 cup	165	15	7	2
caldo de res beef soup	1 cup	143	12	3	2
duck soup	1 cup (8.6 oz)	412	2	tr	tr
egg drop	1 cup	73	1	tr	0
hot & sour	1 serv (14 oz)	173	9	3	3
matzo ball soup	1 cup	118	10	tr	1
minestrone	1 cup	233	22	4	4
miso w/ tofu	1 cup	84	8	2	2
onion soup gratinee	1 serv	492	38	6	4
oxtail	1 cup	68	9	2	1
shark fin	1 bowl (10 oz)	164	9	—	0
shrimp bisque	1 cup	263	13	10	tr
sopa de albondigas	1 cup	171	9	3	1
vietnamese pho beef noodle	1 serv (7.8 oz)	480	78	2	1
wonton soup	1 cup	183	14	tr	1
SOUR CREAM					
Cabot					
Light	2 tbsp	35	2	0	0
No Fat	2 tbsp	20	3	2	0
Sour Cream	2 tbsp	50	1	0	0
Daisy					
No Fat	2 tbsp	20	1	1	0

FOOD	PORTION	CALS	CARB	SUGAR	FIBER
Sour Cream	2 tbsp	60	1	1	0
Friendship					
All Natural	2 tbsp (1 oz)	60	1	1	0
Light	1 tbsp (1 oz)	40	3	1	0
Nonfat	2 tbsp (1 oz)	25	4	2	0
Hood					
Fat Free	2 tbsp	20	4	2	0
Low Fat	2 tbsp	35	3	2	0
Sour Cream	2 tbsp	60	2	1	0
Horizon Organic					
Lowfat	2 tbsp	35	3	2	0
Sour Cream	2 tbsp	60	1	1	0
Land O Lakes					
Fat Free	2 tbsp (1.1 oz)	20	3	2	0
Light	2 tbsp (1.1 oz)	40	2	2	0
Sour Cream	2 tbsp (1.1 oz)	60	2	2	0
Nancy's					
Organic	2 tbsp	60	2	1	0
Organic Valley					
Lowfat	2 tbsp	40	1	1	0

SOUR CREAM SUBSTITUTES
Vegan Gourmet

Alternative Sour Cream	2 tbsp (1 oz)	50	3	0	2

SOY *(see also* CHEESE SUBSTITUTES, ICE CREAM AND FROZEN DESSERTS, MILK SUBSTITUTES, MISO, SMOOTHIES, SOY SAUCE, SOYBEANS, TEMPEH, TOFU, YOGURT FROZEN)

soya cheese	1.4 oz	128	tr	–	0
Bob's Red Mill					
Protein Powder	1 tbsp	20	0	0	0
Good Sense					
Soynuts Honey Roasted	⅓ cup	140	11	4	4
Soynuts Roasted & Salted	⅓ cup	140	10	0	5
Soynuts Roasted w/o Salt	⅓ cup	140	10	0	5
Simple Food					
Soynut Butter Chocolate	2 tbsp	190	8	8	2
Soynut Butter No Sugar No Salt	2 tbsp	200	8	2	2
South Beach					
Soy Nuts Dark Chocolate	1 pkg (0.7 oz)	100	9	6	2

FOOD	PORTION	CALS	CARB	SUGAR	FIBER
Soy Wonder					
Creamy Spread	2 tbsp	170	10	3	1
SoyButter					
Spread	2 tbsp	200	8	4	2

SOY DRINKS *(see MILK SUBSTITUTES, SMOOTHIES)*

SOY SAUCE
Eden					
Organic Shoyu	1 tbsp	15	2	0	0
Organic Shoyu Reduced Sodium	1 tbsp	10	2	0	0
Organic Tamari	1 tbsp	15	2	0	0
House Of Tsang					
Ginger Soy Sauce	1 tbsp	20	4	3	0
Less Sodium	1 tbsp	5	0	0	0
La Choy					
Lite	1 tbsp (0.5 oz)	15	2	2	0
Soy Vay					
Wasablyaki	1 tbsp	35	6	5	0
Tree Of Life					
Organic Shoyu	1 tbsp (0.5 oz)	15	1	1	0
Organic Tamari Wheat Free	1 tbsp (0.5 oz)	15	1	1	0

SOYBEANS
green cooked	½ cup	127	10	–	4
Arrowhead Mills					
Organic Dried not prep	¼ cup	160	11	3	4
C&W					
In the Pod	½ cup	110	12	2	9
Eden					
Organic Blacksoy	½ cup	120	8	1	7
Frieda's					
Edamame	½ cup (2.6 oz)	100	10	2	3
Seapoint Farms					
Edamame Dry Roasted Goji Blend	¼ cup	120	15	5	7
Edamame Dry Roasted Lightly Salted	¼ cup	130	10	1	8
Edamame Dry Roasted Wasabi	¼ cup	130	9	1	7
Edamame In Pods frzn	½ cup	100	9	1	4

FOOD	PORTION	CALS	CARB	SUGAR	FIBER
Edamame In Pods Lightly Salted	½ cup	100	9	1	4
Edamame Shelled	½ cup	100	9	1	4
Organic Edamame In Pods	½ cup	100	9	1	4
Organic Edamame Shelled	½ cup	100	9	1	4
Soyafarm					
Edamame Yuba Sticks	7 pieces (2.5 oz)	123	9	—	4

SPAGHETTI (see PASTA, PASTA DINNERS, PASTA SALAD, SPAGHETTI SAUCE)

SPAGHETTI SAUCE
JARRED
Barilla

FOOD	PORTION	CALS	CARB	SUGAR	FIBER
Arrabbiata Tomato & Spicy Pepper	½ cup	90	11	6	3
Basilico Tomato & Basil	½ cup	70	12	8	3
Campagnola Roasted Garlic & Onion	½ cup	60	11	9	3
Garden Vegetable	½ cup	70	11	6	2
Green & Black Olive	½ cup	80	10	5	4
Mushroom & Garlic	½ cup	70	12	6	2
Rustica Sweet Peppers & Garlic	½ cup	70	11	5	3
Dei Fratelli					
Arrabbiata	½ cup (4.2 oz)	50	8	5	2
Pizza Sauce	¼ cup (2.2 oz)	30	5	4	1
Del Monte					
Garlic & Onion	½ cup	80	16	10	2
DelGrosso					
Aunt Linda's Arrabbiata Memories	½ cup	80	9	6	2
Uncle Bo's Roasted Red Pepper Tour	½ cup	80	9	6	2
Uncle Fred's Fireworks	½ cup	90	9	6	2
Uncle Jim's Late Night Puttanesca	½ cup	70	8	4	2
Eden					
Organic	½ cup	80	12	6	3
Organic No Salt	½ cup	80	12	6	3
Organic Pizza Pasta Sauce	½ cup	65	9	4	5

FOOD	PORTION	CALS	CARB	SUGAR	FIBER
Emeril's					
Homestyle Marinara	½ cup	90	11	7	3
Roasted Gaaahlic	½ cup	70	9	3	2
Sicilian Gravy	½ cup	90	10	1	1
Vodka	½ cup	130	13	2	2
Francesco Rinaldi					
Chunky Garden Tomato Garlic & Onion	½ cup	70	12	11	tr
Hearty Mushroom Pepper & Onion	½ cup	70	11	10	tr
Three Cheese	½ cup	80	15	14	tr
Traditional No Salt Added	½ cup	70	10	9	tr
Hunt's					
Italian Sausage	½ cup	60	10	7	3
Meat	½ cup	60	11	7	3
Traditional	½ cup	50	10	7	2
With Mushrooms	½ cup	45	10	7	3
Joey Pots & Pans					
Arrabbiata	½ cup	100	7	4	1
Marinara	½ cup	50	6	3	1
Vodka Sauce	½ cup	110	6	3	1
Lucini					
Rustic Tomato Basil	½ cup (4.4 oz)	80	8	6	2
Spicy Tuscan	½ cup (4.4 oz)	80	8	5	2
Milo's					
Portobello Shiraz	4 oz	40	8	4	2
Muir Glen					
Organic Chunky Tomato	¼ cup	15	4	2	tr
Organic Garlic Roasted Garlic	½ cup	60	12	4	2
Organic Pizza Sauce	¼ cup	40	6	3	1
Organic Tomato Sauce No Salt Added	¼ cup	25	5	3	1
Newman's Own					
Bambolina	½ cup	90	13	12	tr
Cabernet Marinara	½ cup	70	10	9	2
Five Cheese	½ cup	80	10	0	tr
Italian Sausage & Peppers	½ cup	90	11	9	tr
Marinara	½ cup	70	12	11	tr
Marinara w/ Mushrooms	½ cup	70	12	11	tr
Pesto & Tomato Sauce	½ cup	80	10	9	tr

FOOD	PORTION	CALS	CARB	SUGAR	FIBER
Roasted Garlic & Green Peppers	½ cup	70	11	6	4
Sockarooni	½ cup	70	12	11	tr
Tomato & Roasted Garlic	½ cup	70	11	9	tr
Vodka Sauce	½ cup	110	11	9	0
Pomi					
Marinara	½ cup	80	5	6	3
Prego					
100% Natural Roasted Garlic Parmesan	½ cup	100	20	13	3
Heart Smart Traditional Italian	½ cup	100	15	9	3
Italian	½ cup	70	13	10	3
Italian Marinara	½ cup	100	11	7	4
Italian Meat	½ cup	130	19	12	3
Italian Roasted Red Pepper & Garlic	½ cup	90	13	9	3
Italian Three Cheese	½ cup	80	14	11	3
Italian Tomato Basil & Garlic	½ cup	80	12	9	3
Organic Mushroom	½ cup	90	13	9	4
Progresso					
Lobster Sauce	½ cup (4.3 oz)	100	6	3	2
Red Clam w/ Tomato & Basil	½ cup (4.4 oz)	60	8	4	1
White Clam w/ Garlic & Herb	½ cup (4.4 oz)	120	4	1	1
Robert Rothchild Farm					
Artichoke	½ cup	80	8	7	0
Seeds Of Change					
Balsamic Olive & Onion	½ cup	80	14	8	2
Garden Vegetable	½ cup	70	14	8	2
Mushroom & Onion	½ cup	70	12	7	2
Three Cheese Marinara	½ cup	70	12	8	2
Traditional Herb	½ cup	70	16	9	2
Tuttorosso					
Pasta Sauce Meat	½ cup	90	15	9	3
Vino De Milo					
Mediterranean Pinot Grigio	½ cup	90	12	1	2
Portobella Shiraz	½ cup	40	9	5	2
Tuscan Merlot	½ cup	80	2	13	2
Walnut Acres					
Organic Garlic Garlic	½ cup	125	10	6	1
Organic Marinara & Zinfandel	½ cup	125	9	6	1
Organic Roasted Garlic	½ cup	125	11	7	1

FOOD	PORTION	CALS	CARB	SUGAR	FIBER
Organic Tomato & Basil	½ cup	125	9	7	1
TAKE-OUT					
bolognese	5 oz	195	4	–	tr

SPANISH FOOD
FROZEN
Cedarlane

FOOD	PORTION	CALS	CARB	SUGAR	FIBER
Organic Burrito Low Fat Rice & Cheese	1 (6 oz)	260	48	2	7
Organic Enchilada Low Fat Black Bean & Tofu	1 (9 oz)	220	42	3	6
Roasted Chile Relleno	1 pkg (10 oz)	400	37	12	5
Zone Burrito Beans & Cheese	1 (6 oz)	350	37	3	8
Contessa					
Fajitas Shrimp	2 (8 oz)	230	37	4	5
Paella w/ Chicken & Seafood	1½ cups	200	28	3	2
Seafood Veracruz not prep	1¾ cups	180	27	4	6
El Monterey					
Burrito Bean & Cheese	1 (5 oz)	280	43	1	5
Burrito Beef & Bean	1 (5 oz)	370	42	2	4
Burrito Half Pound Spicy Red Hot Beef & Bean	1 (8 oz)	600	68	3	7
Burrito Supreme Breakfast Egg Cheese & Sausage	1 (4.5 oz)	300	34	1	1
Burrito Supreme Shredded Steak & Cheese	1 (5 oz)	290	41	1	1
Burrito XX Large Bean & Cheese	1 (10 oz)	590	88	2	5
Burrito XX Large Beef & Bean	1 (10 oz)	730	83	2	8
Cruncheros Cheese & Beef	3 (4.5 oz)	330	35	1	2
Cruncheros Taco Beef & Cheese	4 (5.6 oz)	460	38	2	2
Enchiladas Cheese w/ Sauce	1 serv (8 oz)	250	22	1	3
Enchiladas Shredded Beef w/ Sauce	1 serv (4 oz)	140	15	1	2
Quesadillas Chicken & Cheese	2 (6 oz)	380	43	1	2
Quesadillas Steak & Cheese	2 (6 oz)	400	42	2	1
Tamales Chicken	1 (4.5 oz)	240	27	1	2
Tamales Shredded Beef	1 (4.5 oz)	310	27	1	3
Taquitos Corn Shredded Beef	3 (4.5 oz)	300	31	1	1
Taquitos Flour Char-Broiled Chicken Breast	3 (5 oz)	380	36	1	1

FOOD	PORTION	CALS	CARB	SUGAR	FIBER
Taquitos Flour Chicken & Cheese	3 (4.5 oz)	350	36	1	2
Taquitos Southwest Chicken In A Seasoned Batter	2 (2.8 oz)	175	20	0	1
Tornados Apple Cinnamon	1 (3 oz)	180	31	8	0
Tornados Sausage Egg & Cheese	1 (3 oz)	230	23	1	1
Tornados Shredded Beef	1 (3 oz)	210	23	1	1
Tornados Steak Egg & Cheese	1 (3 oz)	170	22	1	0
Tornados Xxl Southwest Chicken	1 (4.2 oz)	210	28	1	1
Health Is Wealth					
Vegetarian Hot Tamale Munchees	6 (3 oz)	160	26	0	3
Healthy Choice					
Enchilada Chicken	1 pkg	300	46	4	6
Helen's Kitchen					
Cheese Enchiladas w/ Tofu Steaks In Spicy Red Sauce	½ pkg (5 oz)	150	20	3	5
Jose Ole					
Burrito Beef & Cheese	1 (5 oz)	300	39	1	2
Burrito Chicken	1 (5 oz)	270	41	tr	2
Chimichanga Chicken & Cheese	1 (5 oz)	330	44	tr	2
Chimichanga Shredded Beef	1 (5 oz)	350	39	1	2
Mini Burrito Chicken & Cheese	3	200	25	tr	1
Mini Chimichanga Beef & Cheddar	3	240	25	tr	1
Mini Quesadilla Grilled Chicken	3	220	28	tr	1
Mini Tacos Beef & Cheese	4	200	19	tr	3
Mini Taquitos Beef & Cheese	4	180	21	tr	2
Soft Taco Beef & Cheese	1 (5 oz)	280	31	1	1
Taquitos Beef & Cheese Flour Tortilla	2	220	24	tr	1
Taquitos Buffalo Chicken Flour Tortilla	2	200	23	tr	tr
Taquitos Chicken Flour Tortilla	3	180	23	0	2
Taquitos Chicken & Cheese Flour Tortilla	2	220	25	1	1
Taquitos Pepperoni Pizza Flour Tortilla	2	240	23	1	1

FOOD	PORTION	CALS	CARB	SUGAR	FIBER
Taquitos Shredded Beef Corn Tortilla	3	180	21	0	2
Patio					
Burrito Bean & Cheese	1 (5 oz)	280	44	4	5
Burrito Beef & Bean Medium	1 (5 oz)	300	44	6	5
Burrito Chicken	1 (5 oz)	280	42	5	2
Stouffer's					
Chicken Enchilada w/ Cheese Sauce & Rice	1 pkg (7.13 oz)	280	30	6	3
Tyson					
Meal Kit Chicken Fajita	1 (3.8 oz)	130	17	3	2
Meal Kit Chicken Quesadilla	1 (4 oz)	250	26	2	3
READY-TO-EAT					
taco shell corn	1 (6.5 inch)	98	13	tr	2
taco shell flour	1 (7 inch)	173	19	tr	1
Ortega					
Tostada Shells	2 (1 oz)	140	19	0	1
SHELF-STABLE					
Fantastic					
Spanish Paella	1 pkg (8 oz)	280	55	2	4
TAKE-OUT					
arroz con coco	1 cup	532	46	5	4
burrito w/ beans	1 med (5 oz)	295	45	1	7
burrito w/ beans & rice	1 (3.5 oz)	221	37	tr	4
burrito w/ beef	1 sm (3.4 oz)	297	25	tr	1
burrito w/ beef & beans	1 med (5 oz)	331	36	1	6
burrito w/ beef beans & cheese	1 med (5 oz)	379	30	1	5
burrito w/ chicken & beans	1 med (5 oz)	295	34	1	5
burrito w/ pork & beans	1 med (5 oz)	320	35	1	6
chiles rellenos meat & cheese filled	1 (5 oz)	213	9	3	2
chimichanga w/ bean cheese lettuce & tomato	1 (4.1 oz)	271	22	2	3
chimichanga w/ beef & rice	1 (10 oz)	634	58	5	5
chimichanga w/ beef beans lettuce & tomato	1 (4.1 oz)	254	22	2	3
chimichanga w/ beef cheese lettuce & tomato	1 (4.1 oz)	337	19	1	1
chimichanga w/ chicken sour cream lettuce & tomato	1 (4 oz)	277	17	1	1

FOOD	PORTION	CALS	CARB	SUGAR	FIBER
empanada fruit filled	1 (3.8 oz)	452	55	25	2
empanada meat & vegetable	1 (7.8 oz)	881	66	1	3
empanada sweet potato	1 (7.8 oz)	546	76	22	4
enchilada w/ beans	1 (4.1 oz)	179	27	2	6
enchilada w/ beans & cheese	1 (4.6 oz)	233	25	2	5
enchilada w/ beef	1 (4 oz)	214	21	2	3
enchilada w/ beef & beans	1 (4 oz)	195	25	2	4
frijoles	1 cup	278	49	6	9
nachos w/ beans & cheese	1 serv (9.4 oz)	616	57	2	13
nachos w/ beef beans cheese & sour cream	1 serv (19 oz)	1620	133	4	19
pupusa meat filled	1 (3.6 oz)	187	26	1	3
quesadilla w/ cheese	1 (5 oz)	498	40	1	3
quesadilla w/ meat & cheese	1 (6.5 oz)	605	40	1	2
taco de jueye w/ crab meat	1 (4.2 oz)	266	18	1	2
taco w/ beans lettuce tomato & salsa	1 (2.8 oz)	117	16	1	4
taco w/ chicken lettuce tomato & salsa	1 (2.5 oz)	114	10	1	1
taco w/ fish lettuce tomato & salsa	1 (2.7 oz)	101	10	1	1
tostada w/ beef lettuce tomato & salsa	1 (2.7 oz)	143	11	1	2

SPICES (see individual names, HERBS/SPICES)

SPINACH
CANNED
drained	1 cup	49	7	1	5
Freshlike					
Cut Leaf	½ cup	45	5	0	3
Popeye					
Leaf Spinach	½ cup	30	4	tr	2
Leaf Spinach No Salt Added	½ cup	40	5	0	2
FRESH					
baby raw	2 cups	20	5	0	3
cooked	1 cup	41	7	1	4
mustard cooked	1 cup	29	5	–	4
raw	1 cup	7	1	tr	1
Fresh Express					
Baby Spinach	3 cups	20	3	0	2

FOOD	PORTION	CALS	CARB	SUGAR	FIBER
Organic Baby Spinach	3 cups	35	9	0	4
FROZEN					
chopped cooked	1 cup	30	5	tr	4
Birds Eye					
Chopped	⅓ cup	20	2	1	2
C&W					
Baby Chopped	1 cup	30	3	tr	1
Creamed	½ cup	100	6	1	4
Cascadian Farm					
Organic Cut	⅓ cup	25	3	tr	1
Cedarlane					
Organic Spanakopita Spinach & Feta Pie	½ pkg (5 oz)	260	38	3	2
Dr. Praeger's					
Spinach Bites	2 (2 oz)	110	17	3	2
Fillo Factory					
Spanakopita Spinach & Cheese Fillo Appetizers	3 (3 oz)	190	20	1	1
Green Giant					
No Sauce	½ cup	25	3	1	1
Health Is Wealth					
Creamed	½ pkg (4.5 oz)	100	27	5	2
Spinach Munchees	6 (3oz)	180	25	1	3
Stouffer's					
Creamed	½ pkg (4.5 oz)	200	8	3	2
Taverna					
Spinach Pie	1 piece (4.8 oz)	190	24	4	5
TAKE-OUT					
indian saag	1 serv	28	2	–	1
spanakopita spinach pie	1 serv (3 oz)	148	8	1	1

SPORTS DRINKS (see ENERGY DRINKS)

SPOT

baked	3 oz	134	0	0	0

SPROUTS
La Choy

Bean Sprouts	⅔ cup	15	3	tr	1

FOOD	PORTION	CALS	CARB	SUGAR	FIBER
SQUAB					
boneless baked	1 (4 oz)	242	0	0	0
SQUASH (see also ZUCCHINI)					
CANNED					
Farmer's Market					
Organic Butternut	½ cup	50	12	4	2
Sunshine					
Slice Yellow	½ cup	25	5	3	2
FRESH					
Frieda's					
Acorn	¾ cup (3 oz)	35	9	3	2
Baby Crookneck	⅔ cup (3 oz)	15	3	2	1
Baby Scallop	⅔ cup (3 oz)	15	3	2	1
Eight Ball	2 (4.4 oz)	18	4	1	1
Hubbard	¾ cup (3 oz)	35	7	3	2
Mini Pumpkin	¾ cup (3 oz)	20	6	4	2
Spaghetti	¾ cup (3 oz)	30	6	3	1
Star Spangled	⅔ cup (3 oz)	20	3	2	1
Turban	¾ cup (3 oz)	30	7	3	1
Glory					
Yellow Sliced	¾ cup	20	3	1	1
FROZEN					
C&W					
Butternut	½ cup	45	10	2	1
McKenzie's					
Southland Butternut	½ cup	70	10	6	1
TAKE-OUT					
fritter	1 (0.8 oz)	81	8	1	1
squash pie	1 slice (5.4 oz)	291	40	24	2
SQUID					
baked	1 cup	192	5	0	0
canned in its own ink	1 can (4 oz)	122	4	0	0
dried	1 sm (1.5 oz)	147	5	0	0
pickled	1 oz	26	1	tr	0
steamed	1 cup	147	5	0	0
Contessa					
Calamari + Sauce	13 pieces + 2 tbsp sauce	160	21	1	1

FOOD	PORTION	CALS	CARB	SUGAR	FIBER
Van de Kamp's					
Fried Calamari	15 pieces (4 oz)	270	26	0	1
TAKE-OUT					
arroz con calamares	1 cup	400	47	2	1
calamari breaded & fried	1 cup	296	17	1	1
SQUIRREL					
roasted	3 oz	147	0	0	0
STARFRUIT					
Frieda's					
Dried	⅓ cup (1.4 oz)	120	29	26	1
STRAWBERRIES					
canned in heavy syrup	½ cup	117	30	28	2
fresh halves	1 cup	49	12	7	3
fresh whole	1 cup	46	11	7	3
fresh whole	1 pint	114	27	17	7
frzn sweetened sliced	½ cup	122	33	31	2
frzn whole sweetened	1 cup	199	54	48	5
frzn whole unsweetened	1 cup	77	20	10	5
organic fresh whole	8 med	45	12	8	4
C&W					
Ultimate Sliced frzn	⅔ cup	50	12	8	1
Chukar Cherries					
Dried	¼ cup	120	29	25	2
Emily's					
Dark Chocolate Covered	6 (1.4 oz)	170	28	22	2
Europe's Best					
Sliced frzn	¾ cup	40	10	7	3
Frieda's					
Dried	½ cup (1.4 oz)	150	34	29	3
LiteHouse					
Glaze Sugar Free	3 tbsp	35	8	0	0
Marie's					
Glaze	2 tbsp	40	10	8	0
Polar					
Strawberries In Syrup	½ cup	90	21	10	1

FOOD	PORTION	CALS	CARB	SUGAR	FIBER
STRAWBERRY JUICE					
Nesquik					
Strawberry Powder not prep	2 tbsp (0.6 oz)	60	15	15	0
STUFFING/DRESSING					
Fresh Gourmet					
All Natural Multi-Grain w/ Cranberries not prep	⅓ cup (1 oz)	110	19	3	1
Organic Seasoned not prep	⅓ cup (1 oz)	110	19	1	1
Kellogg's					
Stuffing Mix as prep	1 cup	240	26	1	1
Pepperidge Farm					
Corn Bread	¾ cup	170	33	2	2
Cube	¾ cup	140	28	2	2
Herb Seasoned	¾ cup	170	33	2	3
One Step Turkey	½ cup	170	23	2	1
Tofurky					
Wild Rice & Mushroom	½ cup	110	21	2	1
Zatarain's					
Creole Chicken as prep	½ cup	100	20	2	1
French Bread as prep	½ cup	100	20	2	1
TAKE-OUT					
bread	1 cup	352	44	5	2
cornbread	½ cup	179	22	0	3
kishke stuffed derma	1 piece (1.3 oz)	166	13	tr	1
oyster	1 cup	304	29	3	2
STURGEON					
broiled	3 oz	115	0	0	0
smoked	1 oz	49	0	0	0
TAKE-OUT					
breaded & fried	4 oz	252	9	1	1
SUCKER					
white baked	3 oz	101	0	0	0
SUGAR (see also FRUCTOSE, SYRUP)					
brown unpacked	1 cup (5.1 oz)	547	141	140	0
brown organic	1 tsp	17	4	4	0
cinnamon sugar	1 tsp	16	4	4	tr
cube	1 (2 g)	9	2	2	0

FOOD	PORTION	CALS	CARB	SUGAR	FIBER
maple	1 piece (1 oz)	99	25	24	0
raw	1 pkg (5 g)	19	5	5	0
sugarcane stem	3 oz	54	14	–	3
white	1 packet (3 g)	12	3	3	0
white	1 tbsp (0.4 oz)	49	13	13	0
Bob's Red Mill					
Date Sugar	1 tsp	11	3	3	0
Turbinado	1 tsp	10	3	3	0
Domino					
Demerara Raw Cane	1 tsp	15	4	4	0
Tree Of Life					
Date Sugar	1 tsp (4 g)	10	3	3	0
Organic Cane Juice Dehydrated	1 tsp (3.5 g)	15	3	3	0
Turbinado	1 tsp (4 g)	15	4	4	0
Wholesome Sweeteners					
Organic Fair Trade Dark Brown Sugar	1 tsp	15	4	4	0
Organic Fair Trade Powdered	¼ cup	120	30	30	0
Organic Fair Trade Sucanat	1 tsp	15	4	4	0
Organic Turbinado	1 tsp	15	4	4	0
SUGAR SUBSTITUTES					
Equal					
Sugar Lite	1 tsp	8	2	2	0
Fructevia					
All Natural	1 tsp (4 g)	5	2	2	0
Nevella					
No Calorie Sweetener	1 tsp	0	tr	0	0
Neway					
Sweet Sensation	¼ tsp	0	tr	0	0
PureVia					
All Natural	1 pkg (2 g)	0	2	tr	0
Splenda					
Brown Sugar Blend	½ tsp (2 g)	10	2	2	0
Cafe Sticks	1 pkg (1 g)	0	tr	0	0
Flavor Accents Sticks	1 pkg (1 g)	0	tr	0	0
Flavors For Coffee	1 pkg (1 g)	0	tr	0	0
No Calorie Granulated	1 tsp (0.5 g)	0	tr	0	0
No Calorie Sweetener w/ Fiber	1 pkg	0	2	0	1
Stevia In The Raw					
100% Natural Sweetener	1 pkg (1 g)	0	0	0	0

FOOD	PORTION	CALS	CARB	SUGAR	FIBER
Steviva					
Blend	1 tbsp (0.4 oz)	2	0	0	0
Sweet Fiber					
All Natural	1 pkg	0	tr	tr	tr
Sweete					
Sugar Free	1 pkg	0	tr	0	0
Truvia					
Calorie Free Sweetener	1 pkg (3.5 g)	0	3	0	0
Whey Low					
Gold	1 tsp	4	4	4	0
Granular	1 tsp	4	4	4	0
Maple Buzz	¼ cup	57	57	57	0
Wholesome Sweeteners					
Organic Zero	1 pkg (6 g)	0	6	0	0
ZSweet					
All Natural	1 pkg (1 g)	0	tr	0	0
SUNCHOKE					
Frieda's					
Sunchoke	½ cup (3 oz)	70	14	0	1
SUNFISH					
pumpkinseed baked	3 oz	97	0	0	0
SUNFLOWER					
seeds dry roasted w/ salt	¼ cup	186	8	1	3
seeds dry roasted w/o salt	¼ cup	186	8	1	4
seeds w/ hulls dried	¼ cup	66	2	tr	1
Arrowhead Mills					
Organic Seeds	¼ cup	170	6	1	3
Bob's Red Mill					
Seeds Roasted & Salted	3 tbsp	186	6	1	5
Dakota Gourmet					
Seeds Honey Roasted	¼ cup (1 oz)	170	8	1	2
Good Sense					
Nuts Honey Roasted	¼ cup	190	7	2	2
Nuts Raw	¼ cup	170	6	0	4
Nuts Roasted & Salted	¼ cup	190	5	1	2
Seeds In Shell Roasted & Salted	½ cup	150	13	0	13
Sunflower Nuts Roasted w/o Salt	¼ cup	190	5	1	2

FOOD	PORTION	CALS	CARB	SUGAR	FIBER
Lance					
Shelled Seeds	1 pkg (1.8 oz)	300	14	1	3
SunButter					
Creamy	2 tbsp	200	7	3	4
Organic	2 tbsp	203	7	4	3
SunGold					
Seeds Roasted Salted	1 oz	172	4	2	2
Tree Of Life					
Seeds Kernels Raw	¼ cup (1.3 oz)	210	7	1	2
SUSHI					
TAKE-OUT					
inari	1 sm	46	9	–	0
roll california	1 (1.2 oz)	48	8	–	tr
roll fresh salmon	4 pieces	250	37	5	3
roll tuna	1 (1.1 oz)	37	6	–	tr
SWAMP CABBAGE					
chopped cooked w/o salt	1 cup	20	4	–	2
SWEET POTATO (see also YAM)					
baked w/ skin w/o salt	1 med (4 oz)	103	24	7	4
baked w/ skin w/o salt	1 lg (6.3 oz)	162	37	12	6
canned in syrup	½ cup	106	25	6	3
canned mashed	½ cup	129	30	7	2
leaves cooked w/o salt	1 cup	22	5	3	1
paste dulce de calabaza	1 oz	82	21	20	tr
Diner's Choice					
Mashed	⅔ cup	160	33	18	2
Dr. Praeger's					
Sweet Potato Bites	2 (2 oz)	110	20	9	1
Farmer's Market					
Organic Puree	½ cup	96	22	15	2
Glory					
Casserole	½ cup	180	43	27	2
Cut Fresh	1 serv (5 oz)	140	36	8	4
Sweet Potatoes	⅔ cup	160	37	17	2
Green Giant					
Candied	¾ cup	240	41	20	3
Health Is Wealth					
Southern Style	½ pkg (5 oz)	190	36	8	2

FOOD	PORTION	CALS	CARB	SUGAR	FIBER
Ian's					
Fries	7 pieces (2.5 oz)	70	13	4	1
Mann's					
Fresh Cubes	1 serv (3 oz)	60	15	3	3
Mrs. Paul's					
Candied	1 serv (5 oz)	300	73	47	3
Princella					
In Light Syrup	⅔ cup	160	39	20	3
Mashed	⅔ cup	120	28	15	3
Royal Prince					
Candied	½ cup	210	50	35	2
Trappey's					
Sugary Sam Cut Sweet	⅔ cup	160	39	20	3
Tree Of Life					
Organic Puree	½ cup (4.5 oz)	130	30	15	2
TAKE-OUT					
white fried batata blanca frita	1 serv (8 oz)	792	129	2	19
SWEETBREAD (PANCREAS)					
beef braised	3 oz	230	0	0	0
lamb braised	3 oz	199	0	0	0
pork braised	3 oz	186	0	0	0
veal braised	3 oz	218	0	0	0
Rumba					
Beef	4 oz	260	0	0	0
SWISS CHARD					
Frieda's					
Bright Lights	1 cup (3 oz)	15	3	1	1
SWORDFISH					
cooked	3 oz	132	0	0	0
raw	3 oz	103	0	0	0
SYRUP					
corn dark & light	¼ cup	240	65	65	0
date syrup	1 tbsp	63	15	–	0
rose hip	1 oz	9	2	2	0
sugar syrup	¼ cup	76	20	20	0
Cary's					
Sugar Free	¼ cup	30	12	0	tr

FOOD	PORTION	CALS	CARB	SUGAR	FIBER
Eden					
Organic Barley Malt	1 tbsp	60	14	8	0
Lundberg					
Organic Sweet Dreams Brown Rice	2 tbsp	110	31	25	0
Navitas Naturals					
Yacon	2 tbsp	90	22	14	0
Nesquik					
Strawberry Calcium Fortified	2 tbsp (1.4 oz)	110	27	27	0
Neway					
Sweet Sensation Luo Han Guo Syrup	1 tsp	8	2	0	0
Wholesome Sweeteners					
Organic Blue Agave	1 tbsp	60	16	16	0
Organic Corn Syrup	2 tbsp	120	30	30	0

TAHINI *(see SESAME)*

TAMARILLOS
Frieda's

FOOD	PORTION	CALS	CARB	SUGAR	FIBER
Gold Or Red	2 (4.2 oz)	40	9	2	4

TAMARIND

FOOD	PORTION	CALS	CARB	SUGAR	FIBER
dried sweetened pulpitas	1 piece (0.8 oz)	56	15	14	1
dried sweetened pulpitas	½ cup	279	73	68	5
fresh	1 (2 g)	5	1	0	tr
fresh cut up	1 cup	143	38	34	3

TAMARIND JUICE

FOOD	PORTION	CALS	CARB	SUGAR	FIBER
nectar	1 cup	143	37	32	1

TANGERINE
CANNED

FOOD	PORTION	CALS	CARB	SUGAR	FIBER
in light syrup	1 cup	154	41	39	2
juice pack	1 cup	92	24	22	2
FRESH					
fresh	1 sm (2.7 oz)	40	10	8	1
fresh	1 med (3.1 oz)	47	12	9	2
fresh	1 lg (4.2 oz)	64	16	13	2
sections	1 cup	103	26	21	4
FRESH					
River Pride					
Sweet	1 (3.8 oz)	50	15	12	3

FOOD	PORTION	CALS	CARB	SUGAR	FIBER
TANGERINE JUICE					
canned sweetened	1 cup	124	30	29	1
fresh	1 cup	106	25	24	1
Odwalla					
100% Juice	8 oz	110	25	25	0
TAPIOCA					
pearl dry	¼ cup (1.3 oz)	136	34	1	tr
Let's Do Organic					
Granulated	1 tbsp	35	9	0	0
Starch	1 tbsp	0	9	0	0
TARO					
Frieda's					
Taro Root	⅔ cup (3 oz)	90	22	1	3
TARPON					
fresh	3 oz	87	0	0	0
TARRAGON					
dried crumbled	1 tsp	2	tr	–	0
ground	1 tsp	5	1	–	tr
TEA/HERBAL TEA *(see also* ICED TEA*)*					
HERBAL					
chamomile brewed	1 cup	2	tr	0	0
Celestial Seasonings					
Chamomile	1 cup	0	0	0	0
Dessert Tea English Toffee	1 cup	0	0	0	0
Moroccan Pomegranate Red	1 cup	0	0	0	0
Peppermint	1 cup	0	0	0	0
Red Safari Spice	1 cup	0	0	0	0
Roastaroma Herb	1 cup	0	0	0	0
Wellness Tea Ginseng Energy	1 tea bag	0	0	0	0
Zinger Acai Mango	1 cup	0	tr	0	0
Zinger Lemon	1 cup	0	0	0	0
Eden					
Organic Genmaicha Tea	1 tea bag	0	0	0	0
Organic Kukicha Tea	1 tea bag	0	0	0	0
Lipton					
Ginger Twist	1 tea bag	0	0	0	0
Mango	1 tea bag	0	0	0	0
Peppermint	1 tea bag	0	0	0	0

FOOD	PORTION	CALS	CARB	SUGAR	FIBER
REGULAR					
Celestial Seasonings					
Black Fast Lane	1 cup	0	0	0	0
Chai White Honey Vanilla	1 tea bag	0	0	0	0
Green Antioxidant	1 cup	0	0	0	0
Green Tropical Acai	1 cup	0	0	0	0
Green Tea	1 cup	0	0	0	0
Morning Thunder	1 cup	0	0	0	0
White Tea Antioxidant Plum	1 tea bag	0	0	0	0
Daily Detox					
Original	1 tea bag	0	0	0	0
Eden					
Organic Bancha Green Tea	1 tea bag	0	0	0	0
Organic Hojicha Tea	1 tea bag	0	0	0	0
Lipton					
Black Tea as prep	1 cup	0	0	0	0
Black Tea French Vanilla	1 tea bag	0	0	0	0
Black Tea Mint	1 tea bag	0	0	0	0
Black Tea Orange & Spice	1 tea bag	0	0	0	0
Decaffeinated Black Tea as prep	1 serv	0	0	0	0
Earl Grey	1 tea bag	0	0	0	0
English Breakfast	1 tea bag	0	0	0	0
English Estate	1 tea bag	0	0	0	0
Green Tea as prep	1 tea bag	0	0	0	0
Green Tea Decaffeinated	1 tea bag	0	0	0	0
Green Tea Lemon Ginseng	1 tea bag	0	0	0	0
Green Tea Mint	1 tea bag	0	0	0	0
Red Rose					
Black Tea Teabag	1	0	0	0	0
English Breakfast Teabag	1 cup	0	0	0	0
TEMPEH					
Lightlife					
Garden Veggie	1 serv (4 oz)	230	14	0	10
Organic Flax	1 serv (4 oz)	230	14	0	11
Organic Grilles Lemon	1 patty (2.7 oz)	140	11	2	0
Organic Grilles Tamari	1 patty (2.7 oz)	130	9	2	0
Organic Soy	1 serv (4 oz)	210	14	0	10
Organic Three Grain	1 serv (4 oz)	240	21	0	8
Organic Wild Rice	1 serv (4 oz)	280	14	0	10

FOOD	PORTION	CALS	CARB	SUGAR	FIBER
Tofurky					
Edamame Veggie	3 oz	145	20	0	7
Five Grain	3 oz	190	20	0	6
Soy	3 oz	160	20	0	7
WildWood					
Organic Nori Seaweed	3 oz	170	16	2	4
TESTICLES					
prairie oysters cooked	1 pair (6.8 oz)	241	0	0	0
THYME					
dried crumbled	1 tsp	3	1	tr	tr
fresh	1 tsp	1	tr	–	tr
ground	1 tsp	4	1	tr	1
TILAPIA					
High Liner					
Loins	1 fillet (4 oz)	110	0	0	0
Van de Kamp's					
Lightly Breaded Fillets	1 (4 oz)	240	17	tr	1
TAKE-OUT					
battered & fried	1 fillet (4 oz)	206	8	tr	tr
breaded & fried	1 fillet (4 oz)	300	16	2	1
broiled w/o fat	1 fillet (3.5 oz)	128	0	0	0
TILEFISH					
cooked	½ fillet (5.3 oz)	220	0	0	0
cooked	3 oz	125	0	0	0
raw	3 oz	81	0	0	0
TOFU					
firm	½ cup	183	5	–	2
okara	½ cup	47	8	–	1
regular	½ cup	94	2	–	1
Eden					
Dried	1 piece (0.4 oz)	50	0	0	2
House					
Atsu-Age Cutlet	1 (2.5 oz)	100	2	0	5
Cut-Age Shredded Fried	1 serv (0.5 oz)	50	0	0	0
Ganmodoki Fritter Small	3 (1.6 oz)	120	2	0	0
Medium Firm	3 oz	60	1	0	tr
Organic Extra Firm	3 oz	90	0	0	0

FOOD	PORTION	CALS	CARB	SUGAR	FIBER
Organic Firm	3 oz	60	0	0	0
Soft Silken	3 oz	50	2	0	tr
Steak Cajun	1 (3 oz)	40	1	0	tr
Steak Grilled	1 (3 oz)	90	2	0	0
Sukui	3 oz	45	2	1	0
Tokusen Kinugoshi	1 piece (5 oz)	90	3	0	tr
Yaki Broiled	3 oz	90	2	0	0
Soyafarm					
Baked Tofu	10 pieces (3.5 oz)	147	6	–	1
Nuggets	4 pieces (3.5 oz)	162	14	–	1
Tofu & Yuba Patties	1 (3.5 oz)	243	12	–	1
Tree Of Life					
Organic Firm	½ block (3.2 oz)	110	4	0	2
WildWood					
Organic Baked Aloha	1 piece (3.5 oz)	180	15	2	3
Organic Calcium Rich Medium	3 oz	70	2	0	1
Organic Golden Pineapple Teriyaki	3 oz	160	5	3	1
Organic High Protein Super Firm	3 oz	100	5	0	1
Organic Smoked Mild Szechuan	3 oz	150	11	4	2
TAKE-OUT					
breaded deep fried w/ soy sauce japanese style	1 piece (0.4 oz)	15	1	0	tr
soy sauce marinated & grilled	1 serv (4 oz)	181	6	–	1
TOMATILLO					
fresh	1 (1.2 oz)	11	2	1	1
fresh chopped	½ cup (2.3 oz)	21	4	3	1
Las Palmas					
Tomatillos Crushed	½ cup	45	7	3	2
TOMATO					
CANNED					
green pickled	½ cup (2.5 oz)	26	6	5	1
green whole pickled	1 (2.6 oz)	27	6	5	1
paste	1 can (6 oz)	139	32	21	7
paste	¼ cup (2.3 oz)	54	12	8	3
paste no salt added	1 can (6 oz)	139	32	21	7

FOOD	PORTION	CALS	CARB	SUGAR	FIBER
puree	1 can (28 oz)	312	74	40	16
puree	1 cup (8.8 oz)	95	22	12	5
puree w/o salt	1 can (28 oz)	312	74	40	16
sauce	1 cup (8.6 oz)	59	13	10	4
sauce no salt added	1 cup (8.6 oz)	102	21	13	4
stewed	1 cup (8.9 oz)	66	16	9	3
Cento					
Crushed	¼ cup	35	7	4	2
Paste	2 tbsp (1.2 oz)	30	7	5	2
Contadina					
Paste Italian Herbs	2 tbsp	35	7	4	1
Petite Cut Diced	½ cup	25	6	4	2
Dei Fratelli					
Chopped Italian Tomatoes	½ cup (4.3 oz)	40	8	5	1
Del Monte					
Diced w/ Garlic & Onion	½ cup	40	8	6	tr
Garden Select Petite Diced	½ cup	15	3	2	tr
Organic Diced	½ cup	25	6	4	2
Organic Diced w/ Basil Garlic & Oregano	½ cup	50	11	8	tr
Organic Tomato Paste	2 tbsp	30	6	3	1
Eden					
Organic Crushed	¼ cup	20	3	2	1
Organic Diced	½ cup	30	6	4	2
Organic Whole Roma	½ cup	30	4	2	1
Hunt's					
Diced w/ Basil Garlic & Oregano	½ cup	35	7	5	2
Muir Glen					
Organic Chunky Tomato & Herb	½ cup	60	11	5	2
Organic Diced Fire Roasted	½ cup	30	6	4	1
Organic Diced w/ Basil & Garlic	½ cup	30	6	4	1
Polar					
Grape	½ cup	50	12	11	2
Pomi					
Chopped	½ cup	20	4	4	3
Progresso					
Crushed w/ Added Puree	¼ cup (2.1 oz)	20	4	2	1
Diced	½ cup (4.4 oz)	25	5	3	1
Puree	¼ cup (2.2 oz)	25	5	3	1

FOOD	PORTION	CALS	CARB	SUGAR	FIBER
Whole Peeled w/ Basil	½ cup (4.2 oz)	20	4	3	1
Redpack					
Crushed In Puree	¼ cup	20	4	2	1
Diced In Juice	½ cup	25	5	3	1
Petite Diced Onion Celery & Green Pepper	½ cup	45	10	7	1
Ro-Tel					
Diced In Sauce	½ cup	40	8	7	tr
Mexican Festival	½ cup	30	6	3	1
Original	½ cup	20	4	3	1
Tillen Farms					
Sunnyside Tomatoes	3 pieces (1 oz)	40	4	3	1
DRIED					
sun dried	1 piece (2 g)	5	1	1	tr
sun dried	¼ cup (0.5 oz)	35	8	5	2
sun dried in oil drained	1 piece (3 g)	6	1	–	tr
sun dried in oil drained	¼ cup (1 oz)	59	6	–	2
tomato powder	1 oz	85	21	12	5
Frieda's					
Red Chopped	⅓ cup (1.1 oz)	100	19	11	2
FRESH					
bruschetta	¼ cup	50	6	4	tr
cherry	1 (0.6 oz)	3	1	tr	tr
cherry	½ cup (2.6 oz)	13	3	2	1
grape tomatoes	20	30	6	4	1
green	1 sm (3.2 oz)	21	5	4	1
green	1 med (4.3 oz)	28	6	5	1
green	1 lg (6.4 oz)	42	9	7	2
green chopped	1 cup (6.3 oz)	41	9	7	2
plum	1 (2.2 oz)	11	2	2	1
red	1 sm (3.2 oz)	16	4	2	1
red	1 med (4.3 oz)	22	5	3	2
red	1 lg (6.4 oz)	33	7	5	2
red chopped	½ cup (3.2 oz)	16	4	2	1
red slice	1 lg (0.9 oz)	5	1	1	tr
roma	1 (2.2 oz)	11	2	2	1
yellow	1 (7.4 oz)	32	6	–	2
yellow chopped	½ cup (2.4 oz)	10	2	–	1
Earthbound Farm					
Organic Roma	1 med (5.2 oz)	35	7	4	1

FOOD	PORTION	CALS	CARB	SUGAR	FIBER
Foxy					
Roma	1 med (5 oz)	35	7	4	1
Frieda's					
Baby Roma	⅔ cup (3 oz)	120	4	2	1
Tear Drop	⅔ cup (3 oz)	20	4	2	1
TAKE-OUT					
aspic	½ cup (4 oz)	32	6	5	tr
broiled slices	2 (2.9 oz)	18	4	3	1
broiled whole	1 med (3.7 oz)	23	5	3	2
bruschetta on toasted italian bread	1 slice	106	18	2	tr
fried slices	2 (2.5 oz)	122	8	2	1
scalloped	½ cup (4 oz)	99	12	5	1
stuffed w/ rice	1 (5.2 oz)	110	20	3	2
stuffed w/ rice & meat	1 (5.2 oz)	142	15	3	2
TOMATO JUICE					
tomato juice	1 cup (8.5 oz)	41	10	9	1
tomato juice w/o added salt	1 cup (8.5 oz)	41	10	9	1
Campbell's					
Healthy Request	8 oz	50	10	8	2
Low Sodium	8 oz	50	10	7	2
Organic	8 oz	50	10	7	2
Dei Fratelli					
Tomato Juice	8 oz	40	10	0	1
Kagome					
Sweet Summer	8 oz	50	11	9	1
Lakewood					
Organic	8 oz	35	7	6	1
TONGUE					
beef simmered	3 oz	241	0	0	0
lamb braised	3 oz	234	0	0	0
pork braised	3 oz	230	0	0	0
veal braised	3 oz	172	0	0	0
Rumba					
Beef	4 oz	250	4	0	0
TORTILLA					
corn	1 (6 in diam)	56	12	–	1
corn w/o salt	1 (6 in diam)	56	12	–	1
flour w/o salt	1 (8 in diam)	114	20	–	1

FOOD	PORTION	CALS	CARB	SUGAR	FIBER
French Meadow Bakery					
Organic Fat Flush	1 (1 oz)	100	18	1	3
La Tortilla Factory					
Carb Cutting Original	1 (1.3 oz)	60	11	0	7
Organic Yellow Corn	2 (2.4 oz)	120	25	0	2
Smart & Delicious Low Fat Low Sodium	1 (2.5 oz)	150	32	1	6
Rudi's Organic Bakery					
Spelt	1 (2 oz)	140	27	1	1
Salba Smart					
Whole Wheat Omega-3 Enriched	1 (1.5 oz)	120	21	1	2
Tumaro's					
Honey Wheat	1 (8 in)	110	23	1	2
Low In Carbs Garden Vegetable	1 (8 in)	100	12	1	8
Low In Carbs Green Onion	1 (8 in)	100	13	0	7
Low In Carbs Multi Grain	1 (8 in)	100	13	1	8
Low In Carbs Salsa	1 (8 in)	100	13	1	8
Pesto & Garlic	1 (8 in)	110	23	1	1
Premium White	1 (8 in)	120	23	1	tr
Soy-full Heart 8 Grain 'N Soy	1 (1.4 oz)	100	14	1	4
Soy-full Heart Apple 'N Cinnamon	1 (1.4 oz)	90	13	1	4
Soy-full Heart Wheat Soy & Flax	1 (1.4 oz)	90	13	1	4
Spinach & Vegetables	1 (8 in)	110	23	1	1

TORTILLA CHIPS *(see CHIPS)*

TRAIL MIX

FOOD	PORTION	CALS	CARB	SUGAR	FIBER
Enjoy Life					
Gluten Free Not Nuts! Beach Bash	1 oz	130	13	9	2
Gluten Free Not Nuts! Mountain Mambo	1 oz	140	12	9	2
Good Sense					
Dietary Snack Mix	¼ cup	130	14	7	2
Organic Tropical	⅓ cup	160	16	11	2
Kopali					
Organic Mix	½ pkg (1 oz)	130	15	7	4
Mrs. May's					
Coconut Almond Crunch	1 oz	183	10	6	2

FOOD	PORTION	CALS	CARB	SUGAR	FIBER
Navitas Naturals					
3 Berry Cacao Nibs & Cashews	1 oz	110	16	8	4
Goji Cacao Nibs & Cashews	1 oz	120	13	7	3
Goji Golden Berry & Mulberry	1 oz	90	19	12	2
Organic Trails					
Summit Blend	¼ cup	150	19	14	2
Planters					
Berry Nut & Chocolate	3 tbsp (1 oz)	120	18	16	1
SunRise					
Honey Coated	3 tbsp (1 oz)	137	14	9	4
W/ Fruit	3 tbsp (1 oz)	130	16	11	2
TRIPE					
beef simmered	3 oz	80	2	0	0
Rumba					
Beef Tripe	4 oz	110	0	0	0
TAKE-OUT					
mondongo w/ potatoes	1 cup	300	26	5	6
TROUT					
baked	3 oz	162	0	0	0
rainbow cooked	3 oz	129	0	0	0
sea trout baked	3 oz	113	0	0	0
TRUFFLES					
fresh	0.5 oz	4	9	–	2
TUNA					
CANNED					
light in oil	1 can (6 oz)	399	0	0	0
light in oil	3 oz	169	0	0	0
light in water	1 can (5.8 oz)	192	0	0	0
light in water	3 oz	99	0	0	0
white in oil	1 can (6.2 oz)	331	0	0	0
white in oil	3 oz	158	0	0	0
white in water	1 can (6 oz)	234	0	0	0
white in water	3 oz	116	0	0	0
Bumble Bee					
Chunk Light In Water	2 oz	60	0	0	0
Chunk Light Touch Of Lemon In Water	¼ cup	60	0	0	0
Chunk Light In Oil	¼ cup	110	0	0	0

FOOD	PORTION	CALS	CARB	SUGAR	FIBER
Chunk White In Water	¼ cup	60	0	0	0
Chunk White In Oil	¼ cup	100	0	0	0
Chunk White In Water Very Low Sodium	¼ cup	70	0	0	0
Light In Oil	¼ cup	110	0	0	0
Sensations Lemon & Pepper w/ Crackers	1 pkg (3.6 oz)	200	13	2	0
Solid White In Oil	¼ cup	90	0	0	0
Solid White In Water	2 oz	70	0	0	0
Tonno In Olive Oil	¼ cup	120	0	0	0
Chicken Of The Sea					
Albacore Solid In Water	2 oz	70	0	0	0
Coral					
Light In Water	¼ cup	60	0	0	0
Polar					
Albacore Solid White In Water	2 oz	70	0	0	0
Chunk Light In Water	2 oz	60	0	0	0
Progresso					
Albacore Solid White Olive Oil	¼ cup (2 oz)	90	0	0	0
Solid Light Olive Oil drained	¼ cup (2 oz)	120	0	0	0
StarKist					
Chunk Light In Water	¼ cup (2 oz)	60	0	0	0
Chunk Light In Water Flavor Pouch	1 pkg (3 oz)	90	0	0	0
Low Sodium Chunk White In Water	¼ cup (2 oz)	60	0	0	0
Solid Light In Water	2 oz	60	0	0	0
Solid White Albacore In Water	2 oz	70	0	0	0
Tuna Creations Hickory Smoked Flavor Pouch	2 oz	60	0	0	0
Tree Of Life					
Wild Light Tongol Chunk In Spring Water No Salt Added	¼ cup (2.4 oz)	50	0	0	0
FRESH					
bluefin cooked	3 oz	157	0	0	0
bluefin raw	3 oz	122	0	0	0
skipjack baked	3 oz	112	0	0	0
yellowfin baked	3 oz	118	0	0	0

FOOD	PORTION	CALS	CARB	SUGAR	FIBER
MIX					
StarKist					
Lunch To-Go Chunk Light	1 pkg	310	27	8	2
Tuna Helper					
Creamy Broccoli as prep	1 cup	310	39	2	2
Creamy Pasta as prep	1 cup	320	39	2	1
Tetrazzini as prep	1 cup	290	33	2	1
SHELF-STABLE					
Bumble Bee					
Steak Entrees Ginger & Soy	1 pkg (4 oz)	170	3	3	0
Steak Entrees Lemon & Cracked Pepper	1 pkg (4 oz)	160	0	0	0
Steak Entrees Mesquite Grilled	1 pkg (4 oz)	150	0	0	0
TURBOT					
european baked	3 oz	104	0	0	0
TURKEY *(see also* TURKEY DISHES, TURKEY SUBSTITUTES*)*					
CANNED					
w/ broth	1 cup	220	0	0	0
Valley Fresh					
Chunk White	2 oz	80	0	0	0
FRESH					
breast pre-basted w/ skin roasted	3.5 oz	126	0	0	0
breast roasted w/ skin	4 oz	212	0	0	0
breast roasted w/o skin	4 oz	175	0	0	0
dark meat w/o skin roasted	1 cup (5 oz)	262	0	0	0
dark meat w/o skin roasted	3 oz	170	0	0	0
ground cooked	3 oz	193	0	0	0
leg w/ skin roasted	1 (19 oz)	1136	0	0	0
light meat w/ skin roasted half turkey	2.3 lbs	2069	0	0	0
light meat w/o skin roasted	4 oz	183	0	0	0
neck simmered	1 (5.3 oz)	274	0	0	0
skin roasted	1 oz	141	0	0	0
skin roasted from half turkey	8.7 oz	1096	0	0	0
tail cooked	1 (2 oz)	197	0	0	0
w/ skin roasted	1 serv (4.2 oz)	249	0	0	0
w/ skin roasted	½ turkey (4 lbs)	3857	0	0	0

FOOD	PORTION	CALS	CARB	SUGAR	FIBER
w/o skin roasted	1 cup (5 oz)	238	0	0	0
w/o skin roasted	1 serv (3.7 oz)	177	0	0	0
wing w/ skin roasted	1 (6.5 oz)	426	0	0	0
wing w/o skin roasted	1	237	0	0	0
Butterball					
Burger Patties	1 (4 oz)	150	0	0	0
Cutlets	4 oz	120	0	0	0
Drumstick	4 oz	170	0	0	0
Ground 7% Fat	4 oz	150	0	0	0
Ground White	4 oz	130	0	0	0
Strips	4 oz	120	0	0	0
Thighs	4 oz	170	0	0	0
Wings	1 (6.3 oz)	380	0	0	0
Empire					
Gound White	4 oz	160	0	0	0
Honeysuckle White					
85% Lean Ground	4 oz	240	0	0	0
93% Lean Patties	1 (4 oz)	160	0	0	0
97% Lean Ground White	4 oz	130	0	0	0
99% Fat Free Breast Tenderloin	4 oz	120	0	0	0
99% Fat Free Breast Cutlets	4 oz	120	0	0	0
Drumettes	4 oz	180	0	0	0
Marinated Strips Asian Grill	4 oz	160	8	5	0
Necks	4 oz	150	0	0	0
Tenderloins Creamy Dijon Mustard	4 oz	140	0	0	0
Tenderloins Homestyle	4 oz	130	0	0	0
Tenderloins Teriyaki	4 oz	140	5	2	0
Thighs	4 oz	190	0	0	0
Whole Honey Roasted	4 oz	180	5	5	0
Wings	4 oz	220	0	0	0
Shady Brook					
Breast Tenderloin	4 oz	130	0	0	0
Breast Tenderloin Creamy Dijon Mustard	4 oz	140	4	0	0
Breast Tenderloin Teriyaki	4 oz	140	5	2	0
Breast Cutlets	4 oz	110	0	0	0
Ground 93% Lean	4 oz	160	0	0	0
Ground 99% Lean	4 oz	120	0	0	0
Marinated Strips Asian Grill	4 oz	160	8	5	0

FOOD	PORTION	CALS	CARB	SUGAR	FIBER
Marinated Strips Mild Herb	4 oz	130	6	1	0
Necks	4 oz	150	0	0	0
Tenderloins Turkey Breast Homestyle	4 oz	130	1	0	0
Thigh	4 oz	145	0	0	0
Wing	4 oz	210	0	0	0
FROZEN					
roast boneless seasoned light & dark meat roasted	3.5 oz	155	3	0	0
Butterball					
Boneless Roast	4 oz	130	0	0	0
Breast Boneless Roast	4 oz	110	1	0	0
Breast Whole	4 oz	110	1	1	0
Breast Whole Smoked Cooked	3 oz	120	1	1	0
Whole Turkey	1 serv (4 oz)	170	0	0	0
Whole Turkey Baked	3.oz	130	0	0	0
Honeysuckle White					
Breast Boneless Roast	4 oz	170	0	0	0
Jennie-O					
Burger	1 (4 oz)	160	0	0	0
Organic Prairie					
Whole Young	4 oz	190	0	0	0
READY-TO-EAT					
bologna	1 slice (1 oz)	59	1	1	tr
breast	1 slice (0.7 oz)	22	1	1	tr
ham	1 slice (1 oz)	35	1	tr	tr
pastrami	2 oz	70	2	2	tr
salami	1 slice (1 oz)	48	tr	tr	0
Applegate Farms					
Organic Herb	2 oz	50	0	0	0
Boar's Head					
Breast 50% Lower Sodium Skin On	2 oz	60	0	0	0
Breast Cracked Pepper Smoked	2 oz	60	1	1	0
Breast Hickory Smoked Black Forest	2 oz	60	0	0	0
Breast Maple Glazed Honey Coat	2 oz	70	2	2	0
Breast Ovengold	2 oz	60	1	0	0
Breast Ovengold Skinless	2 oz	60	0	0	0

FOOD	PORTION	CALS	CARB	SUGAR	FIBER
Breast Roasted Mesquite Smoked Skinless	2 oz	60	1	0	0
Breast Roasted Salsalito	2 oz	60	1	0	0
Butterball					
Breast Honey Roasted Thick Sliced	1 slice (1 oz)	35	2	1	0
Breast Oven Roasted Extra Thin Slice	7 slices (2 oz)	70	3	2	0
Breast Smoked Thin Sliced	4 slices (1.9 oz)	70	4	2	0
Deep Fried Original Thick Sliced	1 slice (1 oz)	30	1	0	0
Honeysuckle White					
Simply Done Whole Breast	4 oz	160	2	0	0
Organic Prairie					
Roasted Breast Slices	2 oz	60	0	0	0
Oscar Mayer					
Breast Smoked Shaved	2 oz	50	2	0	0
Russer					
Turkey Breast Honey Roasted	1 slice (1 oz)	25	1	1	0
Sara Lee					
Breast Cracked Pepper	4 slices (1.8 oz)	50	1	0	0
Breast Hardwood Smoked	4 slices (1.8 oz)	50	1	0	0
Shady Brook					
Turkey Ham Smoked	2 oz	60	0	0	0
Tyson					
Breast Oven Roasted	2 slices (1.6 oz)	40	1	0	0
TURKEY DISHES					
READY-TO-EAT					
Perdue					
Meal Time Starters Turkey Breast Roast W/ Homestyle Gravy	½ cup (4.6 oz)	144	7	1	0
TAKE-OUT					
boneless breast w/ cranberry apple stuffing	1 serv (5 oz)	260	10	2	1
fricassee	1 cup	322	8	tr	tr
salad	1 cup	417	3	1	1
tetrazzini	1 cup	369	29	2	2
turkey a la king	1 cup (8.5 oz)	465	16	4	1
turkey creole w/o rice	1 cup	189	9	5	2
turkey croquette	1 (2 oz)	158	8	2	tr

FOOD	PORTION	CALS	CARB	SUGAR	FIBER
turkey divan	1 cup	321	9	2	3
turkey meatloaf	1 lg slice (5 oz)	243	11	3	1

TURKEY SUBSTITUTES
Lightlife
Smart Deli Roast Turkey	4 slices (2 oz)	80	4	0	1

Tofurky
Deli Slices Cranberry	3 slices (1.8 oz)	98	8	2	3
Deli Slices Hickory Smoked	3 slices (1.8 oz)	100	6	1	3
Deli Slices Italian	3 slices (1.8 oz)	103	7	2	4
Deli Slices Original	3 slices (1.8 oz)	103	6	1	3
Deli Slices Peppered	3 slices (1.8 oz)	103	6	1	3
Deli Slices Philly Steak	3 slices (1.8 oz)	110	7	0	3
Roast	1 serv (4 oz)	190	10	1	2

Worthington
Turkee Slices	3 slices (3.3 oz)	180	5	1	0

Yves
Meatless Ground Turkey	⅓ cup	60	8	0	2
Meatless Deli Turkey Slices	4 slices	100	5	tr	0

TURMERIC
ground	1 tsp	8	1	tr	tr

TURNIPS
fresh greens chopped cooked	½ cup	15	3	—	2
frzn greens cooked	½ cup	24	4	—	2

Allens
Seasoned	½ cup	35	5	1	2

Glory
Greens Fresh	2 cups	20	5	tr	3
Greens Seasoned canned	½ cup	35	4	1	2
Root Cut Fresh	½ cup	20	4	2	1
Sensibly Seasoned Greens	½ cup	20	4	0	2

FOOD	PORTION	CALS	CARB	SUGAR	FIBER
TURTLE					
raw	3.5 oz	85	0	0	0
TUSK FISH					
raw	3.5 oz	79	0	0	0
VANILLA					
vanilla extract	1 tbsp (0.5 oz)	37	2	2	0
vanilla extract	1 tsp (4.2 g)	12	1	1	0
vanilla extract alcohol free	1 tsp (4.2 g)	2	1	1	0
Bob's Red Mill					
Organic Extract	1 tsp	0	0	0	0
VEAL (see also VEAL DISHES)					
breast braised	3 oz	226	0	0	0
chop cooked	1 med (6.5 oz)	230	0	0	0
chop breaded fried	1 med (6.5 oz)	290	13	0	tr
cubed braised	3 oz	160	0	0	0
cutlet cooked	3 oz	141	0	0	0
ground broiled	3 oz	146	0	0	0
leg roasted	3 oz	136	0	0	0
loin roasted	3 oz	184	0	0	0
patty breaded fried	1 (2.8 oz)	211	7	1	tr
shank braised	3 oz	162	0	0	0
VEAL DISHES					
TAKE-OUT					
cordon bleu	1 serv (8 oz)	490	4	2	1
parmigiana	1 serv (6.4 oz)	362	15	3	2
scallopini	1 slice + sauce (3.4 oz)	238	2	1	tr
stew	1 serv (8.8 oz)	192	18	4	3
veal marengo	1 serv (8.8 oz)	274	7	3	1
veal marsala	1 slice + sauce (3.4 oz)	268	6	2	tr
veal paprikash	1 serv (8.6 oz)	280	5	1	1
veal picatta	1 piece + sauce (3.5 oz)	154	2	tr	tr
VEGETABLE JUICE					
low sodium tomato & vegetable juice	1 cup	53	11	9	2
vegetable juice cocktail	8 oz	46	11	8	2

FOOD	PORTION	CALS	CARB	SUGAR	FIBER
Bolthouse Farms					
Vedge Tomato Carrot Celery	8 oz	60	11	9	2
Dei Fratelli					
Vegetable Juice	8 oz	45	11	9	1
Green To Go					
100% Natural Organic as prep	1 pkg (0.3 oz)	32	6	1	tr
Lakewood					
Super Veggie	6 oz	40	9	6	4
V8					
100% Vegetable Essential Antioxidants	8 oz	50	11	6	2
Calcium Enriched	8 oz	50	11	8	2
High Fiber	8 oz	60	13	8	5
Low Sodium	8 oz	50	10	8	2
Organic	8 oz	50	10	8	2
V-Fusion Acai Mixed Berry	8 oz	110	27	26	0
Walnut Acres					
Organic Incredible Vegetable	8 oz	50	12	11	1
VEGETABLES MIXED					
CANNED					
Del Monte					
Savory Sides Homestyle Vegetable Medley	½ cup	70	11	3	2
Savory Sides Rio Grande Vegetables	½ cup	70	14	3	2
Veg-All					
Original Mixed	½ cup	40	8	2	2
DRIED					
Fun-Yums					
Fresh Crispy Mixed Veggies	1 serv (0.9 oz)	114	18	2	1
FRESH					
Mann's					
Broccoli & Cauliflower	1 serv (3 oz)	25	4	2	2
California Stir Fry	1 serv (3 oz)	30	6	3	2
Medley	1 serv (3 oz)	25	5	3	2
Veggies On The Go w/ Dip	1 cup + 1 tbsp dip	100	7	4	2
FROZEN					
mixed vegetables cooked	½ cup	54	12	—	2

FOOD	PORTION	CALS	CARB	SUGAR	FIBER
Birds Eye					
Asparagus Gold & White Corn & Baby Carrots	⅔ cup	70	13	4	1
Italian Herb Harvest Vegetables	1¼ cups	90	6	3	2
Spring Vegetables In Citrus Sauce	1¼ cups	70	8	4	2
Steamfresh Asian Medley	1 cup (3.3 oz)	50	6	3	2
Steamfresh Broccoli Cauliflower & Carrots	¾ cup	30	5	2	2
Steamfresh Broccoli & Cauliflower	1 cup	30	4	2	2
Steamfresh Broccoli Carrots Sugar Snap Peas & Water Chestnuts	¾ cup (2.9 oz)	35	6	3	2
Steamfresh Mixed Vegetables	⅔ cup (3.2 oz)	40	12	4	2
C&W					
Early Harvest Peas & Baby Carrots	⅔ cup	60	10	4	3
Petite Peas & Pearl Onions	⅔ cup	60	11	4	3
Cascadian Farm					
Organic Peas & Carrots	⅔ cup	50	10	4	3
Organic Mixed Vegetables	⅔ cup	60	12	4	2
Europe's Best					
Zen Garden	¾ cup	60	12	3	3
Green Giant					
Broccoli & Carrots w/ Garlic & Herbs as prep	½ cup	40	7	3	2
Garden Vegetable Medley as prep	½ cup	70	14	3	2
Mixed Vegetables as prep	½ cup	50	11	3	2
Southwestern Style as prep	½ cup	90	18	3	4
Szechuan Vegetables as prep	½ cup	50	9	5	2
Health Is Wealth					
Veggie Munchees Vegan	6 (3 oz)	150	26	2	3
La Choy					
Chop Suey Vegetables	½ cup (2.2 oz)	15	3	1	tr
Fancy Chinese Mixed Vegetables	½ cup (2.9 oz)	15	3	0	1
Stir Fry Vegetables	½ cup	15	3	1	2

FOOD	PORTION	CALS	CARB	SUGAR	FIBER
McKenzie's					
Gumbo Mixture	1 serv (2.9 oz)	35	8	3	2
Okra Tomatoes w/ Onions	1 serv (2.8 oz)	20	4	2	2
Melrose Made Gourmet					
Vegetable Souffle Fat Free	1 serv (4 oz)	70	5	2	3
Roast Works					
Flame Roasted Redskins & Vegetables	1 serv (3 oz)	90	14	2	3
Seapoint Farms					
Organic Veggie Blends w/ Edamame Eat Your Greens	¾ cup	60	7	tr	3
Veggie Blends w/ Edamame Garden	¾ cup	60	7	2	3
Veggie Blends w/ Edamame Oriental	¾ cup	60	8	2	3
TAKE-OUT					
buddha's delight	1 serv (16 oz)	174	17	8	3
pakoras	4 (1.7 oz)	57	7	1	2
ratatouille	1 serv (3.5 oz)	96	7	7	4
samosa	1 (2.4 oz)	206	22	1	2
stir fry mix vegetables	1 serv (4 oz)	66	3	2	2
tapenade grilled vegetables	¼ cup	40	4	2	tr
VENISON *(see also JERKY)*					
roasted	4 oz	215	0	0	0
VINEGAR					
cider	1 tbsp	3	tr	tr	0
red wine	1 tbsp	3	tr	0	0
white	1 tbsp	3	tr	tr	0
Carapelli					
Balsamic	1 tbsp	15	4	0	0
Red Wine	1 tbsp	5	0	0	0
White Wine	1 tbsp	5	0	0	0
Eden					
Organic Apple Cider	1 tbsp	0	0	0	0
Organic Brown Rice	1 tbsp	2	0	0	0
Red Wine	1 tbsp	0	0	0	0
Ume Plum	1 tsp	0	0	0	0
Gedney					
Apple Cider	1 tbsp	3	0	0	0

FOOD	PORTION	CALS	CARB	SUGAR	FIBER
Distilled White	1 tbsp	3	0	0	0
Gourme Mist					
Balsamic Of Modena	1 sec spray	1	0	0	0
Balsamic Vinegar + Raspberry	1 sec spray	1	0	0	0
Latino Chef					
Passion Fruit	1 tbsp	40	2	1	tr
Lucini					
Italian Wine Pinot Noir	1 tbsp (0.5 oz)	tr	0	0	0
Newman's Own					
Organic Balsamic	1 tbsp	20	5	5	0

WAFFLES
FROZEN
Aunt Jemima

FOOD	PORTION	CALS	CARB	SUGAR	FIBER
Blueberry	2 (2.5 oz)	190	32	5	1
Low Fat	2 (2.5 oz)	160	30	2	1
Eggo					
Buttermilk	2	180	26	2	1
Homestyle	2	190	29	2	1
Homestyle Minis	12	250	38	3	1
Nutri-Grain Low Fat Whole Wheat	2	140	28	3	3
Special K	3	190	37	5	1
Waf-Fulls Strawberry	1	150	25	10	tr
EnviroKidz					
Organic Gorilla Banana	2 (2.7 oz)	230	34	9	2
Kashi					
Heart To Heart Honey Oat	2 (3 oz)	160	31	6	3
Lifestream					
Organic Fig + Flax	2 (2.8 oz)	210	29	6	6
Organic Pomegran Plus	2 (2.8 oz)	190	31	6	5
Van's					
Belgian Multigrain	2 (2.7 oz)	190	25	3	4
Mini Homestyle	4 (2.8 oz)	210	32	6	1
Organic Flax	2 (2.7 oz)	190	24	3	3
Organic Homestyle	2 (2.7 oz)	200	25	3	2
Original 97% Fat Free	2 (2.7 oz)	140	26	4	3
Original Buttermilk	2 (2.7 oz)	220	31	6	1
Wheat Free Buckwheat	2 (3 oz)	230	36	5	2
Wheat Free Flax	2 (3 oz)	210	33	4	1

FOOD	PORTION	CALS	CARB	SUGAR	FIBER
READY-TO-EAT					
Kashi					
GoLean Blueberry	2 (3 oz)	170	33	4	6
GoLean Original	2 (3 oz)	170	33	4	6
TAKE-OUT					
belgian	1 (4.7 oz)	412	65	6	3
blueberry 9 in sq	1 (7 oz)	556	90	12	5
round 10 in diam	1 (6.8 oz)	598	94	9	5
square 9 in	1 (7 oz)	620	98	9	5
whole wheat 9 in sq	1 (7 oz)	534	67	15	5
WALNUTS					
black chopped	¼ cup	193	3	tr	2
english chopped	¼ cup	191	4	1	2
english ground	¼ cup	131	3	1	1
english halves	14 (1 oz)	185	4	1	2
english in shell	7 (1 oz)	183	4	1	2
honey roasted	¼ cup	172	7	4	2
Diamond					
Chopped	¼ cup	200	4	1	2
Emerald					
Glazed	¼ cup	140	12	9	1
Good Sense					
Organic Raw Walnuts	¼ cup	210	3	0	3
WASABI *(see HORSERADISH)*					
WATER					
ice cubes	3	0	0	0	0
tap water	8 oz	0	0	0	0
Adironack					
Sparkling All Flavors	8 oz	0	0	0	0
Aloe Breeze					
Organic All Flavors	8 oz	0	0	0	0
Aloe Splash					
All Flavors	8 oz	0	0	0	0
Aqua Pacific					
Water	1 liter	0	0	0	0
Aquafina					
Alive Wellness Berry Pomegranate	8 oz	10	2	2	0
Sparkling Citrus Twist	8 oz	0	0	0	0

FOOD	PORTION	CALS	CARB	SUGAR	FIBER
Aroma Water					
All Flavors	8 oz	0	0	0	0
Ayala's					
Herbal All Flavors	1 bottle	0	0	0	0
Bot					
Fortified All Flavors	1 bottle (12 oz)	40	10	9	0
Clearly Canadian					
Zero Sparkling All Flavors	8 oz	0	0	0	0
Crystal Geyser					
Spring Water	8 oz	0	0	0	0
Dasani					
Purified Water	8 oz	0	0	0	0
w/ Lemon	8 oz	2	0	0	0
Eden					
Springs Artesian	8 oz	0	0	0	0
Evian					
Spring Water	1 liter	0	0	0	0
Fiji					
Natural Artesian	1 liter	0	0	0	0
Fruit 2 0					
Grape	8 oz	0	0	0	0
Natural Berry	8 oz	0	0	0	0
Watermelon Kiwi	8 oz	0	0	0	0
Fruit Refreshers					
Lemonade	8 oz	0	0	0	0
Gerolsteiner					
Sparkling Mineral	8 oz	0	0	0	0
H2Odwalla					
Enhanced Tropical Orange	1 bottle (20 oz)	120	33	27	2
Hawaiian Springs					
Naturally Pure	1 liter	0	0	0	0
Highland Spring					
Spring Water	1 liter	0	0	0	0
Hint					
All Flavors	1 bottle (15 oz)	0	0	0	0
Island Chill					
Atresian Water	1 liter	0	0	0	0
Jana					
Natural European Artesian	1 liter	0	0	0	0

FOOD	PORTION	CALS	CARB	SUGAR	FIBER
Klear Splash					
Mini Sip	1 pkg (4 oz)	0	0	0	0
Liquid Salvation					
Ultra Hydrating	1 bottle	0	0	0	0
Nestle					
Pure Life Splash All Flavors	8 oz	0	0	0	0
Nui					
All Natural Kid Water	10 oz	90	21	16	3
O Water					
Hydrate Black Raspberry	8 oz	25	7	7	0
Replenish Lemon Lime	8 oz	25	7	7	0
Vitalize Peach Mango	8 oz	25	7	7	0
San Benedetto					
Sparkling Mineral Water	1 liter	0	0	0	0
Skinny Water					
Hi-Energy Acai Grape Blueberry	8 oz	0	0	0	0
Total-V Passionfruit Lemonade	8 oz	0	0	0	0
SoNu					
Water All Flavors	8 oz	45	13	13	0
Splash					
All Flavors	8 oz	0	0	0	0
TalkingRain					
Ice All Flavors	8 oz	5	1	1	0
Thorpedo					
Ultra Low GI Energy Water	8 oz	45	11	10	0
Tipperary					
Mineral Water	1 liter	0	0	0	0
Trim Water					
Purified	1 bottle (20 oz)	10	3	3	0
Twist					
Organics All Flavors	8 oz	10	2	2	0
Vitamin + Fiber Water					
All Fruit Flavors	8 oz	50	13	12	3
Volvic					
Mineral Water	1 liter	0	0	0	0
Natural Lemon	8 oz	0	1	1	0
Natural Orange	8 oz	30	7	7	0
Wateroos					
All Flavors	1 box (8 oz)	0	0	0	0

FOOD	PORTION	CALS	CARB	SUGAR	FIBER
WaterPlus					
Extra-C Orange Tangerine	8 oz	50	13	13	0
WATER CHESTNUTS					
La Choy					
Sliced	½ cup	25	5	2	1
Polar					
Sliced	2 tbsp	10	3	1	1
WATERCRESS					
cooked w/o fat	1 cup	15	2	tr	1
raw chopped	1 cup	4	tr	tr	tr
Frieda's					
Watercress	1 cup	10	1	0	2
WATERMELON					
cut up	1 cup	46	12	10	1
wedge	1 sm (2.5 oz)	21	5	4	tr
wedge	1 med (10 oz)	86	22	18	1
wedge	1 lg (20 oz)	172	43	35	2
whole melon	1 (9 lb)	1227	309	254	16
Frieda's					
Yellow Seedless	½ cup (3 oz)	25	6	6	0
Sundia					
Fresh	2 cups	80	27	25	2
WATERMELON JUICE					
juice	8 oz	71	18	15	1
Sundia					
100% Natural	8 oz	110	27	24	1
Tang					
Watermelon Wallop	1 box (7 oz)	90	24	24	0
WHALE					
beluga dried	1 oz	92	0	0	0
WHEAT					
sprouted	1 cup (3.8 oz)	214	46	–	1
Arrowhead Mills					
Whole Grain Wheat	¼ cup (1.6 oz)	150	31	0	5
Bob's Red Mill					
Vital Wheat Gluten	¼ cup	120	6	0	0

FOOD	PORTION	CALS	CARB	SUGAR	FIBER
Hodgson Mill					
Vital Wheat Gluten	4 tsp	40	3	0	1
Near East					
Taboule Wheat Salad as prep	⅔ cup (3.5 oz)	120	24	1	5
WHEAT GERM					
plain	¼ cup	108	14	2	4
Bob's Red Mill					
Wheat Germ	2 tbsp	59	7	3	2
Hodgson Mill					
Untoasted	2 tbsp	55	7	0	4
Kretschmer					
Original Toasted	¼ cup (0.6 oz)	35	10	–	7
Tree Of Life					
Toasted	3 tbsp (0.8 oz)	100	12	3	3
WHEY					
acid dry	1 tbsp	10	2	2	0
sweet dry	1 tbsp	26	6	6	0
sweet fluid	½ cup	33	6	6	0
whey cheese	1 oz	126	9	0	0
Bob's Red Mill					
Protein Concentrate	¼ cup	80	1	1	0
Sweet Dairy	1 tbsp	30	6	5	0
Wellements					
Whey Protein Chocolate	1 scoop (1 oz)	120	4	tr	0
Whey Protein Vanilla	1 scoop (1 oz)	120	4	tr	0
WHIPPED TOPPINGS					
Hood					
Light Sugar Free Whipped Cream	2 tbsp	10	tr	0	0
Whipped Light Cream	2 tbsp	20	tr	tr	0
Soyatoo					
Soy Whip	2 tbsp	10	1	1	0
TruWhip					
Whipped Topping	2 tbsp (0.4 oz)	130	3	2	0
WHITEFISH					
baked	3 oz	146	0	0	0
smoked	1 oz	39	0	0	0
smoked	3 oz	92	0	0	0

FOOD	PORTION	CALS	CARB	SUGAR	FIBER
WHITING					
broiled w/o fat	3 oz	99	0	0	0
fillet broiled w/o fat	1 (2.5 oz)	84	0	0	0
fillet steamed w/o fat	1 (2.6 oz)	84	0	0	0
hake raw	3.5 oz	84	0	0	0
TAKE-OUT					
fillet battered & fried	1 (3.1 oz)	157	6	tr	tr
fillet breaded & fried	1 (3.1 oz)	191	7	1	tr
WILD RICE					
cooked	1 cup (5.8 oz)	166	35	1	3
Lundberg					
Organic Quick not prep	¼ cup	150	33	1	2
WINE					
chianti	1 serv (5 oz)	125	4	1	0
chinese cooking	1 bottle (15 oz)	559	3	0	0
cooking	¼ cup (2 oz)	29	4	1	0
haiku	1 serv	93	3	—	0
japanese plum	3 oz	139	16	—	0
japanese sake	2 oz	78	3	0	0
kir	1 serv	78	3	—	0
madeira	3.5 oz	169	10	10	0
nonalcoholic	1 serv (5 oz)	9	2	2	0
port	1 serv (3.5 oz)	165	14	8	0
sake screwdriver	1 serv	175	23	—	tr
sangria	1 serv	88	6	—	tr
sangria blanco	1 serv	155	24	—	3
wassail wine	1 serv	142	22	—	2
white	1 serv (5 oz)	121	4	1	0
wine cooler	1 (7 oz)	116	14	11	0
wine spritzer	1 serv (7 oz)	73	2	1	0
Carlo Rossi					
Cabernet Sauvignon	5 oz	125	5	0	0
WRAPS (see BREAD, SANDWICHES)					
YACON					
Navitas Naturals					
Slices Dried	1 oz	90	22	12	1

FOOD	PORTION	CALS	CARB	SUGAR	FIBER
YAM *(see also* SWEET POTATO*)*					
CANNED					
Bruce's					
In Syrup	⅔ cup	150	36	23	3
Glory					
Candied	½ cup	210	52	38	1
FRESH					
yam cooked w/o salt	1 cup	158	38	1	5
Earthbound Farm					
Organic	1 med (4.6 oz)	130	33	7	4
Frieda's					
Name	¾ cup	100	24	0	3
House					
Black Ita Konnyaku Yam Cake	1 serv (2 oz)	5	1	0	tr
YAUTIA *(see* MALANGA*)*					
YEAST					
baker's compressed	1 cake (0.6 oz)	18	3	0	1
baker's dry	1 pkg (7 g)	21	3	0	2
baker's dry	1 tbsp	35	5	0	3
brewer's dry	1 tbsp	35	5	0	3
Bob's Red Mill					
Active Dry	1 tbsp	25	5	0	2
Hodgson Mill					
Active Dry	1 tsp	30	3	0	1
Fast Rise	1 tsp (9 g)	25	4	0	1
YELLOW BEANS					
fresh cooked w/o salt	1 cup	44	10	2	4
fresh raw	1 cup	34	8	–	4
YELLOWTAIL					
baked	4 oz	199	0	0	0
YOGURT *(see also* YOGURT DRINKS, YOGURT FROZEN*)*					
plain low fat	8 oz	143	16	16	0
plain nonfat	8 oz	127	17	17	0
plain whole milk	8 oz	138	11	11	0
tofu yogurt	1 cup	246	42	3	1
Better Whey					
All Fruit Flavors	1 pkg (6 oz)	145	23	14	3
Plain	1 pkg (6 oz)	130	17	7	3

FOOD	PORTION	CALS	CARB	SUGAR	FIBER
Breyers					
Creme Savers Orange & Creme	1 pkg (8 oz)	240	45	36	0
Creme Savers Raspberries & Creme	1 pkg (8 oz)	240	45	36	0
Light! Probiotic Plus Apple Cinnamon	1 pkg (8 oz)	100	15	10	0
Light! Probiotic Plus Blueberries 'N Cream	1 pkg (8 oz)	110	15	10	0
Light! Probiotic Plus Lemon Chiffon	1 pkg (8 oz)	100	14	9	0
Light! Probiotic Plus Peaches 'N Cream	1 pkg (8 oz)	100	15	10	0
Light! Probiotic Plus Strawberry Banana	1 pkg (8 oz)	110	16	10	0
Light! Probiotic Plus Strawberry Cheesecake	1 pkg (8 oz)	110	16	10	0
Smart! w/DHA Black Cherry	1 pkg (6 oz)	170	35	29	1
Smart! w/ DHA Mixed Berry	1 pkg (6 oz)	170	34	28	1
Smart! w/DHA Peach	6 oz	170	34	28	1
Smart! w/DHA Pineapple	1 pkg (6 oz)	170	34	28	tr
Smart! w/ DHA Strawberry	1 pkg (6 oz)	170	34	28	1
Smart! w/ DHA Strawberry Banana	1 pkg (6 oz)	170	34	27	1
Smooth & Creamy Peaches 'N Cream	1 pkg (8 oz)	240	48	38	0
Smooth & Creamy Strawberry	1 pkg (8 oz)	230	46	36	0
Smooth & Creamy Vanilla Cream	1 pkg (8 oz)	240	47	38	0
YoCrunch Blueberry w/ Granola	1 pkg	240	49	31	2
YoCrunch Cookie N' Cream w/ Oreo	1 pkg	240	41	30	0
YoCrunch Naturals Strawberry Banana w/ Granola	1 pkg	245	50	31	2
YoCrunch Naturals Strawberry w/ Dark Chocolate Chips	1 pkg	280	46	33	2
YoCrunch Raspberry w/ Granola	1 pkg	240	49	31	2
YoCrunch Strawberry w/ Granola	1 pkg	240	49	31	2

FOOD	PORTION	CALS	CARB	SUGAR	FIBER
YoCrunch Vanilla Nestle	1 pkg	260	44	36	0
YoCrunch Vanilla w/ Butterfinger	1 pkg	260	45	34	0
YoCrunch Light Cookies N' Cream w/ Oreo	1 pkg	170	24	11	0
YoCrunch Light Strawberry w/ Granola	1 pkg	170	33	11	2
Cabot					
Greek	1 pkg (6 oz)	210	9	6	0
Greek 2%	1 pkg (6 oz)	160	25	24	0
Non Fat Berry Banana	1 cup	130	24	19	0
Non Fat Black Cherry	1 cup	130	24	19	0
Non Fat Plain	1 cup	100	19	13	0
Non Fat Raspberry	1 cup	130	24	19	0
Chobani					
Greek Yogurt Lowfat Plain	1 pkg (6 oz)	130	7	7	0
Greek Yogurt Nonfat Peach	1 pkg (6 oz)	140	20	19	0
Greek Yogurt Nonfat Plain	1 pkg (6 oz)	100	7	7	0
Greek Yogurt Original Plain	1 pkg (6 oz)	240	6	6	0
Dannon					
Activia Blueberry	1 pkg (4 oz)	110	19	17	0
Activia Mixed Berry	1 pkg (4 oz)	110	19	17	0
Activia Peach	1 pkg (4 oz)	110	19	17	0
Activia Prune	1 pkg (4 oz)	110	19	17	0
Activia Strawberry	1 pkg (4 oz)	110	19	17	0
Activia Vanilla	1 pkg (4 oz)	110	19	17	0
Activia Vanilla Light Fat Free	4 oz	70	13	9	3
All Natural Blended Mini Blueberry	1 (3.3 oz)	110	20	19	0
All Natural Blended Mini Strawberry	1 (3.3 oz)	110	20	19	0
Creamy Fruit Blends Raspberry	6 oz	170	32	29	tr
Fruit On The Bottom Apple Cinnamon	6 oz	150	28	25	tr
Fruit On The Bottom Peach	6 oz	150	28	27	0
Fruit On The Bottom Pineapple	6 oz	150	28	27	0
Fruit On The Bottom Raspberry	6 oz	150	28	26	tr
La Creme Vanilla	4 oz	140	19	18	0
La Creme Mousse French Vanilla	1 (2.6 oz)	110	14	14	0

FOOD	PORTION	CALS	CARB	SUGAR	FIBER
Light & Fit Carb & Sugar Control Blueberries 'N Cream	4 oz	60	3	2	0
Light & Fit Nonfat Cherry Vanilla	6 oz	60	11	8	0
Light & Fit Nonfat Lemon Chiffon	6 oz	60	10	7	0
Light & Fit Nonfat Raspberry	6 oz	60	11	7	0
Light & Fit Nonfat White Chocolate Raspberry	6 oz	90	10	7	0
Fage					
Sheep & Goat's Milk	1 pkg (7 oz)	190	10	10	0
Friendship					
Plain	1 cup	150	18	17	1
Horizon Organic					
Fat Free Peach	1 pkg (6 oz)	140	27	27	1
Fat Free Vanilla	1 cup	180	33	33	0
Kids Strawberry	1 pkg (4 oz)	110	20	20	1
Lowfat Blended Blueberry	1 pkg (6 oz)	160	30	29	2
Tube Lowfat Blueberry	1 (2 oz)	70	12	11	0
Whole Milk Plain	1 cup	160	14	14	0
La Yogurt					
Lowfat Blueberries 'N' Cream	1 pkg (6 oz)	200	39	36	0
Lowfat Fruit On The Bottom Cherry	1 pkg (8 oz)	230	47	46	tr
Lowfat Fruit On The Bottom Probiotic Peach	1 pkg (6 oz)	160	31	29	0
Lowfat Fruit On The Bottom Strawberry	1 pkg (8 oz)	220	43	41	tr
Lowfat Peaches 'N' Cream	1 pkg (6 oz)	200	39	37	0
Lowfat Pina Colada	1 pkg (6 oz)	160	30	26	0
Lowfat Probiotic Pina Colada	1 pkg (6 oz)	160	30	26	0
Lowfat Probiotic Plain	1 pkg (6 oz)	100	12	11	0
Lowfat Probiotic Vanilla	1 pkg (6 oz)	150	26	25	0
Lowfat Vanilla 'N' Cream	1 pkg (6 oz)	200	39	37	0
Nonfat Banana Cream	1 pkg (6 oz)	100	18	14	0
Nonfat Probiotic Cherry	1 pkg (6 oz)	100	17	13	0
Nonfat Probiotic Peach	1 pkg (6 oz)	90	16	12	0
Nonfat Probiotic Raspberry	1 pkg (6 oz)	90	15	11	0
Nonfat Probiotic Vanilla	1 pkg (6 oz)	90	15	10	0

FOOD	PORTION	CALS	CARB	SUGAR	FIBER
Sabor Latino Lowfat Dulce De Leche	1 pkg (6 oz)	190	36	31	0
Sabor Latino Lowfat Guava	1 pkg (6 oz)	190	37	32	0
Sabor Latino Lowfat Horchata	1 pkg (6 oz)	210	41	36	0
Sabor Latino Lowfat Papaya	1 pkg (6 oz)	190	37	32	0
Land O Lakes					
Strawberry Light	1 pkg (8 oz)	80	38	31	0
Strawberry Lowfat	1 pkg (8 oz)	190	36	29	0
Nancy's					
Lowfat Maple	1 pkg (8 oz)	180	26	26	0
Lowfat Plain	1 pkg (8 oz)	150	16	16	0
Lowfat Vanilla	1 pkg (8 oz)	140	15	15	0
Nonfat Fruit On The Top Cherry	1 pkg (8 oz)	140	25	20	1
Nonfat Plain	1 pkg (8 oz)	120	17	17	0
Nonfat Vanilla	1 pkg (8 oz)	220	40	39	0
Organic Soy Kiwi Lime	1 pkg (8 oz)	160	31	21	4
Organic Soy Plain	1 pkg (8 oz)	150	25	15	2
Organic Soy Vanilla	1 pkg (8 oz)	120	19	10	3
Whole Milk Fruit On The Top Peach	1 pkg (8 oz)	220	38	38	1
Whole Milk Honey	1 pkg (8 oz)	170	17	17	0
Oikos					
Organic Greek Vanilla	1 pkg (5.3 oz)	110	12	11	0
Organic Honey	1 pkg (5.3 oz)	120	18	17	0
Organic Plain	1 pkg (5.3 oz)	90	6	6	0
Rachel's					
Essence Berry Jasmine w/ Zinc	1 pkg (6 oz)	160	28	26	2
Essence Plum Honey Lavender	1 pkg (6 oz)	160	28	26	2
Essence Pomegrante Acai	1 pkg (6 oz)	170	29	27	2
Exotic Kiwi Passion Fruit Lime	1 pkg (6 oz)	160	28	26	2
Exotic Orange Strawberry Mango	1 pkg (6 oz)	160	28	27	2
Exotic Pomegranate Blueberry	1 pkg (6 oz)	170	29	27	2
Redwood Hill Farm					
Goat Milk Apricot Mango	1 cup	180	31	22	2
Goat Milk Cranberry Orange	1 cup	180	31	22	2
Goat Milk Plain	1 cup	130	14	4	1
Goat Milk Strawberry	1 cup	180	31	22	2
Goat Milk Vanilla	1 cup	190	31	25	2

FOOD	PORTION	CALS	CARB	SUGAR	FIBER
SoDelicious					
Coconut Milk Plain	1 pkg (6 oz)	130	16	12	3
Coconut Milk Vanilla	1 pkg (6 oz)	150	22	19	2
Dairy Free Cinnamon Bun	1 pkg (6 oz)	160	29	24	3
Dairy Free Raspberry	1 pkg (6 oz)	150	29	22	3
Straus					
Organic Maple Nonfat	1 pkg (8 oz)	170	30	22	0
Organic Maple Whole Milk	1 pkg (8 oz)	210	28	23	0
Organic Plain Lowfat	1 pkg (8 oz)	150	21	10	0
Organic Plain Nonfat	1 pkg (8 oz)	110	16	16	0
Organic Plain Whole Milk	1 pkg (8 oz)	160	13	9	1
Total					
Greek Yogurt 0% Fat	1 pkg (5.3 oz)	80	6	6	0
Greek Yogurt 2% Fat	1 pkg (7 oz)	130	8	8	0
Greek Yogurt Classic	1 pkg (7 oz)	180	6	6	0
Greek Yogurt Light	1 pkg (5.3 oz)	130	5	5	0
Honey	1 pkg (3.5 oz)	250	28	28	0
Wallaby					
Organic Banana Vanilla	1 pkg (6 oz)	150	25	20	0
Organic Lemon	1 pkg (6 oz)	150	25	19	0
Organic Maple	1 pkg (6 oz)	150	26	20	0
Organic Plain	1 cup	150	18	10	0
Organic Raspberry	1 pkg (6 oz)	150	25	19	0
Organic Vanilla	1 pkg (6 oz)	150	25	20	0
Organic Nonfat Mango Lime	1 pkg (6 oz)	140	28	21	0
Organic Nonfat Plain	1 cup	130	19	10	0
Organic Nonfat Vanilla Bean	1 pkg (6 oz)	140	28	22	0
WholeSoy & Co.					
Organic Soy Apricot Mango	1 pkg (6 oz)	160	30	19	2
Organic Soy Lemon	1 pkg (6 oz)	160	29	18	2
Organic Soy Plain	1 pkg (6 oz)	150	27	12	2
Organic Soy Raspberry	1 pkg (6 oz)	170	32	19	2
Organic Soy Vanilla	1 pkg (6 oz)	150	28	12	2
WildWood					
Organic Soyogurt Low Fat Peach	1 pkg (6 oz)	160	29	20	5
Organic Soyogurt Low Fat Vanilla	1 pkg (6 oz)	160	30	21	5
Organic Soyogurt Plain Unsweetened	1 pkg (6 oz)	110	14	4	4

FOOD	PORTION	CALS	CARB	SUGAR	FIBER
Yoplait					
Go-Gurt All Fruit Flavors	1 pkg (2.25 oz)	80	13	11	0
Grande 99% Fat Free All Flavors	1 cup	250	48	42	0
Grande Fat Free Plain	1 cup	90	19	17	0
Kids Banana Vanilla	1 pkg (4 oz)	100	17	13	1
Kids Strawberry Vanilla	1 pkg (4 oz)	100	17	13	1
Light All Fruit Flavors	1 pkg (6 oz)	180	19	14	0
Light Indulgent All Flavors	1 pkg (6 oz)	110	20	15	0
Original All Fruit Flavors	1 pkg (6 oz)	170	33	27	0
Original Coconut Cream	1 pkg (6 oz)	190	34	27	0
Original Lemon Burst	1 pkg (6 oz)	180	36	31	0
Original Pina Colada	1 pkg (6 oz)	170	33	28	0
Trix All Fruit Flavors	1 pkg (4 oz)	120	23	17	0
Yo Plus All Flavors	1 pkg (4 oz)	110	21	16	3
YOGURT DRINKS *(see also* SMOOTHIES*)*					
lassi	7 oz	78	8	8	0
Dahlicious					
Lassi Green Tea	1 bottle	110	21	19	2
Lassi Mango	1 bottle	130	27	24	2
Lassi Plain	1 bottle	110	21	19	2
Dannon					
DanActive Plain	1 bottle (3.3 oz)	90	15	15	0
DanActive Vanilla	1 bottle (3.3 oz)	90	17	17	0
Danimals Rockin' Raspberry	1 bottle (3.1 oz)	70	15	14	0
Danimals Strawberry Explosion	1 bottle (3.1 oz)	70	15	14	0
Danimals Strikin' Strawberry Kiwi	1 bottle (3.1 oz)	70	15	14	0
Frusion Cherry Berry Blend	1 bottle (10 oz)	260	50	47	tr
Frusion Pina Colada	1 bottle (10 oz)	260	50	48	0
Frusion Strawberry Blend	1 bottle (10 oz)	260	50	48	0
Light & Fit Carb & Sugar Control Berries 'N Cream	1 bottle (7 oz)	60	4	3	0

FOOD	PORTION	CALS	CARB	SUGAR	FIBER
Light & Fit Smoothie Peach Passion	1 bottle (7 oz)	70	13	12	0
Light & Fit Smoothie Strawberry Banana	1 bottle (7 oz)	70	13	12	0
Lifeway					
Lassi Lowfat All Flavors	8 oz	174	25	21	3
Promise					
Activ All Flavors	1 bottle (3.5 oz)	70	9	8	tr
Yo On The Go					
All Flavors	1 box (8 oz)	180	31	29	0
Yoplait					
Go-Gurt All Fruit Flavors	1 bottle (5 oz)	120	23	20	0
Light All Flavors	1 bottle (8.3 oz)	90	16	9	3
Nouriche All Fruit Flavors	1 bottle (11 oz)	260	55	42	5
Smoothie All Flavors	1 bottle (8.3 oz)	220	44	33	3
YOGURT FROZEN					
chocolate soft serve	1 cup	230	36	–	3
vanilla soft serve	1 cup	236	35	35	0
Dippin' Dots					
Strawberry Cheesecake	½ cup	100	21	17	1
Hood					
Fat Free Old Fashioned Vanilla	½ cup	110	24	15	tr
Fat Free Strawberry	½ cup	100	23	15	tr
Vanilla Swiss Almond	½ cup	150	25	17	tr
Turkey Hill					
Fudge Ripple	½ cup	100	21	16	0
Neapolitan	½ cup	90	19	14	1
Smoothie Orange Cream Swirl	½ cup	100	22	18	0
Smoothie Peach Mango	½ cup	90	21	17	0
Vanilla Bean	½ cup	100	19	14	0
WholeSoy & Co.					
Organic All Flavors	½ cup	120	25	19	1
ZUCCHINI					
baby raw	1 (0.5 oz)	3	1	–	tr
fresh	1 sm (4.1 oz)	19	4	2	1
pickled	¼ cup	16	4	3	1

FOOD	PORTION	CALS	CARB	SUGAR	FIBER
raw sliced	1 cup	19	4	2	1
sliced cooked w/o salt	1 cup	29	7	3	3
C&W					
Yellow & Green	⅔ cup	20	3	2	tr
Frieda's					
Baby	⅔ cup (3 oz)	20	3	2	0
TAKE-OUT					
breaded & fried	6 slices (3 oz)	141	10	3	1
sticks breaded & fried	6 (2 oz)	90	6	2	1

PART TWO

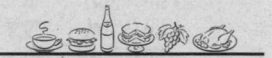

Restaurant Chains

Drop Out of the Clean Plate Club

*When eating out, almost 70% of Americans
eat everything on their plates.
Split an entrée, order an appetizer as a main
course, or order 1 less meal than the number of
people in your group—there will be more than
enough food for everyone and sharing is fun.*

FOOD	PORTION	CALS	CARB	SUGAR	FIBER
A&W					
BEVERAGES					
Coke	1 sm (11 oz)	145	37	37	0
Diet Coke	1 sm (11 oz)	0	0	0	0
Diet Root Beer	1 sm (15 oz)	0	0	0	0
Float Diet Root Beer	1 sm (14 oz)	170	30	17	0
Float Root Beer	1 sm (14 oz)	330	70	57	0
Milkshake Chocolate	1 med	700	100	60	2
Milkshake Strawberry	1 med	670	90	52	0
Milkshake Vanilla	1 med	720	97	57	0
Root Beer	1 sm (15 oz)	220	57	29	0
DESSERTS					
Cone Vanilla	1 med	260	41	29	1
Freeze A&W Root Beer	1 med	480	89	42	0
Polar Swirl M&M	1 med	710	107	93	2
Polar Swirl Oreo	1 med	690	107	79	3
Polar Swirl Reese's	1 med	740	97	85	3
Sundae Caramel	1 med	340	57	13	0
Sundae Chocolate	1 med	320	53	15	0
Sundae Hot Fudge	1 med	350	54	15	4
Sundae Strawberry	1 med	300	47	12	0
Sundae Vanilla	1 med	310	52	18	0
MAIN MENU SELECTIONS					
Cheese Curds	1 serv	570	27	3	2
Cheese Dog	1	320	25	4	1
Cheeseburger Original Bacon	1	570	41	9	2
Cheeseburger Original Bacon Double	1	800	47	10	2
Cheeseburger Original Double	1	720	46	10	2
Chicken Strips	3	500	32	2	7
Chili Bowl	1 serv	190	22	9	5
Coney Chili Dog	1	310	24	5	2
Coney Chili Dog Cheese	1	350	27	5	2
Fries	1 lg	430	61	1	6
Fries Cheese	1 serv	380	50	0	4
Fries Chili	1 serv	370	49	2	5
Fries Chili & Cheese	1 serv	400	51	2	5
Hot Dog Plain	1	280	22	4	1
Onion Rings	1 serv	350	45	3	2
Papa Burger	1	720	46	10	2

FOOD	PORTION	CALS	CARB	SUGAR	FIBER
Sandwich Crispy Chicken	1	590	54	8	3
Sandwich Grilled Chicken	1	440	54	9	2
SAUCES					
Dipping Sauce BBQ	1 serv (1 oz)	40	10	6	0
Dipping Sauce Honey Mustard	1 serv (1 oz)	100	12	6	0
Dipping Sauce Ranch	1 serv (1 oz)	160	2	1	0
Dipping Sauce Sweet & Sour	1 serv (1 oz)	45	12	7	0

ARBY'S
BEVERAGES

FOOD	PORTION	CALS	CARB	SUGAR	FIBER
Dr Pepper	1 (16 oz)	180	52	52	0
Jamocha Shake	1 reg	498	81	78	0
Pepsi	1 (16 oz)	130	34	34	0
Shake Chocolate	1 reg	507	83	81	0
Shake Orange Cream	1 (17 oz)	637	105	100	0
Shake Strawberry	1 reg	498	81	77	0
Shake Strawberry Banana Swirl	1 (17 oz)	567	87	79	0
Shake Vanilla	1 reg	437	66	65	0
Sierra Mist	1 (16 oz)	100	27	27	0

BREAKFAST SELECTIONS

FOOD	PORTION	CALS	CARB	SUGAR	FIBER
Biscuit	1	273	28	3	1
Biscuit Bacon	1	340	29	3	1
Biscuit Bacon Egg & Cheese	1	461	30	4	1
Biscuit Chicken	1	417	39	3	1
Biscuit Ham	1	316	29	4	1
Biscuit Ham Egg & Cheese	1	437	31	4	1
Biscuit Sausage	1	436	26	3	1
Biscuit Sausage Egg & Cheese	1	557	30	3	1
Biscuit Sausage Gravy	1	961	107	19	1
Breakfast Syrup	1 serv (1 oz)	78	20	11	0
Cinnamon Roll Original Gourmet	1	507	73	31	4
Croissant	1	190	21	2	1
Croissant Bacon & Egg	1	337	23	3	1
Croissant Bacon Egg & Cheese	1	378	23	3	1
Croissant Ham & Cheese	1	274	22	3	1
Croissant Ham Egg & Cheese	1	434	26	4	1
Croissant Sausage & Egg	1	433	23	3	1
Croissant Sausage Egg & Cheese	1	475	23	3	1
French Toastix	1 serv	312	44	11	1

FOOD	PORTION	CALS	CARB	SUGAR	FIBER
Muffin Blueberry	1	320	49	26	1
Pecan Sticky Bun	1	688	91	45	5
Sourdough Bacon Egg & Cheese	1	437	40	5	2
Sourdough Egg & Cheese	1	392	40	5	2
Sourdough Ham Egg & Cheese	1	679	42	6	2
Sourdough Sausage Egg & Cheese	1	514	40	5	2
Twist Chocolate	1	250	34	12	2
Twist Cinnamon	1	260	33	11	1
Wrap Bacon Egg & Cheese	1	515	50	2	2
Wrap Ham Egg & Cheese	1	568	51	3	2
Wrap Sausage Egg & Cheese	1	689	50	2	2
CHILDREN'S MENU SELECTIONS					
Kids Meal Chicken Tenders	1 serv	289	21	0	1
Kids Meal Junior Roast Beef Sandwich	1	272	34	5	2
Market Fresh Mini Ham & Cheese Sandwich	1	228	28	6	2
Market Fresh Mini Turkey & Cheese Sandwich	1	235	28	6	2
DESSERTS					
Cookie Chocolate Chip	1 (1.6 oz)	202	26	16	1
Turnover Apple	1	377	65	41	2
Turnover Cherry	1	377	65	41	2
SALAD DRESSINGS AND SAUCES					
Arby's Sauce	1 serv (0.5 oz)	15	4	1	0
Dipping Sauce BBQ	1 pkg (1 oz)	40	11	8	0
Dipping Sauce Bronco Berry	1 serv (2 oz)	122	30	28	0
Dipping Sauce Buffalo	1 serv (1 oz)	10	2	1	0
Dipping Sauce Cool Ranch Sour Cream	1 serv (1.5 oz)	158	2	1	0
Dipping Sauce Honey Mustard	1 serv (1 oz)	129	6	5	0
Dressing Buttermilk Ranch	1 serv (2.2 oz)	325	4	2	0
Dressing Buttermilk Ranch Light	1 serv (2 oz)	112	13	5	1
Dressing Sante Fe Ranch	1 pkg (2.2 oz)	296	4	1	0
Horsey Sauce	1 pkg (0.5 oz)	62	3	0	0
Ketchup	1 pkg	13	3	3	0
Sauce Cheddar Cheese	1 serv (0.7 oz)	30	2	0	0
Sauce Spicy Three Pepper	1 serv (0.5 oz)	22	3	3	0
Sauce Tangy Southwest	1 serv (2 oz)	333	5	4	0

FOOD	PORTION	CALS	CARB	SUGAR	FIBER
SALADS					
Chicken Club	1 serv	487	31	3	4
Martha's Vineyard	1 serv	277	24	17	4
Santa Fe	1 serv	477	42	6	6
SANDWICHES					
Arby's Melt	1	302	36	5	2
Beef 'N Cheddar	1	445	44	8	2
Chicken Bacon & Swiss Crispy	1	624	52	13	2
Chicken Bacon & Swiss Grilled	1	462	38	9	2
Chicken Cordon Bleu Crispy	1	650	49	11	2
Chicken Cordon Bleu Grilled	1	488	35	7	2
Chicken Fillet Crispy	1	576	50	11	3
Chicken Fillet Grilled	1	414	36	7	3
Chicken Salad w/ Pecans	1	769	79	17	9
Corned Beef Reuben	1	606	55	6	3
Fish	1	543	61	9	3
French Dip	1	391	37	2	3
French Dip & Swiss	1	473	28	2	3
Ham & Swiss Melt	1	275	35	6	1
Roast Beef Regular	1	320	34	5	2
Roast Beef Super	1	398	40	10	2
Roast Beef & Swiss	1	777	73	16	5
Roast Beef 'N Cheddar	1	521	45	9	2
Roast Ham & Swiss	1	705	75	19	5
Roast Turkey Ranch & Bacon	1	834	75	17	5
Roast Turkey Reuben	1	611	56	6	3
Roast Turkey & Swiss	1	725	75	17	5
Sourdough Melt Beef	1	355	40	4	2
Sourdough Melt Ham	1	380	39	5	2
Spicy Cajun Fish	1	603	61	9	3
Sub Toasted Classic Italian	1	828	69	5	3
Sub Toasted French Dip & Swiss	1	622	68	2	3
Sub Toasted Philly Beef	1	739	64	4	3
Sub Toasted Turkey Bacon Club	1	619	65	4	3
Swiss Melt	1	303	37	6	2
Ultimate BLT	1	779	75	18	6
Wrap Chicken Salad w/ Pecans	1	638	48	3	8
Wrap Corned Beef Reuben	1	577	42	6	1
Wrap Roast Turkey Ranch & Bacon	1	700	44	3	4

FOOD	PORTION	CALS	CARB	SUGAR	FIBER
Wrap Roast Turkey Reuben	1	581	43	6	1
Wrap Southwest Chicken	1	567	42	3	4
Wrap Ultimate BLT	1	648	45	4	5
SIDES					
Bites Jalapeno	5	305	29	3	2
Bites Loaded Potato	5	353	27	0	2
Cheddar Fries	1 med	465	51	0	5
Chicken Tenders	3 pieces	379	28	0	2
Croutons Cheese & Garlic	1 pkg	77	7	0	0
Curly Fries	1 sm	338	39	0	4
Curly Fries	1 lg	631	73	0	7
Fruit Cup	1 serv	35	9	8	1
Homestyle Fries	1 sm	302	44	1	3
Homestyle Fries	1 lg	566	82	1	6
Mozzarella Sticks	8 pieces	849	75	9	4
Onion Petals	1 reg	331	35	7	2
Popcorn Chicken	1 reg	365	27	0	2
Potato Cakes	2	246	26	0	2
Seasoned Tortilla Strips	1 serv	71	9	0	1

AU BON PAIN
BAKED SELECTIONS

FOOD	PORTION	CALS	CARB	SUGAR	FIBER
Bagel Asiago Cheese	1	360	64	4	3
Bagel Cinnamon Raisin	1	320	67	4	3
Bagel Everything	1	350	64	4	3
Bagel Honey 9 Grain	1	330	68	4	6
Bagel Jalapeno Double Cheddar	1	350	55	4	2
Bagel Onion Dill	1	350	72	5	4
Bagel Plain	1	290	59	4	2
Bagel Poppy Seed	1	290	59	4	2
Bagel Sesame Seed	1	330	61	4	3
Baguette Artisan Honey Multigrain Salad Size	1 (3.5 oz)	240	47	1	4
Baguette Artisan Honey Multigrain Sandwich Size	1 (4.7 oz)	310	62	1	6
Baguette Artisan Salad Size	1 (3.5 oz)	210	44	1	2
Baguette Artisan Sandwich Size	1 (4.7 oz)	290	59	1	2
Blondie	1	330	61	25	3
Bread Artisan Multigrain	1 serv (4 oz)	260	51	0	4
Bread Artisan Sundried Tomato	1 serv (4 oz)	240	49	2	2
Bread Cheese	1 serv (4.8 oz)	290	55	1	3

FOOD	PORTION	CALS	CARB	SUGAR	FIBER
Bread Country White	1 serv (4 oz)	240	50	1	2
Bread Bowl	1 (9.24 oz)	640	127	3	6
Bread Stick Rosemary Garlic	1 (2.3 oz)	200	33	2	2
Brownie Chocolate Chip	1	380	62	41	1
Brownie Hazelnut Mocha	1	430	58	31	3
Brownie Rocky Road	1	410	62	31	2
Ciabatta	1 sm	180	37	2	2
Cinnamon Roll	1	350	53	21	2
Cookie Chocolate Chip	1 (2 oz)	260	37	22	1
Cookie Confetti	1 (2.4 oz)	310	42	25	1
Cookie English Toffee	1 (2 oz)	210	26	15	1
Cookie Gingerbread	1 (2.7 oz)	300	50	21	1
Cookie Hazelnut Fudge	1 (2.25 oz)	290	34	25	3
Cookie Oatmeal Raisin	1 (2 oz)	230	36	23	2
Cookie Shortbread	1 (2.3 oz)	310	34	10	1
Creme De Fleur	1 serv	550	71	32	1
Croissant Almond	1	560	52	16	4
Croissant Apple	1	230	31	11	2
Croissant Chocolate	1	330	42	16	3
Croissant Plain	1 (2.8 oz)	260	28	3	1
Croissant Raspberry Cheese	1	330	41	16	1
Croissant Sweet Cheese	1	320	39	15	1
Danish Cherry	1	370	44	15	1
Danish Sweet Cheese	1	380	44	16	1
Focaccia	1 piece (4.4 oz)	310	57	2	3
Lahvash	1 (4 oz)	320	62	1	2
Macaroon Chocolate Dipped Cranberry Almond	1	320	42	33	3
Mini Loaf Bacon & Cheese	1 (4.8 oz)	540	50	20	1
Muffin Blueberry	1	510	76	33	5
Muffin Carrot Walnut	1	520	66	38	4
Muffin Corn	1	460	69	29	2
Muffin Cranberry Walnut	1	500	61	26	5
Muffin Double Chocolate Chunk	1	590	83	46	5
Muffin Pumpkin	1	490	75	35	2
Muffin Raisin Bran	1	410	74	40	9
Muffin Low Fat Triple Berry	1	290	61	31	2
Pastry Hazelnut Creme	1	540	50	20	3
Poundcake Cappuccino	1 slice (5.2 oz)	530	68	43	1

FOOD	PORTION	CALS	CARB	SUGAR	FIBER
Poundcake Chocolate	1 slice (4.7 oz)	500	58	35	3
Poundcake Lemon	1 slice (4.9 oz)	520	64	40	0
Poundcake Marble	1 slice (4.7 oz)	490	59	35	1
Roll Pecan	1	630	80	38	3
Roll Soft	1 (4.7 oz)	410	65	9	3
Scone Cinnamon	1	430	48	16	1
Scone Orange	1	410	51	16	2
Shortbread Chocolate Dipped	1	350	38	14	1
Toasts Basil Pesto Cheese	3 pieces (2 oz)	140	26	1	1
Tulip Blueberry	1	370	44	25	1
Tulip Chocolate Raspberry	1	430	55	34	1
Tulip Key Lime	1	440	55	33	1
BEVERAGES					
Blast Caramel	1 med (16 oz)	540	104	99	0
Blast Coffee	1 med (16 oz)	440	71	67	0
Blast Mocha	1 med (16 oz)	440	80	74	2
Blast Vanilla	1 med (12 oz)	540	104	99	0
Caffe Americano	1 sm (12 oz)	5	1	1	0
Caffe Latte	1 sm (12 oz)	200	17	17	0
Cappuccino	1 sm (12 oz)	120	10	10	0
Caramel Macchiato	1 sm (12 oz)	350	53	50	0
Chai Latte	1 sm (12 oz)	290	38	26	0
Chocolate Milk	1 (12 oz)	320	54	51	3
Hot Chocolate	1 sm (12 oz)	350	58	54	3
Iced Caffe Latte	1 sm (12 oz)	110	19	10	0
Iced Caramel Macchiato	1 sm (12 oz)	290	49	46	0
Iced Chai Latte	1 sm (12 oz)	190	31	18	0
Iced Mocha Latte	1 sm (12 oz)	210	27	26	1
Iced Tea Peach	1 med (22 oz)	120	30	30	0
Iced Vanilla Latte	1 sm (12 oz)	240	44	44	0
Iced White Chocolate Latte	1 sm (12 oz)	250	35	32	0
Lemonade	1 med (22 oz)	300	72	72	0
Mocha Latte	1 sm (12 oz)	300	35	33	1
Orange Juice	1 (8 oz)	110	26	26	1
Smoothie Peach	1 med (16 oz)	310	69	41	4
Smoothie Strawberry	1 med (16 oz)	310	66	43	3
Vanilla Latte	1 sm (12 oz)	320	50	50	0
White Chocolate Latte	1 sm (12 oz)	310	41	38	0
MAIN MENU SELECTIONS					
Fruit Cup	1 sm (6 oz)	70	16	15	1

FOOD	PORTION	CALS	CARB	SUGAR	FIBER
Harvest Rice Bowl Cajun Shrimp	1 (20 oz)	520	69	8	2
Harvest Rice Bowl Cajun Shrimp w/ Brown Rice	1 (20 oz)	560	73	8	5
Harvest Rice Bowl Mayan Chicken	1 (19.25 oz)	490	67	5	4
Harvest Rice Bowl Mayan Chicken w/ Brown Rice	1 (19.25 oz)	540	71	5	7
Harvest Rice Bowl Steak Teriyaki	1 (19.25 oz)	530	72	11	2
Harvest Rice Bowl Steak Teriyaki w/ Brown Rice	1 (19.25 oz)	570	76	11	5
Macaroni & Cheese	1 med (12 oz)	440	31	4	2
Stew Beef	1 med (12 oz)	300	25	4	3
Stew Chicken Vegetable	1 med (12 oz)	290	26	5	3
SALAD DRESSINGS AND SPREADS					
Artichoke Aioli	1 serv (1 oz)	130	1	0	0
Basil Pesto	1 serv (1 oz)	140	1	0	0
Chili Dijon	1 serv (1 oz)	120	3	2	1
Cream Cheese Honey Pecan	1 serv (2 oz)	120	5	4	0
Cream Cheese Honey Walnut	1 serv (2 oz)	140	12	12	0
Cream Cheese Lite	1 serv (2 oz)	120	5	3	0
Cream Cheese Plain	1 serv (2 oz)	170	4	3	0
Cream Cheese Strawberry	1 serv (2 oz)	180	9	8	0
Cream Cheese Sundried Tomato	1 serv (2 oz)	120	5	4	0
Cream Cheese Vegetable	1 serv (2 oz)	170	3	2	0
Dressing Balsamic Vinaigrette	1 serv (2.25 oz)	190	11	10	0
Dressing Blue Cheese	1 serv (1.75 oz)	230	2	1	0
Dressing Caesar	1 serv (2 oz)	280	4	3	0
Dressing Fat Free Raspberry Vinaigrette	1 serv (2.25 oz)	70	17	16	0
Dressing Light Honey Mustard	1 serv (2.25 oz)	180	21	19	1
Dressing Light Olive Oil Vinaigrette	1 serv (2.25 oz)	130	9	7	0

FOOD	PORTION	CALS	CARB	SUGAR	FIBER
Dressing Light Ranch	1 serv (2.25 oz)	150	3	2	0
Dressing Thai Peanut	1 serv (2.25 oz)	230	24	22	1
Guacamole	1 serv (1 oz)	60	2	0	2
Honey Mustard	1 serv (2.5 oz)	210	23	21	1
Hummus Roasted Red Pepper	1 serv (2 oz)	80	6	0	2
Mayonnaise	1 serv (1 oz)	200	0	0	0
Mayonnaise Herb	1 serv (1 oz)	210	1	1	0
Mayonnaise Jalapeno	1 serv (1 oz)	140	0	0	0
Mayonnaise Tarragon Sauce	1 serv (2 oz)	420	2	2	0
Mustard	1 tsp	0	0	0	0
Spread Herb Bagel	1 serv (2 oz)	130	5	4	0
Spread Sundried Tomato	1 serv (0.53 oz)	70	4	1	0
SALADS					
Caesar Asiago	1 serv	210	18	4	3
Caesar Asiago Grilled Chicken	1 (8.5 oz)	340	19	4	3
Caesar Asiago Side	1 (3.2 oz)	120	12	2	2
Chef's	1 serv	230	7	5	3
Garden	1 (7 oz)	80	14	3	4
Garden Side	1 (3.6 oz)	50	10	2	3
Mediterranean Chicken	1 (9.75 oz)	330	12	1	2
Riviera	1 (9.5 oz)	260	46	31	5
Thai Peanut Chicken	1 (11 oz)	250	22	7	4
Tuna Garden	1 (10.5 oz)	350	14	4	4
Turkey Medallion Cobb	1 (11 oz)	340	15	3	3
Turkey Spinach Sonoma	1 (12.3 oz)	310	22	9	5
SANDWICHES					
Arizona Chicken	1 (12 oz)	750	61	6	4
Baguette Turkey & Swiss	1 (12.3 oz)	770	65	4	3
Baja Turkey	1 (13 oz)	700	61	6	4
Breakfast Asiago Bagel Prosciutto & Egg	1 (9.6 oz)	660	67	4	3
Breakfast Asiago Bagel Sausage Egg & Cheddar	1 (10.2 oz)	770	55	4	0
Breakfast Bagel & Bacon	1 (4.2 oz)	340	56	4	0
Breakfast Egg On A Bagel	1 (6.8 oz)	370	62	5	2
Breakfast Egg On A Bagel w/ Bacon	1 (7.2 oz)	410	58	4	0

FOOD	PORTION	CALS	CARB	SUGAR	FIBER
Breakfast Egg On A Bagel w/ Bacon Cheese	1 (7.9 oz)	500	59	4	0
Breakfast Egg On A Bagel w/ Cheese	1 (7.6 oz)	450	62	5	2
Breakfast Onion Dill Bagel Smoked Salmon & Wasabi	1 (7.1 oz)	490	77	6	3
Caprese	1 (11.8 oz)	700	65	3	4
Chicken Mozzarella	1 (14.5 oz)	800	71	6	2
Chicken Pesto	1 (12.5 oz)	700	62	5	2
Chicken Tarragon	1 (11 oz)	720	61	5	1
Ciabatta Bacon & Egg Melt	1 (7 oz)	400	40	2	2
Ciabatta Ham & Cheddar	1 (12 oz)	650	80	19	4
Club Smoked Turkey	1 (11.6 oz)	780	56	4	2
Croissant Ham & Cheese	1 (4.2 oz)	350	34	4	1
Croissant Spinach & Cheese	1	250	25	3	2
Hot BBQ Chicken On Farmhouse Roll	1 (14.3 oz)	970	78	14	4
Hot Eggplant & Mozzarella	1 (12.4 oz)	710	68	5	6
Hot Steakhouse On Ciabatta	1 (13 oz)	800	70	8	4
Melt Tuna	1 (12.5 oz)	760	60	6	4
Melt Turkey	1 (12.2 oz)	890	70	18	3
Portobello & Goat Cheese	1 (10 oz)	610	61	4	6
Portobello Egg & Cheddar	1 (8.5 oz)	590	42	2	3
Prosciutto Mozzarella	1 (12.7 oz)	880	71	5	4
Spicy Tuna	1 (10.3 oz)	640	57	3	6
The Montana	1 (12.5 oz)	560	62	5	4
Turkey & Cranberry Chutney	1 (10.9 oz)	680	63	25	3
Wrap Chicken Caesar Asiago	1	700	69	6	3
Wrap Chopped Turkey Club	1 (12 oz)	660	70	5	4
Wrap Mediterranean	1 (12.8 oz)	670	80	5	7
Wrap Southwest Tuna	1 (14 oz)	900	72	6	5
Wrap Thai Peanut Chicken	1 (14.5 oz)	660	84	10	4
Wrap Turkey Spinach Sonoma	1 (12 oz)	630	80	12	5
Wrap Hot Cajun Shrimp	1 (14.9 oz)	700	95	8	4
Wrap Hot Mayan Chicken	1 (13.5 oz)	630	92	6	5
Wrap Hot Steak Teriyaki	1 (13.5 oz)	660	93	9	5
SOUPS					
Baked Stuffed Potato	1 med (12 oz)	350	30	6	2
Broccoli Cheddar	1 med (12 oz)	310	20	7	2
Carrot Ginger	1 med (12 oz)	130	21	10	3

FOOD	PORTION	CALS	CARB	SUGAR	FIBER
Chicken Florentine	1 med (12 oz)	240	25	4	1
Chicken & Dumplings	1 med (12 oz)	210	28	6	2
Chicken Noodle	1 med (12 oz)	130	20	2	2
Clam Chowder	1 med (12 oz)	320	27	8	1
Corn & Green Chili Bisque	1 med (12 oz)	250	29	6	3
Corn Chowder	1 med (12 oz)	350	40	10	3
Curried Rice & Lentil	1 med (12 oz)	150	30	4	8
French Moroccan Tomato Lentil	1 med (12 oz)	180	32	7	8
French Onion	1 med (12 oz)	130	19	6	2
Garden Vegetable	1 med (12 oz)	80	14	5	3
Harvest Pumpkin	1 med (12 oz)	190	26	6	2
Hearty Cabbage	1 med (12 oz)	110	14	4	3
Italian Wedding	1 med (12 oz)	170	10	4	2
Jamaican Black Bean	1 med (12 oz)	180	45	4	25
Mediterranean Pepper	1 med (12 oz)	100	18	3	5
Old Fashioned Tomato Rice	1 med (12 oz)	120	24	7	3
Pasta E Fagioli	1 med (12 oz)	240	36	3	9
Portuguese Kale	1 med (12 oz)	120	15	2	3
Potato Cheese	1 med (12 oz)	250	25	4	2
Potato Leek	1 med (12 oz)	300	28	2	2
Red Beans Italian Sausage & Rice	1 med (12 oz)	200	28	3	16
Southern Black Eyed Pea	1 med (12 oz)	180	31	4	12
Southwest Tortilla	1 med (12 oz)	200	24	5	4
Southwest Vegetable	1 med (12 oz)	160	17	3	3
Split Pea	1 med (12 oz)	210	42	3	15
Thai Coconut Curry	1 med (12 oz)	150	20	4	2
Tomato Basil Bisque	1 med (12 oz)	210	29	18	5
Tomato Cheddar	1 med (12 oz)	240	17	7	2
Tomato Florentine	1 med (12 oz)	120	19	6	2
Tuscan Vegetable	1 med (12 oz)	170	24	3	3
Vegetable Beef Barley	1 med (12 oz)	140	21	4	4
Vegetarian Chili	1 med (12 oz)	230	40	7	11
Vegetarian Lentil	1 med (12 oz)	140	32	4	11
Vegetarian Minestrone	1 med (12 oz)	120	21	6	4
Wild Mushroom Bisque	1 med (12 oz)	190	23	6	2
YOGURT					
Blueberry w/ Fruit	1 sm (7.5 oz)	220	44	37	0
Blueberry w/ Granola & Fruit	1 sm (8.5 oz)	310	56	36	2
Strawberry w/ Blueberries	1 sm (7.5 oz)	220	44	37	0

FOOD	PORTION	CALS	CARB	SUGAR	FIBER
Strawberry w/ Granola & Blueberries	1 sm (8.5 oz)	310	56	36	2
Vanilla w/ Blueberries	1 sm (7.5 oz)	190	32	30	0
Vanilla w/ Granola & Blueberries	1 sm (8.5 oz)	310	56	36	2

AUNTIE ANNE'S
BEVERAGES

FOOD	PORTION	CALS	CARB	SUGAR	FIBER
Dutch Ice Blue Raspberry	1 (14 oz)	165	38	35	0
Dutch Ice Grape	1 (14 oz)	180	43	41	0
Dutch Ice Kiwi Banana	1 (14 oz)	190	44	41	0
Dutch Ice Lemonade	1 (14 oz)	315	77	77	0
Dutch Ice Lemonade Strawberry	1 (14 oz)	330	81	81	0
Dutch Ice Mocha	1 (14 oz)	400	74	52	0
Dutch Ice Orange Creme	1 (14 oz)	280	64	59	0
Dutch Ice Pina Colada	1 (14 oz)	220	53	50	0
Dutch Ice Strawberry	1 (14 oz)	220	50	48	0
Dutch Ice Watermelon	1 (14 oz)	200	50	48	0
Dutch Ice Wild Cherry	1 (14 oz)	210	48	45	0
Dutch Latte Caramel	1 (14 oz)	350	49	39	0
Dutch Latte Coffee	1 (14 oz)	290	38	33	0
Dutch Latte Mocha	1 (14 oz)	160	47	37	0
Dutch Shake Chocolate	1 (14 oz)	580	75	67	0
Dutch Shake Coffee	1 (14 oz)	590	77	70	0
Dutch Shake Strawberry	1 (14 oz)	610	78	74	0
Dutch Shake Vanilla	1 (14 oz)	510	58	54	0
Dutch Smoothie Blue Raspberry	1 (14 oz)	230	34	33	0
Dutch Smoothie Grape	1 (14 oz)	230	36	35	0
Dutch Smoothie Kiwi Banana	1 (14 oz)	240	38	35	0
Dutch Smoothie Lemonade	1 (14 oz)	300	53	53	0
Dutch Smoothie Mocha	1 (14 oz)	330	50	39	0
Dutch Smoothie Orange Creme	1 (14 oz)	280	46	44	0
Dutch Smoothie Pina Colada	1 (14 oz)	260	44	41	0
Dutch Smoothie Strawberry	1 (14 oz)	250	40	39	0
Dutch Smoothie Wild Cherry	1 (14 oz)	250	41	39	0
Lemonade	1 (22 oz)	180	43	43	0
Lemonade Strawberry	1 (22 oz)	190	48	48	0

DIPPING SAUCES

FOOD	PORTION	CALS	CARB	SUGAR	FIBER
Caramel Dip	1 serv (1.5 oz)	135	27	21	0

FOOD	PORTION	CALS	CARB	SUGAR	FIBER
Cheese Sauce	1 serv (1.25 oz)	100	4	3	0
Cream Cheese Light	1 serv (1.25 oz)	70	1	1	0
Hot Salsa Cheese	1 serv (1.25 oz)	100	4	4	0
Marinara Sauce	1 serv (1.25 oz)	10	4	2	0
Sweet	1 serv (1.4 oz)	40	10	10	0
Sweet Mustard	1 serv (1.25 oz)	60	8	8	0
PRETZELS					
Almond	1	400	72	15	2
Almond w/o Butter	1	350	72	15	2
Cinnamon Raisin w/o Butter	1	350	74	16	2
Cinnamon Sugar	1	450	83	26	3
Garlic	1	350	68	9	2
Garlic w/o Butter	1	320	66	9	2
Glazin' Raisin	1	510	107	38	4
Glazin' Raisin w/o Butter	1	470	104	37	3
Jalapeno	1	310	59	9	2
Jalapeno w/o Butter	1	270	58	8	2
Original	1	370	72	10	3
Original w/o Butter	1	340	72	10	3
Pretzel Dog	1	290	25	3	1
Sesame	1	410	64	9	7
Sesame w/o Butter	1	350	63	9	3
Sour Cream & Onion	1	340	66	10	2
Sour Cream & Onion w/o Butter	1	310	66	9	2
Stix	6	370	72	10	3
Stix w/o Butter	6	340	72	10	3
Whole Wheat	1	370	72	10	7
Whole Wheat w/o Butter	1	350	72	10	7
BABS DELI					
BAGELS					
Apple Cinnamon	1	332	70	6	4
Banana Nut	1	340	68	4	4
Blueberry	1	330	68	2	4
Blueberry Cobbler	1	392	70	4	2
Cheddar Herb	1	352	60	2	2
Cheddar Nacho	1	352	60	2	4

FOOD	PORTION	CALS	CARB	SUGAR	FIBER
Chocolate Chip	1	348	68	4	4
Cinnamon Apple Pie	1	386	68	4	2
Cinnamon Bun	1	400	70	4	2
Cinnamon Danish	1	396	72	2	4
Cinnamon Raisin	1	336	70	2	4
Cinnamon Sugar	1	350	74	2	2
Cranberry Walnut	1	352	72	6	4
Egg	1	328	66	2	2
Everything	1	336	68	2	4
French Toast	1	372	74	4	2
Garlic	1	330	68	2	4
Honey Oat	1	320	68	2	2
Jalapeno	1	350	30	2	2
Onion	1	336	70	2	4
Plain	1	334	68	2	4
Poppy	1	344	68	2	4
Pumpernickel	1	332	68	2	4
Quiche Lorraine	1	354	54	2	2
Salt	1	324	66	2	2
Sesame	1	358	66	2	4
Spinach	1	356	72	2	4
Strawberry	1	342	72	4	4
Strawberry White Chocolate	1	364	72	8	4
Swiss Melt	1	368	58	2	2
Tomato Basil	1	322	66	2	4
Vegetable	1	318	66	2	4
Wheat	1	330	78	2	4
White Chocolate Swirl	1	396	70	4	2
BEVERAGES					
Americano	1 (16 oz)	12	2	0	0
Cafe Caramello	1 (16 oz)	212	31	26	0
Cappuccino 2% Milk	1 (16 oz)	195	20	0	0
Cappuccino Fat Free Milk	1 (16 oz)	133	18	0	0
Coffee Black Forest	1 (16 oz)	198	37	29	1
Icepresso Caramel Decadence	1 (16 oz)	300	42	28	2
Icepresso Classic	1 (16 oz)	300	52	44	0
Icepresso Java Chip	1 (16 oz)	360	48	38	2
Icepresso Latte	1 (16 oz)	300	42	28	2
Icepresso Mocha	1 (16 oz)	300	42	28	2
Icepresso Strawberry	1 (16 oz)	340	56	48	0

FOOD	PORTION	CALS	CARB	SUGAR	FIBER
Italiano 2% Milk	1 (16 oz)	131	13	0	0
Italiano Fat Free Milk	1 (16 oz)	89	12	0	0
Jittery Monkey 2% Milk	1 (16 oz)	482	82	52	1
Jittery Monkey Fat Free Milk	1 (16 oz)	429	80	52	1
Latte 2% Milk	1 (16 oz)	212	22	0	0
Latte Cinnamon Toast 2% Milk	1 (16 oz)	299	45	26	0
Latte Cinnamon Toast Fat Free Milk	1 (16 oz)	240	44	26	0
Latte Creme Caramel 2% Milk	1 (16 oz)	303	47	27	0
Latte Creme Caramel Fat Free Milk	1 (16 oz)	244	45	27	0
Latte Fat Free Milk	1 (16 oz)	145	20	0	0
Latte Oregon Chai Tea 2% Milk	1 (16 oz)	274	48	34	0
Latte Oregon Chai Tea Fat Free Milk	1 (16 oz)	231	47	34	0
Latte Raspberry Cheesecake 2% Milk	1 (16 oz)	319	51	30	0
Latte Raspberry Cheesecake Fat Free Milk	1 (16 oz)	259	50	30	0
Latte Vanilla Creme 2% Milk	1 (16 oz)	275	39	19	0
Mocha Whipped Cream 2% Milk	1 (16 oz)	454	71	39	2
Mocha Whipped Cream Fat Free Milk	1 (16 oz)	392	70	39	2
Turtle Mocha Fat Free Milk	1 (16 oz)	522	90	62	1
MUFFINS					
My Favorite Banana Nut	2 mini	195	21	12	1
My Favorite Blueberry	2 mini	168	22	12	0
My Favorite Blueberry Cheesecake	2 mini	199	20	9	0
My Favorite Boston Cream Pie	2 mini	176	26	17	0
My Favorite Cherry Cheesecake	2 mini	170	19	10	0
My Favorite Chocolate Cheesecake	2 mini	202	22	11	0
My Favorite Chocolate Chip	2 mini	211	27	16	1
My Favorite Cinnamon Crumb Cake	2 mini	212	21	11	0
My Favorite Cinnamon Swirl Cheesecake	2 mini	214	28	15	0

FOOD	PORTION	CALS	CARB	SUGAR	FIBER
My Favorite Deep Dish Apple	2 mini	177	25	14	0
My Favorite Double Chocolate	2 mini	210	28	17	1
My Favorite Fat Free Blueberry	2 mini	108	26	12	1
My Favorite Fat Free Cherry Pie	2 mini	109	26	14	0
My Favorite Fat Free Chocolate Marble	2 mini	125	29	15	1
My Favorite Fat Free Cinnamon Bun	2 mini	168	42	11	0
My Favorite Fat Free Raspberry Amaretto	2 mini	127	31	18	1
My Favorite Golden Corn Bread	2 mini	197	26	12	1
My Favorite Lemon Poppyseed	2 mini	201	25	14	0
My Favorite Pumpkin Spice	2 mini	181	26	10	0
SALADS					
Calypso Chicken	1 (13.6 oz)	637	34	16	3
Calypso Chicken w/ Lite Italian	1 (13.6 oz)	317	22	10	3
Chicken Caesar	1 (11.5 oz)	524	15	3	3
Chicken Caesar w/ Lite Italian	1 (11.5 oz)	268	17	9	3
Classic Caesar	1 (8.4 oz)	414	12	1	3
Classic Caesar Cafe	1 (4.3 oz)	225	9	1	2
Classic Ceasar w/ Lite Italian	1 (8.4 oz)	158	14	7	3
Garden Mix	1 (12.4 oz)	197	18	5	4
Garden Mix Cafe	1 (6.5 oz)	100	9	3	2
Grilled Chicken Club	1 (17.9 oz)	820	16	5	3
Grilled Chicken Club w/ Lite Italian	1 (17.9 oz)	500	18	7	3
Low Carb Tuna Salad Plate	1 serv (8.9 oz)	356	3	0	1
Mediterranean Bread	1 (18.8 oz)	973	52	1	5
Mediterranean Bread w/ Lite Italian	1 (18.8 oz)	626	55	7	5
SANDWICHES					
Breakfast BLT	1	704	83	5	4
Breakfast Lox & Cream Cheese	1	602	78	3	4
Breakfast Morning Classic	1	486	73	2	3
Breakfast Northern Omelette	1	699	73	2	3
Breakfast So. Tradition w/ Ham	1	547	73	2	3
Breakfast So. Tradition w/ Bacon	1	566	73	2	3
Breakfast So. Tradition w/ Sausage	1	696	73	2	3

FOOD	PORTION	CALS	CARB	SUGAR	FIBER
Build Your Own Ham	1	495	77	1	4
Build Your Own Roast Beef	1	480	77	1	4
Build Your Own Tuna	1	547	77	1	4
Build Your Own Turkey	1	465	77	1	4
Enchilada Bagellata	1	522	84	3	4
Gourmet Classic Turkey	1	552	74	1	4
Gourmet Holey Guacamole	1	476	76	2	4
Gourmet Kick-N Roast Beef	1	579	79	1	4
Gourmet Mediterranean Veg-Out	1	506	90	3	8
Overstuffed Classic Reuben	1	962	57	3	4
Overstuffed Corned Beef	1	661	77	1	3
Overstuffed Ham & Cheese	1	889	79	1	4
Overstuffed Manhattan Club	1	1122	120	6	6
Overstuffed Pastrami	1	661	77	1	3
Overstuffed TD Classic California	1	759	113	2	8
Overstuffed TD Classic Club	1	1110	122	2	5
Overstuffed TD Clubhouse	1	1079	117	2	5
Pizzaah Bruschetta	1 piece	162	7	0	3
Pizzaah Cheese	1 piece	189	23	1	3
Pizzaah Grilled Chicken Bruschetta	1 piece	343	24	1	3
Pizzaah Sausage	1 piece	211	6	1	2
Pizzaah Veggie	1 piece	238	32	1	7
Specialty All American Duo	1	752	78	1	4
Specialty Big Apple Club	1	797	75	2	4
Specialty Chicken Caesar	1	611	78	3	4
Specialty Roma Italian	1	764	76	1	4
Specialty Turkey Club	1	782	75	2	4
Toasted Cafe Chicken Melt	1	815	80	6	4
Toasted Deli Style Turkey	1	732	76	3	4
Toasted Roast Beef Parmesan Grinder	1	583	76	4	4
Toasted Spicy Italian Sub	1	770	77	1	4
Toasted Tuna Melt	1	641	75	2	4
SPREADS					
Cream Cheese	2 tbsp	90	2	1	0
Cream Cheese Cheddar Jalapeno	2 tbsp	90	2	2	0

FOOD	PORTION	CALS	CARB	SUGAR	FIBER
Cream Cheese Garden Vegetable	2 tbsp	90	2	1	0
Cream Cheese Lite	2 tbsp	60	3	3	0
Cream Cheese Onion Chive	2 tbsp	80	2	1	0
Cream Cheese Strawberry	2 tbsp	90	5	5	0
Cream Cheese Whipped	2 tbsp	70	1	1	0
Cream Cheese Whipped Brown Sugar Cinnamon	2 tbsp	70	5	3	0
Cream Cheese Whipped Reduced Fat Spring Veggie	2 tbsp	60	2	1	0

BAJA FRESH
CHILDREN'S MENU SELECTIONS

FOOD	PORTION	CALS	CARB	SUGAR	FIBER
Kid's Mini Burrito Bean & Cheese	1 serv	540	84	–	11
Kid's Mini Burrito Bean & Cheese w/ Chicken	1 serv	590	84	–	12
Kid's Mini Quesadilla Cheese	1 serv	610	72	–	5
Kid's Mini Quesadilla Cheese w/ Chicken	1 serv	650	72	–	5
Kid's Taquitos Chicken	1 serv	630	60	–	4

MAIN MENU SELECTIONS

FOOD	PORTION	CALS	CARB	SUGAR	FIBER
Black Beans	1 serv	360	61	–	26
Burrito Baja Breaded Fish	1 serv	850	78	–	7
Burrito Baja Carnitas	1 serv	830	67	–	8
Burrito Baja Chicken	1 serv	790	65	–	8
Burrito Baja Mahi Mahi	1 serv	780	66	–	7
Burrito Baja Shrimp	1 serv	760	66	–	7
Burrito Baja Steak	1 serv	850	67	–	7
Burrito Bare Carnitas	1 serv	600	99	–	20
Burrito Bare Chicken	1 serv	640	97	–	20
Burrito Bare Steak	1 serv	700	99	–	19
Burrito Bare Veggie & Cheese	1 serv	580	101	–	20
Burrito Bean & Cheese Breaded Fish	1 serv	1030	108	–	20
Burrito Bean & Cheese Carnitas	1 serv	1010	98	–	21
Burrito Bean & Cheese Chicken	1 serv	970	96	–	21
Burrito Bean & Cheese Mahi Mahi	1 serv	960	96	–	20
Burrito Bean & Cheese No Meat	1 serv	840	96	–	20
Burrito Bean & Cheese Shrimp	1 serv	950	96	–	20

FOOD	PORTION	CALS	CARB	SUGAR	FIBER
Burrito Bean & Cheese Steak	1 serv	1030	97	–	20
Burrito Dos Manos Breaded Fish	1 serv	890	107	–	13
Burrito Dos Manos Carnitas	1 serv	780	95	–	14
Burrito Dos Manos Chicken	½ serv	760	94	–	14
Burrito Dos Manos Mahi Mahi	1 serv	780	95	–	13
Burrito Dos Manos Shrimp	1 serv	780	95	–	13
Burrito Dos Manos Steak	½ serv	795	95	–	13
Burrito Grilled Veggie	1 serv	506	94	–	16
Burrito Mexicano Breaded Fish	1 serv	850	129	–	18
Burrito Mexicano Carnitas	1 serv	830	119	–	19
Burrito Mexicano Chicken	1 serv	790	117	–	20
Burrito Mexicano Mahi Mahi	1 serv	790	117	–	18
Burrito Mexicano Shrimp	1 serv	770	117	–	18
Burrito Mexicano Steak	1 serv	860	118	–	18
Burrito Ultimo Breaded Fish	1 serv	940	96	–	8
Burrito Ultimo Carnitas	1 serv	920	86	–	9
Burrito Ultimo Chicken	1 serv	880	84	–	9
Burrito Ultimo Mahi Mahi	1 serv	880	84	–	8
Burrito Ultimo Shrimp	1 serv	860	85	–	8
Burrito Ultimo Steak	1 serv	950	85	–	8
Chips & Guacamole	1 serv	1340	141	–	20
Chips & Salsa Baja	1 serv	810	98	–	14
Fajitas Corn Tortillas Breaded Fish	1 serv	1060	130	–	22
Fajitas Corn Tortillas Carnitas	1 serv	920	108	–	23
Fajitas Corn Tortillas Chicken	1 serv	860	105	–	24
Fajitas Corn Tortillas Mahi Mahi	1 serv	840	105	–	22
Fajitas Corn Tortillas Shrimp	1 serv	840	106	–	22
Fajitas Corn Tortillas Steak	1 serv	960	107	–	22
Fajitas Flour Tortillas Breaded Fish	1 serv	1340	172	–	25
Fajitas Flour Tortillas Carnitas	1 serv	1190	150	–	26
Fajitas Flour Tortillas Chicken	1 serv	1140	147	–	27
Fajitas Flour Tortillas Mahi Mahi	1 serv	1120	147	–	25
Fajitas Flour Tortillas Shrimp	1 serv	1120	148	–	25
Fajitas Flour Tortillas Steak	1 serv	960	170	–	22
Guacamole Side	1 (3 oz)	110	5	–	2
Nachos Breaded Fish	1 serv	2090	176	–	31

FOOD	PORTION	CALS	CARB	SUGAR	FIBER
Nachos Carnitas	1 serv	2060	166	–	32
Nachos Cheese	1 serv	1890	163	–	31
Nachos Chicken	1 serv	2020	164	–	32
Nachos Mahi Mahi	1 serv	2020	164	–	31
Nachos Shrimp	1 serv	2000	164	–	31
Nachos Steak	1 serv	2120	163	–	31
Pico De Gallo Side	1 serv (8 oz)	50	12	–	3
Pinto Beans	1 serv	320	56	–	21
Pronto Guacamole Side	1 serv (6 oz)	560	60	–	8
Quesadilla Breaded Frish	1 serv	1400	96	–	8
Quesadilla Carnitas	1 serv	1370	86	–	9
Quesadilla Cheese	1 serv	1200	84	–	8
Quesadilla Chicken	1 serv	1330	84	–	9
Quesadilla Mahi Mahi	1 serv	1330	84	–	8
Quesadilla Shrimp	1 serv	1310	84	–	8
Quesadilla Steak	1 serv	1430	84	–	8
Quesadilla Veggie	1 serv	1260	96	–	11
Rice	1 serv	280	55	–	4
Rice & Beans Plate	1 serv	420	72	–	18
Salsa Baja Side	1 serv (8 oz)	70	7	–	4
Salsa Roja Side	1 serv (8 oz)	70	13	–	4
Salsa Verde Side	1 serv (8 oz)	50	11	–	3
Soup Tortilla w/ Chicken	1 serv (13.6 oz)	320	29	–	4
Soup Tortilla w/o Chicken	1 serv (12.4 oz)	270	29	–	4
Taco Grilled Mahi Mahi	1 serv	230	26	–	4
Taco Baja Breaded Fish	1 serv	250	27	–	2
Taco Baja Chicken	1 serv	210	28	–	2
Taco Baja Shrimp	1 serv	200	28	–	2
Taco Baja Steak	1 serv	230	28	–	2
Taco Soft Breaded Fish	1 serv	240	23	–	2
Taco Soft Carnitas	1 serv	250	21	–	2
Taco Soft Chicken	1 serv	230	20	–	2
Taco Soft Mahi Mahi	1 serv	240	20	–	2
Taco Soft Shrimp	1 serv	230	21	–	2
Taco Soft Steak	1 serv	260	21	–	2
Taquitos Chicken w/ Beans	3	780	68	–	17
Taquitos Chicken w/ Rice	3	740	66	–	8
Veggie Mix	1 serv	110	24	–	6

FOOD	PORTION	CALS	CARB	SUGAR	FIBER
SALAD DRESSINGS					
Chipotle Vinaigrette	1 serv (2.5 oz)	110	0	0	0
Fat Free Salsa Verde	1 serv (2.5 oz)	15	3	—	1
Olive Oil Vinaigrette	1 serv (2.5 oz)	290	2	—	0
Ranch	1 serv (2.5 oz)	260	4	—	0
SALADS					
Baja Ensalada Chicken	1 serv	310	18	—	7
Baja Ensalada Steak	1 serv	450	18	—	6
Side Salad	1 (6.5 oz)	130	16	—	4
Tostada Breaded Fish	1 serv	1200	111	—	25
Tostada Mahi Mahi	1 serv	1130	99	—	25
BEAR ROCK CAFE					
SANDWICHES					
Colorado Turkey Club	1	855	95	12	5
Coop's Chicken Salad Croissant	1	439	46	12	5
Garden Grill Ciabatta	1	406	55	7	4
Giant Panda Wrap	1	556	68	21	23
Hoot Owl	1	641	32	3	2
Rising Sunflower	1	596	35	6	2
Roast Turkey & Bacon	1	522	31	2	2
Rockslide Focaccia	1	958	57	2	3
The Moose	1	976	64	17	7
BEN & JERRY'S					
FROZEN YOGURT					
Low Fat Cherry Garcia	½ cup	170	32	22	tr
Low Fat Chocolate Fudge Brownie	½ cup	190	35	23	1
Low Fat Half Baked	½ cup	190	35	23	tr
Phish Food	½ cup	220	41	22	1
ICE CREAM					
Bar Cherry Garcia	1	270	29	23	1
Bar Half Baked	1	340	46	36	2
Bar Vanilla	1	300	26	23	1
Bar Vanilla Almond	1	340	30	22	2
Black & Tan	½ cup	230	24	21	1
Brownie Batter	½ cup	310	32	26	1
Butter Pecan	½ cup	280	20	18	1
Cherry Garcia	½ cup	250	26	22	tr
Chocolate	½ cup	260	25	22	2

FOOD	PORTION	CALS	CARB	SUGAR	FIBER
Chocolate Chip Cookie Dough	½ cup	270	32	24	0
Chocolate Fudge Brownie	½ cup	260	32	25	2
Chubby Hubby	½ cup	330	31	24	1
Chunky Monkey	½ cup	300	30	28	1
Coffee	½ cup	240	21	19	0
Coffee Heath Bar Crunch	½ cup	290	29	27	0
Dave Matthews Band Magic Brownies	½ cup	250	29	23	0
Dublin Mudslide	½ cup	270	28	23	tr
Everything But The	½ cup	310	30	27	1
Fossil Fuel	½ cup	280	30	26	1
Fudge Central	½ cup	300	31	27	1
Half Baked	½ cup	280	34	26	tr
In A Crunch	½ cup	350	30	22	1
Karamel Sutra	½ cup	280	32	27	1
Marsha Marsha Marshmallow	½ cup	300	33	24	1
Mint Chocolate Cookie	½ cup	260	26	21	0
Neapolitan Dynamite	½ cup	250	29	26	1
New York Super Fudge Chunk	½ cup	310	29	25	2
Oatmeal Cookie Chunk	½ cup	270	31	24	tr
Organic Chocolate Fudge Brownie	½ cup	270	30	26	2
Organic Strawberry	½ cup	210	21	19	0
Organic Sweet Cream & Cookies	½ cup	250	24	19	0
Organic Vanilla	½ cup	220	18	16	0
Peanut Butter Cup	½ cup	360	27	23	1
Phish Food	½ cup	280	37	22	1
Pistachio Pistachio	½ cup	260	21	18	tr
Sandwich Wich Ice Cream Cookie	1	350	45	30	1
Strawberry	½ cup	230	26	25	0
The Godfather	½ cup	270	32	24	2
Turtle Soup	½ cup	280	30	25	1
Uncanny Cashew	½ cup	290	27	22	0
Vanilla Caramel Fudge	½ cup	280	31	25	0
Vanilla Heath Bar Crunch	½ cup	290	29	27	0
Vermonty Python	½ cup	310	30	26	1
SORBETS					
Berried Treasure	½ cup	110	29	24	1

FOOD	PORTION	CALS	CARB	SUGAR	FIBER
Jamaican Me Crazy	½ cup	130	33	28	4
Strawberry Kiwi Swirl	½ cup	110	28	24	1

BILLY'S BURGER HUT
BEVERAGES

Shake Chocolate	1 (20 oz)	420	63	50	0
Shake Vanilla	1 (20 oz)	320	49	44	0

MAIN MENU SELECTIONS

Big Billy's Roast Beef Sub	1	843	62	12	3
Billyburger	1	426	35	6	3
Billyburger w/ Cheese	1	498	35	8	4
Billy's Best Red Potato Salad	1 serv	190	12	4	3
Billy's Biggest Burger ½ Pounder w/ Everything	1	852	61	15	4
Billy's Famous 7 Layer Salad	1 serv	558	18	9	2
Billy's Seafood Sandwich	1	399	43	9	3
Caesar Side Salad	1 serv	360	12	1	4
Chili w/ Cheese & Onion	1 serv	380	35	8	7
Cowboy Cobb Salad	1 serv	735	25	10	9
Cowboy Coleslaw	1 serv	180	11	4	3
French Fries	1 reg	230	25	7	1
Onion Rings	1 serv	250	37	6	1
Super Billy Burger w/ Bacon	1	663	39	9	4

BOB EVANS
BREAKFAST SELECTIONS

Bacon	1 piece	36	0	0	0
Benedict Ham & Cheese	1 serv	826	44	8	0
Country Benedict Sausage	1 serv	936	40	6	0
Country Benedict Spinach Bacon & Tomato	1 serv	729	42	8	1
Country Biscuit Breakfast	1 serv	659	40	6	1
Egg Beaters	1 serv	173	3	2	0
Egg Hardcooked	1	60	1	0	0
Egg Over Easy	1	101	1	1	0
Eggs Scrambled	1 serv	255	2	0	0
French Toast	1 slice	131	13	3	1
French Toast Stuffed Plain	1 serv	599	53	21	3
Fruit & Yogurt Plate	1 serv	403	93	80	9
Grits	1 serv	178	28	0	2
Ham Smoked	1 slice	87	2	1	0

FOOD	PORTION	CALS	CARB	SUGAR	FIBER
Hotcake Blueberry	1	328	55	17	2
Hotcake Buttermilk	1	318	53	16	2
Hotcake Cinnamon	1	417	66	27	2
Hotcake Multigrain	1	322	52	16	3
Mush	1 serv	79	11	5	2
Oatmeal	1 serv	172	32	1	4
Omelette Bacon & Cheese	1 serv	825	6	2	1
Omelette Border Scramble	1	756	15	6	3
Omelette Egg Beaters Bacon & Cheese	1 serv	615	7	4	1
Omelette Egg Beaters Border Scramble	1 serv	517	16	8	3
Omelette Egg Beaters Farmer's Market	1 serv	569	14	7	2
Omelette Egg Beaters Garden Harvest	1 serv	444	14	7	2
Omelette Egg Beaters Ham & Cheddar	1 serv	426	5	3	1
Omelette Egg Beaters Sausage & Cheddar	1 serv	502	4	2	1
Omelette Egg Beaters Three Cheese	1 serv	435	5	3	1
Omelette Farmer's Market	1	778	13	5	2
Omelette Garden Harvest	1 serv	654	13	5	2
Omelette Ham & Cheddar	1 serv	634	3	0	1
Omelette Sausage & Cheddar	1 serv	741	3	0	1
Omelette Three Cheese	1 serv	645	4	0	1
Omelette Western	1 serv	654	8	3	2
Pot Roast Hash	1 serv	652	34	5	4
Sausage Gravy Bowl	1 serv	268	21	1	0
Sausage Link	1	125	0	0	0
Skillet Sunshine	1 serv	842	36	2	4
Waffles Sweet Cream	1 serv	598	100	30	3
CHILDREN'S MENU SELECTIONS					
Fruit & Yogurt Dippers	1 serv	275	61	54	5
Hotcakes	1 serv	501	79	26	2
Kid's Macaroni & Cheese	1 serv	320	45	11	2
Kid's Pasta	1 serv	113	15	4	1
Mini Cheeseburgers	1 serv	306	21	4	1
Smiley Face Potatoes	1 serv	524	57	2	3

FOOD	PORTION	CALS	CARB	SUGAR	FIBER
Sundae Fudge Blast	1 serv	244	33	25	0
Sundae Reese's I'm Smiling	1 serv	330	41	32	1
MAIN MENU SELECTIONS					
Seniors Chicken Parmesan	1 serv	522	33	7	3
Seniors Garden Vegetable Alfredo	1 serv	363	29	7	5
Seniors Garden Vegetable Alfredo Chicken	1 serv	452	29	7	5
Seniors Steak Tips & Noodles	1 serv	422	23	3	2
Seniors Stir-Fry Chicken	1 serv	368	44	16	5
SOUPS					
Bean	1 cup	144	19	1	3
Cheddar Baked Potato	1 cup	294	19	3	1
Sausage Chili	1 cup	268	18	2	7
Vegetable Beef	1 cup	135	17	2	3

BOJANGLES

FOOD	PORTION	CALS	CARB	SUGAR	FIBER
Biscuit	1	243	29	–	2
Biscuit Sandwich Bacon	1	290	26	–	1
Biscuit Sandwich Bacon Egg Cheese	1	550	27	–	1
Biscuit Sandwich Cajun Filet	1	454	46	–	1
Biscuit Sandwich Country Ham	1	270	26	–	1
Biscuit Sandwich Egg	1	400	26	–	1
Biscuit Sandwich Sausage	1	350	26	–	1
Biscuit Sandwich Smoked Sausage	1	380	27	–	1
Biscuit Sandwich Steak	1	649	37	–	1
Botato Rounds	1 serv	235	31	–	3
Buffalo Bites	1 serv	180	5	–	0
Cajun Pintos	1 serv	110	18	–	6
Cajun Spiced Breast	1 serv	278	12	–	tr
Cajun Spiced Leg	1 serv	264	11	–	tr
Cajun Spiced Thigh	1 serv	310	11	–	tr
Cajun Spiced Wing	1 serv	355	11	–	tr
Chicken Supremes	1 serv	337	26	–	1
Corn On The Cob	1 serv	140	34	–	2
Dirty Rice	1 serv	166	24	–	1
Green Beans	1 serv	25	5	–	2
Macaroni & Cheese	1 serv	198	12	–	tr
Marinated Cole Slaw	1 serv	136	26	–	3

FOOD	PORTION	CALS	CARB	SUGAR	FIBER
Potatoes w/o Gravy	1 serv	80	16	–	1
Sandwich Cajun Filet w/ Mayo	1	437	41	–	3
Sandwich Cajun Filet w/o Mayo	1	337	41	–	3
Sandwich Grilled Filet w/ Mayo	1	335	25	–	2
Sandwich Grilled Filet w/o Mayo	1	235	25	–	2
Seasoned Fries	1 serv	344	39	–	4
Southern Style Breast	1 serv	261	12	–	tr
Southern Style Leg	1 serv	254	11	–	tr
Southern Style Thigh	1 serv	308	14	–	tr
Southern Style Wing	1 serv	337	19	–	tr
Sweet Biscuit Bo Berry	1	320	37	–	1
Sweet Biscuit Cinnamon	1	320	37	–	1

BOSTON MARKET
DESSERTS

FOOD	PORTION	CALS	CARB	SUGAR	FIBER
Apple Pie	1 slice	420	56	24	2
Brownie Chocolate Chip Fudge	1	580	81	61	3
Chocolate Cake	1 serv	600	75	55	2
Cookie Chocolate Chip	1	370	49	28	2
Cornbread	1 piece	180	31	12	0

MAIN MENU SELECTIONS

FOOD	PORTION	CALS	CARB	SUGAR	FIBER
Broccoli w/ Garlic Butter	1 serv	80	6	2	3
Butternut Squash	1 serv	140	25	9	2
Carver Boston Chicken	1	700	68	4	3
Carver Boston Meatloaf	1	940	96	11	6
Carver Boston Sirloin Dip	1	1000	70	4	3
Carver Boston Turkey	1	770	68	3	3
Carver Boston Turkey Dip	1	770	67	2	3
Carver Half Boston Chicken	1	340	29	2	1
Carver Half Boston Sirloin Dip	1	500	35	2	1
Carver Half Boston Turkey	1	390	34	2	2
Cinnamon Apples	1 serv	210	47	42	3
Cranberry Walnut Relish	1 serv	140	30	27	2
Creamed Spinach	1 serv	280	12	1	4
Dip Spinach Artichoke	1 serv	100	3	1	1
Family Meals Boneless Turkey Breast	1 serv (5 oz)	180	0	0	0
Family Meals Roasted Turkey	1 serv (5 oz)	180	0	0	0
Family Meals Rotisserie Chicken	1 serv (6 oz)	290	4	1	0
Family Meals Spiral Sliced Ham	1 serv (8 oz)	450	13	5	0

FOOD	PORTION	CALS	CARB	SUGAR	FIBER
Family Meals Whole Turkey	1 serv (6.7 oz)	310	0	0	0
Fresh Vegetable Stuffing	1 serv	190	25	4	2
Garden Fresh Coleslaw	1 serv	170	21	19	2
Garlic Dill New Potatoes	1 serv	140	24	2	3
Green Bean Casserole	1 serv	60	9	2	2
Green Beans	1 serv	60	7	1	3
Individual Meals ¼ White Rotisserie Chicken	1 serv	290	4	1	0
Individual Meals ¼ White Rotisserie Chicken No Skin	1 serv	210	6	0	0
Individual Meals 1 Thigh & 1 Drumstick	1 serv	300	6	1	0
Individual Meals 3 Piece Dark	1 serv	380	7	1	0
Individual Meals 3 Piece Dark Skinless	1 serv	240	7	1	0
Individual Meals Award Winning Roasted Sirloin	1 serv	290	0	0	0
Individual Meals Meatloaf	1	480	23	6	2
Individual Meals Roasted Turkey	1 serv	180	0	0	0
Macaroni & Cheese	1 serv	330	39	9	1
Mashed Potatoes	1 serv	210	29	2	3
Pot Pie Pastry Topped Chicken	1	780	60	4	4
Poultry Gravy	1 serv (4 oz)	15	4	1	0
Seasonal Fresh Fruit Salad	1 serv	60	15	13	1
Spinach w/ Garlic Butter Sauce	1 serv	130	9	1	5
Squash Casserole	1 serv	320	21	8	3
Steamed Fresh Vegetables	1 serv	60	8	3	3
Sweet Corn	1 serv	170	37	10	2
Sweet Potato Casserole	1 serv	460	77	39	3
SALADS					
Entree Caesar	1	500	12	8	3
Entree Caesar w/o Dressing	1	140	8	6	2
Entree Market Chopped	1	580	30	15	9
Entree Market Chopped w/o Dressing	1	210	28	14	9
Side Caesar	1	400	7	4	2
Side Caesar w/o Dressing	1 serv	40	3	2	1
Side Market Chopped	1	440	12	7	3

FOOD	PORTION	CALS	CARB	SUGAR	FIBER
Side Market Chopped w/o Dressing	1	80	10	5	3
SOUPS					
Chicken Noodle	1 serv	170	17	1	1
Chicken Tortilla w/ Toppings	1 serv	340	24	2	1
Tortilla Soup w/o Toppings	1 serv	80	7	2	1

BOSTON PIZZA
CHILDREN'S MENU SELECTIONS

FOOD	PORTION	CALS	CARB	SUGAR	FIBER
Baked Salmon w/ Ceasar Salad	1 serv	330	13	–	tr
Bug N' Cheese	1 serv	500	73	–	3
Chicken Fingers w/ Fries	1 serv	390	28	–	2
Pizza Pint Size	1	390	64	–	tr
Quesadilla Bacon Double Cheeseburger w/ Caesar Salad	1 serv	540	49	–	3
Reduced Size Fruit Cup	1 serv	80	18	–	tr
Sandwich Grilled Chicken w/ Garden Greens	1 serv	600	45	–	3
Super Spaghetti	1 serv	440	68	–	5
Wrap Ham & Cheese w/ Fries	1 serv	550	60	–	4
DESSERTS					
Blondie Maple	1	850	111	–	1
Blondie Maple Bite Size	1	430	58	–	tr
Brownie Chocolate Addiction	1	490	92	–	2
Brownie Chocolate Addiction Bite Size	1	200	35	–	1
Cheesecake New York	1 slice	620	80	–	0
Cheesecake Vanilla Bean	1 slice	770	70	–	1
Chocolate Explosion	1 serv	890	103	–	4
Tarte Au Sucre	1 serv	310	71	–	1
MAIN MENU SELECTIONS					
Angus Beef Sirloin Steak w/ Spaghetti	1 serv	1260	83	–	8
Baked 3 Cheese Penne	1 half order	460	62	–	4
Baked Seven Cheese Ravioli	1 half order	310	28	–	2
Baked Shrimp & Feta Penne	1 half order	480	54	–	4
Boston's Lasagna	1 half order	340	45	–	3
Boston's Smokey Mountain Spaghetti	1 order	1290	161	–	13
Chicken & Mushroom Fettuccini	1 half order	710	72	–	4
Homestyle Lasagna	1 order	590	37	–	4

FOOD	PORTION	CALS	CARB	SUGAR	FIBER
Jambalaya Fettuccini	1 half order	860	71	–	6
Mama Meata Penne	1 half order	940	66	–	7
Scallop & Prawn Fettuccini	1 half order	710	67	–	5
Sicilian Penne	1 half order	720	55	–	5
Spaghetti w/ Alfredo Sauce	1 half order	440	70	–	3
Spaghetti w/ Bolognese	1 half order	400	73	–	5
Spaghetti w/ Creamy Tomato Sauce	1 half order	410	66	–	4
Spaghetti w/ Pomodoro Sauce	1 half order	450	68	–	5
Spicy Italian Penne	1 half order	980	81	–	5
Starter Baked Raviolo Bites	1 serv	450	45	–	4
Starter Boston's Poutine	1 serv	740	53	–	7
Starter Chicken Fingers	1 serv	360	12	–	0
Starter Chicken Fingers Buffalo Style	1 serv	370	14	–	1
Starter Cracked Pepper Dry Ribs	1 serv	380	3	–	1
Starter Nachos w/ Sour Cream & Salsa	1 serv	1320	126	–	12
Starter Panzerotti Roll	1	820	94	–	3
Starter Potato Skins	1 serv	650	39	–	tr
Starter Quesadilla Oven Roasted Chicken	1 serv	900	96	–	6
Starter Quesadilla Southwest w/ Sour Cream & Salsa	1 serv	770	77	–	4
Starter Shrimp Stuffed Mushroom Caps	1 serv	490	12	–	2
Starter Team Platter w/ Dips & Sauces	1 serv	3030	144	–	12
Starter Thai Chicken Bites	1 serv	540	55	–	2
Tortellini w/ Alfredo Sauce	1 half order	340	37	–	1
Tortellini w/ Bolognese	1 half order	300	40	–	3
Tortellini w/ Creamy Tomato Sauce	1 half order	310	33	–	2
PIZZA					
Bacon Double Cheeseburger Individual	1 pie	1140	94	–	2
Bacon Double Cheeseburger Slice	1 med	280	25	–	tr
BBQ Chicken Individual	1 pie	730	93	–	1
BBQ Chicken Slice	1 med	190	25	–	0

FOOD	PORTION	CALS	CARB	SUGAR	FIBER
Boston Royal Individual	1 pie	840	98	–	3
Boston Royal Slice	1 med	210	26	–	tr
Californian Slice	1 med	280	24	–	0
Clubhouse Individual	1 pie	1040	94	–	3
Deluxe Individual	1 pie	850	94	–	2
Deluxe Slice	1 med	220	25	–	tr
Great White North Individual	1 pie	960	91	–	1
Great White North Slice	1 med	240	24	–	0
Hawaiian Individual	1 pie	780	101	–	2
Hawaiian Slice	1 med	210	27	–	0
La Quebecoise Individual	1 pie	770	93	–	3
La Quebecoise Slice	1 med	200	25	–	tr
Meateor Individual	1 pie	950	91	–	1
Meateor Slice	1 med	260	25	–	0
Pepperoni Individual	1 pie	750	89	–	2
Pepperoni Slice	1 med	200	24	–	0
Pepperoni & Mushroom Individual	1 pie	750	90	–	2
Pepperoni & Mushroom Slice	1 med	200	24	–	tr
Popeye Individual	1 pie	720	93	–	2
Popeye Slice	1 med	200	25	–	tr
Rustic Italian Individual	1 pie	950	102	–	3
Rustic Italian Slice	1 med	260	28	–	tr
Spicy Perogy Individual	1 pie	980	99	–	2
Spicy Perogy Slice	1 med	280	28	–	0
Szechuan Individual	1 pie	750	99	–	1
Szechuan Slice	1 med	200	27	–	0
Tandoori Individual	1 med	730	90	–	2
Tandoori Slice	1 med	200	25	–	tr
Thai Chicken Individual	1 pie	840	108	–	4
Thai Chicken Slice	1 med	240	30	–	1
The Basic Individual	1 pie	620	88	–	1
The Basic Slice	1 med	160	24	–	0
Tropical Chicken Individual	1 pie	970	97	–	tr
Tropical Chicken Slice	1 med	260	26	–	0
Tuscan Individual	1 pie	940	106	–	5
Tuscan Slice	1 med	250	29	–	1
Ultimate Pepperoni Individual	1 pie	870	89	–	2
Ultimate Pepperoni Slice	1 med	230	24	–	tr
Vegetarian Individual	1 pie	680	101	–	4

FOOD	PORTION	CALS	CARB	SUGAR	FIBER
Vegetarian Slice	1 med	180	26	–	1
Zorba The Greek Individual	1 pie	800	97	–	4
Zorba The Greek Slice	1 med	210	26	–	1
SALADS					
Chipotle Chicken & Bacon	1 serv	630	40	–	6
Crispy Chicken Pecan	1 serv	1100	25	–	6
Entree Caesar	1 serv	500	29	–	4
Entree Spinach	1 serv	450	9	–	3
Starter Spinach	1 serv	250	6	–	2
Taco Salad Beef w/o Sour Cream & Salsa	1 serv	610	50	–	6
Taco Salad Chicken w/o Sour Cream & Salsa	1 serv	480	48	–	6
Thai Chicken Salad	1 serv	1060	117	–	12
SANDWICHES					
Beef Dip w/ Fries & Au Jus	1 serv	1340	118	–	5
Boston Cheesesteak w/ Caesar Salad & Au Jus	1 serv	1300	90	–	3
Boston Brute w/ Caesar Salad & Au Jus	1 serv	820	99	–	4
Buffalo Chicken w/ Fries	1 serv	1220	130	–	7
Chicken Parmesan w/ Fries	1 serv	1370	107	–	7
Ciabatta Chicken w/ Caesar Salad	1 serv	920	73	–	4
New York Steak w/ Garden Greens & Au Jus	1 serv	660	32	–	2
Stromboli Bacon Double Cheeseburger w/ Caesar Salad	1 serv	910	111	–	3
Stromboli Chicken Santa Fe w/ Caesar Salad	1 serv	750	106	–	4
Stromboli Smoked Ham & Chicken w/ Caesar Salad	1 serv	880	99	–	1
SOUPS					
Baked French Onion	1 serv	330	40	–	3
Clam Chowder	1 serv	260	18	–	0

BRUEGGER'S BAGELS
BAGELS

FOOD	PORTION	CALS	CARB	SUGAR	FIBER
Asiago Parmesan	1	330	62	8	4
Baked Apple	1	370	77	19	5
Blueberry	1	330	67	14	4

FOOD	PORTION	CALS	CARB	SUGAR	FIBER
Chocolate Chip	1	350	64	14	4
Cinnamon Sugar	1	330	69	17	4
Cranberry Orange	1	330	68	17	4
Everything	1	320	64	8	4
Garlic	1	320	65	8	4
Honey Grain	1	330	65	10	5
Jalapeno Bagel	1	320	64	8	4
Multi-Grain	1	350	68	10	6
Onion	1	320	64	8	4
Plain	1	320	64	8	4
Poppy	1	320	64	8	4
Pumpernickel	1	330	67	11	12
Pumpkin	1	330	68	13	6
Rosemary Olive Oil	1	350	64	10	4
Salt	1	320	64	8	4
Sesame	1	360	68	11	4
Sourdough	1	340	68	8	4
Square Asiago Parmesan	1	360	66	11	4
Square Everything	1	320	64	8	4
Square Plain	1	350	70	11	4
Square Sesame	1	360	68	11	4
Sun Dried Tomato	1	320	64	11	4
Whole Wheat	1	390	73	8	9
DESSERTS					
Brownie Chocolate Chunk	1	330	40	27	2
Cake Lemon Pound	1 slice	320	48	25	tr
Cookie Chocolate Chip	1	500	71	43	3
Cookie Oatmeal Raisin	1	460	71	39	3
Cookie Peanut Butter	1	480	63	38	2
Cookie Triple Chocolate Chunk	1	560	71	44	3
Cookie White Chocolate Macadamia	1	580	70	46	1
Luscious Lemon Bar	1	300	36	24	0
Marshmallow Chew	1	280	55	29	0
Muffin Blueberry	1	450	64	29	3
Muffin Chocolate	1	460	57	38	3
Oreo Dream Bar	1	470	49	35	2
Pecan Chocolate Chunk	1 slice	310	32	16	1
Raspberry Sammies	1 slice	340	44	21	1
Seven Layer Bar	1	650	58	42	5

FOOD	PORTION	CALS	CARB	SUGAR	FIBER
Toffee Almond Bar	1	400	53	34	1
SALADS					
Caesar w/ Dressing	1 serv	270	22	5	2
Tossed Chicken Caesar w/ Dressing	1 serv	370	23	5	2
Tossed Mandarin Medley	1 serv	340	36	27	4
Tossed Sesame Chicken	1 serv	480	30	18	2
SANDWICHES					
BLT w/ Mayo	1	570	72	10	5
Chicken Breast	1	660	87	26	5
Chicken Fajita	1	530	81	16	6
Chicken Salad w/ Mayo	1	630	73	11	5
Cranberry Gobbler	1	620	78	17	5
Cuban Chicken	1	680	74	10	4
Denver Egg	1	460	74	11	5
Egg Cheese	1	420	71	9	4
Egg Cheese Bacon	1	460	65	9	4
Egg Cheese Ham	1	460	73	11	4
Egg Cheese Sausage	1	640	72	10	5
Ham	1	460	76	12	5
Herby Turkey	1	560	78	10	5
Leonardo Da Veggie	1	480	74	11	5
Radishy Roast Beef	1	560	73	11	5
Roadhouse Chicken	1	710	84	22	4
Roast Beef	1	730	71	10	5
Santa Fe Turkey	1	490	75	12	5
Smoked Salmon	1	490	74	10	5
Softwich BLT w/ Mayo	1	600	73	14	5
Softwich Chicken Breast	1	630	81	21	5
Softwich Chicken Fajita	1	570	81	18	6
Softwich Chicken Salad	1	670	76	15	5
Softwich Cranberry Gobbler	1	730	80	20	5
Softwich Cuban Chicken	1	810	77	15	4
Softwich Garden Veggie	1	380	76	15	6
Softwich Ham	1	510	85	25	5
Softwich Herby Turkey	1	580	80	13	5
Softwich Hummus	1	540	85	13	11
Softwich Leonardo Da Veggie	1	550	79	16	6
Softwich Mediterranean	1	790	90	13	11
Softwich Peanut Chicken	1	590	82	18	5

FOOD	PORTION	CALS	CARB	SUGAR	FIBER
Softwich Radishy Roast Beef	1	670	75	14	5
Softwich Roadhouse Chicken	1	670	74	13	4
Softwich Roast Beef	1	750	72	10	5
Softwich Roasted Turkey	1	550	74	13	5
Softwich Smoked Salmon	1	520	76	14	5
Softwich Supreme Club w/o Mayo	1	880	79	18	5
Softwich Tuna Salad	1	720	76	14	5
Softwich Western Wheat	1	820	76	14	8
Supreme Club w/o Mayo	1	470	72	11	5
Tuna Salad	1	620	73	10	5
Turkey	1	510	70	9	5
Wrap Classic w/ Bacon	1	520	52	4	4
Wrap Classic w/ Ham	1	510	54	5	4
Wrap Classic w/ Sausage	1	660	52	3	4
Wrap Rio Grande Bacon	1	560	55	6	4
Wrap Rio Grande Ham	1	630	55	7	4
Wrap Rio Grande Sausage	1	510	53	4	4
Wrap Sesame Chicken Salad	1	770	80	18	5
Wrap Tossed Chicken Caesar	1	660	73	5	5
Wrap Tossed Mandarin Medley Salad	1	630	87	26	7
SOUPS					
Chicken Pot Pie	1 cup	250	12	2	2
Chicken Spaetzle	1 cup	120	12	2	1
Chicken Wild Rice	1 cup	260	16	2	1
Creamy Tomato	1 cup	150	16	11	3
Hearty Mushroom Barley	1 cup	110	18	3	4
Italian Wedding	1 cup	160	15	2	2
Minestrone	1 cup	120	21	3	5
Moroccan Stew	1 cup	140	26	8	4
New England Clam	1 cup	300	23	tr	1
Sweet Potato Cheddar	1 cup	200	20	6	2
SPREADS					
Cream Cheese Bacon Scallion	1 scoop (1.5 oz)	140	5	2	0
Cream Cheese Cucumber Dill	1 scoop (1.5 oz)	140	3	1	0
Cream Cheese Garden Veggie	1 scoop (1.5 oz)	130	5	2	1

FOOD	PORTION	CALS	CARB	SUGAR	FIBER
Cream Cheese Honey Walnut	1 scoop (1.5 oz)	150	8	3	tr
Cream Cheese Jalapeno	1 scoop (1.5 oz)	140	4	2	0
Cream Cheese Light Garden Veggie	1 scoop (1.5 oz)	90	3	2	0
Cream Cheese Light Herb Garlic	1 scoop (1.5 oz)	100	4	2	0
Cream Cheese Light Plain	1 scoop (1.5 oz)	100	4	3	tr
Cream Cheese Olive Pimento	1 scoop (1.5 oz)	140	3	1	0
Cream Cheese Onion & Chive	1 scoop (1.5 oz)	140	3	2	0
Cream Cheese Plain	1 scoop (1.5 oz)	130	6	2	tr
Cream Cheese Pumpkin	1 scoop (1.5 oz)	120	4	3	0
Cream Cheese Strawberry	1 scoop (1.5 oz)	140	4	2	0
Cream Cheese Wildberry	1 scoop (1.5 oz)	140	5	3	0
Hummus	1 scoop (2 oz)	110	10	0	0

BURGER KING
BEVERAGES

FOOD	PORTION	CALS	CARB	SUGAR	FIBER
Chocolate Milk 1% Low Fat	1 (9 oz)	180	31	29	1
Diet Coke	1 sm (16 oz)	0	0	0	0
Iced Coffee Mocha BK Joe	1 (16 oz)	380	66	63	1
Milk 1% Low Fat	1	110	13	12	0
Shake Chocolate	1 sm (16 oz)	470	75	72	1
Shake Oreo Sundae Chocolate	1 sm (16 oz)	680	105	95	2
Shake Oreo Sundae Strawberry	1 sm (16 oz)	660	103	94	1
Shake Oreo Sundae Vanilla	1 sm (16 oz)	610	87	78	1
Shake Strawberry	1 sm (16 oz)	460	73	71	0
Shake Vanilla	1 sm (16 oz)	400	57	55	0
Water Nestle Pure Life	1 bottle (16 oz)	0	0	0	0

BREAKFAST SELECTIONS

FOOD	PORTION	CALS	CARB	SUGAR	FIBER
Biscuit Bacon Egg & Cheese	1	410	31	4	1
Biscuit Ham Egg & Cheese	1	390	31	4	1

FOOD	PORTION	CALS	CARB	SUGAR	FIBER
Biscuit Sausage	1	390	28	2	1
Biscuit Sausage Egg & Cheese	1	530	31	4	1
Croissan'wich Bacon Egg & Cheese	1	340	26	5	tr
Croissan'wich Double w/ Bacon Egg & Cheese	1	430	27	6	tr
Croissan'wich Double w/ Ham Bacon Egg & Cheese	1	420	27	7	1
Croissan'wich Double w/ Ham Egg & Cheese	1	420	27	7	1
Croissan'wich Double w/ Ham Sausage Egg & Cheese	1	550	27	6	1
Croissan'wich Double w/ Sausage Bacon Egg & Cheese	1	550	27	6	1
Croissan'wich Double w/ Sausage Egg & Cheese	1	680	26	6	1
Croissan'wich Egg & Cheese	1	300	26	5	tr
Croissan'wich Ham Egg & Cheese	1	340	26	6	1
Croissan'wich Sausage & Cheese	1	370	23	4	tr
Croissan'wich Sausage Egg & Cheese	1	470	26	5	tr
French Toast Sticks	3 pieces	240	26	6	1
Hash Browns	1 sm	260	25	0	2
Hash Browns	1 lg	620	60	1	6
Omelet Sandwich Enormous	1	730	44	8	2
Omelet Sandwich Ham	1	290	33	8	1
DESSERTS					
Cini-minis	1 serv	390	51	19	2
Dutch Apple Pie	1 serv	300	45	23	1
Hershey Sundae Pie	1	310	32	22	1
MAIN MENU SELECTIONS					
BK Chicken Fries	6 pieces	260	18	1	2
BK Stacker Double	1	610	32	5	1
BK Stacker Quad	1	1000	34	6	1
BK Stacker Triple	1	800	33	5	1
BK Veggie Burger	1	420	46	8	7
Cheeseburger	1	330	31	6	1

FOOD	PORTION	CALS	CARB	SUGAR	FIBER
Cheeseburger Double	1	500	31	6	1
Chicken Sandwich Original	1	660	52	5	4
Chicken Sandwich Tendercrisp	1	790	68	9	5
Chicken Sandwich Tendergrill	1	510	49	7	4
Chicken Tenders	5 pieces	210	13	0	0
Chick'n Crisp Spicy Sandwich	1	480	36	4	1
Double Cheeseburger	1	410	30	6	1
French Fries No Salt Added	1 sm	230	26	1	2
French Fries Salted	1 sm	230	26	1	2
French Fries Salted	1 lg	500	57	1	5
Hamburger	1	290	30	6	1
Onion Rings	1 sm	140	18	2	2
Onion Rings	1 lg	440	53	6	5
Sandwich BK Big Fish	1	640	67	9	3
The Angus Steak Burger	1	640	55	10	3
Whopper	1	670	51	11	3
Whopper Double	1	900	51	11	3
Whopper Double w/ Cheese	1	990	52	11	3
Whopper Jr.	1	370	31	6	2
Whopper Jr. w/ Cheese	1	410	32	6	2
Whopper Triple	1	1130	51	11	3
Whopper Triple w/ Cheese	1	1230	52	11	3
Whopper w/ Cheese	1	760	52	11	3
SALAD DRESSINGS AND TOPPINGS					
Breakfast Syrup	1 serv (1 oz)	80	21	14	0
Croutons Garlic Parmesan	1 serv	60	9	1	0
Dipping Sauce Barbecue	1 serv (1 oz)	40	11	10	0
Dipping Sauce Honey Mustard	1 serv (1 oz)	90	8	7	0
Dipping Sauce Ranch	1 serv (1 oz)	140	1	1	0
Dipping Sauce Sweet And Sour	1 serv (1 oz)	40	11	10	0
Dressing Ken's Creamy Caesar	1 serv (2 oz)	210	4	3	0
Dressing Ken's Fat Free Ranch	1 serv (2 oz)	60	15	5	2
Dressing Ken's Honey Mustard	1 serv (2 oz)	270	15	14	0
Dressing Ken's Ranch	1 serv (2 oz)	190	2	1	0
Jam Grape	1 serv	30	7	6	0
Jam Strawberry	1 serv	30	7	6	0
Ketchup	1 pkg	10	3	2	0
Mayonnaise	1 pkg	80	1	0	0
SALADS					
Chicken Garden Tendercrisp	1	410	26	5	5

FOOD	PORTION	CALS	CARB	SUGAR	FIBER
Chicken Garden Tendergrill w/o Dressing or Croutons	1	240	8	3	4
Side Garden w/o Dressing	1	15	3	1	1

BURGERVILLE
BEVERAGES

Barq's Root Beer	1 (20 oz)	180	49	–	0
Coca-Cola	1 (20 oz)	161	44	–	0
Diet Coke	1 (20 oz)	0	0	–	0
Hot Chocolate Ghirardelli	1 (12 oz)	230	38	–	2
House Coffee	1 (10 oz)	5	1	–	0
Iced Tea	1 (20 oz)	0	0	–	0
Iced Tea Nestea Raspberry	1 (20 oz)	127	34	–	0
Lemonade Odwalla	1 (20 oz)	240	65	–	0
Milk 2%	1 (8 oz)	121	12	–	0
Orange Juice Odwalla	1 (10 oz)	138	31	–	1
Pibb Xtra	1 (20 oz)	163	42	–	0
Sprite	1 (20 oz)	158	42	–	0

BREAKFAST SELECTIONS

Bagel	1	310	63	–	2
Bagel Bacon And Egg	1	490	64	–	2
Bagel Ham And Egg	1	490	65	–	2
Bagel Sausage And Egg	1	640	64	–	2
Breakfast Platter w/ Bacon	1 serv	730	55	–	1
Breakfast Platter w/ Ham	1 serv	725	56	–	1
Breakfast Platter w/ Sausage	1 serv	880	56	–	1
Toaster Biscuit Bacon And Egg	1	450	32	–	1
Toaster Biscuit Ham And Egg	1	440	33	–	1
Toaster Biscuit Sausage And Egg	1	600	32	–	1

MAIN MENU SELECTIONS

Apple Slices	1 serv	29	9	–	2
Cheeseburger	1	350	29	–	2
Cheeseburger Colossal	1	520	31	–	5
Cheeseburger Double Beef	1	430	29	–	2
Cheeseburger Tillamook	1	630	31	–	5
Cheeseburger Tillamook Pepper Bacon	1	690	28	–	5
Chicken Strips	5	320	26	–	0
French Fries	1 serv	410	57	–	6
Gardenburger Spicy Black Bean	1	550	45	–	10
Gardenburger The Original	1	450	52	–	8

FOOD	PORTION	CALS	CARB	SUGAR	FIBER
Halibut	3 pieces	320	24	–	0
Hamburger	1	300	29	–	2
Hamburger Burgerville Classic	1	510	30	–	5
Onion Rings Walla Walla	1 serv	810	83	–	1
Sandwich Crispy Chicken	1	490	59	–	3
Sandwich Deluxe Crispy Chicken	1	590	56	–	3
Sandwich Halibut	1	480	41	–	2
Sandwich Low Fat Grilled Chicken	1	320	44	–	3
Sandwich Nine Grain Turkey Club	1	550	38	–	3
Sweet Potato Fries	1 serv	530	60	–	3
Turkey Burger Seasoned	1	540	33	–	5
Yukon Golds	1 serv	450	59	–	5
SALAD DRESSINGS AND TOPPINGS					
Burgerville Spread Cups	1	280	4	–	0
Cream Cheese	1 serv	100	1	–	0
Cream Cheese Light	1 serv	70	2	–	0
Dip BBQ Sauce	1 serv	60	13	–	0
Dressing Blue Cheese	1 serv	240	3	–	0
Dressing Caesar	1 serv	220	2	–	0
Dressing Honey Mustard	1 serv	210	6	–	0
Dressing Ranch	1 serv	195	2	–	0
Sauce Sweet And Sour	1 serv	90	12	–	0
Tartar Cups	1	260	2	–	0
Vinaigrette Honey Lime	1 serv	250	10	–	0
Vinaigrette Raspberry	1 serv	45	6	–	0
SALADS					
Grilled Chicken	1	430	16	–	7
Rogue River Smokey Blue	1	290	38	–	4
Side Salad	1	50	4	–	2
Wild Smoked Salmon & Hazelnuts	1	440	19	–	7
CAPTAIN D'S SEAFOOD					
Baked Chicken Dinner	1 serv	350	49	4	5
Baked Fish Dinner	1 serv	390	49	4	5
Baked Potato	1 serv	190	44	3	4
Baked Salmon Dinner	1 serv	470	58	12	5
Carb Counter Chicken Dinner	1 serv	320	19	8	6

FOOD	PORTION	CALS	CARB	SUGAR	FIBER
Carb Counter Fish Dinner	1 serv	350	19	8	6
Cole Slaw	1 serv	150	22	0	1
Corn On The Cob	1 serv	150	34	8	2
Fresh Steamed Broccoli	1 serv	25	5	2	3
Green Beans	1 serv	90	15	4	4
Rice Pilaf	1 serv	160	35	2	1
Shrimp Scampi Dinner	1 serv	370	50	4	5
Side Salad w/o Dressing	1	30	6	3	2
Tuscan Style Vegetables	1 serv	30	7	3	2

CARL'S JR.
BEVERAGES

Malt Chocolate	1 (15 oz)	780	98	79	1
Malt Oreo Cookie	1 (15 oz)	790	91	72	1
Malt Strawberry	1 (15 oz)	770	97	83	0
Malt Vanilla	1 (15 oz)	760	99	84	0
Shake Chocolate	1 (14 oz)	710	85	71	1
Shake Oreo Cookie	1 (14 oz)	720	79	64	1
Shake Strawberry	1 (14 oz)	700	84	75	0
Shake Vanilla	1 (14 oz)	710	86	76	0

BREAKFAST SELECTIONS

Breakfast Burger	1	830	65	13	3
Burrito Bacon & Egg	1	570	37	1	1
Burrito Loaded Breakfast	1	820	52	3	2
Burrito Steak & Egg	1	660	44	4	2
French Toast Dips w/o Syrup	5	430	58	15	1
Hash Brown Nuggets	1 serv	330	32	1	3
Sandwich Sourdough Breakfast	1 serv	460	39	4	2
Sunrise Croissant Sandwich	1	560	27	5	1

DESSERTS

Cheesecake Strawberry Swirl	1 serv	290	30	20	0
Chocolate Cake	1 serv	300	48	37	1
Cookie Chocolate Chip	1	350	46	27	1

MAIN MENU SELECTIONS

Burger Jalapeno	1	720	50	10	3
Burger Teriyaki	1	660	61	19	3
Cheeseburger Double Western Bacon	1	970	71	15	3
Cheeseburger Western Bacon	1	710	70	15	3
Chicken Breast Strips	3	420	28	1	1
Chicken Stars	4	170	10	0	1

FOOD	PORTION	CALS	CARB	SUGAR	FIBER
CrissCut Fries	1 serv	410	43	0	4
Famous Star w/ Cheese	1	660	53	10	3
Fish & Chips	1 serv	630	68	4	3
French Fries	1 sm	290	37	0	3
Fried Zucchini	1 serv	320	31	0	0
Hamburger Big	1	470	54	13	3
Hamburger Kid's	1	460	53	13	2
Onion Rings	1 serv	430	53	5	2
Sandwich Bacon Swiss Crispy Chicken	1	720	64	9	3
Sandwich Carl's Catch Fish	1	660	75	14	3
Sandwich Charbroiled BBQ Chicken	1	360	48	12	4
Sandwich Charbroiled Chicken Club	1	550	43	9	4
Sandwich Charbroiled Santa Fe Chicken	1	610	43	10	4
Sandwich Spicy Chicken	1	560	59	7	2
Six Dollar Burger The Bacon Cheese	1	1070	50	10	3
Six Dollar Burger The Guacamole Bacon	1	1140	54	11	6
Six Dollar Burger The Jalapeno	1	1030	52	11	3
Six Dollar Burger The Low Carb	1	490	6	4	2
Six Dollar Burger The Original	1	1010	60	18	3
Six Dollar Burger The Western Bacon	1	1130	83	19	4
Super Star w/ Cheese	1	930	54	10	3
SALAD DRESSINGS					
Blue Cheese	1 serv (2 oz)	320	1	1	0
House	1 serv (2 oz)	220	2	2	0
Low Fat Balsamic	1 serv (2 oz)	35	5	3	0
Thousand Island	1 serv (2 oz)	240	7	3	0
SALADS					
Charbroiled Chicken	1	260	16	8	5
Side	1	50	5	3	2
CARVEL					
Brown Bonnet	1	370	40	29	0
Cake Ice Cream	1 slice	270	33	23	1
Carvelanche Cake Mix	1 reg (16 oz)	720	106	74	0

FOOD	PORTION	CALS	CARB	SUGAR	FIBER
Carvelanche Cookies & Cream	1 reg (16 oz)	550	64	49	0
Carvelanche Triple Fudge Cake Mix	1 reg (16 oz)	900	134	101	4
Chipsters	1	330	44	25	4
Cone Cake Chocolate	1 sm	260	32	25	1
Cone Cake Chocolate	1 lg	600	71	59	3
Cone Cake Vanilla	1 sm	280	31	24	0
Cone Cake Vanilla	1 lg	650	68	57	0
Cone Sugar Chocolate	1 sm	300	40	29	1
Cone Sugar Vanilla	1 sm	320	39	28	0
Cone Waffle Chocolate	1 sm	330	47	31	2
Cone Waffle Chocolate	1 lg	660	86	65	3
Cone Waffle Vanilla	1 sm	350	46	30	1
Cone Waffle Vanilla	1 lg	710	83	63	1
Dashers Banana Barge	1	940	121	86	7
Dashers Bananas Foster	1	600	90	60	2
Dashers Fudge Brownie	1	810	98	80	4
Dashers Mint Chocolate Chip	1	720	85	63	2
Dashers Peanut Butter Cup	1	1090	97	79	4
Dashers Strawberry Shortcake	1	590	78	59	2
Flying Saucer 98% Fat Free Chocolate	1	180	34	19	1
Flying Saucer Chocolate	1	230	33	20	1
Flying Saucer Deluxe Sprinkles	1	330	47	26	1
Flying Saucer Vanilla	1	240	33	19	1
Flying Saucers 98% Fat Free Vanilla	1	180	35	20	1
Ice Cream Chocolate	1 sm (4 oz)	250	29	25	0
Ice Cream Vanilla	1 sm (4 oz)	240	25	21	0
Ice Cream No Fat Chocolate	1 sm (4 oz)	160	37	33	0
Ice Cream No Fat Vanilla	1 sm (4 oz)	160	33	29	0
Sherbet All Flavors	1 sm (4 oz)	180	39	30	0
Sinful Love Bar	1	460	47	28	5
Sprinkle Cup	1	230	28	20	1
Sundae Bittersweet Fudge	1 reg	690	77	64	1
Sundae Caramel	1 reg	670	81	60	0
Sundae Hot Fudge	1 reg	670	73	62	1
Sundae Strawberry	1 reg	580	63	54	1
Sundae Mini Chocolate Syrup	1	200	27	20	0
Thick Shake Chocolate	1 reg (16 oz)	650	93	69	2

FOOD	PORTION	CALS	CARB	SUGAR	FIBER
Thick Shake Vanilla	1 reg (16 oz)	610	81	74	0
Thinny Thin Classic Sundae No Fat Strawberry	1 reg	320	69	59	1
Thinny Thin Classic Sundae No Fat Fudge	1 reg	380	81	46	0
Thinny Thin Minature Sundae No Fat	1	190	45	20	0
Thinny Thin Minature Sundae No Sugar Added	1	200	42	6	0
Thinny Thin No Fat Carvelanche Strawberry	1 (16 oz)	430	91	81	1
Thinny Thin No Fat Chocolate	1 sm	160	37	33	0
Thinny Thin No Fat Vanilla	1 sm	160	33	29	0
Thinny Thin No Sugar Added Vanilla	1 sm	180	34	10	0
Thinny Thin Parfait No Fat	1	190	42	20	0
Thinny Thin Shake No Fat Chocolate	1 (16 oz)	440	104	59	0
Thinny Thin Shake No Fat Mocha	1 (16 oz)	440	97	52	0
Thinny Thin Shake No Fat Vanilla	1 (16 oz)	300	62	55	0

CHIPOTLE

FOOD	PORTION	CALS	CARB	SUGAR	FIBER
Barbacoa	1 serv (4 oz)	228	1	0	0
Black Beans	1 serv (4 oz)	130	22	3	12
Carnitas	1 serv (4 oz)	227	0	0	0
Cheese	1 serv (1 oz)	110	tr	0	0
Chicken	1 serv (4 oz)	219	0	0	0
Chips	1 serv (4 oz)	490	71	1	5
Crispy Taco Shells	3	180	26	0	2
Fajita Vegetables	1 serv (3 oz)	100	6	3	1
Flour Tortilla	1 (13 inch)	330	55	1	5
Flour Tortilla	1 (6 inch)	300	48	0	6
Guacamole	1 serv (4 oz)	170	8	1	5
Lettuce	1 serv (1 oz)	5	tr	0	tr
Pinto Beans	1 serv (4 oz)	138	23	3	10
Rice	1 serv (3.5 oz)	168	28	0	tr
Salsa Corn	1 serv (4 oz)	100	22	3	3
Salsa Tomato	1 serv (4 oz)	25	6	3	1
Sour Cream	1 serv (2 oz)	120	2	2	0

FOOD	PORTION	CALS	CARB	SUGAR	FIBER
Steak	1 serv (4 oz)	230	2	0	0
Tomatillo Green	1 serv (2 oz)	15	3	2	1
Tomatillo Red	1 serv (2 oz)	28	4	1	1
Vinaigrette	1 serv (2 oz)	282	11	25	0

CHURCH'S CHICKEN
DESSERTS

FOOD	PORTION	CALS	CARB	SUGAR	FIBER
Pie Apple	1 pie (3 oz)	280	39	15	1
Pie Edward's Double Lemon	1 pie (3 oz)	300	39	29	0
Pie Edward's Strawberry Cream Cheese	1 pie (2.8 oz)	280	32	22	2

MAIN MENU SELECTIONS

FOOD	PORTION	CALS	CARB	SUGAR	FIBER
Biscuit Honey Butter	1	240	28	4	1
Cajun Rice	1 reg	130	16	0	tr
Chicken Fried Steak w/ White Gravy	1 serv (7.5 oz)	610	31	2	2
Cole Slaw	1 reg	150	15	7	2
Corn On The Cob	1 ear	140	24	2	9
Country Fried Steak w/ White Gravy	1 serv (5.8 oz)	470	36	4	1
Crunchy Tenders	1 (2 oz)	120	6	0	tr
French Fries	1 reg	290	38	1	4
Jalapeno Cheese Bombers	4 (4 oz)	240	29	5	3
Macaroni & Cheese	1 reg	210	23	6	1
Mashed Potatoes & Gravy	1 reg	70	12	2	1
Okra	1 reg	350	36	3	5
Original Breast	1	200	3	0	1
Original Leg	1	110	3	0	0
Original Thigh	1	330	8	0	1
Original Wing	1	300	7	0	3
Sandwich Bigger Better Chicken w/ Cheese	1	510	46	4	4
Sandwich Country Fried Steak	1	490	38	4	2
Sandwich Spicy Fish	1	320	25	3	2
Spicy Breast	1	320	12	0	1
Spicy Crunchy Tenders	1 (2 oz)	135	7	0	4
Spicy Fish Fillet	1 piece (2.3 oz)	160	13	1	1
Spicy Leg	1	180	8	0	1
Spicy Thigh	1	480	20	0	2
Spicy Wing	1	430	17	0	2

FOOD	PORTION	CALS	CARB	SUGAR	FIBER
Sweet Corn Nuggets	1 reg	600	72	14	5
Whole Jalapeno Peppers	2	10	2	tr	1
SAUCES					
BBQ	1 pkg	30	7	2	0
Creamy Jalapeno	1 pkg	100	1	0	0
Honey	1 pkg	27	7	7	0
Honey Mustard	1 pkg	110	4	1	0
Hot Sauce	1 pkg	0	0	0	0
Ketchup	1 pkg	18	5	4	0
Purple Pepper	1 pkg	45	12	6	0
Ranch	1 pkg	130	1	0	0
Sweet & Sour	1 pkg	30	8	2	0

CINNABON

BAKED SELECTIONS

FOOD	PORTION	CALS	CARB	SUGAR	FIBER
Caramel Pecanbon	1	1100	141	47	8
Cinnabon Bites	6	520	78	25	2
Cinnabon Classic	1	813	117	55	4
Cinnabon Stix	1	379	41	14	1
Minibon	1	339	49	22	2
BEVERAGES					
Caramelatta Chill	1 (16 oz)	520	76	73	0
Chillatta Cappuccino	1 (16 oz)	330	56	51	1
Chillatta Caramel	1 (16 oz)	480	72	68	0
Chillatta Chocolate Mocha	1 (16 oz)	460	72	61	3
Chillatta Mango	1 (16 oz)	340	57	47	0
Chillatta Strawberry	1 (16 oz)	330	54	46	0
Chillatta Strawberry Banana	1 (16 oz)	350	58	49	0
Mochalatta Chill	1 (16 oz)	450	66	62	1

COLD STONE CREAMERY

FOOD	PORTION	CALS	CARB	SUGAR	FIBER
Waffle Cone Dipped	1	310	46	31	2
Waffle Cone Dipped w/ Candy	1	390	55	31	2
Waffle Cone Or Bowl	1	160	29	14	0
FROZEN YOGURT					
Cheesecake	1 serv (6 oz)	170	49	33	0
Low Fat Chocolate	1 serv (6 oz)	230	48	29	3
Nonfat Coffee	1 serv (6 oz)	220	45	31	0
Nonfat Sweet Cream	1 serv (6 oz)	220	45	31	0
ICE CREAM					
Amaretto	1 serv (6 oz)	390	40	35	0

FOOD	PORTION	CALS	CARB	SUGAR	FIBER
Banana	1 serv (6 oz)	370	40	34	0
Black Cherry	1 serv (6 oz)	390	43	38	0
Butter Pecan	1 serv (6 oz)	390	40	35	0
Cake A Cheesecake Named Desire	1 slice (5 oz)	410	57	38	0
Cake Butterfinger Bonanza	1 slice (5 oz)	450	58	43	tr
Cake Celebration Sensation	1 slice (4.5 oz)	350	46	34	tr
Cake Chocolate Chipper	1 slice (4.6 oz)	450	50	39	3
Cake Coffeehouse Crunch	1 slice (5 oz)	530	59	36	2
Cake Cookie Dough Delirium	1 slice (4.8 oz)	420	53	34	tr
Cake Cookies & Creamery	1 slice (4.5 oz)	390	48	35	1
Cake Midnight Delight	1 slice (5.3 oz)	510	61	47	4
Cake MMMMMM Chip	1 slice (4.5 oz)	380	46	36	2
Cake Peanut Butter Playground	1 slice (5 oz)	490	54	43	4
Cake Raspberry Truffle Temptation	1 slice (5 oz)	480	57	43	4
Cake Snickers Supreme	1 slice (5 oz)	510	57	46	3
Cake Strawberry Passion	1 slice (5 oz)	380	50	35	1
Cake Zebra Stripes	1 slice (4.8 oz)	400	46	36	1
Cake Batter	1 serv (6 oz)	410	50	36	0
Candy Cane	1 serv (6 oz)	420	48	39	0
Caramel Latte	1 serv (6 oz)	400	47	39	0
Carrot Cake Batter	1 serv (6 oz)	450	54	44	0
Cheesecake	1 serv (6 oz)	390	44	37	0
Chocolate	1 serv (6 oz)	390	39	36	1
Cinnamon	1 serv (6 oz)	400	41	35	tr
Coconut	1 serv (6 oz)	390	39	34	0
Coffee	1 serv (6 oz)	400	40	34	0
Cookie Batter	1 serv (6 oz)	450	53	41	0
Cotton Candy	1 serv (6 oz)	390	41	34	0
Dark Chocolate Peppermint	1 serv (6 oz)	410	41	33	2
Egg Nog	1 serv (6 oz)	400	46	38	0
Expresso	1 serv (6 oz)	350	36	30	0
French Vanilla	1 serv (6 oz)	400	45	39	0
Irish Cream	1 serv (6 oz)	390	40	35	0
Macadamia Nut	1 serv (6 oz)	390	40	35	0
Mango	1 serv (6 oz)	370	40	34	0
Mint	1 serv (6 oz)	400	43	37	0
Mocha	1 serv (6 oz)	390	40	35	1
Oatmeal Batter	1 serv (6 oz)	400	44	34	0

FOOD	PORTION	CALS	CARB	SUGAR	FIBER
Orange Dreamsicle	1 serv (6 oz)	380	41	34	0
Peanut Butter	1 serv (6 oz)	440	39	33	tr
Pecan Praline	1 serv (6 oz)	400	44	37	0
Pistachio	1 serv (6 oz)	390	40	35	0
Pumpkin	1 serv (6 oz)	390	42	36	0
Raspberry	1 serv	390	43	37	0
Sinless Sans Fat Sweet Cream	1 serv (6 oz)	160	41	11	tr
Strawberry	1 serv (6 oz)	380	41	36	0
Sweet Cream	1 serv (6 oz)	390	95	35	0
Vanilla Bean	1 serv (6 oz)	400	39	34	0
White Chocolate	1 serv (6 oz)	390	40	34	0
MIX-INS AND TOPPINGS					
Almond Joy	1 piece	180	20	16	2
Apple Pie Filling	¾ oz	60	16	14	1
Banana	½	60	14	9	1
Black Cherries	¾ oz	80	19	16	0
Blackberries	¾ oz	10	2	2	1
Blueberries	¾ oz	10	2	2	0
Brownies	1 piece	180	29	19	1
Butterfinger	½ bar	140	20	15	1
Butterscotch Fat Free	1 oz	80	19	14	0
Caramel	1 oz	100	22	14	0
Caramel Topping Fat Free	1 oz	110	24	16	0
Cashews	1 oz	170	9	2	1
Chocolate Chips	1 oz	130	15	15	0
Cinnamon	⅛ tsp	15	4	0	3
Coconut	1 oz	80	7	6	1
Cookie Dough	1 piece	180	25	9	1
Fudge	1 oz	100	17	12	0
Fudge Topping Fat Free	1 oz	80	20	16	0
Granola	1 oz	120	23	0	2
Gumballs	1 oz	120	34	24	0
Gummi Bears	1 oz	120	30	13	0
Heath Candy	1 bar	110	12	0	0
Honey	1 oz	90	25	25	0
Kit Kat	½ bar	100	13	9	0
M&M's	1 oz	170	25	22	1
M&M's Peanut	1 oz	150	18	14	1
Macadamia Nuts	1 oz	180	3	1	2
Maraschino Cherry	1	5	1	1	0

FOOD	PORTION	CALS	CARB	SUGAR	FIBER
Marshmallow Creme	1 oz	100	24	20	0
Marshmallows	1 oz	100	24	24	0
Nestle Crunch	½ bar	130	16	14	1
Nilla Wafers	3	70	11	6	0
Oreo Cookies	2	120	17	10	1
Peach Pie Filling	1 oz	60	16	14	1
Peanut Butter	¾ oz	150	5	2	1
Peanuts	1 oz	200	7	0	3
Pecan Pralines	1 oz	210	5	1	2
Pecans	1 oz	140	3	1	1
Pie Crust Graham Cracker	1 oz	110	19	6	1
Pie Crust Oreo	1 oz	180	19	10	0
Pistachio Nuts	1 oz	210	10	1	4
Raisins	1 oz	80	20	16	1
Raspberries	¾ oz	15	4	2	1
Reese's Peanut Butter Cup	1 piece	190	19	16	1
Reese's Pieces	1 oz	170	21	18	1
Roasted Almonds	1 oz	190	5	1	3
Sliced Almonds	1 oz	210	6	0	4
Snickers	½ bar	170	21	17	1
Sprinkles Chocolate	1 oz	25	6	6	0
Sprinkles Rainbow	1 oz	25	6	6	0
Strawberries	¾ oz	20	7	4	1
Toasted Coconut	1 oz	180	13	11	1
Twix	1 cup	150	20	14	0
Walnuts	1 oz	130	4	0	1
Whip Topping	1 serv	45	5	2	0
White Chocolate Chips	1 oz	160	18	18	0
Whoppers	1 oz	100	16	13	0
Yellow Sponge Cake	1 piece	70	15	12	0
York Peppermint Patties	2 pieces	120	24	18	1
SORBET					
Sinless Lemon	1 serv (6 oz)	180	48	41	0
Sinless Raspberry	1 serv (6 oz)	200	50	43	0
Sinless Tangerine	1 serv (6 oz)	200	52	44	0

DAIRY QUEEN
FOOD SELECTIONS

FOOD	PORTION	CALS	CARB	SUGAR	FIBER
Chicken Strip Basket	4 pieces	520	92	7	7
Chili Cheese Dog	1	330	22	4	2

FOOD	PORTION	CALS	CARB	SUGAR	FIBER
DQ Homestyle Bacon Double Cheeseburger	1	610	31	6	2
DQ Homestyle Burger	1	290	29	5	2
DQ Homestyle Cheeseburger	1	340	29	5	2
DQ Homestyle Double Cheeseburger	1	540	30	5	2
DQ Ultimate Burger	1	670	29	6	2
French Fries	1 sm	300	45	tr	3
Grillburger ½ Lb	1	800	41	8	2
Grillburger ½ Lb w/ Cheese	1	930	41	8	2
Grillburger ¼ Lb FlameThrower	1	850	38	6	1
Grillburger Bacon Cheddar	1	710	40	8	1
Grillburger California	1	630	37	5	1
Grillburger Classic	1	540	41	8	2
Grillburger Classic w/ Cheese	1	610	41	8	2
Grillburger Mushroom Swiss	1	700	37	5	1
Hot Dog	1	240	19	4	1
Onion Rings	1 reg	470	45	7	3
Salad Crispy Chicken No Dressing	1 serv	350	21	9	6
Salad Grilled Chicken No Dressing	1 serv	240	17	7	4
Sandwich Crispy Chicken	1	590	50	8	5
Sandwich Grilled Chicken	1	340	26	4	2
Side Salad	1 serv	60	6	4	2
ICE CREAM					
Banana Split	1	510	96	82	3
Blizzard Banana Split	1 sm	460	73	63	tr
Blizzard Chocolate Chip Cookie Dough	1 sm	720	105	78	0
Blizzard Oreo Cookies	1 sm	570	83	64	tr
Blizzard Reese's Peanut Butter Cup	1 sm	600	87	76	0
Blizzard Strawberry Cheesecake	1 sm	530	76	62	tr
Brownie Earthquake	1	740	112	86	0
Buster Bar	1	500	45	37	2
Cake 8 Inch Round	⅛ cake	370	56	42	tr
Cake Blizzard Oreo Cookie	⅛ cake	490	67	51	1

FOOD	PORTION	CALS	CARB	SUGAR	FIBER
Cake Blizzard Reese's Peanut Butter Cup	1/8 cake	490	67	54	1
Cone Chocolate	1 sm	240	37	25	0
Cone Vanilla	1 sm	230	38	27	0
Cone Dipped	1 sm	340	42	31	1
Dilly Bar Chocolate	1	220	25	20	0
DQ Fudge Bar No Sugar Added	1	50	13	3	0
DQ Sandwich	1	200	31	18	1
DQ Soft Serve Chocolate	1/2 cup	150	22	17	0
DQ Soft Serve Vanilla	1/2 cup	140	22	19	0
DQ Vanilla Orange Bar No Sugar Added	1	60	17	2	0
Malt Chocolate	1 sm	640	111	97	1
MooLatte Cappuccino	1 (16 oz)	490	68	60	0
MooLatte Caramel	1 (16 oz)	630	96	85	0
MooLatte French Vanilla	1 (16 oz)	570	87	73	0
MooLatte Mocha	1 (16 oz)	590	80	70	1
Peanut Buster Parfait	1	730	99	85	2
Shake Chocolate	1 sm	560	93	83	1
Slush Arctic Rush	1 sm	220	56	56	0
Starkiss	1	80	21	21	0
Sundae Chocolate	1 sm	280	49	42	0
Sundae Strawberry	1 sm	240	40	35	0
SALAD DRESSINGS					
Blue Cheese	1 serv (2 oz)	210	4	2	0
Honey Mustard	1 serv (2 oz)	260	18	11	0
Italian Fat Free	1 serv (2 oz)	10	3	1	0
Ranch	1 serv (2 oz)	310	3	2	0
D'ANGELO					
CHILDREN'S MENU SELECTIONS					
D'Lite Turkey	1	217	30	2	3
Sub Cheeseburger	1	294	28	2	3
Sub Ham & Cheese	1	227	32	3	1
Sub Kidz Tuna	1	438	30	2	1
Sub Meatball	1	330	37	5	4
SALAD DRESSINGS					
Bleu Cheese	1 serv	152	3	2	0
Caesar	1 serv	397	6	6	0
Caesar Fat Free	1 serv	57	9	9	0
Creamy Italian	1 serv	340	9	6	0

FOOD	PORTION	CALS	CARB	SUGAR	FIBER
Greek w/ Feta Cheese	1 serv	227	6	3	0
Honey Mustard	1 serv	150	7	6	0
Olive Oil Vinaigrette	1 serv	170	9	6	0
Ranch Lite	1 serv	240	6	4	1
SALADS					
Antipasto	1 serv	284	17	7	6
Caesar w/ Dressing	1 serv	474	25	7	4
Chicken Caesar w/ Dressing	1 serv	533	19	8	4
Chicken Stir Fry w/o Dressing	1 serv	168	11	6	4
Cobb w/o Dressing	1 serv	292	11	5	4
Greek	1 serv	290	17	8	4
Lobster w/o Dressing	1 serv	376	12	6	4
Roast Beef w/o Dressing	1 serv	131	10	5	4
Steak Tip Caesar	1 serv	661	21	9	3
Tossed Garden w/o Dressing	1 serv	49	11	5	4
Turkey w/o Dressing	1 serv	157	10	5	4
SANDWICHES					
D'Lite Chicken Caesar Salad	1	374	43	9	4
D'Lite Chicken Stir Fry	1	426	57	8	7
D'Lite Classic Veggie	1	362	63	10	8
D'Lite Fresh Veggie	1	348	62	14	7
D'Lite Grilled Chicken Breast	1	388	52	5	6
D'Lite Roast Beef	1	338	51	5	6
D'Lite Turkey	1	347	51	5	6
D'Lite Turkey Cranberry	1	444	75	22	6
Pokket Big Papi	1	469	53	6	3
Pokket BLT & Cheese	1	397	38	5	3
Pokket Caesar Salad	1	616	54	7	3
Pokket Capacola & Cheese	1	362	35	2	2
Pokket Cheese	1	519	41	6	2
Pokket Cheeseburger	1	459	31	3	2
Pokket Chicken Caesar Salad	1	674	47	7	3
Pokket Chicken Club	1	526	36	3	2
Pokket Chicken Honey Dijon	1	508	40	6	2
Pokket Chicken Salad	1	623	34	3	2
Pokket Chicken Stir Fry	1	380	39	5	2
Pokket Classic Vegetable	1	368	46	8	4
Pokket Classic Veggie No Cheese	1	212	44	7	4
Pokket Greek	1	790	49	8	4

FOOD	PORTION	CALS	CARB	SUGAR	FIBER
Pokket Grilled Chicken	1	303	35	3	2
Pokket Ham	1	229	35	3	2
Pokket Ham & Cheese	1	326	38	5	2
Pokket Ham & Salami	1	386	34	3	12
Pokket Hamburger	1	399	29	2	2
Pokket Italian	1	525	36	4	2
Pokket Lobster	1	530	34	2	2
Pokket Meatball	1	574	52	10	4
Pokket Mortadella & Cheese	1	410	35	2	2
Pokket Number 9	1	407	31	4	2
Pokket Pastrami	1	438	33	1	1
Pokket Pepperoni	1	407	35	3	3
Pokket Roast Beef	1	247	33	2	2
Pokket Salad	1	196	40	6	4
Pokket Salami & Cheese	1	509	33	2	2
Pokket Seafood Salad	1	449	50	7	3
Pokket Steak	1	305	24	1	1
Pokket Steak & Cheese	1	377	26	2	1
Pokket Steak Bomb	1	631	44	4	3
Pokket Steak Tip	1	452	45	12	2
Pokket Tuna	1	664	33	2	2
Pokket Turkey	1	256	33	2	2
Pokket Turkey Club	1	332	32	4	2
Sub Big Papi	1 sm	525	60	7	7
Sub BLT & Cheese	1 sm	463	51	7	6
Sub Capicola & Cheese	1 sm	408	48	4	5
Sub Cheese	1 sm	589	55	8	5
Sub Cheeseburger	1 sm	526	44	5	5
Sub Chicken Club	1	593	49	5	5
Sub Chicken Honey Dijon	1	575	53	8	5
Sub Chicken Salad	1 sm	692	48	5	5
Sub Chicken Stir Fry	1 sm	449	53	7	6
Sub Classic Veggie	1 sm	462	64	10	8
Sub Grilled Chicken	1 sm	369	48	4	5
Sub Ham	1 sm	302	49	6	2
Sub Ham & Cheese	1 sm	395	52	7	2
Sub Ham & Salami	1 sm	456	48	5	2
Sub Hamburger	1 sm	466	42	4	5
Sub Italian	1 sm	614	54	6	3
Sub Lobster	1 sm	598	48	4	5

FOOD	PORTION	CALS	CARB	SUGAR	FIBER
Sub Meatball	1 sm	644	66	12	7
Sub Meatballs & Cheese	1 sm	750	67	13	7
Sub Mortadella & Cheese	1 sm	479	49	4	5
Sub Number 9	1 sm	450	41	5	4
Sub Pastrami	1 sm	613	47	3	5
Sub Pepperoni	1 sm	603	49	6	7
Sub Roast Beef	1 sm	320	48	5	5
Sub Salad	1 sm	281	57	11	8
Sub Salami & Cheese	1 sm	579	47	4	5
Sub Seafood Salad	1 sm	498	61	8	6
Sub Steak	1 sm	373	37	2	4
Sub Steak & Cheese	1 sm	446	40	4	4
Sub Steak Bomb	1 sm	670	52	6	6
Sub Steak Tip	1 sm	545	63	14	3
Sub Tuna	1	685	47	4	2
Sub Turkey Club	1 sm	401	49	6	3
Sub Toasted Italian Bistro	1 sm	585	49	5	5
Sub Toasted Pastrami Ruben	1 sm	750	55	7	7
Sub Toasted Roast Beef & Cheddar	1 sm	564	51	8	5
Sub Toasted Spicy Meatball	1 sm	933	71	17	9
Sub Toasted Tuna & Swiss	1 sm	796	49	6	5
Sub Toasted Turkey Thanksgiving	1 sm	705	80	11	6
Sub Toasted Turkey & Ham	1 sm	532	49	5	5
Wrap Big Papi	1	593	56	3	4
Wrap BLT & Cheese	1	544	54	4	4
Wrap Buffalo Chicken Salad	1	823	67	7	4
Wrap Caesar Salad	1	711	65	7	5
Wrap Capacola & Cheese	1	494	53	2	4
Wrap Cheese	1	675	59	6	4
Wrap Cheeseburger	1	609	48	3	3
Wrap Chicken Caesar Salad	1	830	65	7	5
Wrap Chicken Cobb	1	931	71	17	6
Wrap Chicken Filet & Bacon	1	639	58	4	2
Wrap Chicken Honey Dijon	1	672	43	8	5
Wrap Chicken Salad	1	782	53	3	4
Wrap Chicken Stir Fry	1	535	57	5	4
Wrap Classic Veggie	1	486	68	9	5
Wrap Greek	1	765	44	7	4

FOOD	PORTION	CALS	CARB	SUGAR	FIBER
Wrap Grilled Chicken	1	422	59	4	4
Wrap Ham & Cheese	1	435	60	6	3
Wrap Ham & Salami	1	513	57	4	3
Wrap Hamburger	1	509	50	3	3
Wrap Italian	1	631	59	5	3
Wrap Lobster	1	749	57	3	3
Wrap Meatball	1	687	75	11	5
Wrap Mortadella & Cheese	1	522	58	3	3
Wrap Number 9	1	517	44	4	3
Wrap Pastrami	1	550	55	2	2
Wrap Peppercorn Steak	1	702	45	4	3
Wrap Pepperoni	1	519	57	4	4
Wrap Roast Beef	1	448	58	2	4
Wrap Salad	1	324	66	10	6
Wrap Salami & Cheese	1	605	56	3	3
Wrap Seafood Salad	1	541	69	7	3
Wrap Steak	1	392	41	2	2
Wrap Steak & Cheese	1	464	43	3	2
Wrap Steak Bomb	1	670	52	6	6
Wrap Steak Tip	1	432	41	12	2
Wrap Tuna	1	731	56	4	3
Wrap Turkey	1	369	55	3	3
Wrap Turkey Club	1	415	52	4	3
SOUPS					
Beef Stew	1 sm	220	23	6	2
Broccoli & Cheddar Cheese	1 sm	270	11	3	2
Chicken Noodle	1 sm	110	14	4	1
Hearty Vegetable	1 sm	40	7	4	2
Italian Wedding	1 sm	120	11	3	2
Lobster Bisque	1 sm	360	16	3	1
New England Clam Chowder	1 sm	320	31	1	1
Portuguese Kale	1 sm	130	16	5	3
DELTACO					
BEVERAGES					
Barq's Root Beer	1 sm	278	75	42	0
Classic Coke	1 sm	248	68	68	0
Diet Coke	1 sm	2	0	0	0
Iced Tea	1 sm	0	1	0	0
Light Lemonade Minute Maid	1 sm	13	3	3	0
Milk 2% Low Fat	1 serv	152	15	15	0

FOOD	PORTION	CALS	CARB	SUGAR	FIBER
Mr Pibb Xtra	1 sm	243	65	65	0
Orange Juice	1 serv	140	34	30	1
Shake Chocolate	1 (15 oz)	680	117	101	1
Shake Strawberry	1 (15 oz)	540	100	85	1
Shake Vanilla	1 (15 oz)	550	97	81	0
Sprite	1 sm	243	65	65	0
BREAKFAST SELECTIONS					
Burrito Breakfast	1	250	24	2	1
Burrito Egg & Cheese	1	450	39	2	3
Burrito Macho Bacon & Egg	1	1030	82	6	6
Burrito Steak & Egg	1	580	41	2	3
Hash Brown Sticks	5 pieces	250	20	0	0
Quesadilla Bacon & Egg	1	450	40	2	2
Side of Bacon	2 strips	50	0	0	0
MAIN MENU SELECTIONS					
Beans 'n Cheese Cup	1 serv	260	44	4	16
Bun Taco	1	440	37	3	4
Burrito Del Beef	1	550	42	2	3
Burrito Del Classic Chicken	1	560	41	3	3
Burrito Del Combo	1	530	61	4	11
Burrito Deluxe Combo	1	570	64	5	12
Burrito Deluxe Del Beef	1	590	45	4	4
Burrito Green Bean & Cheese	1	280	36	2	6
Burrito Green Half Pound	1	430	59	4	13
Burrito Macho Beef	1	1170	89	8	7
Burrito Macho Chicken	1	930	111	8	16
Burrito Macho Combo	1	1050	113	9	17
Burrito Red Bean & Cheese	1	270	36	2	6
Burrito Red Half Pound	1	430	65	4	13
Burrito Spicy Chicken	1	480	66	3	8
Burrito Works Chicken	1	520	57	4	4
Burrito Works Steak	1	590	56	4	5
Burrito Works Veggie	1	490	69	5	9
Burritos Crispy Fish	1	497	59	5	2
Cheeseburger	1	330	37	4	3
Cheeseburger Double Del	1	560	35	4	4
Cheeseburger Double Del Bacon	1	610	35	4	4
Chips & Salsa	1 sm	156	22	2	1
Del Cheeseburger	1	430	35	3	4

FOOD	PORTION	CALS	CARB	SUGAR	FIBER
Fries	1 sm	350	34	1	3
Fries Chili Cheese	1 serv	670	51	2	5
Fries Deluxe Chili Cheese	1 serv	710	53	4	6
Hamburger	1	280	37	4	3
Nachos	1 serv	380	40	1	2
Nachos Macho	1 serv	1100	113	7	15
Quesadilla Cheddar	1	500	39	2	2
Quesadilla Spicy Jack	1	490	38	1	2
Quesadilla Spicy Jack Chicken	1	570	40	1	2
Quesadillas Chicken Cheddar	1	580	41	2	2
Rice Cup	1 serv	140	27	1	1
Taco	1	160	11	1	1
Taco Big Fat	1	320	39	3	3
Taco Big Fat Chicken	1	340	38	3	3
Taco Big Fat Steak	1	390	38	3	3
Taco Carne Asada	1	237	22	1	2
Taco Crispy Fish	1	290	30	2	2
Taco Del Carbon Chicken	1	170	19	1	2
Taco Del Carbon Steak	1	220	19	1	2
Taco Macho	1	504	19	2	5
Taco Soft	1	160	16	1	1
Taco Soft Chicken	1	210	16	1	1
SALADS					
Deluxe Chicken Salad	1 serv	740	77	9	15
Taco Salad	1 serv	350	10	3	2
Taco Salad Deluxe	1	780	76	9	14

DESERT MOON CAFE
CHILDREN'S MENU SELECTIONS

FOOD	PORTION	CALS	CARB	SUGAR	FIBER
Burrito Bean & Cheese	1 serv	650	83	2	6
Kids Nachos	1 serv	500	59	0	2
Kids Taco w/ Chicken	1	280	38	1	2
Kids Taco w/ Steak	1	290	38	1	2
Kidsadilla	1 serv	630	70	1	1
MAIN MENU SELECTIONS					
Alamo Burger	1	810	35	8	3
Burrito Adobe Moon w/ Chicken	1	730	85	4	4
Burrito Adobe Moon w/ Steak	1	750	85	4	4
Burrito Black Bean w/ Chicken	1	770	98	6	5
Burrito Black Bean w/ Steak	1	790	98	6	5

FOOD	PORTION	CALS	CARB	SUGAR	FIBER
Burrito Full Moon w/ Chicken	1	620	66	5	7
Burrito Full Moon w/ Steak	1	640	66	5	7
Burrito Get It Smothered	1	120	4	3	0
Burrito Harvest Wrap w/ Chicken	1	620	57	5	6
Burrito Harvest Wrap w/ Steak	1	300	57	5	6
Enchilada Mesa	1	710	74	3	4
Enchilada Queso	1	730	74	6	4
Fajita Platter w/ Chicken	1 serv	1160	109	13	13
Fajita Platter w/ Shrimp	1 serv	1060	109	13	13
Fajita Platter w/ Steak	1	1190	109	13	13
Hell Canyon Chili	1 serv	260	20	12	3
Mucho Nachos	1 serv	800	71	9	5
Mucho Nachos w/ Chicken	1 serv	900	71	9	5
Mucho Nachos w/ Steak	1 serv	920	71	9	5
Pizza Texas BBQ	1	330	68	18	2
Quesadilla Baja Chicken	1	650	53	4	2
Quesadilla Coyote w/ Chicken	1	660	53	3	2
Quesadilla Coyote w/ Steak	1	680	53	3	2
Quesadilla Sonoran	1	660	60	6	5
Rice Bowl Black Bean w/ Chicken	1 serv	790	123	4	4
Rice Bowl Black Bean w/ Steak	1 serv	820	123	4	4
Rice Bowl Chili w/ Chicken	1 serv	760	109	6	2
Rice Bowl Chili w/ Steak	1 serv	790	109	6	2
Rice Bowl Shrimp Creole	1 serv	910	124	13	3
Shrimp Dippers	1 serv	430	50	12	4
Soup Black Bean	1 serv	360	55	7	10
Soup Tortilla	1 serv	330	45	21	5
Taco Acapulco Shrimp	1	230	30	11	2
Taco Classic w/ Chicken	1	190	17	1	2
Taco Classic w/ Steak	1	200	17	1	2
Taco Fajita w/ Chicken	1	200	19	2	2
Taco Fajita w/ Steak	1	210	19	2	2
SALAD DRESSINGS AND SAUCES					
BBQ Sauce	1 serv (1 oz)	50	12	11	0
Buffalo Wing Sauce	1 serv (1 oz)	45	1	0	0
Dressing Bleu Cheese	1 serv (2 oz)	300	2	2	0
Dressing Creamy Caesar	1 serv (2 oz)	320	0	0	0
Dressing Honey Dijon Fat Free	1 serv (2 oz)	80	17	11	2

FOOD	PORTION	CALS	CARB	SUGAR	FIBER
Dressing Lite Ranch	1 serv (2 oz)	150	4	2	0
Dressing Lite Raspberry Vinaigrette	1 serv (2 oz)	150	6	4	0
Dressing Poblano	1 serv (1 oz)	150	2	0	1
Guacamole	1 serv (2 oz)	100	4	1	3
Pepper Cream Sauce	1 serv (2 oz)	100	4	1	0
Pico De Gallo	1 serv (2 oz)	15	3	2	1
Salsa Black Bean	1 serv (2 oz)	20	4	2	1
Salsa Fruit	1 serv (2 oz)	60	12	10	0
Salsa Mild Tomato	1 serv (2 oz)	15	3	3	1
Salsa Rattlesnake	1 serv (2 oz)	15	3	0	1
SALADS W/O TORTILLA BOWL					
Caesar	1 serv	530	15	3	4
Caesar w/ Chicken	1 serv	640	15	3	4
Caesar w/ Shrimp	1 serv	570	15	3	4
Chopped Chicken	1 serv	520	21	10	5
Taco w/ Chicken	1 serv	310	15	10	3
Taco w/ Steak	1 serv	340	15	10	3
DUNKIN' DONUTS					
BAGELS AND CREAM CHEESE					
Bagel Blueberry	1	330	66	10	2
Bagel Cinnamon Raisin	1	330	65	11	3
Bagel Everything	1	370	67	4	3
Bagel Harvest	1	350	61	15	7
Bagel Onion	1	320	61	5	3
Bagel Plain	1	320	62	4	2
Bagel Poppyseed	1	370	65	4	3
Bagel Reduced Carb w/ Cheese	1	380	45	8	14
Bagel Salsa	1	310	60	5	2
Bagel Salt	1	370	62	4	2
Bagel Sesame	1	380	64	4	3
Bagel Wheat	1	330	62	7	4
Cream Cheese Chive	2 oz	170	4	2	2
Cream Cheese Garden Vegetable	2 oz	170	4	2	0
Cream Cheese Lite	2 oz	110	6	0	0
Cream Cheese Plain	2 oz	190	4	2	0
Cream Cheese Salmon	2 oz	170	2	0	0
Cream Cheese Strawberry	2 oz	190	9	9	0

FOOD	PORTION	CALS	CARB	SUGAR	FIBER
BAKED SELECTIONS					
Apple Fritter	1	300	41	12	1
Biscuit	1	250	29	3	1
Bismark Chocolate Iced	1	340	50	31	1
Coffee Roll	1	270	33	10	1
Coffee Roll Chocolate Frosted	1	290	36	12	1
Coffee Roll Maple Frosted	1	290	36	13	1
Coffee Roll Vanilla Frosted	1	290	36	13	1
Cookie Chocolate Chunk	2	220	28	17	1
Cookie Chocolate Chunk w/ Walnuts	2	230	27	16	1
Cookie Oatmeal Raisin Pecan	2	220	29	18	1
Cookie White Chocolate Chunk	2	230	28	19	1
Croissant Plain	1	330	37	3	0
Danish Apple	1	330	32	10	1
Danish Cheese	1	340	30	8	1
Danish Strawberry Cheese	1	320	31	9	1
Donut Apple Crumb	1	230	34	12	1
Donut Apple Crumb Cake	1	290	41	22	1
Donut Apple N' Spice	1	200	29	7	1
Donut Bavarian Kreme	1	210	30	9	1
Donut Black Raspberry	1	210	32	10	1
Donut Blueberry	1	290	35	16	1
Donut Blueberry Crumb	1	240	36	15	1
Donut Boston Kreme	1	240	36	14	1
Donut Bow Tie	1	300	34	10	1
Donut Chocolate Coconut	1	300	31	12	1
Donut Chocolate Frosted	1	360	40	15	1
Donut Chocolate Glazed	1	290	33	14	1
Donut Chocolate Kreme Filled	1	270	35	16	1
Donut Cinnamon	1	330	34	14	1
Donut Double Chocolate	1	310	37	18	2
Donut Frosted Lemon	1	240	28	17	0
Donut Glazed	1	180	25	6	1
Donut Glazed Gingerbread	1	260	35	18	1
Donut Glazed Lemon	1	240	28	16	0
Donut Jelly Filled	1	210	32	14	1
Donut Lemon Burst	1	300	35	25	3
Donut Maple Frosted	1	210	30	12	1
Donut Marble Frosted	1	200	29	11	1

FOOD	PORTION	CALS	CARB	SUGAR	FIBER
Donut Old Fashioned	1	300	28	9	1
Donut Powdered	1	330	36	17	1
Donut Strawberry	1	210	32	11	1
Donut Strawberry Frosted	1	210	30	12	1
Donut Sugar Raised	1	170	22	4	1
Donut Vanilla Kreme Filled	1	270	36	17	1
Donut Whole Wheat Glazed	1	310	32	14	2
Eclair	1	270	39	17	1
English Muffin	1	160	31	1	2
French Cruller	1	150	17	8	1
Fritter Glazed	1	260	31	7	1
Muffin Banana Walnut	1	540	69	31	3
Muffin Blueberry	1	470	73	38	2
Muffin Chocolate Chip	1	630	89	49	2
Muffin Coffee Cake	1	580	78	40	1
Muffin Corn	1	510	77	32	1
Muffin Cranberry Orange	1	440	66	30	3
Muffin Honey Bran Raisin	1	480	79	43	5
Muffin Reduced Fat Blueberry	1	400	78	33	3
Munchkins Chocolate Glazed	3	200	26	13	1
Munchkins Cinnamon	4	270	31	14	1
Munchkins Glazed	3	280	38	22	1
Munchkins Jelly Filled	5	210	30	15	1
Munchkins Lemon Filled	4	170	23	9	0
Munchkins Plain	4	270	27	9	1
Munchkins Powdered	4	270	31	15	1
Munchkins Sugar Raised	7	220	26	5	1
Stick Cinnamon	1	450	42	17	1
Stick Glazed	1	490	51	26	1
Stick Glazed Chocolate	1	470	49	24	2
Stick Jelly	1	530	61	32	1
Stick Plain	1	420	35	12	1
Stick Powdered	1	450	42	18	1
BEVERAGES					
Cappuccino	1 (10 oz)	60	7	7	0
Cappuccino w/ Soy Milk	1 (10 oz)	70	6	5	1
Cappuccino w/ Soy Milk Sugar	1 (10 oz)	120	20	19	1
Cappuccino w/ Sugar	1 (10 oz)	130	21	20	0
Coffee Blueberry	1 (10 oz)	20	4	0	0
Coffee Caramel	1 (10 oz)	20	4	0	0

FOOD	PORTION	CALS	CARB	SUGAR	FIBER
Coffee Chocolate	1 (10 oz)	20	4	0	0
Coffee Cinnamon	1 (10 oz)	20	4	0	0
Coffee Coconut	1 (10 oz)	20	4	0	0
Coffee French Vanilla	1 (10 oz)	20	4	0	0
Coffee Hazelnut	1 (10 oz)	20	4	0	0
Coffee Marshmallow	1 (10 oz)	20	4	0	0
Coffee Regular	1 (10 oz)	15	3	0	0
Coffee Toasted Almond	1 (10 oz)	20	4	0	0
Coffee w/ Cream	1 (10 oz)	70	3	0	0
Coffee w/ Cream Sugar	1 (10 oz)	120	15	12	0
Coffee w/ Milk	1 (10 oz)	35	4	2	0
Coffee w/ Milk Sugar	1 (10 oz)	80	16	13	0
Coffee w/ Skim Milk	1 (10 oz)	25	4	1	0
Coffee w/ Skim Milk Sugar	1 (10 oz)	70	16	13	0
Coffee w/ Sugar	1 (10 oz)	60	15	12	0
Coolatta Lemonade	1 (16 oz)	240	59	56	0
Coolatta Strawberry Fruit	1 (16 oz)	290	72	65	1
Coolatta Tropicana Orange	1	370	92	87	3
Coolatta Vanilla Bean	1 (16 oz)	440	70	69	1
Coolatta Coffee w/ 2% Milk	1 (16 oz)	190	41	40	0
Coolatta Coffee w/ Cream	1 (16 oz)	350	40	35	0
Coolatta Coffee w/ Milk	1 (16 oz)	210	42	40	0
Coolatta Coffee w/ Skim Milk	1 (16 oz)	170	41	40	0
Dunkaccino	1 (10 oz)	230	35	25	0
Espresso	1 (2 oz)	0	1	1	0
Espresso w/ Sugar	1 (2 oz)	30	7	7	0
Hot Chocolate	1 (10 oz)	220	38	28	2
Iced Coffee	1 (16 oz)	15	3	0	0
Iced Coffee w/ Cream	1 (16 oz)	70	4	0	0
Iced Coffee w/ Cream Sugar	1 (16 oz)	120	16	12	0
Iced Coffee w/ Milk	1 (16 oz)	35	4	2	0
Iced Coffee w/ Milk Sugar	1 (16 oz)	80	16	13	0
Iced Coffee w/ Skim Milk	1 (16 oz)	25	4	0	0
Iced Coffee w/ Skim Milk Sugar	1 (16 oz)	70	16	12	0
Iced Coffee w/ Sugar	1 (16 oz)	60	15	12	0
Iced Latte	1 (16 oz)	120	11	10	0
Iced Latte Caramel Creme	1 (16 oz)	260	40	40	0
Iced Latte Caramel Swirl	1 (16 oz)	240	37	36	0
Iced Latte Caramel Swirl w/ Skim Milk	1 (16 oz)	180	36	35	0

FOOD	PORTION	CALS	CARB	SUGAR	FIBER
Iced Latte Lite	1 (16 oz)	80	13	10	0
Iced Latte Mocha Almond	1 (16 oz)	290	46	45	1
Iced Latte Mocha Swirl	1 (16 oz)	240	38	36	1
Iced Latte Mocha Swirl w/ Skim Milk	1 (16 oz)	180	37	35	1
Iced Latte w/ Skim Milk	1 (16 oz)	70	11	10	0
Iced Latte w/ Skim Milk Sugar	1 (16 oz)	120	23	22	0
Iced Latte w/ Sugar	1 (16 oz)	170	23	21	0
Latte	1 (10 oz)	120	10	9	0
Latte Caramel Creme	1 (10 oz)	260	40	40	0
Latte Caramel Swirl	1 (10 oz)	230	36	35	0
Latte Caramel Swirl w/ Soy Milk	1 (10 oz)	210	34	32	1
Latte Lite	1 (10 oz)	70	11	9	0
Latte Mocha Almond	1 (10 oz)	290	46	45	1
Latte Mocha Swirl	1 (10 oz)	230	37	35	1
Latte Mocha Swirl w/ Soy Milk	1 (10 oz)	210	35	32	2
Latte Soy Milk	1 (10 oz)	90	8	6	1
Latte Soy Milk Sugar	1 (10 oz)	150	22	20	1
Latte Sugar	1 (10 oz)	160	22	21	0
Smoothie Mango Passion Fruits	1 (16 oz)	360	79	68	2
Smoothie Reduced Calorie Berry	1 sm (16 oz)	250	49	41	0
Smoothie Strawberry Banana	1 (16 oz)	360	79	69	2
Smoothie Wildberry	1 (16 oz)	360	79	70	1
Tea Regular Or Decaffeinated	1 (10 oz)	0	1	0	0
Tea w/ Milk	1 (10 oz)	25	2	2	0
Tea w/ Milk Sugar	1 (10 oz)	70	14	13	0
Tea w/ Skim Milk	1 (10 oz)	25	4	1	0
Tea w/ Skim Milk Sugar	1 (10 oz)	60	14	13	0
Tea w/ Sugar	1 (10 oz)	50	13	12	0
Turbo Ice	1 (16 oz)	120	14	13	0
Vanilla Chai	1 (10 oz)	230	40	32	0
SANDWICHES					
Bagel Bacon Egg Cheese	1	540	69	11	2
Bagel Egg Cheese	1	470	65	10	2
Bagel Ham Egg Cheese	1	510	65	10	2
Bagel Sausage Egg Cheese	1	660	63	8	3
Biscuit Egg Cheese	1	410	32	9	1
Biscuit Sausage Egg Cheese	1	610	32	9	1
Croissant Bacon Egg Cheese	1	520	40	9	0

FOOD	PORTION	CALS	CARB	SUGAR	FIBER
Croissant Egg Cheese	1	550	41	9	0
Croissant Ham Egg Cheese	1	520	40	9	0
Croissant Sausage Egg Cheese	1	490	40	8	0
English Muffin Bacon Egg Cheese	1	360	36	8	1
English Muffin Egg Cheese	1	280	34	3	1
English Muffin Ham Egg Cheese	1	310	34	3	1
English Muffin Sausage Egg Cheese	1	530	37	8	1
Flatbread Egg White Turkey	1	280	37	5	3
Flatbread Egg White Veggie	1	290	39	4	3
Panini Meatball	1	480	56	6	3
Panini Southwestern Chicken	1	420	57	4	3
Panini Steak	1	450	56	4	3

EDDIE'S PIZZA

FOOD	PORTION	CALS	CARB	SUGAR	FIBER
Bar Pie	1 pie	350	27	–	8
Bar Pie No Fat Cheese	1 pie	270	27	–	8

EL POLLO LOCO
DESSERTS

FOOD	PORTION	CALS	CARB	SUGAR	FIBER
Caramel Flan	1 serv (5.5 oz)	290	41	39	0
Churros	2	300	32	10	2
Cone Vanilla	1	330	55	47	0
Soft Serve Vanilla	1 cup (5 oz)	300	48	47	0

MAIN MENU SELECTIONS

FOOD	PORTION	CALS	CARB	SUGAR	FIBER
BBQ Black Beans	1 serv (6 oz)	200	38	16	4
Bowl The Original Pollo	1 serv	540	85	1	11
Burrito BRC	1 (7.5 oz)	390	61	0	6
Burrito Classic Chicken	1 (10.3 oz)	500	63	0	6
Burrito Twice Grilled	1 (15 oz)	830	58	2	5
Burrito Ultimate Grilled	1 (13.6 oz)	650	80	1	8
Chicken Breast	1 (4.3 oz)	220	0	0	0
Chicken Breast Skinless	1 (4 oz)	180	0	0	0
Chicken Leg	1 (1.8 oz)	90	0	0	0
Chicken Thigh	1 (3.1 oz)	220	0	0	0
Chicken Wing	1 (1.3 oz)	90	0	0	0
Cole Slaw	1 serv (6 oz)	120	8	6	2
Corn Cobbette	1 (5 oz)	90	19	3	2
French Fries	1 serv (5.5 oz)	440	57	0	6
Fresh Vegetables w/ Margarine	1 serv (4.1 oz)	60	8	3	3

FOOD	PORTION	CALS	CARB	SUGAR	FIBER
Fresh Vegetables w/o Margarine	1 serv (4 oz)	35	8	3	3
Gravy	1 serv (1 oz)	10	2	0	0
Loco Nachos	1 serv	170	7	2	1
Macaroni & Cheese	1 serv (5.5 oz)	280	28	3	6
Mashed Potatoes	1 serv (5 oz)	100	20	tr	2
Pinto Beans	1 serv (6 oz)	140	25	0	7
Quesadilla Cheese	1 (4.5 oz)	420	35	0	2
Refried Beans w/ Cheese	1 serv (6.3 oz)	270	36	2	10
Skinless Breast Meal	1 serv	310	17	6	5
Soup Chicken Tortilla w/o Tortilla Strips	1 serv (10 oz)	140	8	2	2
Spanish Rice	1 serv (4.5 oz)	160	34	0	1
Taco Al Carbon	1 (3.1 oz)	150	17	tr	1
Taco Soft Chicken	1 (4.5 oz)	270	19	0	2
Taquito Chicken	1	190	18	0	1
Tortilla Chips	1 serv (1.5 oz)	210	28	tr	3
Tortilla Corn 6 Inches	2	120	24	0	2
Tortilla Flour 6.5 Inches	2	210	30	2	2
SALAD DRESSINGS AND TOPPINGS					
Creamy Cilantro	1 serv (1.5 oz)	220	1	1	0
Creamy Cilantro Light	1 pkg	70	6	3	0
Guacamole	1 serv (1 oz)	45	4	tr	tr
Hot Sauce Jalapeno	1 pkg	5	1	0	0
Jack & Poblano Queso	1 serv (1.8 oz)	100	4	1	0
Ketchup	1 pkg	10	2	2	0
Light Italian	1 pkg	20	2	2	0
Pico De Gallo Medium	1 serv (1 oz)	10	1	tr	0
Ranch	1 pkg	230	2	2	0
Salsa Avocado Hot	1 serv (1 oz)	30	1	0	tr
Salsa Chipotle Hot	1 serv (1 oz)	5	1	tr	0
Salsa House Mild	1 serv (1 oz)	5	1	tr	0
Sour Cream	1 serv (1 oz)	60	1	0	0
Thousand Island	1 pkg	220	6	6	0
SALADS					
Caesar Pollo	1 (11.4 oz)	520	17	6	4
Ceasar Pollo w/o Dressing	1 (9.4 oz)	220	15	4	4
Garden	1 (4.8 oz)	120	9	3	2
Tostada Chicken	1 (17.3 oz)	840	76	4	7
Tostada Chicken w/o Shell	1 (14.7 oz)	410	42	3	5

FOOD	PORTION	CALS	CARB	SUGAR	FIBER
EMERALD CITY SMOOTHIE					
Apple Andie	1 (11 oz)	230	46	37	2
Berry Berry	1 (13 oz)	350	77	47	9
Blueberry Blast	1 (13 oz)	380	78	51	9
Coconut Passion	1 (11 oz)	600	80	58	11
Cranberry Delight	1 (10 oz)	550	127	114	2
Energizer	1 (10 oz)	350	62	36	7
Fruity Supreme	1 (9 oz)	280	59	34	6
Grape Escape	1 (10 oz)	480	109	102	2
Guava Sunrise	1 (13 oz)	366	80	67	6
Kiwi Kic	1 (11 oz)	400	88	81	2
Lean Body	1 (11 oz)	330	24	6	8
Lean Out	1 (11 oz)	600	35	21	5
Low Carb	1 (10 oz)	350	27	17	2
Mango Mania	1 (8 oz)	370	82	78	2
Marionberry Fuel	1 (13 oz)	380	81	50	10
Mega Mass	1 (14 oz)	610	103	55	7
Mini Mass	1 (13 oz)	520	79	53	6
Mocha Bliss	1 (10 oz)	550	63	58	1
Nutty Banana	1 (11 oz)	720	97	72	9
Orange Twister	1 (10 oz)	140	31	24	2
Pacific Splash	1 (12 oz)	240	58	34	6
PB&J	1 (14 oz)	630	77	43	12
Peach Pleasure	1 (12 oz)	270	54	41	5
Peanut Passion	1 (11 oz)	580	61	31	10
Pineapple Bliss	1 (12 oz)	210	45	35	4
Power Fuel	1 (11 oz)	450	66	29	6
Quick Start	1 (10 oz)	280	46	27	4
Raspberry Dream	1 (13 oz)	410	80	48	10
Rejuvenator	1 (10 oz)	340	62	35	7
Sambazon	1 (15 oz)	410	92	69	8
Slim N Fit	1 (10 oz)	350	60	35	6
The Builder	1 (18 oz)	1270	144	73	10
Zesty Lemon	1 (14 oz)	430	67	46	5
Zip Zip	1 (10 oz)	240	35	24	3
Zone Zinger	1 (14 oz)	430	76	53	4
EVOS					
BEVERAGES					
Shake Mango Guava	1 reg (16 oz)	180	48	44	2
Shake Multi-Berry	1 reg (20 oz)	200	52	35	1

FOOD	PORTION	CALS	CARB	SUGAR	FIBER
Shake Strawberry Banana	1 reg (16 oz)	190	47	38	1
Shake Organic Cappuccino	1 reg (16 oz)	230	47	44	0
Shake Organic Vanilla	1 reg (16 oz)	180	30	30	0
CHILDREN'S MENU SELECTIONS					
Kids Champion Burger	1	400	48	3	7
Kids Chicken Strips	1 serv	130	13	0	0
Kids Freerange Steakburger	1	390	39	2	2
Kids Good Corn Dog	1	150	27	4	3
MAIN MENU SELECTIONS					
Airbaked Chicken Strips	1 serv	260	26	0	0
Airfries	1 reg	230	35	1	3
American Champion	1	420	53	7	6
American DeLite	1	330	53	6	7
Burger Bun	1	190	39	2	2
Cheddar Cheese Slice	1	80	0	0	0
Crispy Mesquite Chicken	1 serv	330	53	3	2
Freerange Steakburger	1	400	42	4	3
Fresh Fruit Bowl	1 serv	200	52	47	4
Good Corn Dog	1	150	22	4	3
Herb Crusted Trout	1 serv	440	62	7	3
Honey Mesquite Chicken	1 serv	290	41	3	2
Spicy Chipotle Turkey	1 serv	370	42	3	3
Veggie Chili	1 reg	110	20	3	5
Veggie Garden Grill Italian	1	350	54	4	8
Wraps Avocado Turkey	1	480	51	5	4
Wraps Crispy Buffalo Chicken	1	440	64	5	5
Wraps Crispy Thai Trout	1	660	96	6	5
Wraps Freerange Beef Taco	1	600	53	6	5
Wraps Honey Wheat	1	300	49	4	4
Wraps Southwest Soy Taco	1	500	58	6	10
Wraps Spicy Thai Chicken	1	510	76	3	4
Wraps Spinach Herb	1	310	52	3	3
Wraps Tomato Basil Chicken	1	520	82	3	4
SALAD DRESSINGS AND TOPPINGS					
Balsamic Vinegar	1 serv (0.5 oz)	5	2	2	0
Crispy Noodles	1 serv (7 g)	35	5	0	0
Croutons Multi-Grain	1 serv (7 g)	30	4	0	0
Dressing Avocado	1 serv (3 oz)	190	5	1	2
Dressing Caesar	1 serv (1.7 oz)	300	2	0	0
Dressing Fat Free Vinaigrette	1 serv (1 oz)	5	2	1	0

FOOD	PORTION	CALS	CARB	SUGAR	FIBER
Dressing Raspberry	1 serv (2 oz)	50	14	12	0
Dressing Spicy Thai	1 serv (1.4 oz)	150	15	12	0
Extra Virgin Olive Oil	1 serv (1 oz)	250	0	0	0
Herb Spread	1 serv (0.7 oz)	30	2	0	0
Ketchup Cayenne Firewalker	1 serv (1.2 oz)	35	9	8	0
Ketchup Garlic Garvity	1 serv (1.2 oz)	35	9	8	0
Ketchup Mesquite Magic	1 serv (1.2 oz)	35	9	8	0
Mustard	1 serv (0.5 oz)	10	1	0	0
Mustard Mesquite Honey	1 serv (0.7 oz)	80	3	2	0
Southwest Sour Cream	1 serv (1.4 oz)	60	4	2	0
Spicy Chipotle Mayo	1 serv (0.7 oz)	30	2	0	0
Tomato Basil Sauce	1 serv (1.4 oz)	150	5	2	0
SALADS					
Bordeaux Bistro w/o Dressing	1	260	7	2	3
For Salads Chicken Strips	1 serv (3 oz)	130	13	0	0
For Salads Grilled Chicken	1 serv (3 oz)	90	1	0	0
Mediterranean Summer w/o Dressing	1	200	22	11	6
Santa Ana Caesar w/o Dressing	1	20	4	1	2
Side Salad w/o Dressing	1	35	8	3	2
Spicy Thai w/o Dressing	1	35	7	4	2
SUPPLEMENTS					
Fat Burner	1 serv (5 g)	16	4	0	0
Go Energy	1 serv (5 g)	15	4	0	0
Mega Protein	1 serv (0.5 oz)	45	0	0	0
Multi-Vitamin	1 serv (5 g)	10	3	0	0

FAZOLI'S
BEVERAGES

FOOD	PORTION	CALS	CARB	SUGAR	FIBER
Lemon Ice All Flavors	1	360	90	90	0
Lemon Ice Original	1 reg	180	45	45	0
Lemon Ice Strawberry	1	320	81	81	0
CHILDREN'S MENU SELECTIONS					
Fettuccine Alfredo	1 serv	290	50	4	2
Meat Lasagna	1 serv	260	21	4	2
Ravioli w/ Marinara	1 serv	290	43	5	3
Spaghetti w/ Meat Sauce	1 serv	300	53	5	4
Spaghetti w/ Meatballs	1 serv	350	55	5	4
Ziti w/ Meat Sauce	1 serv	190	25	4	3
DESSERTS					
Cheesecake Original	1 slice	290	17	17	0

FOOD	PORTION	CALS	CARB	SUGAR	FIBER
Cheesecake Turtle	1 slice	450	43	31	2
Cookie Chocolate Chunk	1	510	68	39	3
MAIN MENU SELECTIONS					
Breadstick	1	100	20	1	0
Breadstick Garlic	1	150	20	1	1
Fettuccine Alfredo	1 sm	520	83	8	4
Fettuccine w/ Marinara	1 serv	450	88	10	7
Fettuccine w/ Meat Sauce	1 serv	500	87	9	7
Oven Baked Chicken Parmesan	1 serv	960	117	12	9
Oven Baked Meat Lasagna	1 serv	510	43	7	5
Oven Baked Rigatoni Romano	1 serv	1090	101	13	11
Oven Baked Spaghetti	1 serv	680	90	10	7
Oven Baked Spaghetti w/ Meatballs	1 serv	940	100	12	9
Panini Four Cheese & Tomato	1	510	53	4	3
Panini Grilled Chicken	1	540	56	4	3
Panini Smoked Turkey	1	620	54	5	3
Penne w/ Alfredo	1 serv	520	83	8	4
Penne w/ Marinara	1 serv	450	88	10	7
Penne w/ Meat Sauce	1 serv	500	87	9	7
Pizza Slice Cheese	1	270	31	2	2
Pizza Slice Pepperoni	1	310	31	2	2
Platter Ultimate Sampler	1	980	134	17	11
Platter Classic Sampler	1	810	110	13	8
Ravioli w/ Marinara	1 serv	500	71	10	7
Ravioli w/ Meat Sauce	1 serv	300	42	5	3
Ravioli w/ Meat Sauce	1 serv	550	71	10	7
Spaghetti w/ Alfredo	1 serv	520	83	8	4
Spaghetti w/ Marinara	1 sm	450	88	10	7
Spaghetti w/ Meat Sauce	1 sm	500	87	9	7
Submarinos Club	half	973	65	6	3
Submarinos Ham n'Swiss	1	680	65	6	3
Submarinos Italian Beef	half	660	68	7	3
Submarinos Original	half	940	68	6	4
Topping Broccoli	1 serv	25	5	1	3
Topping Broccoli & Tomatoes	1 serv	30	6	2	3
Topping Garlic Shrimp	1 serv	160	3	0	1
Topping Italian Sausage	1 serv	240	3	0	1
Topping Meat Balls	1 serv	160	6	1	1
Topping Peppery Chicken	1 serv	70	1	0	0

FOOD	PORTION	CALS	CARB	SUGAR	FIBER
Ziti w/ Meat Sauce	1 serv	480	65	9	6
SALAD DRESSINGS					
Caesar	1 serv	220	1	0	0
Fat Free Honey Mustard	1 serv	60	15	14	1
Fat Free Italian	1 serv	25	6	3	0
Honey French	1 serv	220	14	13	0
Italian	1 serv	160	7	7	0
Ranch	1 serv	220	2	2	0
Ranch Lite	1 serv	120	2	1	0
SALADS					
Chicken & Fruit	1	220	28	20	4
Chicken & Pasta Caesar	1	440	41	8	4
Chicken BLT Ranch	1	270	13	5	4
Parmesan Chicken	1	360	31	5	4
Side Caesar	1	40	4	1	2
Side Garden	1	25	4	2	3
Side Pasta	1 serv	320	41	7	1
FRESHENS					
PRETZELS					
Bites	1 serv (3 oz)	255	48	8	2
Gourmet	1 (6 oz)	510	98	16	4
FRUITFULL					
BREADS					
Almond Cherry	½ slice	226	29	17	1
Apple Spice	½ slice	186	29	18	1
Banana	½ slice	165	24	11	1
Cappuccino Chocolate Chip	½ slice	229	27	16	1
Carrot	½ slice	190	24	12	0
Chocolate	½ slice	120	26	16	2
Lemon Blueberry	½ slice	120	27	14	1
Old Fashion Pound Cake	½ slice	227	25	14	0
Orange Cranberry	½ slice	130	28	12	0
Pumpkin	½ slice	150	32	12	0
Sweet Potato	½ slice	176	28	17	1
Zucchini	½ slice	190	24	13	1
SNACKS					
All About Almonds	1 pkg (1 oz)	170	5	–	4
Buzzworthy Banana	1 pkg (1.1 oz)	140	17	–	2
Calypso Cashews	1 pkg (1.1 oz)	170	7	–	1

FOOD	PORTION	CALS	CARB	SUGAR	FIBER
Chocolate Twisted Bliss	1 pkg (1.4 oz)	190	27	–	1
Debbie Loves Fruit	1 pkg (1 oz)	110	23	–	1
Got Nuts?	1 pkg (1.1 oz)	180	9	–	2
Hit The Road Jack	1 pkg (1.1 oz)	130	19	–	2
Honey I Ate The Peanuts	1 pkg (1 oz)	160	8	–	1
Jamaican Me Crazy Cranberry Mix	1 pkg (1.1 oz)	100	24	–	2
Judy's Apple Crisps	1 pkg (1 oz)	140	20	–	2
Nacho Chips They're Mine	1 pkg (1.1 oz)	120	25	–	0
Nature Lover's Choice	1 pkg (1.1 oz)	140	15	–	2
Power Pistachios	1 pkg (1.1 oz)	100	14	–	2
Reggae Rice Crackers	1 pkg (1.1 oz)	120	26	–	0
Rockin' Raisins	1 pkg (1.4 oz)	170	28	–	1
Rocky Mountain Munch	1 pkg (1.1 oz)	120	22	–	1
Sour Wiggle Giggle	1 pkg (1.5 oz)	150	9	–	0
Soy Glad You're Healthy	1 pkg (1.1 oz)	160	9	–	4
Survivor Snacks	1 pkg (1.1 oz)	140	15	–	2
Swinging Sesame Stix	1 pkg (1.1 oz)	180	12	–	2
Tammy's Flax Snacks	1 pkg (1.1 oz)	170	10	–	3
Whassup Wasabi!	1 pkg (1.1 oz)	150	17	–	2
Yogurt Twisted Bliss	1 pkg (1.4 oz)	190	28	–	1
You've Got Trail	1 pkg (1.1 oz)	150	17	–	2
Yummy Gummy In My Tummy	1 pkg (1.4 oz)	150	33	–	0
Zydeco Cajun Mix	1 pkg (1.1 oz)	108	15	–	1

GODFATHER'S PIZZA

FOOD	PORTION	CALS	CARB	SUGAR	FIBER
Breadstick	1	80	14	–	1
Golden All Meat Combo	1 med slice	300	27	–	1
Golden Apple Dessert	⅙ sm	202	37	–	1
Golden Bacon Cheeseburger	1 med slice	270	26	–	1
Golden Cheese	1 med slice	220	26	–	1
Golden Cherry Dessert	⅙ sm	206	38	–	1
Golden Cinnamon Streusel	⅙ sm	226	39	–	1
Golden Combo	1 med slice	290	28	–	2
Golden Hawaiian	1 med slice	240	29	–	1
Golden Hot Stuff	1 med slice	290	27	–	1
Golden Humble Pie	1 med slice	310	27	–	1
Golden M&M Streusel Dessert	⅙ sm	249	42	–	1
Golden Pepperoni	1 med slice	260	26	–	1
Golden Super Combo	1 med slice	320	13	–	2
Golden Super Hawaiian	1 med slice	250	27	–	1

FOOD	PORTION	CALS	CARB	SUGAR	FIBER
Golden Super Taco	1 med slice	330	28	–	2
Golden Taco	1 med slice	300	27	–	2
Golden Veggie	1 med slice	230	27	–	2
Monkey Bread	⅙	120	23	–	1
Original All Meat Combo	1 med slice	370	35	–	2
Original Bacon Cheeseburger	1 med slice	330	35	–	2
Original Cheese	1 med slice	260	34	–	1
Original Combo	1 med slice	350	37	–	3
Original Hawaiian	1 med slice	280	38	–	1
Original Hot Stuff	1 med slice	360	35	–	2
Original Humble Pie	1 med slice	380	35	–	2
Original Pepperoni	1 med slice	290	34	–	1
Original Super Combo	1 med slice	390	37	–	3
Original Super Hawaiian	1 med slice	280	37	–	1
Original Super Taco	1 med slice	390	36	–	2
Original Taco	1 med slice	360	36	–	2
Original Veggie	1 med slice	270	36	–	2
Potato Wedges	1 serv (4 oz)	192	24	–	4
Thin All Meat Combo	1 med slice	280	20	–	1
Thin Bacon Cheeseburger	1 med slice	250	20	–	1
Thin Cheese	1 med slice	180	16	–	1
Thin Combo	1 med slice	250	18	–	1
Thin Hawaiian	1 med slice	200	19	–	1
Thin Hot Stuff	1 med slice	270	20	–	1
Thin Humble Pie	1 med slice	270	17	–	1
Thin Pepperoni	1 med slice	220	16	–	1
Thin Super Combo	1 med slice	300	21	–	2
Thin Super Hawaiian	1 med slice	230	21	–	1
Thin Super Taco	1 med slice	310	21	–	2
Thin Taco	1 med slice	260	17	–	1
Thin Veggie	1 med slice	190	18	–	1

HARDEE'S
BEVERAGES

FOOD	PORTION	CALS	CARB	SUGAR	FIBER
Barq's Root Beer	1 sm (20 oz)	290	79	79	0
Cherry Coke	1 sm (20 oz)	260	70	70	0
Coca-Cola	1 sm (20 oz)	260	71	71	0
Coffee Black	1 sm (12 oz)	5	1	0	0
Diet Coke	1 sm (20 oz)	0	0	0	0
Dr Pepper	1 sm (20 oz)	260	68	68	0
Hi-C Fruit Punch	1 sm (20 oz)	260	70	70	0

FOOD	PORTION	CALS	CARB	SUGAR	FIBER
Hi-C Orange	1 sm (20 oz)	280	76	76	0
Lemonade Minute Maid	1 sm (20 oz)	250	70	70	0
Mello Yellow	1 sm (20 oz)	265	72	72	0
Milk 2%	1 (10 oz)	150	18	18	0
Orange Juice	1 serv (10 oz)	150	37	35	0
Shake Chocolate	1 (16 oz)	700	85	55	1
Shake Strawberry	1 (16 oz)	700	86	76	0
Shake Vanilla	1 (16 oz)	710	87	73	0
Sprite	1 sm	260	68	68	0
BREAKFAST SELECTIONS					
Big Country Breakfast Platter Bacon	1 serv	980	90	13	3
Big Country Breakfast Platter Breaded Pork Chop	1 serv	1220	102	13	4
Big Country Breakfast Platter Chicken	1 serv	1140	105	12	4
Big Country Breakfast Platter Country Ham	1 serv	970	90	12	3
Big Country Breakfast Platter Country Steak	1 serv	1150	98	12	4
Big Country Breakfast Platter Grilled Pork Chop	1 serv	1130	92	13	3
Big Country Breakfast Platter Sausage	1 serv	1060	91	13	4
Biscuit Bacon	1 serv	430	35	4	0
Biscuit Bacon Egg Cheese	1	560	37	4	0
Biscuit Breaded Pork Chop	1 serv	690	48	4	1
Biscuit Chicken Fillet	1 serv	600	50	3	1
Biscuit Cinnamon 'N' Raisin	1	280	40	17	0
Biscuit Country Ham	1	440	36	3	0
Biscuit Country Steak	1 serv	620	44	3	0
Biscuit Country Steak & Egg	1 serv	690	44	4	0
Biscuit Egg	1 serv	450	35	4	0
Biscuit Ham Egg Cheese	1	560	37	5	0
Biscuit Loaded Omelet	1 serv	640	37	5	0
Biscuit Made From Scratch	1	370	35	3	0
Biscuit 'N' Gravy	1	530	47	6	0
Biscuit Sausage	1	530	36	4	0
Biscuit Sausage Egg	1	610	36	4	0

FOOD	PORTION	CALS	CARB	SUGAR	FIBER
Breakfast Bowl Loaded Biscuit 'N' Gravy	1 serv	770	49	7	1
Breakfast Bowl Low Carb	1 serv	620	6	2	2
Burrito Loaded Breakfast	1	780	38	2	2
Burrito Steak 'N' Egg Breakfast	1	470	38	1	1
Folded Egg	1 serv	80	1	0	0
Frisco Breakfast Sandwich	1	410	39	4	2
Grits	1 serv	110	16	0	0
Hash Rounds	1 sm	260	25	1	2
Loaded Omelet	1	270	2	2	0
Pancake Platter	1 serv	300	55	12	2
Scrambled Egg	1 serv	160	1	1	0
Sunrise Croissant	1	210	26	4	0
Sunrise Croissant w/ Bacon	1	450	28	5	0
Sunrise Croissant w/ Ham	1	430	28	5	0
Sunrise Croissant w/ Sausage	1	550	29	5	0
CHILDREN'S MENU SELECTIONS					
French Fries	1 serv	250	32	0	3
Kids Meal Cheeseburger	1 serv	600	68	8	4
Kids Meal Chicken Strips	1 serv	500	50	1	3
Kids Meal Hamburger	1 serv	560	67	8	6
DESSERTS					
Apple Turnover	1	290	36	11	1
Cone Single Scoop	1	285	37	26	0
Cookie Chocolate Chip	1	290	44	26	0
Ice Cream Bowl Single Scoop	1 serv	235	27	22	0
Peach Cobbler	1 serv	280	56	45	1
MAIN MENU SELECTIONS					
Burger Six Dollar	1	1060	60	18	3
Cheeseburger	1	680	52	11	2
Cheeseburger Double	1	510	38	9	1
Chicken Strips	3 pieces	380	27	1	1
Cole Slaw	1 serv	170	20	10	2
Crispy Curls	1 sm	340	43	0	4
French Fries	1 sm	390	51	1	4
Fried Chicken Breast	1 piece	370	29	0	0
Fried Chicken Leg	1 piece	170	15	0	0
Fried Chicken Thigh	1 piece	330	30	0	0
Fried Chicken Wing	1 piece	200	23	0	0
Grilled Onions	1 serv	35	2	2	0

FOOD	PORTION	CALS	CARB	SUGAR	FIBER
Hamburger	1	310	36	8	1
Hamburger Double	1	420	37	9	1
Hot Dog	1	420	22	4	1
Hot Ham 'N' Cheese	1	420	39	4	2
Hot Ham 'N' Cheese Big	1	520	40	4	2
Mashed Potatoes	1 sm	90	17	1	0
Roast Beef Big	1	470	38	3	2
Roast Beef Regular	1	330	29	2	2
Sandwich Big Chicken Fillet	1	850	76	9	3
Sandwich Charbroiled Chicken Club	1	560	33	8	3
Sandwich Fish Supreme	1	500	38	5	1
Thickburger	1	850	54	12	3
Thickburger Bacon Cheese	1	910	50	11	3
Thickburger Double	1	1240	55	13	3
Thickburger Double Bacon Cheese	1	1300	51	11	3
Thickburger Low Carb	1	420	5	3	2
Thickburger Monster	1	1410	47	9	2
Thickburger Mushroom 'N Swiss	1	720	48	7	2
SAUCES AND SPREADS					
Au Jus Sauce	1 serv (3 oz)	10	2	1	0
Chicken Gravy	1 serv (1.5 oz)	20	3	1	0
Dipping Sauce BBQ	1 serv (0.5 oz)	15	3	3	0
Dipping Sauce Honey Mustard	1 serv (1 oz)	110	6	4	0
Dipping Sauce Ranch Dressing	1 serv (1 oz)	160	2	1	0
Dipping Sauce Sweet N Sour	1 serv (1 oz)	45	10	9	0
Gravy Biscuit	1 serv (5 oz)	160	12	3	0
Horseradish Sauce	1 pkg	25	1	1	0
Hot Sauce	1 pkg	0	0	0	0
Jam Grape	1 serv	10	2	2	0
Jam Strawberry	1 serv	35	9	9	0
Ketchup	1 pkg	10	2	2	0
Mayonnaise	1 pkg	90	1	0	0
Pancake Syrup	1 serv (1 oz)	90	21	16	0

HUNGRY HOWIE'S PIZZA
OTHER MENU SELECTIONS

FOOD	PORTION	CALS	CARB	SUGAR	FIBER
Cajun Bread	¼ bread	300	46	–	1
Chicken Tenders	2	140	11	–	0

FOOD	PORTION	CALS	CARB	SUGAR	FIBER
Cinnamon Bread	¼ bread	313	59	–	1
Howie Bread	¼ bread	300	46	–	1
Howie Wings	5	180	0	0	0
Sub Deluxe Italian	½ sub	506	61	–	2
Sub Ham & Cheese	½ sub	475	61	–	2
Sub Pizza	½ sub	689	67	–	3
Sub Pizza Special	½ sub	606	68	–	3
Sub Steak & Cheese	½ sub	491	64	–	2
Sub Turkey	½ sub	466	63	–	2
Sub Turkey Club	½ sub	556	63	–	2
Sub Vegetarian	½ sub	530	64	–	3
Three Cheeser Bread	¼ bread	370	47	–	1
PIZZA					
Cheese Slice	1 sm	161	20	–	1
Cheese Slice	1 med	191	23	–	1
Cheese Slice	1 lg	208	25	–	1
Cheese Slice	1 extra lg	395	42	–	2
Cheese Slice Thin	1 med	111	10	–	tr
Cheese Slice Thin	1 lg	124	11	–	1
Medium Topping Anchovies	1 serv	44	0	0	0
Medium Topping Bacon	1 serv	32	tr	–	0
Medium Topping Banana Peppers	1 serv	6	1	–	0
Medium Topping Beef	1 serv	30	tr	–	tr
Medium Topping Black Olives	1 serv	7	tr	–	tr
Medium Topping Ham	1 serv	7	0	–	0
Medium Topping Mushrooms	1 serv	2	tr	–	tr
Medium Topping Pepperoni	1 serv	22	0	–	0
Medium Topping Pineapple	1 serv	5	2	–	1
Medium Topping Sausage	1 serv	27	tr	–	tr
SALAD DRESSINGS AND SAUCES					
Dressing Blue Cheese	1 serv (1 oz)	150	1	–	0
Dressing Creamy Italian	1 serv (1 oz)	120	2	–	0
Dressing Fat Free Italian	1 serv (1.5 oz)	25	5	–	0
Dressing Fat Free Ranch	1 serv (1.5 oz)	45	10	–	1
Dressing French Style	1 serv (1 oz)	30	7	–	0
Dressing Greek	1 serv (1 oz)	110	2	–	0
Dressing Italian	1 serv (1 oz)	80	2	–	0
Dressing Ranch	1 serv (1 oz)	180	1	–	0
Dressing Thousand Island	1 serv (1 oz)	140	4	–	0

FOOD	PORTION	CALS	CARB	SUGAR	FIBER
Sauce Dipping	1 serv (3 oz)	45	9	–	1
SALADS					
Antipasto	1 sm	115	3	–	2
Chef	1 sm	114	4	–	2
Garden	1 sm	20	3	–	2
Greek	1 sm	126	8	–	2

IN-N-OUT BURGER
BEVERAGES

FOOD	PORTION	CALS	CARB	SUGAR	FIBER
Coca-Cola	1 (16 oz)	198	54	54	0
Coffee Black	1 (10 oz)	5	1	0	0
Diet Coca-Cola	1 (16 oz)	0	0	0	0
Dr Pepper	1 (16 oz)	180	52	52	0
Iced Tea	1 (16 oz)	0	0	0	0
Lemonade	1 (16 oz)	180	40	38	0
Milk	1 (10 oz)	108	18	18	0
Root Beer	1 (16 oz)	222	60	60	0
Seven-Up	1 (16 oz)	200	54	54	0
Shake Chocolate	1 (15 oz)	690	83	62	0
Shake Strawberry	1 (15 oz)	690	91	75	0
Shake Vanilla	1 (15 oz)	680	78	57	0

MAIN MENU SELECTIONS

FOOD	PORTION	CALS	CARB	SUGAR	FIBER
Cheeseburger w/ Onions	1	480	39	10	3
Cheeseburger w/ Onions Lettuce Bun	1	330	11	7	3
Cheeseburger w/ Onions Mustard Ketchup No Spread	1	400	41	10	3
French Fries	1 serv (4.4 oz)	400	54	0	2
Hamburger Double Double w/ Onions	1	670	39	10	3
Hamburger Double Double w/ Onions Lettuce Bun	1	520	11	7	3
Hamburger Double Double w/ Onions Mustard Ketchup No Spread	1	590	41	10	3
Hamburger w/ Onions	1	390	39	10	3
Hamburger w/ Onions Lettuce Bun	1	240	11	7	3
Hamburger w/ Onions Mustard Ketchup No Spread	1	310	41	10	3

FOOD	PORTION	CALS	CARB	SUGAR	FIBER
JACK IN THE BOX					
BEVERAGES					
Barq's Root Beer	1 (20 oz)	180	50	50	0
Chocolate Milk Low Fat Chug	1 (3.5 oz)	200	34	33	1
Coca-Cola Classic	1 (20 oz)	170	46	46	0
Coffee Regular & Decaf	1 (11 oz)	5	1	0	0
Diet Coke	1 (20 oz)	0	0	0	0
Dr Pepper	1 (20 oz)	150	42	42	0
Fanta Orange	1 (20 oz)	150	41	41	0
Fanta Strawberry	1 (20 oz)	150	41	41	0
Iced Tea	1 (20 oz)	5	2	0	0
Lemonade	1 (20 oz)	160	42	42	0
Orange Juice	1 (10 oz)	140	32	27	2
Reduced Fat Milk Chug	1 (3.5 oz)	130	13	13	0
Shake Chocolate	1 (16 oz)	880	107	94	1
Shake Oreo	1 (16 oz)	910	102	80	1
Shake Strawberry	1 (16 oz)	880	105	88	0
Shake Vanilla	1 (16 oz)	790	83	70	0
Sprite	1 (20 oz)	160	42	42	0
BREAKFAST SELECTIONS					
Biscuit Bacon Egg Cheese	1	430	34	3	1
Biscuit Chicken	1	450	42	2	2
Biscuit Sausage	1	440	32	3	2
Biscuit Sausage Egg Cheese	1	740	35	3	2
Biscuit Spicy Chicken	1	460	44	2	2
Breakfast Sandwich Ciabatta	1	710	63	4	3
Breakfast Sandwich Ultimate	1	570	49	8	2
Breakfast Jack	1	290	39	4	1
Breakfast Jack Bacon	1	300	29	4	1
Breakfast Jack Sausage	1	450	29	4	1
Burrito Hearty Breakfast	1	480	29	1	2
Burrito Sirloin Steak & Egg w/o Salsa	1	790	52	2	6
Croissant Sausage	1	580	37	5	2
Croissant Supreme	1	450	36	5	1
French Toast Sticks	4 (4.2 oz)	470	58	14	4
French Toast Sticks Blueberry	4	450	59	15	3
Hash Browns	1 serv	150	13	0	2
Sandwich Extreme Sausage	1	670	31	5	2

FOOD	PORTION	CALS	CARB	SUGAR	FIBER
DESSERTS					
Cake Chocolate Overload	1 serv (3.2 oz)	300	57	34	2
Cheesecake	1 serv (3.6 oz)	310	34	23	0
MAIN MENU SELECTIONS					
Bacon Cheddar Potato Wedges	1 serv (9 oz)	720	52	2	4
Cheeseburger Bacon Ultimate	1	1090	53	12	2
Cheeseburger Junior Bacon	1	430	30	6	1
Cheeseburger Sourdough Ultimate	1	950	36	7	2
Cheeseburger Ultimate	1	1010	53	12	2
Chicken Fajita Pita	1	280	30	3	2
Chicken Sandwich	1	400	38	4	2
Chicken Strips Crispy	4	500	36	1	3
Chicken Strips Grilled	4 (5 oz)	180	3	2	0
Ciabatta Chipotle w/ Grilled Chicken	1	690	65	6	4
Ciabatta Chipotle w/ Spicy Crispy Chicken	1	750	75	5	5
Ciabatta Sirloin Steak 'N' Cheddar	1	770	65	5	4
Ciabatta Burger Bacon 'N Cheese	1	1120	66	9	4
Ciabatta Burger Single Bacon 'N' Cheese	1	870	66	8	4
Club Sourdough Grilled Chicken	1	530	34	5	3
Curly Fries Seasoned	1 sm (3 oz)	270	30	1	3
Dipping Sauce Barbeque	1 serv (1 oz)	45	11	4	0
Egg Rolls	1	130	15	1	2
Fish & Chips	1 serv (7.6 oz)	570	58	1	4
Fries Natural Cut	1 sm	340	41	1	5
Fruit Cup	1 serv	90	22	18	2
Hamburger	1	310	30	6	1
Hamburger Deluxe	1	370	31	6	2
Hamburger Deluxe w/ Cheese	1	460	33	7	2
Hamburger w/ Cheese	1	350	31	7	1
Jack's Spicy Chicken	1 serv	620	61	8	4
Jack's Spicy Chicken w/ Cheese	1	700	62	8	4
Jumbo Jack	1	600	51	11	3
Jumbo Jack w/ Cheese	1	690	54	12	3
Mozzarella Cheese Sticks	3	240	21	1	1

FOOD	PORTION	CALS	CARB	SUGAR	FIBER
Onion Rings	8 (4.2 oz)	500	51	3	3
Sampler Trio	1 serv	750	65	4	5
Sandwich Bacon Chicken	1	440	39	4	2
Sirloin Burger w/ American Cheese & Red Onion	1	1120	63	11	4
Sirloin Burger w/ Swiss & Grilled Onions	1	1070	61	10	4
Sirloin Steak Melt	1	640	34	4	2
Sourdough Jack	1	710	36	7	3
Spicy Chicken Bites	1 serv	290	21	1	3
Stuffed Jalapeno	3 (2.5 oz)	230	22	2	2
Taco Monster Beef	1	240	20	4	3
Taco Regular Beef	1	160	15	4	2
SALAD DRESSINGS AND TOPPINGS					
Asian Sesame	1 serv (2.5 oz)	230	20	13	0
Bacon Ranch	1 serv (2.5 oz)	320	4	2	0
Creamy Southwest	1 serv (2.5 oz)	270	4	1	0
Dipping Sauce Buttermilk House	1 serv (0.9 oz)	130	3	0	0
Dipping Sauce Frank's Red Hot Buffalo	1 serv (1 oz)	10	2	0	0
Dipping Sauce Sweet & Sour	1 serv (1 oz)	45	11	6	0
Dipping Sauce Teriyaki	1 serv (1 oz)	60	13	11	0
Dipping Sauce Zesty Marinara	1 serv (0.8 oz)	15	4	2	0
Low Fat Balsamic	1 serv (2.5 oz)	40	6	3	0
Mayo Onion Sauce	1 serv (0.5 oz)	90	4	2	0
Ranch	1 serv (2.5 oz)	390	4	2	0
Ranch Lite	1 serv (2.5 oz)	190	3	2	0
Soy Sauce	1 serv (0.3 oz)	5	1	0	0
Syrup Log Cabin	1 serv (2 oz)	190	49	18	0
Taco Sauce	1 serv (0.3 oz)	0	0	0	0
Tartar Sauce	1 serv (1.5 oz)	210	2	1	0
SALADS					
Asian w/ Crispy Chicken w/o Dressing	1 (13.8 oz)	330	34	11	7
Asian w/ Grilled Chicken w/o Dressing	1 (12.8 oz)	160	18	11	5
Chicken Club w/ Crispy Chicken w/o Dressing	1 (14 oz)	480	26	5	6

FOOD	PORTION	CALS	CARB	SUGAR	FIBER
Chicken Club w/ Grilled Chicken w/o Dressing	1 (13 oz)	320	11	5	4
Side w/o Dressing	1 (4.3 oz)	50	5	2	2
Southwest Crispy Chicken w/o Dressing	1 (16 oz)	480	44	5	9
Southwest w/ Grilled Chicken w/o Dressing	1 (15 oz)	320	27	5	7
JAMBA JUICE					
Acai Supercharger Original	1 (24 oz)	420	86	74	5
Aloha Pineapple Original	1 (26 oz)	500	117	110	4
Banana Berry Original	1 (25 oz)	480	112	99	4
Berry Fulfilling Original	1 (24 oz)	290	62	45	8
Berry Lime Sublime Original	1 (26 oz)	460	106	84	5
Caribbean Passion Original	1 (26 oz)	440	102	92	4
Chocolate Moo'd Original	1 (24 oz)	680	138	126	2
Citrus Squeeze Original	1 (26 oz)	470	110	103	4
Coldbuster Original	1 (25 oz)	430	100	94	5
Grape Escape Original	1 (24 oz)	300	74	68	5
Mango Mantra Original	1 (25 oz)	310	71	63	6
Mango-A-Go-Go Original	1 (24 oz)	440	104	93	4
Matcha Green Tea Blast Original	1 (24 oz)	440	97	87	1
Matcha Green Tea Mist Original	1 (24 oz)	280	60	54	1
Mega Mango Original	1 (24 oz)	330	80	69	5
Mighty Cherry Charger Original	1 (24 oz)	490	103	85	3
Orange Berry Blitz Original	1 (26 oz)	410	94	88	5
Orange Dream Machine Original	1 (24 oz)	540	111	105	tr
Orange-A-Peel Original	1 (25 oz)	440	102	92	5
Passion Berry Breeze Original	1 (24 oz)	270	60	51	5
Peach Pleasure Original	1 (25 oz)	460	108	90	4
Peanut Butter Moo'd Original	1 (24 oz)	840	139	122	7
Peenya Kowlada Original	1 (26 oz)	690	152	143	3
Protein Berry Pizazz Original	1 (24 oz)	440	92	79	5
Raspberry Rainbow Original	1 (24 oz)	300	73	56	6
Razzmatazz Original	1 (26 oz)	480	112	92	4
Strawberries Wild Original	1 (25 oz)	450	105	92	4
Strawberry Nirvana Original	1 (25 oz)	280	64	53	7
Strawberry Surf Rider Original	1 (25 oz)	490	119	107	4
Strawberry Whirl Original	1 (24 oz)	310	76	64	6

FOOD	PORTION	CALS	CARB	SUGAR	FIBER

JIMMY JOHN'S
BEVERAGES

FOOD	PORTION	CALS	CARB	SUGAR	FIBER
Coke	1 sm	248	68	–	0
Diet Coke	1 sm	0	0	0	0
Iced Tea	1 sm	3	1	–	0
Iced Tea Raspberry	1 sm	195	53	–	0
Lemonade	1 sm	243	65	–	0
Lemonade Light	1 sm	13	3	–	0
Sprite	1 sm	243	65	–	0

SANDWICHES

FOOD	PORTION	CALS	CARB	SUGAR	FIBER
Giant Club Beach	1	798	78	–	2
Giant Club Billy	1	867	77	–	1
Giant Club Bootlegger	1	720	74	–	1
Giant Club Country	1	840	75	–	1
Giant Club Gourmet Smoked Ham	1	851	76	–	1
Giant Club Gourmet Veggie	1	856	77	–	2
Giant Club Hunter's	1	854	76	–	1
Giant Club Italian Night	1	975	77	–	1
Giant Club Lulu	1	790	74	–	1
Giant Club Tuna	1	719	77	–	2
Giant Club Ultimate Porker	1	843	73	–	6
Slim Double Provolone	1	588	71	–	0
Slim Ham & Cheese	1	534	72	–	0
Slim Salami Capicola Cheese	1	624	72	–	0
Slim Tuna Salad	1	577	72	–	1
Slim Turkey Breast	1	407	70	–	0
Sub Big John	1	564	54	–	1
Sub J.J.B.L.T.	1	662	54	–	1
Sub Pepe	1	684	55	–	1
Sub Totally Tuna	1	502	57	–	2
Sub Turkey Tom	1	555	54	–	1
Sub Vegetarian	1	640	57	–	2
Sub Vito	1	579	56	–	1
The J.J. Gargantuan	1	1008	60	–	1
Unwich Hunter's Club	1	520	8	–	2
Unwich The J.J. Gargantuan	1	769	11	–	2

SIDES

FOOD	PORTION	CALS	CARB	SUGAR	FIBER
Cookie Chocolate Chunk	1	421	62	–	1
Cookie Raisin Oatmeal	1	421	65	–	4

FOOD	PORTION	CALS	CARB	SUGAR	FIBER
Jimmy Chips	1 pkg	160	18	–	0
Jimmy Chips BBQ	1 pkg	160	17	–	0
Jimmy Chips Jalapeno	1 pkg	150	18	–	0
Jimmy Chips Sea Salt & Vinegar	1 pkg	140	16	–	0
Pickle Spear	1	4	1	–	tr
Pickle Whole	1	15	3	–	1

KENTUCKY FRIED CHICKEN
BEVERAGES

FOOD	PORTION	CALS	CARB	SUGAR	FIBER
Diet Pepsi	1 med (14 oz)	0	0	0	0
Mt. Dew	1 med (14 oz)	190	54	54	0
Pepsi	1 med (14 oz)	180	47	47	0

DESSERTS

FOOD	PORTION	CALS	CARB	SUGAR	FIBER
Cake Double Chocolate Chip	1 slice	330	41	26	1
Cookie Sweet Life Chocolate Chip	1 (1.2 oz)	160	23	14	1
Cookie Sweet Life Oatmeal Raisin	1 (1.2 oz)	150	24	12	1
Cookie Sweet Life Sugar	1 (1.2 oz)	160	23	10	0
Lil' Bucket Chocolate Cream	1	280	38	21	3
Lil' Bucket Lemon Creme	1 serv	410	61	53	2
Lil' Bucket Strawberry Short Cake	1 serv	210	33	25	1
Pie Mini's Apple	3 (4 oz)	370	44	19	2
Teddy Graham Cinnamon Snacks	1 serv	90	15	5	1

MAIN MENU SELECTIONS

FOOD	PORTION	CALS	CARB	SUGAR	FIBER
Baked Beans	1 serv	220	45	20	7
Biscuit	1 (2 oz)	220	24	2	1
Bowl Chicken & Biscuit	1	870	88	5	7
Bowl Mashed Potato w/ Gravy	1	740	80	6	7
Bowl Rice w/ Gravy	1	620	67	7	6
Chicken Pot Pie	1 (15 oz)	770	70	2	5
Cole Slaw	1 serv	180	22	18	3
Corn On The Cob	1 ear (3 inch)	70	13	5	3
Crispy Strips	2 (3.5 oz)	240	11	0	0
Extra Crispy Breast	1 (5.7 oz)	440	15	0	0
Extra Crispy Drumstick	1 (2 oz)	160	6	0	0
Extra Crispy Thigh	1 (4 oz)	370	12	0	0
Extra Crispy Whole Wing	1 (1.8 oz)	170	6	0	1
Green Beans	1 serv	50	7	2	2

FOOD	PORTION	CALS	CARB	SUGAR	FIBER
KFC Snacker	1	290	29	5	2
KFC Snacker Buffalo	1	260	31	4	1
KFC Snacker Fish	1	330	31	6	1
KFC Snacker Fish w/o Sauce	1	290	29	4	1
KFC Snacker Honey BBQ	1	210	32	12	2
KFC Snacker Ultimate Cheese	1	280	30	5	1
Macaroni & Cheese	1 serv	180	18	3	0
Mashed Potatoes w/ Gravy	1 serv	140	20	1	1
Mashed Potatoes w/o Gravy	1 serv	110	17	0	1
Original Recipe Breast	1 (5.6 oz)	360	7	0	0
Original Recipe Breast w/o Skin Or Breading	1 (3.8 oz)	140	1	0	0
Original Recipe Drumstick	1 (2 oz)	130	2	0	0
Original Recipe Thigh	1 (4.4 oz)	330	8	0	0
Original Recipe Whole Wing	1 (1.6 oz)	130	4	0	0
Popcorn Chicken	1 reg (4 oz)	400	22	0	3
Potato Salad	1 serv	180	22	6	2
Potato Wedges	1 serv	260	33	0	3
Sandwich Crispy Twister	1	550	49	5	3
Sandwich Double Crunch	1	470	38	4	2
Sandwich Honey BBQ	1	280	40	16	3
Sandwich Tender Roast	1	380	29	4	2
Sandwich Tender Roast w/o Sauce	1	300	28	3	2
Seasoned Rice	1 serv	180	32	1	2
Twister Oven Roasted	1	420	40	6	3
Twister Oven Roasted w/o Sauce	1	330	39	5	3
Wings Fiery Buffalo	5	380	19	1	2
Wings Honey BBQ	5	390	23	9	3
Wings Hot	5	350	14	0	2
Wings Hot & Spicy	5	400	24	13	2
Wings Teriyaki	5	480	40	30	2
Wings Boneless Fiery Buffalo	5	420	33	1	3
Wings Boneless Honey BBQ	5	450	41	11	4
Wings Boneless Sweet & Spicy	5	440	38	11	3
Wings Boneless Teriyaki	5	500	50	24	3
SALAD DRESSINGS					
Creamy Parmesan Caesar	1 serv (2 oz)	260	4	2	0
Golden Italian Light	1 serv (1.5 oz)	45	6	5	0

FOOD	PORTION	CALS	CARB	SUGAR	FIBER
Ranch	1 serv (2 oz)	200	3	1	0
Ranch Fat Free	1 serv (1.5 oz)	35	8	2	0
SALADS					
Crispy BLT w/o Dressing	1 (12 oz)	330	18	5	4
Crispy Caesar w/o Dressing & Croutons	1 (11 oz)	350	16	3	3
Croutons Parmesan Garlic	1 pkg	60	8	1	0
Roasted BLT w/o Dressing	1 (12 oz)	200	8	5	4
Roasted Caesar w/o Dressing & Croutons	1 (11 oz)	220	6	3	3
Side Caesar w/o Dressing & Croutons	1 (3 oz)	50	2	1	1
Side House w/o Dressing	1 (3 oz)	15	2	2	1

KOO-KOO-ROO
MAIN MENU SELECTIONS

FOOD	PORTION	CALS	CARB	SUGAR	FIBER
Baked Yam	1 serv (6 oz)	197	47	–	7
Black Beans	1 serv (6 oz)	125	23	–	6
Buffalo Wings	6	606	42	–	2
Burrito California Chicken	1	810	60	–	4
Burrito Fajita Chicken	1	750	70	–	4
Burrito Original Chicken	1	709	71	–	5
Butternut Squash	1 serv (6 oz)	66	17	–	3
Chicken Bowl Spicy Garlic Ginger w/o Sauce	1	485	63	–	2
Chicken Bowl w/o Sauce Chargrilled	1	569	57	–	4
Creamed Spinach	1 serv (8 oz)	100	10	–	3
Italian Vegetable	1 serv (5.5 oz)	47	9	–	2
Kernel Corn	1 serv (4.5 oz)	105	26	–	3
Mashed Potatoes	1 serv (6.5 oz)	188	32	–	3
Original Breast	1 (4.1 oz)	187	tr	–	0
Original Chicken Dark	3 pieces (5 oz)	320	5	–	0
Roasted Garlic Potatoes	1 serv (5 oz)	133	21	–	2
Rotisserie Chicken Breast & Wing	1 serv (6.5 oz)	355	1	–	tr
Rotisserie Chicken Leg & Thigh	1 serv (4.8 oz)	300	1	–	tr
Rotisserie Half Chicken	1 serv (11.3 oz)	655	2	–	tr
Sandwich BBQ Chicken	1	562	71	–	3
Sandwich Chicken Caesar	1	781	63	–	2

FOOD	PORTION	CALS	CARB	SUGAR	FIBER
Sandwich Original Chicken	1	661	63	–	3
Sandwich Turkey Hand Carved	1	599	31	–	5
Southwestern Bowl w/o Sauce	1	570	67	–	8
Tostada Bowl w/o Sauce w/o Shell	1	528	45	–	7
Traditional Turkey Dinner	1 serv	692	67	–	8
Turkey Breast Sliced	1 serv	182	0	0	0
Turkey Pot Pie	1	883	83	–	6
Wrap Caesar Chicken	1	757	59	–	4
Wrap Chipotle Chicken	1	924	89	–	6
SALADS					
BBQ Chicken w/o Dressing	1	365	22	–	6
Canteloupe & Honeydew	1 serv (5 oz)	50	12	–	1
Chicken Caesar w/o Dressing	1	286	13	–	4
Chinese Chicken w/o Dressing	1	550	39	–	10
Creamy Coleslaw	1 serv (5 oz)	238	14	–	2
Cucumber	1 serv (4.5 oz)	41	9	–	2
House	1	113	16	–	5
Tangy Tomato	1 serv (4.5 oz)	60	6	–	1
Tossed w/ Dressing	1 serv (3 oz)	16	3	–	1
SOUPS					
Chicken Noodle	1 serv (5 oz)	71	4	–	tr
Chicken Tortilla	1 serv (5 oz)	112	7	–	1
Ten Vegetable	1 serv (5 oz)	94	16	–	4

KRISPY KREME
BEVERAGES

FOOD	PORTION	CALS	CARB	SUGAR	FIBER
Chillers Fruity Orange You Glad	1 (12 oz)	180	43	43	0
Chillers Fruity Very Berry	1 (12 oz)	170	43	43	0
Chillers Kremey Berries & Kreme	1 (12 oz)	620	92	71	tr
Chillers Kremey Chocolate Chocolate	1 (12 oz)	970	104	62	2
Chillers Kremey Lemon Sherbert	1 (12 oz)	630	95	71	tr
Chillers Kremey Lotta Latte	1 (12 oz)	670	49	60	tr
Chillers Kremey Mocha Dream	1 (12 oz)	670	105	58	1
Chillers Kremey Oranges & Kreme	1 (12 oz)	630	92	71	tr
DOUGHNUTS					
Apple Fritter	1	380	47	24	2

FOOD	PORTION	CALS	CARB	SUGAR	FIBER
Caramel Kreme Crunch	1	380	40	30	tr
Chocolate Iced Cake	1	280	36	20	tr
Chocolate Iced Custard Filled	1	300	36	19	tr
Chocolate Iced Glazed	1	250	33	21	tr
Chocolate Iced Kreme Filled	1	350	39	23	tr
Chocolate Iced w/ Sprinkles	1	270	38	24	tr
Cinnamon Apple Filled	1	290	32	14	tr
Cinnamon Bun	1	260	28	13	tr
Cinnamon Twist	1	240	23	7	tr
Dulce De Leche	1	300	31	14	tr
Glazed Chocolate Cake	1	300	42	27	2
Glazed Cinnamon	1	210	24	12	tr
Glazed Creme Filled	1	340	39	23	tr
Glazed Cruller	1	240	26	14	tr
Glazed Cruller Chocolate	1	290	37	25	tr
Glazed Lemon Filled	1	290	36	18	tr
Glazed Pumpkin Spice	1	300	42	27	tr
Glazed Raspberry Filled	1	300	36	20	tr
Glazed Sour Cream	1	300	43	28	tr
Holes Glazed Blueberry	4	220	27	13	tr
Holes Glazed Cake	4	210	29	17	tr
Holes Glazed Chocolate Cake	4	210	29	17	tr
Holes Glazed Original	4	200	25	15	tr
Holes Glazed Pumpkin Spice	4	210	29	17	tr
Maple Iced Glazed	1	240	32	20	tr
New York Cheesecake	1	340	34	17	tr
Original Glazed	1	200	22	10	tr
Powdered Strawberry Filled	1	290	33	13	tr
Powdered Cake	1	290	37	19	tr
Sugar	1	200	21	10	0
Traditional Cake	1	230	25	9	tr

KRYSTAL
BEVERAGES

Coca-Cola Classic	1 sm (16 oz)	129	40	40	0
Coca-Cola Classic frzn	1 (16 oz)	130	36	36	0
Diet Coke	1 sm (16 oz)	tr	tr	0	0
Sprite	1 sm (16 oz)	126	39	39	0

BREAKFAST SELECTIONS

4 Carb Scrambler Bacon	1 serv	370	4	0	1
4 Carb Scrambler Sausage	1 serv	600	3	1	2

FOOD	PORTION	CALS	CARB	SUGAR	FIBER
Biscuit Bacon Egg Cheese	1	390	33	2	0
Biscuit Chik	1	360	40	2	0
Biscuit & Gravy	1	280	34	2	0
Biscuit Plain	1	270	33	2	0
Biscuit Sausage	1	480	33	2	0
Country Breakfast	1 serv	660	46	3	8
Kryspers	1 serv	190	17	0	2
Krystal Sunriser	1	240	14	1	2
Scrambler	1 serv	440	33	tr	3
DESSERTS					
Fried Apple Turnover	1	220	31	7	2
Lemon Icebox Pie	1 serv	260	41	37	2
MAIN MENU SELECTIONS					
BA Burger	1	470	39	6	2
BA Burger Cheese	1	530	40	6	2
BA Burger Double Bacon Cheese	1	800	41	6	2
Chik'n Bites	1 sm	310	16	0	1
Chik'n Bites Salad	1 serv	290	12	1	4
Fries	1 reg	470	53	0	7
Fries Chili Cheese	1 serv	540	59	1	6
Krystal	1	160	17	1	1
Krystal Bacon Cheese	1	190	16	2	2
Krystal Cheese	1	180	17	1	2
Krystal Chik	1	240	24	1	2
Krystal Chili	1 serv	200	22	2	7
Krystal Double	1	260	24	2	2
Krystal Double Cheese	1	310	26	2	tr
Pup Chili Cheese	1	210	17	2	2
Pup Corn	1	260	19	5	1
Pup Plain	1	170	15	–	1
MARBLE SLAB CREAMERY					
Cone Honey Wheat	1	130	24	12	tr
Cone Sugar	1	130	23	12	0
Cone Vanilla Cinnamon	1	130	24	12	tr
Frozen Yogurt Nonfat	½ cup	100	22	17	tr
Frozen Yogurt Nonfat No Sugar Added	½ cup	90	17	6	tr
Ice Cream Reduced Fat	1 serv (6.75 oz)	390	47	45	0

FOOD	PORTION	CALS	CARB	SUGAR	FIBER
Ice Cream Superpremium	1 serv (6.75 oz)	450	44	43	0
Sorbet	½ cup	90	22	19	0

MAUI WOWI
SMOOTHIES

Fresh Fruit Banana Banana	1 (12 oz)	210	50	36	2
Fresh Fruit Black Raspberry	1 (12 oz)	240	59	46	0
Fresh Fruit Kiwi Lemon Lime	1 (12 oz)	180	42	34	0
Fresh Fruit Lemon Wave	1 (12 oz)	415	108	108	tr
Fresh Fruit Mango Orange Banana	1 (12 oz)	240	57	43	tr
Fresh Fruit Passion Papaya	1 (12 oz)	220	54	38	tr
Fresh Fruit Pina Colada	1 (12 oz)	240	57	46	0

MAX & ERMA'S

Black Bean Roll Up	1 serv	577	95	–	10
Caribbean Chicken Lunch Portion	1 serv	536	59	–	3
Fruit Smoothie	1	124	29	–	1
Garlic Breadstick	1	156	21	–	0
Hula Bowl w/ Fat Free Honey Mustard Dressing w/o Breadsticks	1 serv	823	79	–	6
Salad Baby Greens w/o Breadstick	1 serv	119	6	–	2
Salad Shrimp Stack	1 serv	322	116	–	3
Salad Dressing French Fat Free	2 tbsp	126	31	–	2
Salad Dressing Honey Mustard Fat Free	2 tbsp	60	14	–	0
Salad Dressing Tex Mex Low Fat	2 tbsp	23	2	–	tr

MCALISTER'S DELI
CHILDREN'S MENU SELECTIONS

Kid's Nacho	1 serv	734	74	2	3
Mac's Dog	1	307	24	2	1
Pita Pizza	1	503	54	5	3
Sandwich Ham & Cheese	1	455	39	5	4
Sandwich PB&J	1	714	86	46	7
Sandwich Toasted Cheese	1	620	40	5	4
Sandwich Turkey & Cheese	1	451	39	4	4

FOOD	PORTION	CALS	CARB	SUGAR	FIBER
DESSERTS					
Brownie Chocolate	1 (3.5 oz)	424	59	48	3
Brownie Delight	1 (11 oz)	917	111	81	4
Chocolate Loving Spoon Cake	1 (4 oz)	538	54	26	2
Ice Cream Vanilla Bean	1 scoop (5 oz)	160	19	16	0
Kentucky Pie	1 slice (12 oz)	807	110	32	1
New York Cheesecake	1 slice (5 oz)	505	37	34	2
Sundae Topping Caramel	2 tbsp	100	20	20	0
Sundae Topping Chocolate	1 tbsp	110	21	21	0
MAIN MENU SELECTIONS					
Appetizers Chips & Salsa	1 serv (5 oz)	87	9	0	0
Appetizers Dip Cheese & Chili	1 serv (5 oz)	572	54	1	3
Appetizers Dip Cheese & Veggie Chili	1 serv (5 oz)	552	58	3	5
Appetizers Nacho Basket	1 serv (6 oz)	579	61	2	3
Appetizers Nacho Chili	1 serv (6 oz)	564	46	2	4
Appetizers Nacho Veggie Chili	1 serv (6 oz)	537	52	4	6
Chicken Cordon Bleu	1 serv	810	53	11	2
Chili Vegetarian	1 serv (8 oz)	133	28	4	15
Cole Slaw	1 serv (4 oz)	190	14	10	7
Fruit Cup	1 serv (4 oz)	98	12	19	2
Giant Spud Cheese	1 (27 oz)	930	139	11	19
Giant Spud Grilled Chicken	1 (27 oz)	839	99	14	19
Giant Spud Just A Spud	1 (26 oz)	604	123	12	18
Giant Spud Ole	1 (30 oz)	1252	110	14	18
Giant Spud Ole w/ Chili	1 (33 oz)	1512	134	13	21
Giant Spud Ole w/ Veggie Chili	1 (33 oz)	1457	146	18	24
Giant Spud Veggie	1 (28 oz)	668	99	11	18
Macaroni & Cheese	1 serv (4 oz)	200	17	1	1
Mashed Potatoes	1 serv (4 oz)	136	19	1	2
Meatloaf w/ Gravy	1 serv	340	21	0	1
Open-Faced Roast Beef	1 serv	751	88	6	6
Pot Roast Spud	1 serv	906	121	12	17
Potato Salad	1 serv (4 oz)	200	22	3	3
Salmon Filet	1 serv	235	3	1	1
Steamed Vegetables	1 serv (4 oz)	43	7	4	3
SALAD DRESSINGS AND SAUCES					
Au Jus	1 serv (4 oz)	10	2	0	0
Comeback Gravy	1 serv (4 oz)	37	6	0	0
Dressing Blue Cheese	2 tbsp	140	1	1	0

FOOD	PORTION	CALS	CARB	SUGAR	FIBER
Dressing Greek	2 tbsp	90	2	1	0
Dressing Parmesan Peppercorn	2 tbsp	150	2	1	0
Dressing Ranch	2 tbsp	100	1	1	0
Dressing Tomato Basil	2 tbsp	30	6	6	0
Dressing Lite Olive Oil Vinaigrette	2 tbsp	60	3	2	0
Dressing Lite Ranch	2 tbsp	100	1	1	0
Dressing Low Calorie Italian	2 tbsp	25	2	2	0
SALADS					
Caesar w/ Salmon	1 (17 oz)	800	42	3	5
Chicken Fiesta	1 (20 oz)	493	34	14	8
Chicken Grill	1 (21 oz)	840	47	8	4
Garden	1 (15 oz)	264	21	8	4
Garden w/ Chicken Salad	1 (18 oz)	537	14	16	5
Garden w/ Salmon	1 (17 oz)	315	28	4	6
Garden w/ Tuna Salad	1 (18 oz)	373	21	8	5
Greek Chicken	1 (19 oz)	584	32	8	7
Side Caesar	1 (6 oz)	328	19	3	1
Side Garden	1 (8 oz)	138	11	4	2
Taco	1 (26 oz)	641	33	12	11
Taco w/ Veggie Chili	1 (26 oz)	641	33	17	15
SANDWICHES					
BLT	1	654	50	11	6
Chicken Salad	1	677	58	19	2
Deli Corned Beef On Wheat	1	369	39	4	4
Deli Ham On Wheat	1	350	43	7	5
Deli Pastrami On Wheat	1	371	36	4	4
Deli Roast Beef On Wheat	1	398	49	6	5
Deli Salami On Wheat	1	565	43	6	5
Deli Turkey On Wheat	1	342	43	6	5
French Dip	1	676	50	3	2
Grilled Chicken Breast	1	751	56	21	2
Grilled Chicken Club	1	1234	87	27	7
Ham Melt	1	700	52	6	4
McAlisters Club	1	1225	86	27	7
Meatloaf Parmesan	1	708	49	6	5
Memphian	1	585	48	6	4
Muffuletta	¼ (8 oz)	615	40	0	2
New Yorker	1	628	50	4	4
Orange Cranberry Club	1	954	62	18	6

FOOD	PORTION	CALS	CARB	SUGAR	FIBER
Reuben On Rye	1	492	35	8	2
Roast Beef Melt	1	635	48	6	4
Salmon	1	608	66	10	3
Submarine	1	833	53	9	3
Sweetberry Chicken On Wheatberry	1	701	67	8	5
Tuna Salad On Wheat	1	452	47	7	5
Turkey Melt	1	700	52	6	4
Veggie On Pita	1	522	33	5	2
Wrap Greek Chicken	1	630	57	3	14
Wrap Grilled Chicken Caesar	1	533	46	4	13
SOUPS					
Asiago Cheese Bisque	1 (8 oz)	240	17	1	0
Broccoli Cheddar	1 (8 oz)	213	13	4	0
Cheddar Potato	1 (8 oz)	213	19	0	1
Cheesy Chicken Tortilla	1 (8 oz)	150	13	4	0
Chicken & Sausage Gumbo	1 (8 oz)	150	17	3	2
Clam Chowder	1 (8 oz)	200	09	4	0
Country Potato	1 (8 oz)	173	23	4	0
Country Vegetable	1 (8 oz)	93	17	4	3
French Onion	1 (8 oz)	80	11	5	1
Red Beans & Rice	1 (8 oz)	107	25	3	11
Southwest Roasted Corn	1 (8 oz)	90	20	4	3

MCDONALD'S
BEVERAGES

FOOD	PORTION	CALS	CARB	SUGAR	FIBER
Apple Juice	1 box (6.8 oz)	90	23	21	0
Chocolate Milk 1% Low Fat	8 oz	170	26	25	1
Coca-Cola Classic	1 sm (16 oz)	150	40	40	0
Coffee	1 sm (12 oz)	0	0	0	0
Diet Coke	1 sm (16 oz)	0	0	0	0
Half & Half Creamer	1 pkg	20	0	0	0
Hi-C Orange Lavaburst	1 sm (16 oz)	160	44	44	0
Iced Coffee Caramel	1 sm (16 oz)	130	21	20	1
Iced Coffee Hazelnut	1 sm (16 oz)	130	21	21	0
Iced Coffee Regular	1 sm (16 oz)	140	22	22	0
Iced Coffee Vanilla	1 sm (16 oz)	130	21	21	0
Iced Tea	1 sm (16 oz)	0	0	0	0
Milk Lowfat 1%	1 pkg	100	12	12	0
Orange Juice	1 sm (12 oz)	140	33	29	0
Powerade Mountain Blast	1 sm (16 oz)	100	27	21	0

FOOD	PORTION	CALS	CARB	SUGAR	FIBER
Shake Triple Thick Chocolate	1 sm (12 oz)	440	76	63	1
Shake Triple Thick Strawberry	1 sm (12 oz)	420	73	63	0
Shake Triple Thick Vanilla	1 sm (16 oz)	420	72	54	0
Sprite	1 sm (16 oz)	150	39	39	0
BREAKFAST SELECTIONS					
Big Breakfast Regular Biscuit	1 serv	720	49	3	3
Biscuit	1 reg	250	32	2	2
Biscuit Regular Bacon Egg Cheese	1	450	36	3	2
Biscuit Regular Sausage	1	410	33	2	2
Biscuit Regular Sausage w/ Egg	1	500	35	2	2
Burrito Sausage	1	300	26	2	1
Deluxe Breakfast Regular Biscuit w/o Syrup & Margarine	1 serv	1070	109	17	6
English Muffin	1	160	27	2	2
Hash Browns	1 serv	140	15	0	2
Hotcake Syrup	1 pkg (2 oz)	180	45	32	0
Hotcakes & Sausage w/o Syrup & Margarine	1 serv	520	61	14	3
Hotcakes w/o Syrup & Margarine	1 serv	350	60	14	3
McGriddles Bacon Egg Cheese	1	460	48	16	2
McGriddles Sausage	1	420	44	15	2
McGriddles Sausage Egg & Cheese	1	560	48	15	2
McMuffin Sausage	1	370	29	2	2
McMuffin Sausage w/ Egg	1	250	30	2	2
McSkillet Burrito w/ Sausage	1	610	44	4	3
McSkillet Burrito w/ Steak	1	570	44	4	3
Sausage Patty	1	170	1	0	0
Scrambled Eggs	2	170	1	0	0
DESSERTS					
Apple Dippers	1 pkg	35	8	6	0
Apple Pie Baked	1	270	36	14	4
Caramel Dip Low Fat	1 pkg	70	15	9	0
Cinnamon Melts	1 serv	460	66	32	3
Cookie Chocolate Chip	1	180	22	15	1
Cookie Oatmeal	1 (1.1 oz)	150	22	13	1
Cookie Sugar	1 (1.1 oz)	150	21	11	0
Cookies McDonaldland	1 pkg (2 oz)	250	42	14	1

FOOD	PORTION	CALS	CARB	SUGAR	FIBER
Cookies McDonaldland Chocolate Chip	1 pkg	270	39	19	1
Fruit 'n Yogurt Parfait	1 serv	160	31	21	1
Ice Cream Cone Reduced Fat Vanilla	1	150	24	18	0
Kiddie Cone	1	45	8	6	0
McFlurry M&M's	1 (12 oz)	620	96	85	1
McFlurry Oreo	1 (12 oz)	560	88	71	0
Peanuts For Sundae	1 serv	45	2	0	1
Sundae Hot Caramel	1	340	60	44	1
Sundae Hot Fudge	1	330	54	48	2
Sundae Strawberry	1	280	49	45	1
MAIN MENU SELECTIONS					
Apple Sauce Strawberry	1 serv	90	23	21	tr
Big Mac	1	540	45	9	3
Big N' Tasty	1	460	37	8	3
Big N' Tasty w/ Cheese	1	510	38	8	3
Cheeseburger	1	300	33	6	2
Cheeseburger Double	1	440	34	7	2
Cheesy Tots	6 pieces	210	20	1	2
Chicken McNuggets	4 pieces	170	10	0	0
Chicken Selects	3 pieces	380	28	0	0
Filet-O-Fish	1	380	38	5	2
French Fries	1 sm	250	30	0	3
French Fries	1 lg	570	70	0	7
Hamburger	1	250	31	6	2
McChicken	1	360	40	5	1
McRib	1	500	44	11	3
Onion Rings	1 sm	140	18	2	2
Quarter Pounder	1	410	37	8	3
Quarter Pounder Double w/ Cheese	1	740	40	9	3
Quarter Pounder w/ Cheese	1	510	40	9	3
Sandwich Chicken Classic Crispy	1	500	61	10	3
Sandwich Chicken Classic Grilled	1	420	51	11	3
Sandwich Club Chicken Crispy	1	660	63	11	4
Sandwich Club Chicken Grilled	1	570	52	12	4

FOOD	PORTION	CALS	CARB	SUGAR	FIBER
Sandwich Ranch BLT Chicken Crispy	1	600	64	12	3
Sandwich Ranch BLT Chicken Grilled	1	520	53	13	3
Snack Wrap Grilled w/ Chipotle BBQ	1	260	28	5	1
Snack Wrap Grilled w/ Honey Mustard	1	260	27	4	1
Snack Wrap Grilled w/ Ranch	1	270	26	2	1
Snack Wrap w/ Chipotle BBQ	1	320	35	4	2
Snack Wrap w/ Honey Mustard	1	320	34	4	1
Snack Wrap w/ Ranch	1	140	32	2	2
SALAD DRESSINGS AND SAUCES					
Dipping Sauce Buffalo	1 serv (1 oz)	80	2	1	0
Dipping Sauce Zesty Onion Ring	1 serv (1 oz)	150	3	2	tr
Dressing Ken's Light Italian	1 pkg (2 oz)	120	5	4	0
Dressing Newman's Own Creamy Caesar	1 pkg (2 oz)	170	4	2	0
Dressing Newman's Own Creamy Southwest	1 pkg (1.5 oz)	100	11	3	0
Dressing Newman's Own Low Fat Balsamic Vinaigrette	1 pkg (1.5 oz)	40	4	3	0
Dressing Newman's Own Low Fat Family Recipe Italian	1 pkg (1.5 oz)	60	8	1	0
Dressing Newman's Own Low Fat Sesame Ginger	1 pkg (1.5 oz)	90	15	1	0
Dressing Newman's Own Ranch	1 pkg (2 oz)	170	9	4	0
Honey	1 pkg (0.5 oz)	50	12	11	0
Ketchup	1 pkg	15	3	2	0
Sauce Barbecue	1 pkg (1 oz)	50	12	10	0
Sauce Creamy Ranch	1 pkg (1.5 oz)	200	2	1	0
Sauce Hot Mustard	1 pkg (1 oz)	60	9	6	2
Sauce Southwestern Chipotle Barbeque	1 pkg (1.5 oz)	70	18	13	1
Sauce Spicy Buffalo	1 pkg (1.5 oz)	60	1	0	2
Sauce Sweet'N Sour	1 pkg (1 oz)	50	12	10	0
Sauce Tangy Honey Mustard	1 pkg (1.5 oz)	70	13	0	0
SALADS					
Asian w/ Crispy Chicken w/o Dressing	1 serv	380	33	12	5

FOOD	PORTION	CALS	CARB	SUGAR	FIBER
Asian w/ Grilled Chicken w/o Dressing	1 serv	300	23	12	5
Asian w/o Chicken & Dressing	1 serv	150	15	9	5
Bacon Ranch w/ Crispy Chicken	1 serv	350	23	4	3
Bacon Ranch w/ Grilled Chicken w/o Dressing	1 serv	260	12	5	3
Bacon Ranch w/o Chicken	1 serv	140	10	4	3
Caesar w/ Crispy Chicken	1 serv	300	22	4	3
Caesar w/ Grilled Chicken	1 serv	220	12	5	3
Caesar w/o Chicken	1 serv	90	9	4	3
Croutons Butter Garlic	1 pkg	60	10	0	1
Fruit & Walnut Snack Size	1 serv	210	31	25	2
Side Salad	1 serv	20	4	2	1
Southwest w/ Crispy Chicken w/o Dressing	1 serv	400	41	10	7
Southwest w/ Grilled Chicken	1 serv	320	30	11	7
Southwest w/o Chicken & Dressing	1 serv	140	20	5	6

MIMIS CAFE
CHILDREN'S MENU SELECTIONS

FOOD	PORTION	CALS	CARB	SUGAR	FIBER
Chicken Fingers	1 serv	408	21	2	1
Grilled Cheese	1 serv	273	14	1	0
Macaroni & Cheese	1 serv	353	48	10	2
Mini Burger	1 serv	554	48	5	3
Mini Corn Dogs	1 serv	460	35	8	0
Pancakes Chocolate Chip	1 serv	563	71	33	3
Pancakes Mimi Mouse	1 serv	477	69	23	1
PB&J Soldiers	1 serv	730	78	29	4
Pepperoni Pizzadillas	1 serv	617	39	7	3
Scrambled Eggs & Bacon	1 serv	216	1	1	0
Spaghetti	1 serv	343	62	17	5
Turkey Dinner	1 serv	337	25	1	3

DESSERTS

FOOD	PORTION	CALS	CARB	SUGAR	FIBER
Bread Pudding	1 serv	819	69	1	

MAIN MENU SELECTIONS

FOOD	PORTION	CALS	CARB	SUGAR	FIBER
Appetizer Dip Spinach & Artichoke	1 serv	2459	191	9	11
Appetizer Fried Chicken Tenders	1 serv	800	60	19	3
Appetizer Jazz Fest	1 serv	1252	108	9	8

FOOD	PORTION	CALS	CARB	SUGAR	FIBER
Appetizer Zucchini Parmesan	1 serv	626	73	12	7
Blackened Soul w/ Shrimp Creole	1 serv	852	59	–	9
Broiled Flat Iron Steak	1 serv	1026	58	–	9
Burger Half Pound	1	684	48	–	3
Cafe Fish & Chips	1 serv	1290	119	–	10
Cajun Blackened Salmon	1 serv	919	55	–	9
Cheeseburger BBQ Ranch	1	999	62	–	3
Cheeseburger Half Pound	1	855	49	–	3
Chicken Feta Penne	1 serv	1879	158	–	12
Ciabatta Chicken	1	1251	81	–	4
Club Cafe	1	1132	73	–	4
Crab Cake Dinner	1 serv	1662	129	–	9
Dip Classic Beef	1	521	43	–	5
Fillet Of Soul	1 serv	636	56	–	7
French Quarter	1	1480	68	–	7
Garlic Shrimp Spaghettini	1 serv	860	109	–	7
Grilled Chicken Tuscan Style	1 serv	880	80	–	12
Hibachi Salmon	1 serv	846	75	–	8
Original Patty Melt	1	976	62	–	6
Parmesan Crusted Chicken Breast	1 serv	1820	211	–	15
Pasta Jambalaya	1 serv	1223	113	–	8
Pot Pie Chicken	1 serv	1403	86	–	11
Reuben West Coast	1	2015	120	–	11
Sandwich 5 Way Grilled Cheese	1	703	49	–	2
Sandwich Bacon Lettuce & Tomato	1	586	48	–	7
Sandwich Fresh Roasted Turkey Breast	1	532	28	–	1
Sandwich Turkey Walnut Salad On Raisin Bread	1	549	36	–	3
Sandwich Veggie Stack	1	836	93	–	6
Small Bites Black & Blue Quesadilla	1 serv	1241	60	13	7
Small Bites Chicken & Fruit	1 serv	460	21	17	3
Small Bites Citrus Salmon	1 serv	699	37	21	10
Small Bites Crab Cakes	1 serv	412	27	6	2
Small Bites Smokey Chicken Enchiladas	1 serv	1154	68	16	8

FOOD	PORTION	CALS	CARB	SUGAR	FIBER
Small Bites Sweet & Sour Coconut Shrimp	1 serv	608	79	38	4
Small Bites Thai Chicken Wrap	1 serv	1004	106	16	7
SOUPS					
Broccoli Cheddar	1 serv	270	18	4	2
Chicken Gumbo	1 serv	235	25	4	2
Clam Chowder	1 serv	240	21	2	2
Corn Chowder	1 serv	196	28	6	3
Cream Of Chicken	1 serv	337	19	3	1
French Market Onion	1 serv	207	16	4	2
Red Bean & Andouille Sausage	1 serv	256	30	4	5
Split Pea	1 serv	194	29	5	11
Vegetarian Vegetable	1 serv	60	12	5	2

NOAH'S BAGELS
BAGELS AND BREADS

FOOD	PORTION	CALS	CARB	SUGAR	FIBER
Bagel Asiago Cheese Topped	1 (4.2 oz)	330	57	5	2
Bagel Blueberry	1 (3.7 oz)	270	59	11	3
Bagel Candy Cane	1 (3.7 oz)	270	54	5	2
Bagel Cheddar Stick	1 (4.2 oz)	330	57	5	2
Bagel Chocolate Chip	1 (3.7 oz)	290	60	12	3
Bagel Chopped Garlic	1 (3.9 oz)	290	58	5	2
Bagel Cinnamon Raisin	1 (3.7 oz)	270	58	11	3
Bagel Cinnamon Sugar	1 (4.1 oz)	310	64	11	2
Bagel Cracked Pepper	1 (3.7 oz)	280	55	6	2
Bagel Cranberry Orange	1 (3.5 oz)	250	54	6	3
Bagel Dutch Apple	1 (5 oz)	340	72	14	3
Bagel Egg	1 (3.7 oz)	290	57	5	2
Bagel Everything	1 (3.9 oz)	280	57	5	2
Bagel Good Grains	1 (3.9 oz)	280	58	6	4
Bagel Jalapeno Cheddar	1 (4.9 oz)	350	58	5	2
Bagel Onion	1 (3.7 oz)	270	57	5	3
Bagel Plain	1 (3.7 oz)	270	57	5	2
Bagel Poppyseed	1 (3.9 oz)	290	57	5	2
Bagel Power	1 (4 oz)	310	61	16	4
Bagel Pumpernickel	1 (3.7 oz)	260	57	4	3
Bagel Sesame Seed	1 (3.9 oz)	290	57	5	2
Bagel Six Cheese	1 (4.5 oz)	340	57	5	2
Bagel Spinach Florentine	1 (4.9 oz)	350	58	6	2
Bagel Sun Dried Tomato	1 (3.7 oz)	270	57	6	3
Bagel Whole Wheat	1 (3.7 oz)	260	57	6	4

FOOD	PORTION	CALS	CARB	SUGAR	FIBER
Bagel Whole Wheat Sesame & Sunflower Seeds	1 (4.4 oz)	370	61	6	6
Bialy	1 (5.3 oz)	380	77	5	4
Bread Ciabatta	1 serv (4.25 oz)	290	60	1	2
Bread Corn Meal Rye	1 slice (2 oz)	150	31	1	2
Bread Harvest Grain	1 slice (2.3 oz)	180	36	7	4
Bread Marble Rye	1 slice (1.7 oz)	160	30	1	1
Bread Potato	1 slice (1.7 oz)	140	28	3	1
Challah Braided	1 serv (2 oz)	160	29	4	1
Challah Roll	1 (3 oz)	230	44	6	2
Pizza Bagel Artichoke Tomato & Red Onion	1 (11.1 oz)	550	67	8	5
Pizza Bagel Artichoke & Spinach	1 (12 oz)	670	70	7	5
Pizza Bagel Cheese	1 (6.2 oz)	420	60	6	3
Pizza Bagel Cheesy Garlic & Herb	1 (6.2 oz)	500	62	6	2
Pizza Bagel Pepperoni	1 (6.8 oz)	500	60	6	3
Pizza Bagel Spinach & Mushroom	1 (9.5 oz)	580	68	8	4
Pizza Bagel Tomato & Rosemary	1 (8.7 oz)	540	63	7	4
BEVERAGES AND EXTRAS					
Cafe Latte Low Fat	1 reg (12 oz)	160	17	17	0
Cafe Latte Nonfat	1 reg (12 oz)	110	17	17	0
Cafe Latte Whole	1 reg (12 oz)	200	16	16	0
Cappuccino Low Fat	1 reg (12 oz)	120	13	13	0
Cappuccino Nonfat	1 reg (12 oz)	90	13	13	0
Cappuccino Whole	1 reg (12 oz)	150	13	13	0
Chai Tea Low Fat Milk	1 reg (12 oz)	220	47	45	0
Chai Tea Non Fat Milk	1 reg (12 oz)	210	47	45	0
Chai Tea Whole Milk	1 reg (12 oz)	230	47	45	0
Coca-Cola	8 oz	99	27	27	0
Coca-Cola Cherry	8 oz	104	28	28	0
Coffee Iced Americano	8 oz	0	0	0	0
Coffee Regular & Decaf	1 (12 oz)	0	0	0	0
Diet Coke	8 oz	1	0	0	0
Espresso	1 reg (2 oz)	0	0	0	0
Fanta Orange	8 oz	106	29	29	0
Frozen Drinks Cafe Caramel	1 (18 oz)	620	100	66	0

FOOD	PORTION	CALS	CARB	SUGAR	FIBER
Frozen Drinks Cafe Mocha	1 (18 oz)	510	102	64	0
Frozen Drinks Strawberry Cream	1 (18 oz)	450	75	64	3
Frozen Drinks Wild Berry Fat Free	1 (18 oz)	270	62	48	5
Half & Half Creamer	1 oz	40	1	1	0
Hi-C Fruit Punch	8 oz	104	28	28	0
Hot Chocolate Nonfat	1 reg (12 oz)	220	37	36	1
Hot Chocolate Whole	1 reg (12 oz)	290	35	34	1
Iced Cappuccino Nonfat	1 reg (12 oz)	90	13	13	0
Iced Mocha Low Fat	1 reg (12 oz)	230	39	34	0
Iced Tea Raspberry	8 oz	78	21	21	0
Iced Tea Unsweetened	8 oz	1	0	0	0
Lemonade	1 (16 oz)	200	24	24	0
Lemonade Blackberry	1 (16 oz)	310	74	74	0
Macchiato Nonfat	1 reg (12 oz)	230	49	44	0
Macchiato Whole	1 reg (12 oz)	290	47	42	0
Milk Low Fat	8 oz	120	12	11	0
Milk Skim	8 oz	80	15	13	0
Milk Whole	8 oz	150	11	11	0
Mocha Low Fat	1 reg (12 oz)	230	39	34	0
Mocha Nonfat	1 reg (12 oz)	190	39	34	0
Mocha Whole	1 reg (12 oz)	270	38	33	0
Mr. Pibb	8 oz	97	26	26	0
On Top Reduced Fat Topping	2 tbsp (0.3 oz)	20	2	2	0
Orange Juice	1 (10 oz)	143	34	31	2
Sprite	8 oz	97	26	26	0
Syrup Blackberry	2 tbsp (1 oz)	100	25	25	0
Syrup Caramel	2 tbsp (1 oz)	70	18	17	0
Syrup Hazelnut	2 tbsp (1 oz)	100	25	25	0
Syrup Vanilla	2 tbsp (1 oz)	100	25	25	0
Syrup Vanilla Sugar Free	2 tbsp (1 oz)	116	0	0	0
Tea Hamey & Sons All Flavors	8 oz	0	0	0	0
Whipped Cream Light	2 tbsp (1 oz)	36	2	2	0
CREAM CHEESE AND SPREADS					
Butter	1 tbsp (0.5 oz)	110	0	0	0
Cream Cheese Whipped Onion & Chive	2 tbsp (0.7 oz)	70	3	1	0
Cream Cheese Whipped Plain	2 tbsp (0.7 oz)	70	1	1	0

FOOD	PORTION	CALS	CARB	SUGAR	FIBER
Cream Cheese Whipped Reduced Fat Blueberry	2 tbsp (0.7 oz)	70	6	5	0
Cream Cheese Whipped Reduced Fat Garden Vegetable	2 tbsp (0.7 oz)	60	3	1	0
Cream Cheese Whipped Reduced Fat Garlic Herb	2 tbsp (0.7 oz)	60	3	1	0
Cream Cheese Whipped Reduced Fat Honey Almond	2 tbsp (0.7 oz)	70	6	4	0
Cream Cheese Whipped Reduced Fat Jalapeno Salsa	2 tbsp (0.7 oz)	60	3	1	0
Cream Cheese Whipped Reduced Fat Plain	2 tbsp (0.7 oz)	60	2	1	0
Cream Cheese Whipped Reduced Fat Strawberry	2 tbsp (0.7 oz)	60	2	1	0
Cream Cheese Whipped Reduced Fat Sun Dried Tomato & Basil	2 tbsp (0.7 oz)	60	2	1	0
Cream Cheese Whipped Smoked Salmon	2 tbsp (0.7 oz)	60	2	1	0
Deli Mustard	1 tsp (5 g)	0	0	0	0
Garlic Mayo	1 serv (1.5 oz)	270	8	1	0
Grape Jam	1 serv (1 oz)	110	28	26	0
Honey	1 serv (1 oz)	90	23	22	0
Hummus	1 serv (2 oz)	90	11	1	2
Mayo	1 tbsp (0.5 oz)	110	0	0	0
DESSERTS					
Cinnamon Twists	1 serv (3.8 oz)	370	41	18	2
Coffee Cake Apple Cinnamon	1 serv (6.6 oz)	700	108	57	1
Coffee Cake Chocolate Chip	1 serv (6.1 oz)	760	110	58	2
Coffee Cake Mixed Berry	1 serv (6.9 oz)	710	110	59	2
Cookie Chocolate Mudslide	1 (2.75 oz)	320	46	38	1
Cookie Chocolate Chip	1 (2.8 oz)	360	48	29	2
Cookie Iced Sugar	1 (3.7 oz)	480	76	46	1
Cookie Oatmeal Raisin	1 (2.8 oz)	320	54	31	2
Cookie Snickerdoodle	1 (2.8 oz)	400	56	32	1
Cookie Mini Chocolate Mudslide	1 (1.38 oz)	160	23	19	1
Cookie Mini Chocolate Chip	1 (1.38 oz)	180	24	14	1
Cookie Mini Iced Sugar	1 (1.87 oz)	230	39	24	1
Cookie Mini Oatmeal Raisin	1 (1.38 oz)	160	27	16	1

FOOD	PORTION	CALS	CARB	SUGAR	FIBER
Marshmallow Crispy Treat	1 (3.9 oz)	410	86	37	0
Muffin Blueberry	1 (5 oz)	480	65	36	2
Muffin Cranberry Orange	1 (4.6 oz)	460	63	39	2
Muffin Strawberry White Chocolate	1 (5.5 oz)	550	78	49	1
Strudel Cinnamon Walnut	1 serv (5.4 oz)	630	56	20	4
SALAD DRESSINGS					
Caesar	2 tbsp (1 oz)	150	1	1	0
Harvest Chicken Salad	2 tbsp (1 oz)	90	3	2	0
Raspberry Vinaigrette	2 tbsp	160	8	8	0
SALADS					
Caesar	1 (10.5 oz)	600	23	4	6
Caesar Side	1 (4.5 oz)	280	7	2	2
Ceasar Chicken	1 (14 oz)	720	23	6	4
City	1 (11.5 oz)	830	39	29	7
City w/ Chicken	1 (15 oz)	950	40	30	8
Southwestern Chicken	1 (15.2 oz)	710	54	14	10
SANDWICHES					
Bagel & Lox	1 (11.2 oz)	520	65	11	4
Bagel Dog Asiago	1 (7.1 oz)	510	59	6	2
Bagel Dog Everything	1 (7.1 oz)	510	59	6	2
Bagel Dog Original	1 (6.9 oz)	490	59	6	2
Bagel Plain w/ Peanut Butter & Jelly	1 (6.2 oz)	550	90	31	4
Breakfast Wrap Santa Fe	1 (14.5 oz)	750	77	8	9
Breakfast Wrap Veggie	1 (15.6 oz)	810	77	7	10
California Chicken	1 (9.9 oz)	360	49	8	3
Club Blackened Chicken	1 (10.4 oz)	630	53	8	2
Club Deli Pesto Turkey	1 (10.9 oz)	670	47	9	2
Deli Chicken Salad	1 (11 oz)	1150	61	5	5
Deli Cornbeef	1 (14 oz)	740	61	5	4
Deli Egg Salad Kosher	1 (11.5 oz)	650	68	6	5
Deli Pastrami	1 (14 oz)	750	62	6	5
Deli Roast Beef	1 (14 oz)	730	60	5	4
Deli Tuna Salad	1 (13 oz)	740	53	9	5
Deli Turkey	1 (14.5 oz)	720	67	6	5
Deli Whitefish	1 (12.2 oz)	850	68	9	6
Deli Melts Hummus	1 (10.2 oz)	570	76	7	6
Deli Melts Pastrami	1 (9.6 oz)	530	61	7	3
Deli Melts Roast Beef	1 (9.6 oz)	530	60	6	3

FOOD	PORTION	CALS	CARB	SUGAR	FIBER
Deli Melts Tuna	1 (11.6 oz)	700	82	7	3
Deli Melts Turkey	1 (9.6 oz)	500	60	7	3
Deli Melts Veggie	1 (12.3 oz)	590	70	10	5
Egg Mit Artichoke & Tomato	1 (12 oz)	620	67	10	4
Egg Mit Bacon & Cheddar	1 (9.2 oz)	620	61	8	2
Egg Mit Cheese & Tomato	1 (10 oz)	530	61	8	3
Egg Mit Lox & Chives	1 (8.8 oz)	490	59	8	2
Egg Mit Plain	1 (7.9 oz)	450	59	7	2
Egg Mit Spinach Mushroom & Swiss	1 (9.8 oz)	530	61	8	3
Egg Mit Turkey Sausage	1 (9.9 oz)	590	61	8	2
Egg Mit w/ Cheese	1 (8.5 oz)	520	60	7	2
Kosher Vegetarian On Plain Bagel	1 (13.9 oz)	860	79	9	4
Panini Albacore Tuna	1 (13.6 oz)	750	62	2	6
Panini Egg Spinach Bacon	1 (11.8 oz)	790	65	4	5
Panini Egg Vegetarian Omelet	1 (13.8 oz)	670	66	5	6
Panini Italian Chicken	1 (12.5 oz)	810	67	3	5
Panini Mediterranean	1 (10.6 oz)	550	77	3	9
Panini Tomato Mozzarella	1 (7.9 oz)	440	59	1	6
Panini Turkey Club	1 (12.3 oz)	610	64	4	6
Sandwich Rachel	1 (13.9 oz)	1030	53	14	2
Sandwich Reuben	1 (13.9 oz)	770	47	8	3
Sandwich Veg Out	1 (10.1 oz)	490	75	9	4
Wrap Alabacore Tuna	1 (12.3 oz)	600	57	5	8
Wrap Chicken Caesar	1 (12.6 oz)	790	62	7	7
Wrap Southwestern Turkey	1 (13.5 oz)	750	74	12	9
Wrap Veggie	1 (9.8 oz)	460	64	6	9
SIDES					
Cole Slaw	1 serv (3 oz)	120	15	2	2
Egg Salad	1 serv (5 oz)	330	3	2	0
Fresh Fruit Cup	1 (11 oz)	140	36	31	3
Fruit & Yogurt Parfait	1 (12 oz)	220	43	25	3
Kosher Pickle	1	5	1	1	0
Macaroni & Cheese	1 serv (6 oz)	340	32	–	1
Redskin Potato Salad	1 serv (3 oz)	160	13	1	1
Tuna Salad	1 serv (5 oz)	280	3	1	1
SOUPS					
Broccoli Cheese	1 cup (8.7 oz)	290	16	6	2
Chicken Noodle	1 cup (8.7 oz)	110	13	1	1

FOOD	PORTION	CALS	CARB	SUGAR	FIBER
Italian Wedding	1 cup (8.7 oz)	160	15	2	2
Tortilla	1 cup (8.7 oz)	300	19	6	3
Turkey Chili	1 cup (8.7 oz)	220	24	5	5

PACIUGO GELATO

FOOD	PORTION	CALS	CARB	SUGAR	FIBER
Milk Base Amarena Black Cherry Swirl	1 scoop (3.5 oz)	160	30	30	tr
Milk Base Banana Creme Pie	1 scoop (3.5 oz)	80	14	13	tr
Milk Base Cheesecake	1 scoop (3.5 oz)	90	12	12	tr
Milk Base Chocolate	1 scoop (3.5 oz)	80	14	13	tr
Milk Base Chocolate Cookies'N Milk	1 scoop (3.5 oz)	90	16	13	tr
Milk Base Coconut	1 scoop (3.5 oz)	80	13	12	tr
Milk Base Coffee	1 scoop (3.5 oz)	75	12	11	tr
Milk Base Fiordilatte	1 scoop (3.5 oz)	75	13	13	tr
Milk Base French Vanilla Bean	1 scoop (3.5 oz)	80	13	13	tr
Milk Base Green Tea	1 scoop (3.5 oz)	70	12	12	tr
Milk Base Hazelnut	1 scoop (3.5 oz)	85	11	11	tr
Milk Base Lemon Custard	1 scoop (3.5 oz)	75	12	12	tr
Milk Base Mascarpone Chocolate Rum	1 scoop (3.5 oz)	95	11	10	tr
Milk Base Pannacotta Wedding Cake	1 scoop (3.5 oz)	75	13	13	tr
Milk Base Peppermint	1 scoop (3.5 oz)	75	14	13	1
Milk Base Rose	1 scoop (3.5 oz)	70	12	12	tr
Milk Base Tiramisu	1 scoop (3.5 oz)	80	12	12	tr
Milk Base Zabajone	1 scoop (3.5 oz)	80	12	12	tr

FOOD	PORTION	CALS	CARB	SUGAR	FIBER
No Sugar Added Chocolate	1 scoop (3.5 oz)	28	9	3	1
No Sugar Added Mint	1 scoop (3.5 oz)	25	9	3	1
No Sugar Added Mocha	1 scoop (3.5 oz)	28	9	3	1
No Sugar Added Strawberry Milk	1 scoop (3.5 oz)	23	8	3	1
Soy Banana	1 scoop (3.5 oz)	40	6	6	1
Soy Blueberry	1 scoop (3.5 oz)	40	6	6	1
Soy Chocolate	1 scoop (3.5 oz)	38	5	5	1
Soy Coffee	1 scoop (3.5 oz)	35	5	5	1
Soy Hazelnut	1 scoop (3.5 oz)	35	5	5	1
Soy Strawberry	1 scoop (3.5 oz)	38	6	6	1
Soy Wild Berries	1 scoop (3.5 oz)	40	6	6	1
Water Base Blackberry	1 scoop (3.5 oz)	28	7	7	tr
Water Base Ginger Lemon	1 scoop (3.5 oz)	25	7	7	tr
Water Base Green Apple	1 scoop (3.5 oz)	28	7	7	tr
Water Base Lemon Sage	1 scoop (3.5 oz)	25	7	7	tr
Water Base Lychee	1 scoop (3.5 oz)	25	6	6	tr
Water Base Orange Vidalia	1 scoop (3.5 oz)	25	7	7	0
Water Base Passion Fruit	1 scoop (3.5 oz)	23	6	6	0
Water Base Pineapple	1 scoop (3.5 oz)	28	7	7	tr
Water Base Strawberry Port	1 scoop (3.5 oz)	25	6	6	tr

FOOD	PORTION	CALS	CARB	SUGAR	FIBER
Water Base Watermelon	1 scoop (3.5 oz)	25	7	7	tr

PANDA EXPRESS
MAIN MENU SELECTIONS

BBQ Pork	1 serv	350	13	5	tr
Beef & Broccoli	1 serv	150	9	2	1
Beef w/ String Beans	1 serv	170	11	0	2
Black Pepper Chicken	1 serv	180	10	2	2
Chicken w/ Mushrooms	1 serv	130	7	2	2
Chicken w/ Potato	1 serv	220	17	1	1
Chicken w/ String Beans	1 serv	170	12	2	3
Egg Roll Chicken	1 (3 oz)	190	21	tr	3
Fried Shrimp	6 pieces	260	26	0	tr
Mandarin Chicken	1 serv	250	8	2	2
Mixed Vegetables	1 serv	70	8	1	1
Orange Chicken	1 serv	480	50	5	2
Spicy Chicken w/ Peanuts	1 serv	200	17	2	4
Spring Roll Veggie	1 (1.7 oz)	80	14	0	tr
Steamed Rice	1 serv	330	74	0	2
String Beans w/ Fried Tofu	1 serv	180	11	3	3
Sweet & Sour Chicken	1 serv	310	28	0	2
Sweet & Sour Pork	1 serv	410	17	0	3
Vegetable Chow Mein	1 serv	330	48	6	4
Vegetable Fried Rice	1 serv	390	61	0	2
SAUCES					
Hot	2 tsp	10	2	1	0
Hot Mustard	1 serv	18	1	0	0
Mandarin	1 serv	70	16	14	0
Soy	1 tbsp	16	2	2	0
Sweet & Sour	1 serv	60	15	13	0

PEI WEI ASIAN DINER
CHILDREN'S MENU SELECTIONS

Kid's Wei Honey Seared Chicken w/o Noodles Or Rice	1 serv	290	19	8	0
Kid's Wei Lo Mein Chicken w/o Noodles Or Rice	1 serv	180	7	3	0
Kid's Wei Teriyaki Chicken w/o Noodles Or Rice	1 serv	240	20	18	0

FOOD	PORTION	CALS	CARB	SUGAR	FIBER
DESSERTS					
Cookie Chocolate Chip	1	342	53	37	2
Cookie Fortune	1	30	7	3	0
MAIN MENU SELECTIONS					
Bowl w/ Brown Rice Japanese Teriyaki Beef	1 serv	580	66	21	4
Bowl w/ Brown Rice Japanese Teriyaki Chicken	1 serv	460	64	21	4
Bowl w/ Brown Rice Japanese Teriyaki Shrimp	1 serv	410	64	21	4
Bowl w/ Brown Rice Japanese Teriyaki Vegetables & Tofu	1 serv	410	71	24	7
Bowl w/ White Rice Japanese Teriyaki Beef	1 serv	560	62	21	3
Bowl w/ White Rice Japanese Teriyaki Chicken	1 serv	440	60	21	3
Bowl w/ White Rice Japanese Teriyaki Shrimp	1 serv	390	61	21	3
Bowl w/ White Rice Japanese Teriyaki Vegetables & Tofu	1 serv	390	68	24	5
Crispy Potstickers	4	130	10	1	0
Edamame	1 serv	156	12	4	5
Fried Rice Beef	1 serv	630	68	9	3
Fried Rice Chicken	1 serv	525	68	9	3
Fried Rice Shrimp	1 serv	475	67	9	3
Fried Rice Vegetable & Tofu	1 serv	440	73	12	5
Ginger Broccoli Beef	1 serv	450	19	11	2
Ginger Broccoli Chicken	1 serv	300	19	11	2
Ginger Broccoli Shrimp	1 serv	230	18	11	2
Ginger Broccoli Vegetables & Tofu	1 serv	170	23	14	4
Honey Seared Chicken	1 serv	420	45	17	0
Honey Seared Shrimp	1 serv	370	43	17	0
Hot & Sour Soup	1 cup	150	11	0	2
Lemon Pepper Beef	1 serv	550	32	18	2
Lemon Pepper Chicken	1 serv	440	34	18	2
Lemon Pepper Shrimp	1 serv	380	34	18	2
Lemon Pepper Vegetables & Tofu	1 serv	230	29	19	4
Maindarin Kung Pao Chicken	1 serv	450	28	10	3

FOOD	PORTION	CALS	CARB	SUGAR	FIBER
Mandarin Kung Pao Beef	1 serv	610	31	10	3
Mandarin Kung Pao Shrimp	1 serv	400	28	10	3
Mandarin Kung Pao Vegetables & Tofu	1 serv	290	23	10	4
Minced Chicken w/ Cool Lettuce Wraps w/o Rice Sticks	1 serv	250	31	15	3
Mongolian Beef	1 serv	420	14	8	1
Mongolian Chicken	1 serv	280	14	8	1
Mongolian Shrimp	2 serv	210	12	8	1
Mongolian Vegetables & Tofu	2 serv	180	19	11	3
Noodles Dan Dan Chicken	1 serv	390	54	9	3
Noodles Lo Mein Beef	1 serv	570	61	9	5
Noodles Lo Mein Chicken	1 serv	460	61	9	5
Noodles Lo Mein Shrimp	1 serv	400	60	9	5
Noodles Lo Mein Vegetables & Tofu	1 serv	400	66	11	7
Noodles Thai Blazing Beef	1 serv	630	55	11	4
Noodles Thai Blazing Chicken	1 serv	520	55	11	4
Noodles Thai Blazing Shrimp	1 serv	482	55	11	4
Noodles Thai Blazing Vegetables & Tofu	1 serv	430	59	14	6
Noodles Egg	1 serv	210	39	0	2
Noodles Rice	1 serv	130	32	0	0
Orange Peel Beef	1 serv	660	52	33	3
Orange Peel Chicken	1 serv	520	52	33	3
Orange Peel Shrimp	1 serv	460	51	33	3
Orange Peel Vegetables & Tofu	1 serv	330	46	33	4
Pad Thai Beef	1 serv	670	63	19	2
Pad Thai Chicken	1 serv	560	61	19	2
Pad Thai Shrimp	1 serv	490	60	19	2
Pei Wei Spicy Beef	1 serv	480	25	8	2
Pei Wei Spicy Chicken	1 serv	330	25	8	2
Pei Wei Spicy Shrimp	1 serv	300	29	8	2
Rice Brown	1 serv	170	37	0	3
Rice Fried	1 serv	260	44	5	2
Rice Sticks	1 cup	130	33	0	0
Rice White	1 serv	200	44	0	1
Spicy Korean Beef	1 serv	490	26	12	3
Spicy Korean Chicken	1 serv	350	26	12	3
Spicy Korean Shrimp	1 serv	280	24	12	3

FOOD	PORTION	CALS	CARB	SUGAR	FIBER
Spicy Korean Vegetables & Tofu	1 serv	240	27	14	4
Spring Rolls	2	90	11	3	1
Sweet & Sour Chicken	1 serv	440	61	30	2
Sweet & Sour Shrimp	1 serv	390	59	30	2
Thai Coconut Curry Beef	1 serv	550	20	10	2
Thai Coconut Curry Chicken	1 serv	380	23	10	2
Thai Coconut Curry Shrimp	1 serv	300	18	10	2
Thai Coconut Curry Vegetables & Tofu	1 serv	220	19	11	2
Thai Dynamite Chicken	1 serv	390	20	7	2
Thai Dynamite Shrimp	1 serv	280	20	9	2
Thai Dynamite Vegetables & Tofu	1 serv	220	15	9	3
Wontons Crab	4	190	9	0	0
SALAD DRESSINGS AND SAUCES					
Dressing Sesame Ginger	1 serv (2 oz)	170	5	4	0
Lime Vinaigrette	1 serv (2 oz)	230	13	11	0
Sauce Lettuce Wrap	1 serv (2 oz)	70	2	1	0
Sauce Sweet Chili	1 serv (2 oz)	140	34	28	2
Sauce Thai Peanut	1 serv (2 oz)	168	15	11	1
SALADS					
Asian Chopped Chicken w/ Dressing	1 serv	280	13	4	2
Asian Chopped Chicken w/o Dressing	1 serv	200	10	2	2
Pei Wei Spicy Chicken w/ Dressing	1 serv	350	28	8	2
Pei Wei Spicy Chicken w/o Dressing	1 serv	210	23	3	2
Vietnamese Chicken Salad Rolls	3	53	5	3	1
PINKBERRY					
Frozen Yogurt Coffee	½ cup	90	24	19	0
Frozen Yogurt Green Tea	½ cup	50	10	10	0
Frozen Yogurt Original	½ cup	70	14	12	0
POLLO TROPICAL					
DESSERTS					
Flan	1 serv (4 oz)	390	59	54	1
Key Lime	1 serv (3.9 oz)	210	26	25	0
Tres Leches	1 serv (5.4 oz)	410	76	68	0

FOOD	PORTION	CALS	CARB	SUGAR	FIBER
MAIN MENU SELECTIONS					
Balsamic Tomato	1 combo	88	7	5	1
Balsamic Tomato	1 sm	176	14	11	2
Bananas Tropical	1 serv	437	89	28	9
Beef Skewers	1 (1 oz)	77	1	tr	tr
Black Beans	1 combo	90	18	0	7
Black Beans	1 sm	203	41	0	16
Boiled Yuca	1 combo	188	51	0	4
Boiled Yuca	1 sm	251	68	0	5
Caesar Salad	1 combo	130	4	0	1
Caesar Salad	1 sm	207	6	0	1
Chicken Boneless Breast	2 pieces	240	0	0	0
Chicken ¼ Dark Meat	1 serv	291	0	0	0
Chicken ¼ Dark Meat No Skin	1 serv	191	0	0	0
Chicken ¼ White Meat	1 serv	323	0	0	0
Chicken ¼ White Meat No Skin	1 serv	204	0	0	0
Chicken Caesar Salad	1 serv	669	13	0	3
Corn	1 combo	121	19	3	5
French Fries	1 sm	311	40	0	4
Ribs	½ rack (4 oz)	400	2	2	0
Ribs	¼ rack (2 oz)	200	1	1	0
Roast Pork	1 serv	392	0	0	0
Sandwich Chicken Caesar	1	881	71	12	5
Sandwich Grilled Chicken	1	827	84	22	6
Sandwich Roast Pork	1	773	83	20	5
Steak & Chicken Dark Meat	1 serv	437	2	tr	tr
TropiChop Chicken w/ Yellow Rice & Vegetables	1 serv	341	50	0	2
TropiChop Chicken w/ White Rice & Black Beans	1 serv	564	95	0	11
TropiChop Grilled Chicken Deluxe	1 serv	409	52	1	3
TropiChop Pork w/ White Rice & Black Beans	1 serv	714	97	2	12
TropiChop Pork w/ Yellow Rice & Vegetables	1 serv	480	91	2	5
TropiChop Ropa Vieja	1 serv	618	98	5	13
TropiChop Shrimp Creole	1 serv	506	75	0	3
TropiChop Vegetarian	1 serv	580	109	4	16

FOOD	PORTION	CALS	CARB	SUGAR	FIBER
TropiChop Max Chicken w/ Yellow Rice & Vegetables	1 serv	864	93	0	4
TropiChop Max Chicken w/ White Rice & Black Beans	1 serv	1117	144	0	16
TropiChop Max Grilled Chicken Deluxe	1 serv	753	91	1	5
TropiChop Max Pork w/ White Rice & Black Beans	1 serv	1273	147	2	18
TropiChop Max Pork w/ Yellow Rice & Vegetables	1 serv	1020	96	2	6
TropiChop Max Ropa Vieja	1 serv	1160	161	10	20
TropiChop Max Shrimp Creole	1 serv	1102	129	0	7
TropiChop Max Vegetarian	1 serv	950	177	7	26
White Rice	1 combo	203	40	0	1
White Rice	1 sm	339	66	0	2
Wrap Chicken Ceasar	1	901	64	2	4
Wrap Chicken Classic	1	694	68	12	5
Wrap Curry Chicken	1	930	94	34	6
Wrap Steak	1	993	106	5	6
Yellow Rice w/ Vegetables	1 combo	163	31	0	1
Yellow Rice w/ Vegetables	1 sm	245	47	0	2
Yucatan Fries	1 serv	497	69	0	3
SALAD DRESSINGS AND SAUCES					
BBQ Sauce	1 serv (1.8 oz)	83	20	12	0
BBQ Sauce Guava	1 serv (1.8 oz)	83	22	8	0
Dressing Caesar	1 serv (1 oz)	161	1	0	0
Guacamole Sauce	1 serv (1.8 oz)	75	3	0	3
Mojo Sauce	1 serv (0.9 oz)	97	3	0	tr
Mustard Curry Sauce	1 serv (1.8 oz)	265	0	0	0
Salsa	1 serv (1.8 oz)	8	2	0	0
SOUPS					
Caribbean Chicken	1 sm (8 oz)	121	21	2	3
Tropical Shrimp	1 sm (8 oz)	134	18	1	0
POPEYE'S					
Buttermilk Biscuit	1	240	25	2	1
Cajun Rice	1 reg	180	23	1	2
Coleslaw	1 serv	230	20	15	9
Collard Greens	1 serv	50	7	1	3
Corn On The Cob	1	220	48	7	4
Etouffee Chicken	1 serv	223	35	1	2

FOOD	PORTION	CALS	CARB	SUGAR	FIBER
Etouffee Crawfish	1 serv	200	26	0	2
French Fries	1 serv	261	34	1	3
Fried Catfish	1 serv	300	19	0	0
Fried Crawfish	1 serv	370	27	0	tr
Green Beans	1 serv	40	6	1	2
Jambalaya Chicken Sausage	1 serv	257	26	3	1
Mashed Potatoes & Gravy	1 serv	120	18	0	2
Mashed Potatoes No Gravy	1 serv	100	17	3	tr
Mild Breast	1	510	18	0	0
Mild Breast Skinless	1	280	7	0	0
Mild Leg	1	200	7	0	0
Mild Leg Skinless	1	110	2	0	0
Mild Strips	2	280	21	0	tr
Mild Strips No Breading	2	200	12	0	0
Mild Thigh	1	390	12	0	0
Mild Thigh Skinless	1	210	6	0	0
Mild Wing	1	220	10	0	0
Mild Wing Skinless	1	130	4	0	tr
Naked Chicken Strips	3	170	2	0	0
Popcorn Shrimp	1 serv	280	22	0	tr
Red Beans & Rice	1 reg	340	33	29	16
Sandwich Catfish Fully Dressed	1	640	59	7	5
Sandwich Deluxe Tame w/ Mayo	1	728	63	5	3
Sandwich Deluxe Tame w/o Mayo	1	530	63	5	3
Sandwich Shrimp Fully Dressed	1	740	741	5	8
Smothered Chicken	1 serv	210	24	0	1
Spicy Breast	1	530	13	0	1
Spicy Breast Skinless	1	290	7	0	tr
Spicy Leg	1	190	5	0	0
Spicy Leg Skinless	1	120	2	0	0
Spicy Strips	2	310	24	0	tr
Spicy Strips No Breading	2	190	11	0	0
Spicy Thigh	1	390	10	0	0
Spicy Thigh Skinless	1	200	2	0	0
Spicy Wing	1	220	7	0	0
Spicy Wing Skinless	1	140	5	0	tr
Turnover Cinnamon Apple	1	250	37	11	2

FOOD	PORTION	CALS	CARB	SUGAR	FIBER
PRETZELMAKER					
Bites	1 med (7.4 oz)	640	112	21	4
Bites	1 sm (5.3 oz)	450	80	15	3
Bites Cinnamon Sugar	1 serv (5.8 oz)	520	95	28	3
Breezer Coffee	1 (20 oz)	640	107	106	0
Breezer Mocha	1 (20 oz)	620	106	104	0
Breezer Peach	1 (20 oz)	650	117	115	0
Breezer Raspberry	1 (20 oz)	650	117	112	0
Breezer Strawberry Banana	1 (20 oz)	650	115	108	0
Caramel Nut	1 (4.5 oz)	390	74	17	2
Cinnamon Sugar	1 (4.3 oz)	370	68	17	2
Cream Cheese	1 serv (1.5 oz)	200	4	2	0
Diet Coke	1 sm (20 oz)	0	0	0	0
Garlic	1 (4.1 oz)	350	64	12	2
Icing Cream Cheese	1 serv (1.5 oz)	180	22	21	0
Ketchup	2 pkg (0.6 oz)	20	4	4	0
Lemonade	1 sm (20 oz)	160	92	87	0
Mustard	2 pkg (0.4 oz)	5	1	0	0
Original	1 (4 oz)	340	61	11	2
Parmesan	1 (4.2 oz)	360	61	11	2
Plain	1 (4 oz)	209	61	11	2
PT Pretzel Dog	1 (6 oz)	440	34	8	1
Ranch	1 (4.1 oz)	240	63	11	2
Sauce Caramel	1 serv (1.5 oz)	140	35	27	0
Sauce Cheddar Cheese	1 serv (1.5 oz)	70	6	2	0
Sauce Nacho Cheese	1 serv (1.5 oz)	80	7	2	0
Sauce Pizza	1 serv (1.5 oz)	30	6	3	2
QUIZNO'S					
COOKIES					
Dark Chocolate Chunk	1	380	58	32	1
Double Chocolate Chip	1	370	58	34	3
Oatmeal Raisin	1	340	59	36	2
Snickerdoodle	1	400	59	36	0
SANDWICHES					
Breakfast Bacon Egg Cheddar	1	380	36	2	4
Breakfast Black Angus Steak & Cheddar	1 sm	330	36	2	3
Breakfast Egg & Cheddar	1	240	35	2	3
Breakfast Garden Vegetable Cheddar	1	250	38	3	4

FOOD	PORTION	CALS	CARB	SUGAR	FIBER
Breakfast Ham Egg Cheddar	1	290	37	3	4
Deli Honey Ham & Swiss	1	260	38	5	4
Deli Oven Roasted Turkey & Cheese	1	250	39	4	4
Deli Roast Beef & Cheddar	1	230	37	3	4
Deli Tuna Melt	1	500	37	3	4
Sammie Alpine Chicken	1	200	24	1	1
Sammie Balsamic Chicken	1	170	24	1	1
Sammie Bistro Steak Melt	1	180	25	1	1
Sammie Black Angus Steak	1	180	24	1	1
Sammie Italiano	1	240	24	1	1
Sammie Sonoma Turkey	1	160	25	1	1
Sub Baja Chicken w/ Bacon	1 sm	320	37	2	4
Sub Black Angus Steak On Rosemary Parmesan	1 sm	380	46	3	5
Sub Chicken Carbonara w/ Bacon	1 sm	360	42	3	3
Sub Classic Club w/ Bacon	1 sm	320	39	5	5
Sub Classic Italian	1 sm	360	38	4	4
Sub Honey Bacon Club	1 sm	320	39	5	5
Sub Honey Bourbon Chicken	1 sm	260	38	3	4
Sub Honey Mustard Chicken w/ Bacon	1 sm	330	38	4	4
Sub Mesquite Chicken w/ Bacon	1 sm	330	38	4	4
Sub Prime Rib Cheesesteak	1 sm	360	40	4	4
Sub Prime Rib & Peppercorn	1 sm	380	46	3	5
Sub Steakhouse Beef Dip	1 sm	260	37	3	4
Sub The Traditional	1 sm	260	39	5	5
Sub Turkey Bacon Guacamole	1 sm	360	43	6	6
Sub Turkey Ranch & Swiss	1 sm	250	39	4	5
Sub Tuscan Turkey On Rosemary Parmesan	1 sm	300	47	5	4
Sub Veggie	1 sm	270	41	5	6
SOUPS					
Bread Bowl Chili	1 serv	730	104	7	8
Bread Bowl Country French	1 serv	720	100	7	5
Broccoli Cheese	1 cup	150	10	5	2
Chicken Noodle	1 cup	130	18	1	0
Chili	1 cup	140	12	4	4

FOOD	PORTION	CALS	CARB	SUGAR	FIBER
RANCH 1					
BEVERAGES					
Barq's Root Beer	1 sm (16 oz)	167	45	45	0
Coca-Cola	1 sm (16 oz)	150	40	40	0
Diet Coke	1 sm (16 oz)	2	0	0	0
Sprite	1 sm (16 oz)	150	40	40	0
CHILDREN'S MENU SELECTIONS					
Kids Meal Chicken Tenders	1 (2 oz)	111	9	0	0
Kids Meal Fries	1 serv (4 oz)	279	31	1	4
Kids Meal Popcorn Chicken	1 (2 oz)	112	10	0	0
MAIN MENU SELECTIONS					
Bowl Chicken Teriyaki	1 (19.3 oz)	504	78	10	1
Chicken Crispy	1 serv (5 oz)	326	22	1	1
Chicken Grilled	1 serv (3.9 oz)	146	0	0	0
Chicken On Mixed Greens	1 serv (21 oz)	340	17	9	7
Chicken Popcorn	1 serv (5.5 oz)	325	30	0	1
Chicken Tenders	1 serv (5.6 oz)	387	32	1	1
Fajita Mix Tomatoes Onion & Carrot	1 serv (3.2 oz)	20	5	3	1
Fajitas Chicken	1 serv (10 oz)	540	53	4	3
Fries	1 med	381	43	2	6
Fries Cheese	1 reg	493	54	2	6
Green Mix For Sandwiches	1 serv (2.5 oz)	31	2	1	1
Peppers & Onions	1 serv (1.6 oz)	27	3	2	1
Platter Chicken Rice	1 (10.9 oz)	273	28	4	3
Popcorn Chicken	1 sm	325	30	0	1
Rice	1 serv (4 oz)	97	21	0	0
Sandwich Chicken & Cheese	1 (11.2 oz)	389	39	5	2
Sandwich Chicken Philly	1 (9.2 oz)	410	40	4	2
Sandwich Crispy Chicken	1 (11.4 oz)	711	60	4	3
Sandwich Crispy Spicy Chicken	1 (11.4 oz)	543	68	7	3
Sandwich Grilled Spicy Chicken	1 (10.3 oz)	363	46	7	2
Sandwich Ranch 1 Classic	1 (9.4 oz)	683	37	3	2
Steamed Vegetables	1 serv (3 oz)	27	6	2	2
Wrap Grilled Chicken Caesar	1 (13.2 oz)	746	55	2	4
SALAD DRESSINGS AND SAUCES					
Dressing Balsamic Vinaigrette	1 oz	71	1	0	0
Dressing Classic Caesar	1 oz	103	1	0	0
Dressings Salad	1 oz	201	0	0	0
Sauce Ancho Chili Pepper	1 oz	134	1	1	0

FOOD	PORTION	CALS	CARB	SUGAR	FIBER
Sauce BBQ	1 oz	84	12	8	0
Sauce Honey Mustard	1 oz	110	9	6	0
Sauce Pepper & Onion Saute	1 oz	143	1	0	0
Sauce Teriyaki	1 oz	24	5	5	0
SALADS					
Caesar	1 (7 oz)	34	7	2	4
Caesar Grilled Chicken	1 (11.3 oz)	223	13	2	5
Crispy Chicken Club	1 (13.6 oz)	495	29	4	4
Mandarin Chicken	1 (14.5 oz)	553	62	19	14
Mixed Greens w/o Cheese	1 (17 oz)	194	17	9	7
Salad Blend	1 serv (10.3 oz)	45	9	4	5
Southwest Chicken Chop	1 (17.6 oz)	681	44	7	7
RED MANGO					
Blenders Blueberry Moon	1 cup	150	33	28	1
Blenders Captain Berry	1 cup	140	31	25	2
Blenders Green Tea Blueberry	1 cup	130	29	25	1
Blenders Green Tea Honeydew	1 cup	130	29	25	0
Blenders Mango Island	1 cup	150	31	26	1
Blenders Pina Colada	1 cup	160	30	25	1
Blenders Tri-Berry	1 cup	130	30	25	2
Blenders Watermelon Breeze	1 cup	130	29	25	0
Frozen Yogurt All Flavors	½ cup	90	19	15	0
RITA'S					
Cream Ice	1 reg	312	70	66	1
Cream Ice Kids	1 serv	193	44	40	0
Custard	1 reg	385	43	37	1
Custard Kids	1 serv	285	32	27	1
Gelati w/ Chocolate Custard	1 reg	351	60	55	1
Gelati w/ Vanilla Custard	1 reg	120	59	53	0
Gelati w/ Cream Ice w/ Chocolate Custard	1 reg	368	60	55	1
Gelati w/ Cream Ice w/ Vanilla Custard	1 reg	392	61	54	0
Ice	1 reg	263	69	67	0
Ice Kids	1 serv	165	43	42	0
Misto w/ Chocolate Custard	1 reg	409	90	85	1
Misto w/ Vanilla Custard	1 reg	420	90	85	0
Misto w/ Cream Ice w/ Chocolate Custard	1 reg	463	90	84	1

FOOD	PORTION	CALS	CARB	SUGAR	FIBER
Misto w/ Cream Ice w/ Vanilla Custard	1 reg	473	90	83	0
Sugar Free Gelati w/ Chocolate Custard	1 reg	268	45	22	1
Sugar Free Gelati w/ Vanilla Custard	1 reg	288	45	21	0
Sugar Free Ice	1 reg	160	39	0	0
Sugar Free Ice Kids	1 serv	63	24	0	0
Sugar Free Misto w/ Chocolate Custard	1 reg	233	56	13	1
Sugar Free Misto w/ Vanilla Custard	1 reg	245	57	12	0

ROBEKS
FREEZES AND SHAKES

FOOD	PORTION	CALS	CARB	SUGAR	FIBER
800 Lb Gorilla	12 oz	375	50	38	2
Freeze Lemon	12 oz	279	60	57	0
Freeze Orange	12 oz	242	56	49	1
Shake Bananasplit	12 oz	302	69	54	2
Shake P-Nut Power	12 oz	422	52	37	4

SMOOTHIES

FOOD	PORTION	CALS	CARB	SUGAR	FIBER
Acai Energizer	12 oz	167	36	31	2
Awesome Acai	12 oz	183	42	34	2
Banzai Blueberry	12 oz	175	38	34	3
Berry Brilliance	12 oz	194	45	40	2
Big Wednesday	12 oz	172	40	36	1
Cardio Cooler	12 oz	215	44	38	3
Citrus Stinger	12 oz	194	40	36	2
Cranberry Quest	12 oz	173	40	37	1
Dr. Robeks	12 oz	181	40	35	3
Guava Lava	12 oz	180	42	38	2
Hummingbird	12 oz	185	44	40	1
Infinite Orange	12 oz	181	42	36	3
Mahalo Mango	12 oz	174	42	39	1
Malibu Peach	12 oz	153	36	33	1
Outrageous Raspberry	12 oz	174	39	36	2
Passionfruit Cove	12 oz	168	38	35	1
Pina Koolada	12 oz	261	46	39	3
Polar Pineapple	12 oz	164	38	36	1
Pomegranate Passion	12 oz	196	48	44	1
Pomegranate Power	12 oz	211	50	46	1

FOOD	PORTION	CALS	CARB	SUGAR	FIBER
Pro Arobek	12 oz	265	54	43	3
Raspberry Romance	12 oz	172	42	35	2
Robeks MuscleMax	12 oz	202	38	32	2
Robeks Rejuvenator	12 oz	193	43	39	2
South Pacific Squeeze	12 oz	188	42	38	3
Strawnana Berry	12 oz	179	44	38	2
Venice Burner	12 oz	231	46	39	4
Zen Berry	12 oz	190	45	29	5

SALADWORKS
SALAD DRESSINGS

FOOD	PORTION	CALS	CARB	SUGAR	FIBER
Balsamic Vinaigrette	1 serv (2 oz)	192	9	9	0
Blue Cheese	1 serv (2 oz)	192	3	2	0
Creamy Italian	1 serv (2 oz)	232	5	4	0
Dijon Honey	1 serv	272	00	8	0
Fat Free Balsamic w/ Sundried Tomatoes	1 serv (2 oz)	28	2	1	0
French	1 serv (2 oz)	266	16	13	0
Herbal Ranch	1 serv (2 oz)	198	5	2	0
Italian Vinaigrette	1 serv (2 oz)	255	5	4	0
Lowfat Ranch	1 serv (2 oz)	34	4	2	0
Oriental Sesame	1 serv (2 oz)	147	21	19	0
Royal Caesar	1 serv (2 oz)	266	4	2	0
Russian	1 serv (2 oz)	221	8	5	0

SALADS

FOOD	PORTION	CALS	CARB	SUGAR	FIBER
B.L.T.	1 serv	262	9	4	4
Bently	1 serv	340	7	4	3
Caesar	1 serv	283	32	4	4
Caesar Chicken	1 serv	423	32	4	4
Caesar Shrimp	1 serv	350	32	4	4
Fiesta	1 serv	460	26	4	6
Garden	1 serv	58	12	5	5
Mandarin Chicken	1 serv	589	63	40	6
Newport	1 serv	184	8	3	4
Nicoise	1 serv	407	50	6	6
Spinach	1 serv	433	29	3	2
Tivoli	1 serv	563	50	6	5
Turkey Club	1 serv	720	90	8	6

FOOD	PORTION	CALS	CARB	SUGAR	FIBER
SAMURAI SAM'S					
BOWLS					
Low Carb	1 reg	230	16	9	5
Spicy Beef 'N Broccoli	1 reg	620	97	20	3
Spicy Beef 'N Broccoli Brown Rice	1 reg	580	85	19	7
Sumo Brown Rice	1	1022	111	28	9
Sumo White Rice	1	1083	128	28	3
Sweet & Sour Dark Chicken	1 reg	610	96	24	6
Sweet & Sour Dark Chicken Brown Rice	1 reg	570	84	24	9
Sweet & Sour White Chicken	1 reg	580	96	24	6
Sweet & Sour White Chicken Brown Rice	1 reg	540	85	24	9
Teriyaki Dark Chicken	1 reg	540	79	13	2
Teriyaki Dark Chicken Brown Rice	1 reg	500	68	11	12
Teriyaki Dark Chicken & Shrimp	1 reg	492	78	12	2
Teriyaki Dark Chicken & Shrimp Brown Rice	1 reg	451	67	12	5
Teriyaki Dark Chicken & Steak	1 reg	540	83	13	2
Teriyaki Dark Chicken & Steak Brown Rice	1 reg	490	71	13	5
Teriyaki Salmon	1 reg	643	121	20	3
Teriyaki Shrimp Brown Rice	1 reg	407	65	10	5
Teriyaki Steak	1 reg	530	86	13	2
Teriyaki Steak Brown Rice	1 reg	490	74	13	5
Teriyaki Steak & Shrimp	1 reg	483	77	12	2
Teriyaki Steak & Shrimp Brown Rice	1 reg	442	66	12	5
Teriyaki Veggie	1 reg	363	81	13	3
Teriyaki Veggie Brown Rice	1 reg	323	69	13	7
Teriyaki White Chicken	1 reg	520	79	13	2
Teriyaki White Chicken Brown Rice	1 reg	470	68	13	5
Teriyaki White Chicken & Shrimp	1 reg	478	78	12	2
Teriyaki White Chicken & Shrimp Brown Rice	1 reg	437	67	12	5
Teriyaki White Chicken & Steak	1 reg	520	83	13	2

FOOD	PORTION	CALS	CARB	SUGAR	FIBER
Teriyaki White Chicken & Steak Brown Rice	1 reg	480	71	13	5
Yakisoba Dark Chicken	1	842	114	24	6
Yakisoba Dark Chicken & Steak	1	825	113	25	6
Yakisoba Shrimp	1	677	110	21	6
Yakisoba Steak	1	809	112	26	6
Yakisoba Veggie	1	509	110	21	6
Yakisoba White Chicken	1	794	114	25	6
Yakisoba White Chicken & Steak	1	801	113	25	6
SALADS AND SIDES					
Crab Rangoon	1 serv	210	20	12	1
Dressing Chinese Ginger	1 serv (1 oz)	85	9	9	0
Dressing Oriental	1 serv (1 oz)	70	12	12	0
Egg Roll Grilled Chicken	1	150	17	7	1
Salad Oriental Chicken	1 serv	220	9	5	3
Salad Side	1	10	2	1	1
Salad Toss Sesame Chicken	1	490	57	33	8
Soup Asian Noodle	1 serv	89	14	6	1
Teriyaki Sauce	1 serv (1 oz)	40	9	8	0
WRAPS					
Teriyaki Dark Chicken	1	670	95	13	8
Teriyaki Dark Chicken Brown Rice	1	650	90	13	9
Teriyaki Steak	1	650	101	14	8
Teriyaki Steak Brown Rice	1	630	95	13	9
Teriyaki Veggie	1	510	94	12	8
Teriyaki Veggie Brown Rice	1	490	89	12	10
Teriyaki White Chicken	1	640	96	13	8
Teriyaki White Chicken Brown Rice	1	620	90	13	9
Teriyaki White Chicken & Steak	1	649	95	13	8
Teriyaki White Chicken & Steak Brown Rice	1	628	89	13	9

SBARRO
MAIN MENU SELECTIONS

FOOD	PORTION	CALS	CARB	SUGAR	FIBER
Baked Ziti w/ Sauce	1 serv (14 oz)	700	43	–	4
Calzone Cheese	1 (12 oz)	770	87	–	3
Chicken Francese	1 serv (11 oz)	640	8	–	2
Chicken Parmesan	1 serv (11 oz)	520	16	–	2
Chicken Portofino	1 serv (12 oz)	730	7	–	1

FOOD	PORTION	CALS	CARB	SUGAR	FIBER
Chicken Vesuvio	1 serv (11 oz)	690	8	—	1
Eggplant Rollatini w/ Cheese	1 serv (11 oz)	580	40	—	4
Garlic Roll	1 (2.2 oz)	170	28	—	tr
Meat Lasagna	1 serv (13 oz)	650	36	—	3
Meatballs	1 serv (3.7 oz)	140	10	—	1
Mixed Vegetables	1 serv (7 oz)	190	14	—	4
Penne w/ Sausage & Peppers	1 serv (14 oz)	710	33	—	4
Pizza Cheese	1 slice	460	60	—	3
Pizza Chicken Vegetable	1 slice	530	69	—	5
Pizza Fresh Tomato	1 slice	450	60	—	3
Pizza Mushroom	1 slice	460	62	—	4
Pizza Pepperoni	1 slice	730	61	—	3
Pizza Sausage	1 slice	670	60	—	3
Pizza Sauteed Spinach & Yellow Pepper	1 slice	670	86	—	5
Pizza Supreme	1 slice	630	63	—	3
Pizza White	1 slice	570	59	—	2
Pizza Gourmet Broccoli & Spinach	1 slice	720	88	—	6
Pizza Gourmet Cheese	1 slice	660	84	—	4
Pizza Gourmet Ham Pineapple & Bacon	1 slice	680	88	—	4
Pizza Gourmet Meat Delight	1 slice	780	84	—	4
Pizza Gourmet Mushroom	1 slice	610	85	—	5
Pizza Gourmet Mushroom & Spinach	1 slice	710	87	—	6
Pizza Gourmet Tomato & Basil	1 slice	700	87	—	5
Pizza Stuffed Pepperoni	1 slice	960	89	—	4
Pizza Stuffed Philly Cheesesteak	1 slice	830	94	—	5
Pizza Stuffed Spinach & Broccoli	1 slice	790	89	—	5
Sausage & Peppers	1 serv (10 oz)	410	19	—	4
Spaghetti w/ Chicken Francese	1 serv (15 oz)	800	64	—	5
Spaghetti w/ Chicken Parmesan	1 serv (15 oz)	930	75	—	6
Spaghetti w/ Chicken Vesuvio	1 serv (15 oz)	850	64	—	4
Spaghetti w/ Meatballs	1 serv (18 oz)	680	96	—	9
Spaghetti w/ Sauce	1 serv (20 oz)	820	120	—	10
Stromboli Pepperoni	1 (10 oz)	890	82	—	3
Stromboli Spinach Tomato Broccoli	1 (10 oz)	680	84	—	5

FOOD	PORTION	CALS	CARB	SUGAR	FIBER
SALADS					
Caesar	1 serv (8 oz)	80	6	–	1
Cucumber & Tomato	1 serv (8 oz)	130	9	–	2
Fruit Salad	1 serv (12 oz)	130	32	–	3
Greek	1 serv (8 oz)	60	3	–	tr
Mixed Garden	1 serv (8 oz)	35	7	–	3
Pasta Primavera	1 serv (8 oz)	190	21	–	2
Stringbean & Tomato	1 serv (8 oz)	100	9	–	2
SEASON 52					
CHILDREN'S MENU SELECTIONS					
Children's Chicken	1 serv	344	21	–	4
Children's Flatbread	1	468	50	–	1
Children's Pasta	1 serv	177	31	–	2
DESSERTS					
Boston Cream Pie	1 serv	188	30	–	0
Carrot Cake	1 serv	320	42	–	2
Chocolate & Peanut Butter Harlequin	1 serv	330	40	–	0
Fresh Spring Fruit	1 serv	35	8	–	3
Key Lime Pie	1 serv	283	37	–	0
Pecan Pie	1 serv	263	29	–	2
Sorbet w/ Fruit	1 serv	213	50	–	7
Strawberry Shortcake	1 serv	154	22	–	0
Strawberry Mango Cheesecake	1 serv	226	20	–	1
Toasted Almond Amaretto	1 serv	324	38	–	1
FLATBREADS					
Artichoke & Goat Cheese	1	469	59	–	4
Garlic Chicken	1	474	52	–	2
Parmesan Crispbread	1	363	50	–	1
Spicy Shrimp	1	474	61	–	3
Steak & Mushroom	1	474	52	–	2
Tomato	1	460	57	–	3
MAIN MENU SELECTIONS					
Appetizer Goat Cheese Ravioli	1 serv	473	39	–	2
Appetizer Grilled Artichokes	1 serv	185	32	–	10
Appetizer Grilled Asparagus	1 serv	186	17	–	5
Appetizer Roasted Potato Wedges	1 serv	333	68	–	6
Appetizer Shrimp Cocktail	1 serv	221	14	–	1

FOOD	PORTION	CALS	CARB	SUGAR	FIBER
Appetizer Shrimp Stuffed Mushrooms	1 serv	302	15	–	1
Appetizer Steak Skewers w/ Thai Salad	1 serv	438	39	–	6
Appetizer Steamed Mussels	1 serv	472	51	–	4
Cedar Salmon	1 serv	472	32	–	6
Chicken Boccone Pasta	1 serv	434	54	–	8
Chicken Breast	1 serv	403	31	–	5
Filet Mignon	1 serv	473	37	–	5
Grilled Rainbow Trout	1 serv	410	33	–	5
Grilled Scallops	1 serv	471	58	–	10
Pork Tenderloin	1 serv	392	23	–	4
Sandwich Chicken Breast	1	472	49	–	5
Sandwich Fresh Fish	1	437	55	–	6
Sandwich Grilled Steak	1	463	46	–	4
Sandwich Vegetable Stack	1	461	57	–	8
Shrimp Stuffed w/ Crab	1 serv	470	43	–	3
Soup Chicken Tortilla	1 serv (8 oz)	181	23	–	3
Soup Vegetable	1 serv (8 oz)	153	27	–	3
Spring Vegetable Plate	1 serv	465	74	–	17
Tuna w/o Soy Sauce	1 serv	175	13	–	2
Turkey Skewer	1 serv	404	41	–	5
Yellowfin Tuna	1 serv	466	49	–	10
SALADS					
Chicken Cobb	1 entree	474	19	–	4
Greek	1 entree	478	27	–	6
Mesclun Greens	1 side	315	37	–	3
Portobello & Romaine	1 entree	270	20	–	4
Salmon	1 entree	470	22	–	5
Spinach	1 side	272	19	–	4
Spring Greens	1 side	240	16	–	4
Tabbouleh	1 side	417	60	–	12
Tomato & Blue Cheese Stack	1 side	352	20	–	5
SIZZLER					
Grilled Salmon w/ Broccoli	1 serv	393	14	–	7
Hibachi Chicken w/ Broccoli	1 serv	290	15	–	6
Petite Steak w/ Broccoli	1 serv	520	11	–	6

FOOD	PORTION	CALS	CARB	SUGAR	FIBER
SOUPER SALAD					
BEVERAGES					
Lemonade	1 (24 oz)	190	49	46	0
Lemonade Mango	1 (24 oz)	220	58	55	0
Lemonade Raspberry	1 (24 oz)	220	58	54	0
Lemonade Strawberry	1 (24 oz)	220	57	53	0
Smoothie Mango	1 tall	250	64	62	0
Smoothie Peach	1 tall	230	62	60	0
Smoothie Raspberry	1 tall	230	62	58	0
Smoothie Strawberry	1 tall	230	60	55	0
DESSERTS					
Blueberry Bread	1 piece	150	29	13	1
Brownies	2 pieces	120	21	14	0
Cornbread	1 piece	170	30	9	1
Cottage Cheese	½ cup	90	5	4	0
Gingerbread	1 piece	180	30	14	1
Peaches	½ cup	70	17	13	0
Pineapple Tidbits	¼ cup	60	15	13	1
Pudding Banana	½ cup	160	26	19	0
Pudding Chocolate	½ cup	170	30	23	0
Soft Serve Cone Chocolate	1	120	22	16	0
Soft Serve Cone Vanilla	1	120	22	14	0
Sponge Cake	4 pieces	80	14	8	0
Strawberry Parfait	½ cup	100	19	18	0
Vanilla Wafers	4	70	13	6	0
Whipped Topping	½ cup	100	8	8	0
PASTA AND PIZZA					
Chicken Alfredo	1 cup	320	40	3	1
Macaroni & Cheese	1 cup	380	38	2	1
Pizza Slice Cheese	1	70	8	1	0
Pizza Slice Garden	1	80	9	1	1
Pizza Slice Pepperoni	1	90	8	1	0
Pizza Slice Sausage	1	80	9	1	1
Spaghetti & Meatballs	1 cup	280	38	2	4
SALAD DRESSINGS AND SAUCES					
Balsamic Vinegar	1 oz	60	15	15	0
Bleu Cheese	2 oz	220	1	1	0
Caesar	2 oz	280	4	4	0
Chipotle Ranch	2 oz	280	8	4	0
Fat Free French	2 oz	60	18	10	1

FOOD	PORTION	CALS	CARB	SUGAR	FIBER
Fat Free Italian w/ Cheese	2 oz	30	6	4	0
Green Goddess	2 oz	260	4	4	0
Honey Mustard	2 oz	240	2	1	0
Mayonnaise	2 tbsp	200	20	0	0
Olive Oil	1 oz	240	0	0	0
Peppercorn Ranch	2 oz	220	2	2	0
Pesto Basil	1 tbsp	45	0	0	0
Ranch	2 oz	220	2	2	0
Reduced Calorie Ranch	2 oz	120	3	2	0
Sauce Alfredo	1 ½ tbsp	45	2	1	0
Sauce Chipotle Pepper	¼ tsp	0	0	0	0
Sauce Cholula Hot	¼ tsp	0	0	0	0
Sauce Jalapeno Cheese	1 serv (2 oz)	35	5	0	1
Sauce Marinara	1 ½ tbsp	10	2	1	0
Sauce Meaty Marinara	1 ½ tbsp	40	2	1	0
Sauce Sriracha Hot	¼ tsp	0	0	0	0
Sour Cream Light	2 tbsp	40	3	2	0
Tangy Oriental	2 oz	160	10	8	0
Thousand Island	1 oz	300	6	4	0
Vinaigrette Cranberry	2 oz	100	24	20	0
Vinaigrette House	2 oz	220	4	4	0
SALADS					
Apple Walnut	1 cup	130	7	5	1
Asian Chicken	1 cup	80	10	7	2
Asian Shrimp	1 cup	100	13	7	2
Buffalo Chicken	1 cup	70	3	2	1
Caesar Chicken	1 cup	90	4	1	1
Caesar Chicken Salsa	1 cup	80	4	1	1
Caesar Shrimp	1 cup	90	3	1	1
California Chicken Salad	⅓ cup	80	4	3	0
Capri	1 cup	50	8	3	0
Chicago Chopped	1 cup	120	3	2	1
Chickpea	⅓ cup	110	11	1	4
Cobb	1 cup	100	2	2	1
Coleslaw Broccoli	⅓ cup	80	6	4	1
Edamame	⅓ cup	70	4	2	2
Fisherman's Kettle Shrimp & Crab	⅓ cup	120	15	9	1
Gazpacho	⅓ cup	30	3	2	1
Green Goddess Crab	1 cup	70	4	2	1

FOOD	PORTION	CALS	CARB	SUGAR	FIBER
Italian Antipasto	1 cup	70	3	2	1
Mango Berry	1 cup	110	13	11	1
Marinated Mushrooms	⅓ cup	60	1	0	0
Marinated Oriental Cucumber	⅓ cup	10	2	1	0
Marinated Tomato	1 cup	60	11	10	1
Melon Couscous	⅓ cup	50	10	4	1
Mustard Potato	⅓ cup	80	7	1	1
Paco's Taco	⅓ cup	100	12	1	2
Pasta De Garden	⅓ cup	80	8	1	0
Pasta Fettuccine	⅓ cup	100	11	1	1
Pasta Primavera	⅓ cup	45	4	1	0
Pasta Thai Chicken	⅓ cup	100	11	2	1
Pasta Tuna Skroodle	⅓ cup	130	10	1	1
Red Potato	⅓ cup	50	5	1	1
Rice Florentine	⅓ cup	90	11	0	0
Roasted Mushrooms & Artichokes w/ Feta Cheese	⅓ cup	40	3	1	1
Roasted Vegetables	⅓ cup	20	2	1	1
Salad Of The Sea	⅓ cup	50	6	1	0
Salmon Medley	1 cup	70	10	8	1
Santa Fe Corn	⅓ cup	100	13	2	3
Shrimp & Crab Louie	1 cup	130	5	2	1
Southwest Chicken Chipotle	1 cup	90	4	2	1
Sweet Garden Slaw	⅓ cup	35	4	3	1
Tropical Tuxedo	⅓ cup	60	7	2	0
Tuna Fish	⅓ cup	70	1	1	0
SOUPS					
Adobe Rice & Chicken	1 (5 oz)	100	10	2	1
Alaskan Salmon Chowder	1 (5 oz)	70	9	1	1
Beef Mushroom Barley	1 (5 oz)	80	11	1	2
Beef Noodle	1 (5 oz)	80	10	2	1
Beef Shellini	1 (5 oz)	90	11	3	1
Beef Stroganoff	1 (5 oz)	120	13	2	1
Black Bean	1 (5 oz)	80	20	2	11
Broccoli Cheese	1 (5 oz)	70	10	2	1
Cajun Gumbo	1 (5 oz)	110	13	1	1
Cauliflower Cheese	1 (5 oz)	70	11	2	1
Cheddar Chicken Broccoli Stew	1 (5 oz)	140	15	3	2
Cherokee Joe Cornbread	1 (5 oz)	70	13	5	2
Chicken Creole	1 (5 oz)	100	12	3	1

FOOD	PORTION	CALS	CARB	SUGAR	FIBER
Chicken Enchilada	1 (5 oz)	180	13	3	1
Chicken Gumbo	1 (5 oz)	90	10	2	1
Chicken Mushroom Barley	1 (5 oz)	80	9	2	1
Chicken Noodle	1 (5 oz)	80	9	2	1
Chicken Tetrazini	1 (5 oz)	120	13	2	1
Chicken Tortilla	1 (5 oz)	60	7	2	1
Cream Of Asparagus	1 (5 oz)	140	7	3	1
Cream Of Broccoli	1 (5 oz)	60	9	2	1
Cream Of Cauliflower	1 (5 oz)	60	10	2	1
Cream Of Chicken	1 (5 oz)	100	9	2	1
Cream Of Mushroom	1 (5 oz)	80	10	1	1
Holiday Harvest	1 (5 oz)	90	5	1	0
Vegan Split Pea	1 (5 oz)	90	16	2	5
Vegetable Beef	1 (5 oz)	80	11	3	2
Vegetable Cheese	1 (5 oz)	80	12	2	1
Vegetable Lentil	1 (5 oz)	70	16	2	5
Vegetarian Butter Bean	1 (5 oz)	70	21	2	10
Vegetarian Vegetable	1 (5 oz)	50	11	2	2

SOUTHERN TSUNAMI SUSHI BAR
SALADS

FOOD	PORTION	CALS	CARB	SUGAR	FIBER
Calamari	1 serv (4 oz)	148	22	8	1
Edamame	1 serv (4 oz)	124	9	7	1
Harusame	1 serv (5 oz)	148	33	8	0
Seabreeze	1 serv (4 oz)	113	23	23	0

SUSHI

FOOD	PORTION	CALS	CARB	SUGAR	FIBER
California Roll	1 (0.8 oz)	31	6	1	tr
Cream Cheese Roll w/ Salmon	1 piece (0.8 oz)	43	5	1	tr
Crunchy Shrimp Roll	1 piece (0.9 oz)	42	5	1	tr
Dragon Roll	1 piece (0.8 oz)	42	6	1	1
Freshwater Eel Roll	1 piece (0.8 oz)	41	5	1	tr
Green Horseradish	1 tsp	7	1	0	0
Inari	1 piece (1.9 oz)	105	18	2	0
Nigiri Cuttlefish	1 piece (1 oz)	42	9	1	0
Nigiri Egg Cake	1 piece (1.4 oz)	73	13	5	0
Nigiri Fish Roe	1 piece (1.4 oz)	61	9	1	0
Nigiri Fresh Salmon	1 piece (1.3 oz)	68	9	1	0
Nigiri Fresh Water Eel	1 piece (1.6 oz)	108	11	2	0
Nigiri Octopus	1 piece (1.1 oz)	57	9	1	0
Nigiri Sea Eel	1 piece (1.6 oz)	90	11	2	0
Nigiri Shrimp	1 piece (1.1 oz)	44	8	1	0

FOOD	PORTION	CALS	CARB	SUGAR	FIBER
Nigiri Smoked Salmon	1 piece (1.3 oz)	68	9	1	0
Nigiri Tilapia	1 piece (1.2 oz)	49	8	1	0
Nigiri Tuna	1 piece (1.3 oz)	60	8	1	0
Nigiri Yellowtail	1 piece (1.2 oz)	54	8	1	0
Ocean Crab Roll	1 piece (0.8 oz)	33	5	1	tr
Orange Roll	1 piece (0.8 oz)	32	6	1	tr
Pickled Ginger	1 tbsp	9	2	1	0
Rainbow Roll	1 piece (1 oz)	41	6	1	tr
Sea Eel Roll	1 piece (0.8 oz)	36	6	1	tr
Soy Sauce	1 pkg	16	2	0	0
Spicy Roll Salmon	1 piece (0.8 oz)	40	5	1	tr
Spicy Roll Shrimp	1 piece (0.8 oz)	31	5	1	tr
Spicy Roll Tuna	1 piece (0.8 oz)	37	5	1	tr
Tempura Roll	1 piece (0.9 oz)	44	7	2	tr
Tofu Roll	1 piece (0.8 oz)	27	5	1	tr
Tsunami Roll Crab & Fish Roe	1 piece (0.8 oz)	39	6	1	tr

STARBUCKS
BAKED SELECTIONS

FOOD	PORTION	CALS	CARB	SUGAR	FIBER
Apple Fritter	1	480	64	27	1
Bagel French Toast	1	280	62	10	2
Bagel Multigrain	1	280	60	12	4
Bagel Plain	1	280	62	8	2
Bar Cranberry Bliss	1	320	41	28	1
Bar Toffee Almond	1	400	53	34	1
Brownie Espresso	1	340	40	27	2
Cinnamon Roll	1	470	56	29	1
Cocoa Crispy Square	1	420	66	30	1
Cookie Chocolate Chunk	1	420	56	28	6
Cookie Coffee Ginger	1	470	70	40	3
Cookie Penguin	1	370	50	31	tr
Cookie Rainbow	1	420	61	33	1
Cookies Mini Black & White	2	240	32	22	1
Croissant Butter	1	370	35	4	3
Dougnut Glazed	1	490	65	39	1
Loaf Banana Nut	1 serv	470	56	32	2
Loaf Iced Lemon	1 serv	500	78	53	1
Loaf Marble	1 serv	410	52	31	tr
Loaf Pumpkin	1 serv	380	59	36	2
Mallorca Sweet Bread	1	420	43	14	2
Muffin Blueberry	1	310	55	31	1

FOOD	PORTION	CALS	CARB	SUGAR	FIBER
Muffin Pumpkin Cream Cheese	1	490	63	42	1
Muffin Reduced Fat Chocolate	1	290	53	31	2
Muffin Walnut Bran	1	430	62	26	4
Reduced Fat Coffee Cake Banana Chocolate Chip	1	390	76	50	3
Reduced Fat Coffee Cake Blueberry	1 serv	320	54	33	1
Reduced Fat Coffee Cake Cinnamon Swirl	1 serv	290	52	33	1
Reduced Fat Coffee Cake Pumpkin Chocolate Chip	1	300	58	36	3
Rustic Apple Tart	1	190	37	30	3
Scone Blueberry	1	480	64	24	2
Scone Cran Apple Crumb	1	490	74	30	4
Scone Raspberry	1	470	64	25	2
BEVERAGES					
Apple Juice	1 grande	250	64	57	0
Cafe Americano	1 grande	15	3	0	0
Cafe Au Lait Nonfat Milk	1 grande	70	10	10	0
Caffe Mocha No Whip Nonfat Milk	1 grande	220	42	32	2
Caffe Mocha Whip Nonfat Milk	1 grande	290	44	34	2
Cappuccino Nonfat Milk	1 grande	80	12	10	0
Caramel Macchiato Nonfat Milk	1 grande	190	35	32	0
Caramel Apple Cider Whip	1 grande	380	76	68	0
Caramel Apple Spice No Whip	1 grande	310	74	66	0
Chocolate Milk Nonfat	1 grande	280	53	45	2
Cinnamon Dolce Creme No Whip Nonfat Milk	1 grande	220	41	41	0
Cinnamon Dolce Whip Nonfat Milk	1 grande	290	43	43	0
Coffee Of The Week	1 grande	5	0	0	0
Coffee Of The Week Decaf	1 grande	5	0	0	0
Frappuccino Blended Coffee Cafe Vanilla Whip Nonfat Milk	1 grande	430	70	60	0
Frappuccino Blended Coffee Cafe Vanilla Whip Soy	1 grande	430	70	60	0
Frappuccino Blended Coffee Cafe Vanilla No Whip Soy	1 grande	310	67	58	0

FOOD	PORTION	CALS	CARB	SUGAR	FIBER
Frappuccino Blended Coffee Caffe Vanilla No Whip Nonfat Milk	1 grande	310	67	58	0
Frappuccino Blended Coffee Caramel No Whip Nonfat Milk	1 grande	270	53	45	0
Frappuccino Blended Coffee Caramel No Whip Soy	1 grande	270	53	45	0
Frappuccino Blended Coffee Caramel Whip Soy	1 grande	380	57	48	0
Frappuccino Blended Coffee Cinnamon Dolce No Whip Nonfat Milk	1 grande	260	52	45	0
Frappuccino Blended Coffee Cinnamon Dolce No Whip Soy	1 grande	260	52	45	0
Frappuccino Blended Coffee Cinnamon Dolce Whip Soy	1 grande	370	55	47	0
Frappuccino Blended Coffee Coffee Whip Nonfat Milk	1 grande	380	57	48	0
Frappuccino Blended Coffee Espresso Nonfat Milk	1 grande	190	38	31	0
Frappuccino Blended Coffee Java Chip No Whip Nonfat Milk	1 grande	340	64	52	2
Frappuccino Blended Coffee Java Chip No Whip Soy	1 grande	190	38	31	0
Frappuccino Blended Coffee Java Chip Whip Nonfat Milk	1 grande	460	67	55	2
Frappuccino Blended Coffee Java Chip Whip Soy	1 grande	460	67	55	2
Frappuccino Blended Coffee Mocha No Whip Nonfat Milk	1 grande	260	54	45	0
Frappuccino Blended Coffee Mocha No Whip Soy	1 grande	260	54	45	0
Frappuccino Blended Coffee Mocha Whip Nonfat Milk	1 grande	380	57	47	0
Frappuccino Blended Coffee Pumpkin Spice No Whip Nonfat Milk	1 grande	290	59	51	0
Frappuccino Blended Coffee Pumpkin Spice No Whip Soy	1 grande	290	59	51	0

FOOD	PORTION	CALS	CARB	SUGAR	FIBER
Frappuccino Blended Coffee Pumpkin Spice Whip Nonfat Milk	1 grande	400	62	53	0
Frappuccino Blended Coffee Pumpkin Spice Whip Soy	1 grande	400	62	53	0
Frappuccino Blended Coffee Whip Nonfat Milk	1 grande	370	55	47	0
Frappuccino Blended Coffee White Chocolate Mocha No Whip Nonfat Milk	1 grande	300	59	51	0
Frappuccino Blended Coffee White Chocolate Mocha No Whip Soy	1 grande	300	59	51	0
Frappuccino Blended Coffee White Chocolate Mocha Whip Nonfat Milk	1 grande	410	62	54	0
Frappuccino Blended Coffee White Chocolate Mocha Whip Soy	1 grande	410	62	54	0
Frappuccino Blended Creme Tazo Chai No Whip Nonfat Milk	1 grande	330	67	56	0
Frappuccino Blended Creme Tazo Chai Whip Nonfat Milk	1 grande	570	95	83	1
Frappuccino Blended Creme Vanilla Bean No Whip Nonfat Milk	1 grande	350	72	60	0
Frappuccino Blended Creme Vanilla Bean Whip Nonfat Milk	1 grande	470	75	62	0
Frappuccino Light Blended Coffee Cafe Vanilla Nonfat Milk	1 grande	190	42	32	3
Frappuccino Light Blended Coffee Caramel	1 grande	160	30	21	3
Frappuccino Light Blended Coffee Cinnamon Dolce Nonfat Milk	1 grande	140	29	21	3
Frappuccino Light Blended Coffee Java Chip Nonfat Milk	1 grande	200	36	24	4
Frappuccino Light Blended Coffee Mocha Nonfat Milk	1 grande	140	29	19	3

FOOD	PORTION	CALS	CARB	SUGAR	FIBER
Frappuccino Light Blended Coffee Nonfat Milk	1 grande	130	25	16	3
Frappuccino Light Blended Coffee Pumpkin Spice Nonfat Milk	1 grande	150	31	22	3
Frappuccino Light Blended Creme Double Chocolaty Chip Whip Nonfat Milk	1 grande	510	78	59	2
Frappuccino Light Blended Creme Pumpkin Spice No Whip Nonfat Milk	1 grande	360	71	61	0
Frappuccino Light Blended Creme Pumpkin Spice Whip Nonfat Milk	1 grande	470	74	63	0
Frappuccino Light Blended Creme Tazo Green Tea No Whip Nonfat Milk	1 grande	380	78	67	1
Frappuccino Light Blended Creme Tazo Green Tea Whip Nonfat Milk	1 grande	440	71	59	0
Frappuccino Light Blended Creme Tazo Green Tea Whip Nonfat Milk	1 grande	490	82	69	1
Frappuccino Light Blended Creme White Chocolate No Whip Nonfat Milk	1 grande	480	89	77	0
Frappuccino Light Blended Creme White Chocolate Whip Nonfat Milk	1 grande	610	92	79	0
Frappuccino Light Espresso Nonfat Milk	1 grande	110	20	12	2
Hot Chocolate No Whip Nonfat Milk	1 grande	240	48	40	2
Hot Chocolate Whip Nonfat Milk	1 grande	320	50	41	2
Iced Brewed Coffee	1 grande	90	21	20	0
Iced Cafe Mocha Whip Nonfat Milk	1 grande	290	39	29	2
Iced Caffe Americano	1 grande	15	3	0	0
Iced Caffe Latte Nonfat Milk	1 grande	90	13	11	0

FOOD	PORTION	CALS	CARB	SUGAR	FIBER
Iced Caffe Mocha No Whip Nonfat Milk	1 grande	170	36	26	2
Iced Caramel Macchiato Nonfat Milk	1 grande	190	34	31	0
Iced Latte Pumpkin Spice No Whip Nonfat Milk	1 grande	220	44	42	0
Iced Latte Pumpkin Spice Whip Nonfat Milk	1 grande	330	48	44	0
Iced Latte Skinny Cinnamon Dolce No Whip Nonfat Milk	1 grande	80	12	10	0
Iced Latte Sugar Free Flavored Syrup Nonfat Milk	1 grande	80	12	10	0
Iced Latte Syrup Flavored Nonfat Milk	1 grande	160	31	28	0
Iced Latte Vanilla Nonfat Milk	1 grande	160	31	28	0
Iced Peppermint White Chocolate Mocha No Whip Nonfat Milk	1 grande	370	72	68	0
Iced Peppermint White Chocolate Mocha Whip Nonfat Milk	1 grande	490	75	71	0
Iced Tazo Latte Black Tea Nonfat Milk	1 grande	170	35	34	0
Iced Tazo Latte Black Tea Soy	1 grande	200	38	34	1
Iced Tazo Latte Chai Nonfat Milk	1 grande	200	44	42	0
Iced Tazo Latte Green Tea Nonfat Milk	1 grande	220	45	43	1
Iced Tazo Latte Green Tea Soy	1 grande	260	48	44	2
Iced Tazo Latte Red Tea	1 grande	200	38	34	1
Iced Tazo Latte Red Tea Nonfat Milk	1 grande	170	35	34	0
Iced White Chocolate Mocha No Whip Nonfat Milk	1 grande	310	55	52	0
Iced White Chocolate Mocha Whip Nonfat Milk	1 grande	430	59	55	0
Latte Caffe Nonfat Milk	1 grande	130	19	18	0
Latte Cinnamon Dolce No Whip Nonfat Milk	1 grande	210	41	39	0
Latte Cinnamon Dolce w/ Sugar Free Syrup Nonfat Milk	1 grande	130	19	17	0

FOOD	PORTION	CALS	CARB	SUGAR	FIBER
Latte Cinnamon Dolce Whip Nonfat Milk	1 grande	280	43	40	0
Latte Pumpkin Spice No Whip Nonfat Milk	1 grande	260	50	48	0
Latte Pumpkin Spice Whip Nonfat Milk	1 grande	330	52	50	0
Latte Skinny Caramel No Whip Nonfat Milk	1 grande	130	19	17	0
Latte Skinny Cinnamon Dolce No Whip Nonfat Milk	1 grande	130	19	17	0
Latte Skinny Cinnamon Dolce No Whip Nonfat Milk	1 grande	130	19	17	0
Latte Skinny Hazelnut No Whip Nonfat Milk	1 grande	130	19	17	0
Latte Skinny Vanilla No Whip Nonfat Milk	1 grande	130	19	17	0
Latte Syrup Flavored Nonfat Milk	1 grande	200	37	35	0
Milk Nonfat	1 grande	180	26	26	0
Peppermint White Chocolate Mocha No Whip Nonfat Milk	1 grande	420	78	75	0
Peppermint White Chocolate Mocha Whip Nonfat Milk	1 grande	490	80	76	0
Pumpkin Spice Creme No Whip Nonfat Milk	1 grande	270	51	51	0
Pumpkin Spice Creme Whip Nonfat Milk	1 grande	340	53	52	0
Shaken Black Iced Tea & Lemonade	1 grande	130	33	33	0
Shaken White Iced Tea Blueberry	1 grande	80	21	20	0
Steamed Apple Juice	1 grande	230	56	50	0
Tazo Black Shaken Iced Tea & Lemonade	1 grande	130	33	33	0
Tazo Chai Latte Iced Tea Soy	1 grande	230	47	43	1
Tazo Chai Latte Nonfat Milk	1 grande	200	44	42	0
Tazo Chai Latte Soy	1 grande	230	47	42	1
Tazo Latte Black Tea Soy	1 grande	190	36	32	1
Tazo Latte Black Tea Nonfat Milk	1 grande	170	34	32	0

FOOD	PORTION	CALS	CARB	SUGAR	FIBER
Tazo Latte Green Tea Nonfat Milk	1 grande	200	42	41	1
Tazo Latte Green Tea Soy	1 grande	220	44	40	2
Tazo Latte Red Tea Nonfat Milk	1 grande	170	34	32	0
Tazo Latte Red Tea Soy	1 grande	190	36	32	1
Tazo Shaken Iced Tea Green	1 grande	80	21	20	0
Tazo Shaken Iced Tea Green & Lemonade	1 grande	130	33	33	0
Tazo Shaken Iced Tea Orange Passion	1 grande	70	19	18	0
Tazo Shaken Iced Tea Passion	1 grande	80	21	20	0
Tazo Shaken Iced Tea Passion & Lemonade	1 grande	130	33	33	0
Tazo Tea	1 grande	0	0	0	0
Vanilla Creme Whip Nonfat Milk	1 grande	270	39	38	0
Vanilla Creme No Whip Nonfat Milk	1 grande	200	37	37	0
Vivanno Blend Banana Chocolate	1 grande (20 oz)	85	44	28	6
Vivanno Blend Organe Mango Banana	1 grande (20 oz)	250	47	32	5
White Chocolate Mocha No Whip Nonfat Milk	1 grande	360	62	61	0
White Chocolate Mocha Whip Nonfat Milk	1 grande	430	64	62	0
SALADS					
Fiesta	1 (9.4 oz)	320	44	12	8
Fruit & Cheese Plate	1 (8.6 oz)	400	44	26	2
Vegetable Vinaigrette	1 (10.7 oz)	310	40	8	10
SANDWICHES					
Club Chicken Cheddar Bacon w/ Mayo	1	480	48	8	2
Club Turkey & Avocado	1	390	33	5	7
Egg Salad On Multigrain	1	470	53	11	2
Turkey & Swiss w/ Mayo	1	310	26	3	2
TOPPINGS					
Caramel	1 tbsp	15	2	2	0
Chocolate	1 tsp	5	1	1	0
Flavored Sugar Free Syrup	1 pump	0	0	0	0
Flavored Syrup	1 pump	20	5	5	0

FOOD	PORTION	CALS	CARB	SUGAR	FIBER
Mocha Syrup	1 pump	25	5	4	0
Sprinkles	1 serv	0	0	0	0

SUBWAY
ADD-ONS AND SALAD DRESSINGS

FOOD	PORTION	CALS	CARB	SUGAR	FIBER
American Cheese	1 serv (0.4 oz)	40	1	0	0
Bacon Strips	2	45	0	0	0
Banana Pepper Slices	3	0	0	0	0
Cheddar	1 serv (0.5 oz)	60	0	0	0
Fat Free Italian	1 serv (2 oz)	35	7	4	0
Fat Free Red Wine Vinaigrette	1 serv (0.7 oz)	30	6	3	0
Jalapeno Pepper Slices	3	<5	0	0	0
Mayonnaise	1 tbsp	110	0	0	0
Mayonnaise Light	1 tbsp	50	tr	0	0
Monterey Cheddar Shredded	1 serv (0.5 oz)	50	1	0	0
Mustard Yellow or Deli	2 tsp	5	tr	0	0
Olive Oil Blend	1 tsp	45	0	0	0
Pepperjack Cheese	1 serv (0.5 oz)	50	0	0	0
Provolone	1 serv (0.5 oz)	50	0	0	0
Ranch	1 serv (2 oz)	320	3	2	0
Red Wine Vinaigrette	1 serv (2 oz)	80	17	7	0
Sauce Chipotle Southwest	1.5 tbsp	100	1	1	0
Sauce Fat Free Honey Mustard	1.5 tbsp	30	7	6	0
Sauce Fat Free Sweet Onion	1.5 tbsp	40	9	8	0
Swiss	1 serv (0.5 oz)	50	0	0	0
Vinegar	1 tsp	0	0	0	0

BREADS

FOOD	PORTION	CALS	CARB	SUGAR	FIBER
Hearty Italian	6 inch	220	41	5	2
Honey Oat	6 inch	250	48	9	5
Italian	6 inch	200	38	5	1
Italian Herb & Cheese	6 inch	250	40	5	2
Italian White	1 mini	140	26	3	1
Monterey Cheddar	6 inch	240	39	5	1
Parmesan Oregano Bread	6 inch	220	40	5	2
Wheat	1 mini	140	27	3	2
Wheat	6 inch	200	40	5	4
Wrap	1	190	33	1	1

DESSERTS

FOOD	PORTION	CALS	CARB	SUGAR	FIBER
Apple Slices	1 pkg	35	9	7	2
Cookie Chocolate Chip	1	210	30	18	1

FOOD	PORTION	CALS	CARB	SUGAR	FIBER
Cookie Chocolate Chip w/ M&M's	1 (1.6 oz)	210	32	18	tr
Cookie Chocolate Chunk	1	220	30	17	tr
Cookie Double Chocolate Chip	1 (1.6 oz)	210	30	20	1
Cookie Oatmeal Raisin	1	200	30	17	1
Cookie Peanut Butter	1	220	26	16	1
Cookie Sugar	1	220	28	14	tr
Cookie White Chip Macadamia Nut	1	220	29	18	tr
Raisins	1 pkg	150	33	30	2
SALADS					
Ham w/o Dressing & Croutons	1 serv	120	14	6	4
Oven Roasted Chicken Breast w/o Dressing & Croutons	1 serv	140	11	5	4
Roast Beef w/o Dressing & Croutons	1 serv	120	12	6	4
Subway Club w/o Dressing & Croutons	1 serv	150	14	7	4
Sweet Onion Chicken Teriyaki w/o Dressing & Croutons	1 serv	210	26	17	4
Turkey Breast	1 serv	110	13	6	4
Turkey Breast & Ham w/o Dressing & Croutons	1 serv	120	14	6	4
Veggie Delight w/o Dressing & Croutons	1 serv	60	11	5	4
SANDWICHES					
6 Inch Chicken & Bacon Ranch	1	580	47	7	6
6 Inch Cold Cut Combo	1	410	47	8	5
6 Inch Double Stacked Cold Cut Combo	1	550	49	8	5
6 Inch Double Stacked Italian BMT	1	630	49	10	5
6 Inch Double Stacked Steak & Cheese	1	540	49	12	7
6 Inch Double Stacked Subway Club	1	420	50	10	5
6 Inch Double Stacked Sweet Onion Chicken Teriyaki	1	480	65	23	6
6 Inch Double Stacked Turkey Breast	1	330	48	8	5

FOOD	PORTION	CALS	CARB	SUGAR	FIBER
6 Inch Ham	1	290	47	8	5
6 Inch Italian BMT	1	450	47	8	5
6 Inch Meatball Marinara	1	560	63	13	8
6 Inch Oven Roasted Chicken Breast	1	310	48	9	6
6 Inch Roast Beef	1	290	45	8	5
6 Inch Spicy Italian	1	480	45	8	5
6 Inch Steak & Cheese	1	400	48	9	6
6 Inch Subway Club	1	320	47	8	5
6 Inch Subway Melt	1	380	48	8	5
6 Inch Sweet Onion Chicken Teriyaki	1	370	59	19	5
6 Inch Tuna	1	530	44	7	5
6 Inch Turkey Breast	1	280	46	7	5
6 Inch Turkey Breast & Ham	1	290	47	8	5
6 Inch Veggie Delite	1	230	44	7	5
Mini Sub Ham	1	180	30	5	4
Mini Sub Roast Beef	1	190	30	5	4
Mini Sub Tuna w/ Cheese	1	320	30	5	4
Mini Sub Turkey Breast	1	190	30	5	4
Softwich Santa Fe Turkey	1	520	78	17	5

TACO BELL

FOOD	PORTION	CALS	CARB	SUGAR	FIBER
Border Bowl Southwest Steak	1 serv	600	68	3	9
Border Bowl Zesty Chicken	1 serv	640	60	4	10
Border Bowl Zesty Chicken w/o Dressing	1 serv	440	57	3	10
Burrito 7 Layer	1	490	65	5	9
Burrito Bean	1	350	54	4	8
Burrito Chili Cheese	1	370	40	3	3
Burrito Grilled Stuft Chicken	1	640	73	6	7
Burrito Grilled Stuft Steak	1	630	72	5	7
Burrito Supreme Beef	1	420	51	5	7
Burrito ½ Lb Beef & Potato	1	530	68	4	6
Burrito ½ Lb Combo Beef	1	440	51	4	8
Burrito Fiesta Chicken	1	360	47	4	3
Burrito Fiesta Steak	1	370	49	4	4
Burrito Supreme Chicken	1	400	49	5	6
Burrito Supreme Steak	1	390	49	5	6
Chalupa Baja Beef	1	410	30	4	4
Chalupa Baja Chicken	1	390	29	4	3

FOOD	PORTION	CALS	CARB	SUGAR	FIBER
Chalupa Baja Steak	1	390	28	3	3
Chalupa Nacho Cheese Beef	1	370	32	4	3
Chalupa Nacho Cheese Chicken	1	360	30	4	2
Chalupa Nacho Cheese Steak	1	340	30	4	2
Chalupa Supreme Beef	1	380	30	4	3
Chalupa Supreme Chicken	1	360	29	4	2
Chalupa Supreme Steak	1	360	28	4	2
Cheesy Fiesta Potatoes	1 serv	290	29	2	2
Cinnamon Twists	1 serv	170	26	12	1
Crunchwrap Supreme	1	560	68	7	5
Crunchwrap Supreme Spicy Chicken	1	540	67	7	4
Crunchy Taco	1	170	13	1	3
Crunchy Taco Supreme	1	210	15	2	3
Empanada Caramel Apple	1	290	37	13	1
Enchirito Beef	1	360	34	3	7
Enchirito Chicken	1	340	33	3	6
Fresco Border Bowl Zesty Chicken w/o Dressing	1 serv	350	51	4	10
Fresco Burrito Bean	1	330	54	4	9
Fresco Burrito Fiesta Chicken	1	330	48	4	3
Fresco Burrito Supreme Chicken	1	330	49	5	7
Fresco Burrito Supreme Steak	1	330	48	5	7
Fresco Crunchy Taco	1	150	13	1	3
Fresco Soft Taco Beef	1	180	21	2	3
Fresco Soft Taco Grilled Steak	1	160	20	3	2
Fresco Soft Taco Ranchero Chicken	1	170	21	3	3
Gordita Baja Beef	1	340	29	8	4
Gordita Baja Chicken	1	320	28	6	3
Gordita Baja Steak	1	320	27	5	3
Gordita Nacho Cheese Beef	1	300	31	6	3
Gordita Nacho Cheese Chicken	1	280	29	6	2
Gordita Nacho Cheese Steak	1	270	29	6	2
Gordita Supreme Beef	1	310	29	6	3
Gordita Supreme Chicken	1	290	28	6	2
Gordita Supreme Steak	1	290	28	6	2
Guacamole Side	1 serv	70	5	1	2
Mexican Pizza	1	530	46	3	6

FOOD	PORTION	CALS	CARB	SUGAR	FIBER
Mexican Rice	1 serv	180	23	0	1
MexiMelt	1 serv	260	22	2	3
Nacho Supreme	1 serv	440	41	3	7
Nachos	1 serv	330	32	3	2
Nachos Bellgrande	1 serv	770	77	5	12
Pintos 'n Cheese	1 serv	160	19	1	7
Quesadilla Cheese	1	470	39	4	2
Quesadilla Chicken	1	520	40	4	3
Quesadilla Steak	1	520	39	4	3
Salsa Side	1 serv	15	3	2	0
Soft Taco Grande	1	430	43	5	5
Soft Taco Grilled Steak	1	270	20	3	2
Soft Taco Ranchero Chicken	1	270	21	3	2
Soft Taco Supreme Beef	1	250	23	3	3
Sour Cream Side	1 serv	80	3	2	0
Taco Double Decker	1	320	38	2	6
Taco Double Decker Supreme	1	370	40	4	7
Taco Spicy Chicken	1	170	20	2	2
Taco Salad Express	1	610	56	8	14
Taco Salad Fiesta	1	840	80	10	15
Taco Salad Fiesta Chicken	1	790	77	10	13
Taco Salad Fiesta Chicken w/o Shell	1	430	38	9	11
Taco Salad w/o Shell Fiesta	1	470	41	9	13
Taquitos Grilled Chicken	1 serv	310	37	3	2
Taquitos Steak Grilled	1 serv	310	36	3	2
Tostada	1	240	27	2	7

TACO BUENO
MAIN MENU SELECTIONS

FOOD	PORTION	CALS	CARB	SUGAR	FIBER
Bueno Chilada Beef	1 (7.9 oz)	523	42	6	2
Bueno Chilada Beef w/o Chili	1 (5.5 oz)	412	29	6	1
Bueno Chilada Beef w/o Queso	1 (5.6 oz)	337	36	2	2
Bueno Chilada Chicken	1 (7.4 oz)	477	43	7	2
Bueno Chilada Chicken w/o Chili	1 (5 oz)	366	30	6	1
Bueno Chilada Chicken w/o Queso	1 (5.1 oz)	290	30	2	2
Burrito Bean	1 (6.4 oz)	490	45	1	5
Burrito Bean w/o Cheddar Cheese	1 (5.9 oz)	412	44	1	5

FOOD	PORTION	CALS	CARB	SUGAR	FIBER
Burrito Bean w/o Chili	1 (5.2 oz)	434	39	1	4
Burrito Beef	1 (6.9 oz)	510	41	1	3
Burrito Beef Potato	1 (4.8 oz)	350	32	3	3
Burrito Beef Potato w/o Queso	1 (4.1 oz)	305	30	1	3
Burrito Beef Potato w/o Sour Cream	1 (4.3 oz)	330	31	2	3
Burrito Beef w/o Cheddar Cheese	1 (6.4 oz)	432	40	1	3
Burrito Beef w/o Chili	1 (5.7 oz)	455	36	1	2
Burrito Big Ol' Beef	1 (10.6 oz)	772	57	2	3
Burrito Big Ol' Beef w/o Cheddar Cheese	1 (9.6 oz)	615	56	2	3
Burrito Big Ol' Beef w/o Chili	1 (9.4 oz)	716	51	2	2
Burrito Big Ol' Beef w/o Sour Cream	1 (9.6 oz)	715	55	1	3
Burrito Big Ol' Chicken	1 (8.4 oz)	607	53	3	5
Burrito Big Ol' Chicken w/o Cheddar Cheese	1 (7.4 oz)	450	52	3	2
Burrito Big Ol' Chicken w/o Sour Cream	1 (7.4 oz)	551	51	2	2
Burrito Chicken Potato	1 (4.5 oz)	327	33	3	3
Burrito Chicken Potato w/o Queso	1 (3.8 oz)	274	31	2	3
Burrito Chicken Potato w/o Sour Cream	1 (4 oz)	299	32	2	3
Burrito Combination	1 (6.8 oz)	507	43	1	4
Burrito Combination w/o Cheddar Cheese	1 (6.3 oz)	429	42	1	4
Burrito Combination w/o Chili	1 (5.6 oz)	452	37	1	3
Burrito Combination w/o Refried Beans	1 (5.7 oz)	440	40	1	3
Burrito Party	1 (4 oz)	298	29	1	3
Burrito Party w/o Cheddar Cheese	1 (3.8 oz)	259	29	1	3
Chimichanger Cheesecake	1 (2 oz)	210	24	4	1
Cinnamon Chips	1 serv (4.5 oz)	676	95	54	4
Corn Tortilla Chips	1 serv (1.5 oz)	219	27	1	4
Guacamole	1 serv (0.9 oz)	55	2	0	1
Jalapenos	1 serv (0.7 oz)	3	1	0	1
Mexican Rice	1 serv (4.2 oz)	469	83	4	2

FOOD	PORTION	CALS	CARB	SUGAR	FIBER
Muchaco Beef	1 (5.2 oz)	449	40	2	3
Muchaco Beef w/o Cheddar Cheese	1 (4.9 oz)	410	40	2	3
Muchaco Beef w/o Refried Beans	1 (4.2 oz)	392	38	2	2
Muchaco Chicken	1 (4.6 oz)	387	40	2	2
Muchaco Chicken w/o Cheddar Cheese	1 (4.4 oz)	348	39	2	2
Nachos Cheese	1 serv (5.5 oz)	572	47	8	6
Quesadilla Cheese	1 (6.5 oz)	709	48	1	2
Quesadilla Chicken	1 (7.9 oz)	761	50	1	2
Quesadilla Kids Cheese	1 (2.2 oz)	219	23	1	1
Quesadilla Mini Cheese	1 (2.7)	274	23	1	1
Quesdadilla Beef	1 (8.5 oz)	823	49	1	2
Refried Beans Powdered	1 serv (6.3 oz)	406	17	1	5
Refried Beans w/o Cheddar Cheese	1 serv (5.8 oz)	327	16	1	5
Refried Beans w/o Chili	1 serv (5.1 oz)	360	11	0	4
Salsa Red	1 serv (2 oz)	14	3	0	1
Soup Tortilla	1 bowl	237	19	3	2
Soup Tortilla w/o Tortilla Strips & Cheese	1 bowl	148	11	3	2
Sour Cream	1 serv (1 oz)	57	2	1	0
Taco Party	1 (1.9 oz)	143	5	0	0
Taco w/o Cheddar Cheese	1 (1.5 oz)	104	5	0	0
Taco Crispy Beef	1 (2.6 oz)	200	7	0	0
Taco Crispy Chicken	1 (1.9 oz)	140	8	1	0
Taco Crispy Chicken w/o Cheddar Cheese	1 (1.7 oz)	100	7	1	0
Taco Crispy w/o Cheddar Cheese	1 (2.4 oz)	161	6	0	0
Taco Soft Beef	1 (3.5 oz)	245	18	0	1
Taco Soft Beef w/o Cheddar Cheese	1 (3.2 oz)	206	17	0	1
Taco Soft Chicken	1 (2.9 oz)	184	19	1	1
Taco Soft Chicken w/o Cheddar Cheese	1 (2.5 oz)	145	18	1	1
Tostada	1 (4.1 oz)	324	18	1	3
Tostada w/o Cheddar Cheese	1 (3.3 oz	207	17	1	3
Tostada w/o Chili	1 (2.9 oz)	269	12	0	3

FOOD	PORTION	CALS	CARB	SUGAR	FIBER
Tostada w/o Refried Beans	1 (2.5 oz)	234	15	1	2
SALADS					
Nacho Beef	1 (9.3 oz)	759	58	6	8
Nacho Beef w/o Cheddar Cheese	1 (8.8 oz)	681	57	6	8
Nacho Beef w/o Chili	1 (6.9 oz)	648	45	5	6
Nacho Chicken	1 (8.9 oz)	713	59	7	8
Nacho Chicken w/o Cheddar Cheese	1 (8.4 oz)	634	58	7	8
Nacho Chicken w/o Chili	1 (6.5 oz)	601	46	6	6
Taco Beef	1 (12.7 oz)	1043	58	2	12
Taco Beef w/o Cheddar Cheese	1 (11.7 oz)	886	56	2	12
Taco Beef w/o Chili	1 (11.5 oz)	987	51	2	12
Taco Beef w/o Guacamole	1 (11.7 oz)	988	56	2	11
Taco Beef w/o Sour Cream	1 (11.7 oz)	986	56	2	12
Taco Beef w/o Tortilla Bowl	1 (9.7 oz)	564	15	2	2
Taco Chicken	1 (9.6 oz)	838	53	3	12
Taco Chicken w/o Cheddar Cheese	1 (8.6 oz)	680	52	3	12
Taco Chicken w/o Guacamole	1 (8.6 oz)	783	51	3	11
Taco Chicken w/o Sour Cream	1 (8.6 oz)	781	51	2	12
Taco Chicken w/o Tortilla Bowl	1 (6.6 oz)	359	10	2	1

TACOTIME
DESSERTS

FOOD	PORTION	CALS	CARB	SUGAR	FIBER
Churro Plain	1 (1.5 oz)	205	16	4	0
Churro w/ Cinnamon & Sugar	1 (2 oz)	245	26	14	0
Crustos	1 serv	294	58	19	3
Empanada Apple	1 (4 oz)	234	40	10	2
Empanada Cherry	1 (4 oz)	240	41	4	2
Empanada Pumpkin	1 (4 oz)	256	42	16	2
MAIN MENU SELECTIONS					
Burrito Big Juan Chicken	1 (13 oz)	594	68	5	10
Burrito Big Juan Seasoned Ground Beef	1 (13 oz)	651	71	6	12
Burrito Big Juan Shredded Beef	1 (13 oz)	633	67	5	10
Burrito Casita Chicken	1 (12 oz)	494	43	4	5
Burrito Casita Seasoned Ground Beef	1 (12 oz)	552	46	5	6
Burrito Casita Shredded Beef	1 (12 oz)	533	42	4	5
Burrito Chicken & Black Bean	1 (10 oz)	478	51	3	9

FOOD	PORTION	CALS	CARB	SUGAR	FIBER
Burrito Chicken BLT	1 (10 oz)	721	44	4	8
Burrito Chicken Ranchero	1 (10.8 oz)	654	52	3	7
Burrito Crisp Chicken	1 (5.5 oz)	336	32	0	2
Burrito Crisp Meat	1 (5.8 oz)	450	36	1	4
Burrito Crisp Pinto Bean	1 (6 oz)	394	50	1	6
Burrito Soft Meat	1 (6.7 oz)	426	43	2	8
Burrito Soft Pinto Bean	1 (6.7 oz)	377	54	1	10
Burrito Veggie	1 (11 oz)	534	74	4	12
Cheddar Fries	1 sm (6 oz)	374	29	1	3
Cheddar Melt	1 (2.8 oz)	250	25	0	4
Mexi-Fries	1 sm (5 oz)	290	29	1	2
Mexi-Rice	1 serv (4 oz)	87	19	1	0
Nachos Grande	1 serv (16.5 oz)	1132	114	8	11
Refritos w/ Chips	1 serv (7 oz)	304	35	2	6
Refritos w/o Chips	1 serv (6.7 oz)	285	32	2	6
Stuffed Fries	1 sm (5 oz)	321	29	3	3
Taco Crisp Seasoned Ground Beef	1 (4.3 oz)	225	12	1	2
Taco Super Soft Chicken	1 (11 oz)	540	56	3	10
Taco Super Soft Seasoned Ground Beef	1 (11 oz)	598	59	4	12
Taco Super Soft Shredded Beef	1 (11 oz)	579	55	3	10
Taco Value Soft	1 (5.3 oz)	314	28	2	6
Taco ½ Lb Shredded Beef	1 (9 oz)	440	42	3	7
Taco ½ Lb Soft Chicken	1 (9 oz)	401	43	3	7
Taco ½ Lb Soft Seasoned Ground Beef	1 (9 oz)	459	46	4	9
Taco Chips	1 serv (2 oz)	150	27	0	1
SALAD DRESSINGS AND TOPPINGS					
Cheddar Cheese	1 serv (2 oz)	223	1	0	0
Dressing Chipotle Ranch	1 serv (1 oz)	165	1	1	0
Dressing Thousand Island	1 serv (1 oz)	132	5	3	0
Guacamole	1 serv (1 oz)	50	2	1	1
Salsa Nuevo	1 serv (1 oz)	8	2	1	0
Salsa Verde	1 serv (1 oz)	6	2	0	0
Sour Cream	1 serv (1.5 oz)	85	1	1	0
SALADS					
Taco Chicken	1 reg (9.2 oz)	351	24	4	2
Taco Seasoned Ground Beef	1 reg (7.8 oz)	396	24	3	4

FOOD	PORTION	CALS	CARB	SUGAR	FIBER
Taco Shredded Beef	1 reg (7.8 oz)	377	21	2	2
Tostada Delight Chicken	1 (10.5 oz)	565	36	3	4
Tostada Delight Seasoned Ground Beef	1 (10.5 oz)	623	39	4	6
Tostada Delight Shredded Beef	1 (10.5 oz)	604	35	3	5

TCBY
FROZEN YOGURT AND SORBET

FOOD	PORTION	CALS	CARB	SUGAR	FIBER
Hand Scooped Butter Pecan Perfection	½ cup	110	14	11	tr
Hand Scooped Chocolate Chocolate Swirl	½ cup	120	19	16	tr
Hand Scooped Chocolate Chunk Cookie Dough	½ cup	160	24	18	0
Hand Scooped Cookies & Cream	½ cup	140	22	17	0
Hand Scooped Cotton Candy	½ cup	120	20	16	0
Hand Scooped Mint Chocolate Chunk	½ cup	140	22	18	0
Hand Scooped Mocha Almond	½ cup	150	22	18	tr
Hand Scooped No Sugar Added Chocolate Chocolate Swirl	½ cup	90	23	5	6
Hand Scooped No Sugar Added Vanilla	½ cup	80	19	6	5
Hand Scooped No Sugar Added Vanilla Fudge Brownie	½ cup	100	22	5	5
Hand Scooped Pralines & Cream	½ cup	140	23	19	0
Hand Scooped Psychedelic Sorbet	½ cup	290	75	55	0
Hand Scooped Rainbow Cream	½ cup	120	20	16	0
Hand Scooped Rocky Road	½ cup	220	36	27	1
Hand Scooped Strawberries & Cream	½ cup	120	21	18	0
Hand Scooped Vanilla Chocolate Chunk	½ cup	140	22	18	0
Hand Scooped Vanilla Bean	½ cup	120	19	16	0
Soft Serve Frozen Yogurt All Flavors 96% Fat Free	½ cup	140	23	20	0
Soft Serve Frozen Yogurt All Flavors Low Carb	½ cup	110	16	3	7

FOOD	PORTION	CALS	CARB	SUGAR	FIBER
Soft Serve Frozen Yogurt All Flavors Nonfat	½ cup	110	23	20	0
Soft Serve Frozen Yogurt All Flavors Nonfat No Sugar Added	½ cup	90	20	7	0
Soft Serve Sorbet All Flavors Nonfat Nondairy	½ cup	100	24	19	0
SMOOTHIES					
Berrylicious	1 (16 oz)	290	65	54	3
Black 'N Blueberry	1 (16 oz)	280	63	54	2
Mando Mango	1 (16 oz)	310	70	63	2
Mango Tango	1 (16 oz)	330	76	66	2
Mangolada	1 (16 oz)	340	70	60	2
Pina Paradise	1 (16 oz)	350	58	48	1
Pink Pineapple	1 (16 oz)	340	63	52	2
Straight Up Strawberry	1 (16 oz)	280	44	54	1
Strawberry Bonanza	1 (16 oz)	320	74	61	2
Strawberry Fling	1 (16 oz)	340	78	67	2
TIM HORTONS					
BAKED SELECTIONS					
Bagel Blueberry	1	270	55	7	2
Bagel Cinnamon Raisin	1	270	55	12	3
Bagel Everything	1	280	53	7	3
Bagel Flax Seed	1	290	53	4	4
Bagel Onion	1	260	53	8	3
Bagel Plain	1	260	52	7	2
Bagel Poppy Seed	1	270	53	7	3
Bagel Sesame Seed	1	270	53	7	3
Bagel Sun Dried Tomato	1	310	59	4	2
Bagel Twelve Grain	1	330	52	5	6
Cinnamon Roll Frosted	1	470	57	20	2
Cinnamon Roll Glazed	1	420	50	15	2
Cookie Caramel Chocolate Pecan	1	230	32	17	1
Cookie Chocolate Chip	1	230	34	19	1
Cookie Oatmeal Raisin Spice	1	220	35	21	1
Cookie Peanut Butter Chocolate Chunk	1	260	28	18	2
Cookie Triple Chocolate	1	250	31	20	2

FOOD	PORTION	CALS	CARB	SUGAR	FIBER
Cookie White Chocolate Macadamia Nut	1	240	31	17	1
Croissant Butter	1	340	38	7	1
Croissant Cheese	1	370	37	6	0
Danish Cherry Cheese	1	330	46	24	1
Danish Chocolate	1	430	51	27	1
Danish Maple Pecan	1	380	46	21	1
Donut Apple Fritter	1	300	49	16	2
Donut Chocolate Dip	1	210	30	8	1
Donut Chocolate Glazed	1	260	39	20	2
Donut Honey Dip	1	210	33	11	1
Donut Maple Dip	1	210	31	9	1
Donut Old Fashion Glazed	1	320	35	22	1
Donut Old Fashion Plain	1	260	20	7	1
Donut Sour Cream Plain	1	270	27	10	1
Donut Walnut Crunch	1	360	35	19	1
Donut Filled Angel Cream	1	310	46	21	1
Donut Filled Blueberry	1	230	36	11	1
Donut Filled Boston Cream	1	250	38	12	1
Donut Filled Canadian Maple	1	260	41	16	1
Donut Filled Strawberry	1	230	36	12	1
Honey Cruller	1	320	37	23	0
Muffin Blueberry	1	330	54	27	2
Muffin Blueberry Bran	1	300	53	25	5
Muffin Carrot Wheat	1	400	55	26	4
Muffin Chocolate Chip	1	430	69	40	2
Muffin Cranberry Blueberry Bran	1	290	51	24	5
Muffin Cranberry Fruit	1	350	59	31	2
Muffin Fruit Explosion	1	360	61	32	2
Muffin Raisin Bran	1	360	65	37	6
Muffin Strawberry Sensation	1	350	61	31	1
Muffin Low Fat Blueberry	1	290	62	32	2
Muffin Low Fat Cranberry	1	290	62	31	2
Tea Biscuit Plain	1	250	35	4	1
Tea Biscuit Raisin	1	290	45	12	2
Timbits Apple Fritter	1	50	9	4	0
Timbits Chocolate Glazed	1	70	10	5	0
Timbits Honey Dip	1	60	9	4	0
Timbits Old Fashion Plain	1	70	5	2	0

FOOD	PORTION	CALS	CARB	SUGAR	FIBER
Timbits Filled Banana Cream	1	60	9	3	0
Timbits Filled Lemon	1	60	9	4	0
Timbits Filled Strawberry	1	60	10	4	0
Timbits Filled Strawberry	1	60	10	4	0
BEVERAGES					
Cafe Mocha	1 (10 oz)	160	25	21	1
Cappuccino Iced	1 (12 oz)	300	41	40	0
Coffee Decaffeinated + Sugar & Cream	1 (10 oz)	75	9	9	0
Coffee + Sugar & Cream	1 (10 oz)	75	9	9	0
English Toffee	1 (10 oz)	220	40	30	0
Flavor Shot	1 serv	5	1	0	0
French Vanilla	1 (10 oz)	240	39	31	0
Hot Chocolate	1 (10 oz)	240	45	35	2
Hot Smoothie	1 (10 oz)	260	39	28	2
Iced Cappuccino w/ Milk	1 (12 oz)	180	39	35	0
Tea + Sugar & Milk	1 (10 oz)	50	10	10	0
CREAM CHEESE					
Garden Vegetable	1.5 oz	120	3	2	1
Light Plain	1.5 oz	60	3	3	0
Plain	1.5 oz	130	2	2	0
Strawberry	1.5 oz	120	6	6	0
SANDWICHES					
B.L.T.	1	450	53	9	2
Breakfast Bacon Egg Cheese	1	410	31	4	1
Breakfast Egg Cheese	1	360	30	3	1
Breakfast Sausage Egg Cheese	1	520	30	3	1
Chicken Salad	1	380	55	6	3
Egg Salad	1	390	52	7	2
Ham & Swiss	1	440	56	7	3
Toasted Chicken Club	1	460	70	14	2
Turkey Breast	1	390	59	6	4
SOUPS					
Beef Stew	1 serv (10 oz)	236	25	3	3
Chicken Noodle	1 serv (10 oz)	120	18	2	1
Chili	1 serv (10 oz)	300	18	5	5
Country Field Mushroom	1 serv (10 oz)	150	28	3	1
Cream Of Broccoli	1 serv (10 oz)	160	16	6	1
Hearty Vegetable	1 serv (10 oz)	70	14	2	3
Minestrone	1 serv (10 oz)	120	24	4	2

FOOD	PORTION	CALS	CARB	SUGAR	FIBER
Potato Bacon	1 serv (10 oz)	180	30	5	2
Split Pea w/ Ham	1 serv (10 oz)	150	27	3	5
Turkey Rice	1 serv (10 oz)	120	21	2	1
Vegetable Beef Barley	1 serv (10 oz)	110	21	2	2
YOGURT					
Low Fat Creamy Vanilla w/ Berries	1 (6 oz)	160	32	26	2
Low Fat Strawberry w/ Berries	1 (6 oz)	150	28	23	2
TJ CINNAMONS					
Chocolate Twist	1	250	34	12	2
Cinnamon Twist	1	280	33	11	1
Mocha Chill w/ Whipped Cream	1 (12.5 oz)	306	48	48	1
Mocha Chill w/o Whipped Cream	1 (12.5 oz)	264	48	44	1
Original Roll w/o Icing	1	507	73	31	4
Pecan Sticky Bun	1	688	91	45	5
TJ Icing	1 serv (1 oz)	117	18	16	0
WENDY'S					
BEVERAGES					
Chocolate Milk 1%	8 oz	170	28	26	0
Coca-Cola	1 med (12 oz)	140	37	37	0
Dasani Water	1 bottle	0	0	0	0
Diet Coke	1 med (11 oz)	0	0	0	0
Frosty	1 sm (8 oz)	330	56	42	0
Milk 2%	8 oz	120	13	12	0
Sprite	1 med (12 oz)	130	34	34	0
CHILDREN'S MENU SELECTIONS					
French Fries	1 serv (3.2 oz)	280	37	0	3
Kid's Meal Cheeseburger	1	320	34	6	1
Kid's Meal Chicken Nuggets	4 pieces	180	10	1	0
Kid's Meal Ham & Cheese	1 serv	240	32	5	1
Kid's Meal Hamburger	1	270	33	6	1
Kid's Meal Turkey & Cheese	1 serv	250	34	5	1
SALAD DRESSINGS AND TOPPINGS					
Ancho Chipotle Ranch	1 pkg	110	4	2	0
Blue Cheese	1 pkg	260	3	1	0
Buttery Best Spread	1 pkg	50	0	0	0
Caesar	1 pkg	120	1	0	0
Cheddar Cheese Shredded	2 tbsp	70	1	0	0

FOOD	PORTION	CALS	CARB	SUGAR	FIBER
Creamy Ranch	1 pkg	230	5	3	0
Creamy Ranch Reduced Fat	1 pkg	100	6	3	1
Crispy Noodles	1 pkg	60	10	1	0
Croutons Homestyle Garlic	1 pkg	70	9	0	0
Dipping Sauce Deli Honey Mustard	1 pkg	170	6	5	0
Dipping Sauce Heartland Ranch	1 pkg	200	1	1	0
Dipping Sauce Spicy Southwest Chipotle	1 pkg	150	5	1	0
Dipping Sauce Sweet & Sour Hawaiian	1 pkg	70	17	13	0
Dipping Sauce Wild Buffalo Ranch	1 pkg	180	2	1	0
French Fat Free	1 pkg	80	19	16	0
Granola Topping	1 pkg	110	15	6	1
Honey Mustard	1 pkg	280	11	10	0
Honey Mustard Low Fat	1 pkg	110	21	16	0
Hot Chili Seasoning	1 pkg	5	2	1	0
Italian Vinaigrette	1 pkg	140	9	8	0
Ketchup	1 tsp	7	2	1	0
Mayonnaise	1 tsp	30	1	0	0
Mustard	½ tsp	5	0	0	0
Nuggets Sauce Barbeque	1 pkg	45	10	8	0
Nuggets Sauce Honey Mustard	1 pkg	130	6	5	0
Nuggets Sauce Sweet & Sour	1 pkg	50	13	11	0
Oriental Sesame	1 pkg	190	21	19	0
Roasted Almonds	1 pkg	130	4	1	2
Saltines	2	25	4	0	0
Sour Cream Reduced Fat	1 pkg	45	2	1	0
Thousand Island	1 pkg	260	8	7	0
Tortilla Strips	1 pkg	110	13	0	1
SALADS					
Caesar Chicken w/o Dressing & Croutons	1 serv	180	9	4	4
Ceasar Side w/o Dressing & Croutons	1 serv	70	3	1	2
Chicken BLT w/o Dressing & Croutons	1 serv	340	12	6	4
Mandarin Chicken w/o Dressing	1 serv	170	18	13	3
Side Salad w/o Dressing	1	35	8	4	2

FOOD	PORTION	CALS	CARB	SUGAR	FIBER
Southwest Taco w/o Dressing Tortilla Strip & Sour Cream	1 serv	440	32	10	9
SANDWICHES AND SIDES					
Baked Potato Plain	1	270	61	3	7
Baked Potato w/ Sour Cream & Chives	1 serv	320	63	4	7
Big Bacon Classic	1	580	46	11	3
Chicken Nuggets	5 pieces	220	13	1	0
Chili	1 sm (8 oz)	220	23	6	5
Classic Single w/ Everything	1	420	37	8	2
French Fries	1 med (5 oz)	440	58	0	5
Frescata Black Forest Ham & Swiss	1	480	50	8	4
Frescata Club	1	440	50	5	4
Frescata Roasted Turkey & Basil Pesto	1	420	50	4	4
Frescata Roasted Turkey & Swiss	1	490	52	5	4
Hamburger	1	280	34	7	1
Homestyle Chicken Strips	3 pieces	410	33	0	0
Jr. Bacon Cheeseburger	1	370	34	6	2
Jr. BBQ Cheeseburger	1	330	36	8	1
Jr. Cheeseburger	1	320	34	7	1
Jr. Cheeseburger Deluxe	1	360	37	8	2
Mandarin Orange Cup	1 serv	80	19	17	1
Sandwich Crispy Chicken	1	380	43	5	1
Sandwich Spicy Chicken Fillet	1	510	57	8	2
Sandwich Ultimate Chicken Grill	1	360	44	10	2
Yogurt Low Fat Strawberry	1 pkg	140	27	11	0

WHATABURGER
BEVERAGES

FOOD	PORTION	CALS	CARB	SUGAR	FIBER
Barq's Root Beet	1 sm (16 oz)	220	61	61	0
Cherry Coke	1 sm (16 oz)	210	56	56	0
Coca-Cola	1 sm (16 oz)	207	56	56	0
Coffee	1 sm (8 oz)	5	1	0	0
Coffee Decaf	1 sm (8 oz)	5	1	0	0
Diet Coke	1 sm (16 oz)	0	0	0	0
Dr Pepper	1 sm (16 oz)	190	51	51	0
Fanta Orange	1 sm (16 oz)	210	56	56	0
Fanta Strawberry	1 sm (16 oz)	230	61	61	0

FOOD	PORTION	CALS	CARB	SUGAR	FIBER
Iced Tea Sweetened	1 (34 oz)	430	114	114	0
Iced Tea Unsweetened	1 sm (19 oz)	0	0	0	0
Lemonade Hi-C Poppin' Pink	1 sm (16 oz)	200	51	51	0
Malt Chocolate	1 sm (16 oz)	670	123	115	2
Malt Strawberry	1 sm (16 oz)	670	123	117	0
Malt Vanilla	1 sm (16 oz)	600	98	92	0
Milk Reduced Fat	8 oz	120	11	11	0
Orange Juice Tropicana	1 (10 oz)	140	33	28	0
Powerade Fruit Punch	1 sm (16 oz)	130	33	28	0
Shake Chocolate	1 sm (16 oz)	630	111	103	2
Shake Strawberry	1 sm (16 oz)	630	111	105	0
Shake Vanilla	1 sm (16 oz)	560	87	80	0
Sprite	1 sm (16 oz)	200	51	51	0
CHILDREN'S MENU SELECTIONS					
Kid's Meal Chicken Strips	1 serv	770	53	0	2
Kid's Meal Justaburger	1 serv	570	60	2	3
DESSERTS					
Apple Pie A La Mode	1 serv	520	75	43	2
Apple Pie Hot	1	230	29	1	2
Cinnamon Roll	1	400	80	16	2
Cookie Chocolate Chunk	1 (2 oz)	230	33	21	1
Cookie White Chocolate Chunk Macadamia	1 (2 oz)	250	30	20	0
Peach Pie A La Mode	1 serv	570	82	52	2
MAIN MENU SELECTIONS					
Biscuit	1	300	32	2	1
Biscuit Honey Butter Chicken	1	610	51	9	1
Biscuit Sandwich Bacon Egg & Cheese	1	500	33	2	1
Biscuit Sandwich Egg & Cheese	1	450	33	2	1
Biscuit Sandwich Sausage Egg & Cheese	1	690	33	2	1
Biscuit w/ Bacon	1	355	32	2	1
Biscuit w/ Gravy	1	530	52	7	1
Biscuit w/ Sausage	1	540	32	2	1
Breakfast Platter w/ Bacon	1 serv	730	53	3	2
Breakfast Platter w/ Sausage	1 serv	930	53	3	2
Breakfast On A Bun w/ Bacon	1	380	29	2	1
Breakfast On A Bun w/ Sausage	1	570	29	2	1
Chicken Strip w/ Gravy	4	840	53	2	0

FOOD	PORTION	CALS	CARB	SUGAR	FIBER
Chicken Strips	1	200	11	0	0
French Fries	1 sm	260	31	0	2
Gravy White Peppered	1 serv	60	8	2	0
Hashbrown Sticks	4	200	20	0	1
Justaburger	1	329	30	2	1
Onion Rings	1 med	420	36	17	3
Pancakes Plain	1 serv	580	112	27	5
Pancakes w/ Bacon	1 serv	630	112	27	5
Pancakes w/ Sausage	1 serv	820	112	27	5
Sandwich Chicken Strip Honey BBQ	1	1110	102	16	3
Sandwich Chicken Strip Junior Honey BBQ	1	720	59	9	1
Sandwich Egg	1	330	29	2	1
Sandwich Grilled Chicken	1	450	45	8	6
Taquito w/ Bacon & Egg	1	370	27	2	3
Taquito w/ Bacon Egg & Cheese	1	420	27	2	3
Taquito w/ Potato & Egg	1	430	37	2	3
Taquito w/ Potato Egg & Cheese	1	470	37	2	3
Taquito w/ Sausage & Egg	1	410	27	2	3
Taquito w/ Sausage Egg & Cheese	1	450	27	2	3
Texas Toast	1 slice	180	25	3	1
Whataburger	1	640	61	10	3
Whataburger Double Meat	1	890	61	10	3
Whataburger Jr.	1	330	32	3	1
Whataburger Triple Meat	1	1140	61	10	3
Whataburger w/ Bacon & Cheese	1	800	62	10	3
Whatacatch	1	480	42	3	2
Whatacatch Dinner	1 serv	1095	161	88	8
Whatachick'n	1	530	61	8	7
SALADS					
Chicken Strips	1 serv	570	34	6	4
Garden Salad	1	60	12	6	4
Grilled Chicken	1 serv	230	19	6	4

WHITE CASTLE
BEVERAGES

FOOD	PORTION	CALS	CARB	SUGAR	FIBER
Barq's Red Cream Soda	1 sm (21 oz)	260	69	69	0
Barq's Root Beer	1 sm (21 oz)	250	68	68	0

FOOD	PORTION	CALS	CARB	SUGAR	FIBER
Coca-Cola	1 sm (21 oz)	220	61	61	0
Coffee Black	1 sm (12 oz)	<5	1	0	0
Crave Cooler Coke	1 sm (21 oz)	150	41	41	0
Diet Coke	1 sm (21 oz)	0	0	0	0
Fanta Orange	1 sm (21 oz)	240	64	64	0
Hi-C Flashing Fruit Punch	1 sm (21 oz)	240	63	63	0
Hot Chocolate	1 sm (12 oz)	220	40	32	tr
Hot Tea	1 sm (12 oz)	0	0	0	0
Ice Tea Unsweetened	1 sm (21 oz)	0	0	0	0
Iced Tea Sweetened w/ Lemon	1 sm (16 oz)	170	46	46	0
Iced Tea Sweetened w/ Lemon	1 sm (21 oz)	170	46	46	0
Lemonade Raspberry	1 sm (21 oz)	290	78	73	0
Pibb Xtra	1 sm (21 oz)	220	59	59	0
Powerade Mountain Blast	1 sm (21 oz)	140	38	33	0
Sprite	1 sm (21 oz)	220	59	59	0
MAIN MENU SELECTIONS					
Cheeseburger	1	170	15	2	tr
Cheeseburger Bacon	1	200	15	2	tr
Cheeseburger Bacon Double	1	370	23	4	1
Cheeseburger Double	1	300	23	4	1
Cheeseburger Jalapeno	1	180	15	2	tr
Cheeseburger Jalapeno Double	1	320	23	4	1
Chicken Rings	6	210	15	0	0
Clam Strips	1 reg	250	5	1	0
Fish Nibblers	1 reg	280	24	0	5
French Fries	1 reg	310	39	1	4
Mozzarella Cheese Sticks	3	250	22	2	1
Onion Chips	1 reg	480	62	9	2
Sandwich Chicken Breast w/ Cheese	1	200	21	2	1
Sandwich Chicken Ring	1	180	19	2	tr
Sandwich Chicken Ring w/ Cheese	1	200	19	2	tr
Sandwich Fish w/ Cheese	1	180	19	2	tr
White Castle	1	140	14	2	tr
White Castle Double	1	250	22	4	1
SAUCES AND SPREADS					
Dressing Ranch	1 serv (1 oz)	150	0	0	0
Ketchup	1 pkg	10	3	2	0
Lemon Juice	1 pkg	0	0	0	0

FOOD	PORTION	CALS	CARB	SUGAR	FIBER
Mayonnaise	1 pkg	60	0	0	0
Sauce BBQ	1 serv (1 oz)	35	8	7	0
Sauce Hot	1 pkg	0	0	0	0
Sauce Marinara	1 serv (1 oz)	15	4	3	0
Sauce Seafood	1 serv (1 oz)	30	7	6	0
Sauce Tartar	1 pkg	30	2	1	0
Sauce Zesty Zing	1 serv (1 oz)	110	3	3	0
Sauce Fat Free Honey Mustard	1 serv (1 oz)	50	12	10	0

WORLD WRAPPS
SIDES AND SOUPS

FOOD	PORTION	CALS	CARB	SUGAR	FIBER
Chips & Mango Salsa	1 serv	224	34	–	4
Chips & Tomato Corn Salsa	1 serv	184	82	–	4
Potstickers	3	170	24	–	1
Soup Tortilla	1 cup	191	26	–	6
Yogurt Parfait	1 serv	281	41	–	4

SMOOTHIES

FOOD	PORTION	CALS	CARB	SUGAR	FIBER
Blue Mango Boost	1 (16 oz)	295	70	–	5
Caribbean C	1 (16 oz)	276	64	–	3
Strawberry Orange Banana	1 (16 oz)	268	61	–	5
Tropical Storm	1 (16 oz)	309	72	–	3

WRAPS

FOOD	PORTION	CALS	CARB	SUGAR	FIBER
Baja Veggie w/ Cheese Sour Cream Avocados	1 sm	541	89	–	11
Barcelona	1 sm	460	65	–	4
Bean & Cheese	1 sm	452	67	–	11
Bombay Curry Veggie	1 sm	495	81	–	23
Buffalo w/ Shrimp	1 sm	422	65	–	7
Burrito w/ Chicken Cheese Sour Cream Avocado	1 sm	576	66	–	10
Burrito w/ Steak Cheese Sour Cream Avocado	1 sm	573	66	–	7
Caribbean Sole	1 sm	523	80	–	3
Chicken Caesar	1 sm	547	44	–	5
Chicken Parmesan	1 sm	495	53	–	2
Portobello & Goat Cheese	1 sm	391	55	–	5
Samurai Salmon	1 sm	543	65	–	2
Spicy Southwest Shrimp	1 sm	460	75	–	8
Tequila Lime Shrimp	1 sm	422	65	–	7
Teriyaki Chicken	1 sm	482	73	–	8
Teriyaki Steak	1 sm	497	69	–	8

FOOD	PORTION	CALS	CARB	SUGAR	FIBER
Teriyaki Tofu & Mushroom	1 sm	387	58	–	5
Texas Roadhouse BBQ Chicken	1 sm	512	64	–	4
Texas Roadhouse BBQ Steak	1 sm	569	64	–	4
Thai Chicken	1 sm	508	58	–	4

YOGEN FRUZ

FOOD	PORTION	CALS	CARB	SUGAR	FIBER
Blend It No Sugar Added Vanilla	1 sm	110	24	8	0
Blend It Probiotic Low Fat Chocolate	1 sm	121	22	21	0
Blend It Probiotic Low Fat Vanilla	1 sm	121	22	21	4
Blend It Probiotic Non Fat Vanilla	1 sm	110	24	21	0
Smoothie Dairy Blueberry Breeze	1 sm	180	45	36	2
Smoothie Dairy Peach Berry Sunset	1 sm	150	36	30	2
Smoothie Dairy Strawberry Banana	1 sm	180	42	33	3
Smoothie Non Dairy Raspberry Blast	1 sm	208	51	45	3
Smoothie Non Dairy Tropical Storm	1 sm	224	56	46	2
Smoothie Non Dairy Very Berry	1 sm	192	50	40	3
Top It Probiotic Soft Serve	1 sm	132	28	25	0

YOGURTLAND

FOOD	PORTION	CALS	CARB	SUGAR	FIBER
Arctic Vanilla	½ cup (3 oz)	108	24	14	0
Blueberry Tart	½ cup (3 oz)	127	16	15	0
Cafe Con Leche	½ cup (3 oz)	108	24	14	0
Chocolate Mint	½ cup (3 oz)	100	23	15	0
Double Cookies & Cream	½ cup (3 oz)	121	27	14	0
Dutch Chocolate	½ cup (3 oz)	118	27	14	0
Fresh Strawberry	½ cup (3 oz)	108	24	14	0
Green Tea	½ cup (3 oz)	107	24	15	0
Heath Bar	½ cup (3 oz)	132	25	14	0
Mango	½ cup (3 oz)	96	22	16	0
Mango Tart	½ cup (3 oz)	127	16	15	0
No Sugar Added French Vanilla	½ cup (3 oz)	89	19	9	0
NY Cheesecake	½ cup (3 oz)	100	23	16	0

FOOD	PORTION	CALS	CARB	SUGAR	FIBER
Peach	½ cup (3 oz)	100	23	15	0
Peach Tart	½ cup (3 oz)	127	16	15	0
Peanut Butter	½ cup (3 oz)	119	24	14	0
Pineapple Tart	½ cup (3 oz)	127	16	15	0
Pistachio	½ cup (3 oz)	100	22	16	0
Plain Tart	½ cup (3 oz)	108	19	19	0
Strawberry Tart	½ cup (3 oz)	127	16	15	0
Taro	½ cup (3 oz)	102	23	14	0

ZOUP!
DESSERTS

FOOD	PORTION	CALS	CARB	SUGAR	FIBER
Cookie Chocolate Chunk	1	410	57	–	1
Cookie Peanut Butter	1	420	43	–	1

SANDWICHES

FOOD	PORTION	CALS	CARB	SUGAR	FIBER
Pesto Three Cheese	1	720	42	–	2
Tuna Melt	1	600	42	–	2
Wrap American Farm	½	435	30	–	5
Wrap Asian	½	615	54	–	7
Wrap Chicken Caesar w/o Dressing	½	505	43	–	5
Wrap Greek w/o Dressing	½	485	33	–	6
Wrap Tuna	½	365	35	–	4

SOUPS

FOOD	PORTION	CALS	CARB	SUGAR	FIBER
Chicken & Dumplings	1 (8 oz)	130	22	–	1
Chicken Potpie	1 (8 oz)	200	21	–	3
Italian Wedding w/ Turkey Meatballs	1 (8 oz)	120	13	–	1
Jamaican Bay Gumbo	1 (8 oz)	140	20	–	2
Lobster Bisque	1 (8 oz)	260	14	–	0
Pepper Steak	1 (8 oz)	160	19	–	1
Potato Cheddar	1 (8 oz)	210	16	–	1
Sesame Noodle Bowl	1 (8 oz)	80	7	–	1
Shrimp & Crawfish Etouffee	1 (8 oz)	130	17	–	1
Sicilian Pizza	1 (8 oz)	150	18	–	2
Spicy Crab & Rice	1 (8 oz)	110	21	–	1
Turkey Chili	1 (8 oz)	120	19	–	3
Wild Mushroom Barley	1 (8 oz)	108	18	–	2